Accident and Emergency

re

(

Accident and Emergency

Theory into Practice

Edited by

Brian Dolan MSc(Oxon) MSc(Lond) BSc(Hons) RMN RGN CHSM

Nursing Research Fellow, King's A&E Primary Care Service, London, UK;
Editor, *Emergency Nurse*

Lynda Holt RGN EN(G) DipHS

A&E Clinical Manager, South Warwickshire General Hospitals NHS Trust, Warwick, UK;
Chair, Royal College of Nursing A&E Nursing Association, UK

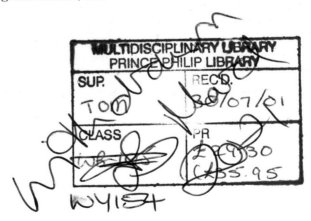
Baillière Tindall
PUBLISHED IN ASSOCIATION WITH THE RCN

Royal College
of Nursing

EDINBURGH LONDON NEW YORK PHILADELPHIA ST LOUIS SYDNEY TORONTO 2000

BAILLIÈRE TINDALL   ·

An imprint of Harcourt Publishers Limited

© Harcourt Publishers Limited 2000

⚜ is a registered trademark of Harcourt Publishers Limited

First published 2000
  Reprinted 2000 (twice)

ISBN 0 7020 2239 X

British Library Cataloguing in Publication Data
A catalogue record for this book is available from the British Library

Library of Congress Cataloging in Publication Data
A catalog record for this book is available from the Library of Congress

Note
Nursing and medical knowledge is constantly changing. As new information becomes available, changes in treatment, procedures, equipment and the use of drugs become necessary. The editors, contributors and publishers have, as far as it is possible, taken care to ensure that the information given in this text is accurate and up to date. However, readers are strongly advised to confirm that the information, especially with regard to drug usage, complies with the latest legislation and standards of practice.

The photographs on the front cover are reproduced with permission from Nursing Standard.

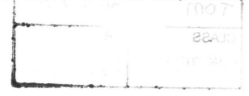

Printed in China

Contents

Contributors   ix

Preface   xi

Introduction: Nursing in Accident and Emergency   *Gary Jones*   1
The coming of casualty; From casualty to accident and emergency; Patient attendance; A&E nursing today;
Models of nursing; The nurse/patient relationship; Patient assessment; Waiting times; Clinical practice;
Towards a Faculty of Emergency Nursing; Conclusion

Part 1   Trauma Management   13

1   Pre-hospital Care   *Tim Kilner*   15
Introduction; Major incidents; Equipping the mobile team; Inadequate training and experience;
Defining the role of the mobile medical and nursing team; Non-major incidents; Delivery of care;
Patient assessment; Unique role played by nurses in providing pre hospital care; Conclusion

2   Trauma Life Support   *Lisa Hadfield-Law*   25
Introduction; Preparation; Primary survey; Secondary survey; Trauma in children; Definitive care; Conclusion

3   Major Incident Planning   *Andrew Whitfield & Tim Kilner*   33
Introduction; Definition; Planning; Exercise and training; The hospital's response to a major incident alert;
Medicolegal issues; Aftermath; Conclusion

Part 2   Trauma Care   43

4   Head Injuries   *Deborah Dawson & Karen Sanders*   45
Introduction; Anatomy and physiology; Physiology of raised intracranial pressure; Classification of head
injuries; Assessment of head injury; Management of serious injury; Transfer to a specialist neurosurgical unit;
Brain stem death; Management of minor injury; Conclusion

5   Skeletal Injuries   *Lynda Holt*   67
Introduction; Anatomy and physiology; Pelvic injury; Hip injury; Limb injury; Femoral fractures; Lower leg
injury; Ankle fractures; Foot fractures; Injury to the shoulder; Upper arm injury; Elbow injury; Forearm injury;
The wrist; The hand; Soft tissue injuries; Conclusion

6   Spinal Injuries   *Mike Paynter*   109
Introduction; Anatomy and physiology; Pathophysiology; History-taking; Examination; Cervical spine fractures;
Thoracolumbar spine fractures; Spinal cord injury; Conclusion

7   Thoracic Injuries   *Karen Castille & Lynda Holt*   119
Introduction; Mechanism of injury; Anatomy of the chest; The physiology of respiration; Principles of care;
Immediately life-threatening injuries; Serious chest injury; Sternum, ribs and scapular injuries; Conclusion

8   Abdominal Injuries   *Paul Gee*   137
Introduction; Anatomy and pathophysiology; Types and patterns of injury; Uncontrolled haemorrhage;
Assessment of abdominal trauma; Abdominal injuries in children; Conclusion

9 Facial Injuries   *Elspeth Richie*   147
   Introduction; Anatomy and physiology; Mechanism of injury; Assessment; Le Fort fractures;
   Mandibular fractures; Orbit floor fractures (blow-out fracture); Temporomandibular joint (jaw) dislocation;
   Frontal sinus fractures; Nasal fractures; Facial wounds; Conclusion

10 Burns   *Steve Harulow & Lynda Holt*   159
   Introduction; Assessment; Specific burns injuries; Burn wound care; Pain control; Escharotomies;
   Psychological considerations; Transfer to specialist units; Minor burn wound care; Conclusion

Part 3 Psychological Dimensions   **173**

11 Aggression   *Barbara Neades*   175
   Introduction; Why aggression occurs in A&E; Prevention of aggression in A&E; Recognising potential
   aggression; Diffusing aggression in A&E; Managing the violent individual; Follow-up care after an aggressive
   violent incident; Conclusion

12 Stress and Distress   *Bob Wright*   183
   Introduction; Coping; Distress in A&E nursing; Approaches to support and care; Defusion; Demobilisation;
   Critical incident stress debriefing; Responses to burn-out; Conclusion

13 Care of the Bereaved   *Brian Dolan*   189
   Introduction; Background; Preparing for receiving the patient and relatives; Witnessed resuscitation;
   Breaking bad news; Viewing the body; Organ donation; Legal and ethical issues; Sudden infant death
   syndrome; Staff support; Conclusion

14 Psychiatric Emergencies   *Barbara Warncken & Brian Dolan*   199
   Introduction; Aetiology of mental illness; Assessment of psychiatric patients in A&E; Acute organic reactions;
   Acute psychotic episode; Anxiety states; Alcohol-related emergencies; Munchausen's syndrome and
   Munchausen's syndrome by proxy; Suicide and deliberate self-harm (parasuicide); Individual at odds with
   society; Learning disability clients and mental health problems; Elderly clients presenting to A&E with mental
   health problems; Child and adolescent psychiatry; Patients attending A&E with eating disorders;
   Social problems; Iatrogenic drug-induced psychosis; Monoamine oxidase inhibitors; Conclusion

Part 4 Life Continuum   **215**

15 Infants   *Cathryn Bird & Lindsey Lorkin*   217
   Introduction; Assessment; The critically ill infant and child; Causes of respiratory difficulty;
   The febrile infant; Meningitis; Dehydration in infants; Failure to thrive; The vomiting infant;
   The injured infant; Sudden infant death syndrome; Conclusion

16 Pre-school Children   *Lynne Poucher & Lynda Holt*   233
   Introduction; Normal development; The child under stress; Understanding illness; Asthma;
   Acute laryngotracheobronchitis (viral croup); Epiglottitis; Accidental injury; Accidental poisoning;
   Non-accidental injuries (child abuse); Sexual abuse; Munchausen's syndrome by proxy; Conclusion

17 Age 5 to Puberty   *Anita Tyler*   251
   Introduction; Child development; Environment; Pain relief; Fractures; Sports injury; Abdominal pain;
   Consent; Health promotion; Conclusion

18 Adolescence   *Lynda Holt*   257
   Introduction; Adolescent development; Caring for the adolescent in A&E; Personal fable; Risk-taking behaviour;
   Substance misuse; Overdose; Conclusion

19 Young Adults   *Judy Davies*   269
   Introduction; Sporting injuries; Road traffic accidents; Alcohol-related attendances; Accidents related to sexual
   activity; Psychological illness in young adults; Conclusion

20 Middle Years *Grant Williams*   275
Introduction; Chest pain; Pancreatitis; Epigastric pain; Homelessness; Conclusion

21 The Elderly *Brian Dolan*   283
Introduction; Physiology of old age; Assessing the elderly person in A&E; Hypothermia; Elder abuse;
Confusion; Falls; Conclusion

Part 5   Physiology for A&E Practice   **293**

22 Physiology for Practice *Marion Richardson*   295
Introduction; Homeostasis; Oxygen transport; Carbon dioxide transport; Oxygen/carbon dioxide homeostasis;
Oxygen therapy; Flight physiology; Temperature control; Fluid and electrolyte balance; Haemostasis; Shock;
Conclusion

23 Wound Care *Lynda Holt*   307
Introduction; Anatomy of the skin; Wound healing; Wound assessment; Wound cleansing; Wound closure;
Wound infection; Managing bite wounds; Tetanus prophylaxis; Discharge information; Conclusion

24 Pain Management *Brian Dolan*   325
Introduction; Physiology of pain; Pain theories; Assessing pain; Pharmacological pain management;
Non-pharmacological pain management; Conclusion

25 Local and Regional Anaesthesia *Bernie Edwards*   333
Introduction; Pharmacology of local anaesthetics; Classification of local anaesthetics; Benefits of local
anaesthetics; Disadvantages and limitations of local anaesthetics; Types and uses of anaesthesia;
Nursing implications of procedures involving local anaesthetics; Conclusion

Part 6   Emergency Care   **339**

26 Cardiac Emergencies *Jamie Walthall*   341
Introduction; Related anatomy and physiology; The cardiac cycle; Assessment; Basic ECG interpretation;
Cardiac arrest; Rhythm disturbances; Heart block; Pacing; Acute chest pain; Acute cardiac failure;
Viral/inflammatory conditions; Conclusion

27 Medical Emergencies *Tim Kilner & Rosie Wilkinson*   371
Introduction; Respiration; Asthma; Pulmonary chronic obstructive disease; Pulmonary oedema;
Pulmonary embolism; Anaphylaxis; Near drowning; Carbon monoxide poisoning; Renal disorders;
Urinary tract disease; Dehydration — fluid volume deficit; Thermoregulation; Nervous system;
Glucose regulation; Haematology; Conclusion

28 Surgical Emergencies *Peter Dowds*   393
Introduction; Anatomy and physiology of the abdomen; Nursing assessment of the acute abdomen;
Acute abdominal emergencies; Vascular disorders; Genitourinary disorders; Preoperative preparation;
Conclusion

29 Gynaecological and Obstetric Emergencies *Lynda Holt & Orla Devereux*   411
Introduction; Anatomy and physiology; Emergency care of the non-pregnant woman; Sexual assault;
Emergency care of the pregnant woman; Conclusion

30 Ophthalmic Emergencies *Janet Marsden*   429
Introduction; Anatomy and physiology of the eye; Assessing ophthalmic conditions; Ocular burns;
Penetrating trauma; Major closed trauma; Minor trauma; Eyepads; Eyedrops; Red eye; Health promotion;
Conclusion

31 Ear, Nose and Throat Emergencies *Tim Kilner, Philip Docking & Elaine Hayward*   447
Introduction; The ear; Infections of the ear; Mechanical obstruction; Foreign bodies; Perforation of the
tympanic membrane; The nose; Foreign bodies; Epistaxis; Nasal fracture; Rhinorrhea; Allergic rhinitis;
Sinusitis; The throat; Oral cavity; Pharynx; Conclusion

Part 7 Practice Issues in A&E

459

32 Primary Care; the A&E Dimension *Robert Crouch* 461

Introduction; Legitimacy of attendance; A&E – the primary care role; Providing for primary care in A&E;
Developing the primary care role of A&E nurses; Bridging the gaps between A&E and primary care;
Changing the culture; Nurse practitioners; Telephone consultation – extending the primary care role;
Future implications – out-of-hours care delivery; Conclusion

33 Health Promotion *Stewart Piper* 469

Introduction; Health persuasion techniques; Legislative action for health; Community development;
Personal counselling for health; Conclusion

34 Nurse Triage *Cherine Woolwich* 475

Introduction; The concept of nurse triage; Direct nurse triage; Providing a nurse triage system;
Patient assessment; The triage decision; Documentation; Training; Audit; A national triage scale; Conclusion

35 Nurse Practitioners *Stuart Cable & Brian Dolan* 485

Introduction; Development of the nurse practitioner role in A&E; The activities of nurse practitioners;
Education needs of nurse practitioners; Audit and evaluation; Conclusion

Part 8 Professional Issues in A&E

495

36 Clinical Leadership and Supervision *Andrew Cook & Lynda Holt* 497

Introduction; Clinical leadership; Clinical supervision; Conclusion

37 Clinical Reasoning *Bernie Edwards* 505

Introduction; Nursing process; Intuitive reasoning; Hypothetico-deductive approach; Conclusion

38 Ethical Issues *Kevin Kendrick* 513

Introduction; Duty as a moral endeavour; Applying the imperative to practice; Duty as a moral problem; Above
all, do no harm; Consent as an ethical process; Conclusion

39 Law *Ann Young* 521

Introduction; An outline of law in the UK; Classification of law; Attendance; Assessment; Treatment and care;
Death and organ donation; Patient property; Consent to treatment; Detention of patients; Confidentiality, the
police and the press; Staff health and safety; Conclusion

40 Maintaining a Safe Environment *Sheelagh Brewer* 529

Introduction; Preventing accidents; Legislation; Legislation since 1992; Infection control; Working time;
Framework for maintaining a safe environment; Conclusion

Appendix 539
Normal physiological values

Index 541

Contributors

Cathryn Bird BSc(Hons) RGN RSCN DipNursePractitioner
Nurse Practitioner, Primary Care

Sheelagh Brewer BA MIPD
Senior Employment Relations Adviser,
Royal College of Nursing

Stuart Cable MSc BA(Hons) RGN
Researcher/Lecturer, School of Nursing and Midwifery,
University of Dundee, Dundee

Karen Castille MSc PGDip RN RM
Senior Nurse, A&E
Royal Bolton Hospital

Andrew L. Cook BSc(Hons) RGN
Accident and Emergency Senior Nurse Manager,
East Surrey Hospital, Redhill

Robert Crouch RGN
Research Fellow (A&E) and Co-director,
Emergency Care Clinical Academic Unit,
EIHMS, University of Surrey, Guildford

Judy Davies MA SRN
Senior Nurse, A&E Department,
Norfolk and Norwich Hospital

Deborah Dawson BSc(Hons) RGN
Lead Nurse, ICU,
St George's Hospital, London

Orla Devereux RGN RM
Staff Nurse, ICU/CCU,
Mayo General Hospital, Castlebar, Ireland

Philip Docking MSc RGN RNT
formerly Lecturer,
University of Luton, Luton

Brian Dolan MSc(Oxon) MSc(Lond) BSc(Hons) RMN
RGN CHSM
Nursing Research Fellow, King's A&E Primary Care Service,
London; Editor, *Emergency Nurse*

Peter Dowds MSc RGN
Consultant Nurse, Cheshire

Bernie Edwards BSc(Hons) RGN DipN RNT
Senior Lecturer, Institute of Health and Community Studies,
Bournemouth University, Bournemouth

Paul Gee RN OHND
Occupational Health Adviser, London

Lisa Hadfield-Law RGN
Management Consultant, Oxford

Steve Harulow BA(Hons) MA RGN
Freelance Writer, Melbourne, Australia
formerly Clinical Coordinator, Burns Unit,
The Royal London Hospital, London

Elaine F. Hayward MSc RGN DMS
Service Development Manager,
Corby Primary Care Group, Northants
formerly Clinical Nurse Specialist, A&E Department,
Kettering NHS Trust, Kettering

Lynda Holt RGN EN(G) DipHS
A&E Clinical Manager, South Warwickshire General
Hospitals NHS Trust, Warwick;
Chair, Royal College of Nursing A&E Nursing Association,
UK

Gary J. Jones RGN OND DipN(Lond) FETC
Fellow, Florence Nightingale Foundation;
A&E Nurse Consultant/Lecturer and Expert Witness

Kevin Kendrick MSc BA(Hons) DipSocAdmin RGN OTN
EN(G)
Assistant Director of Teaching and Learning,
Division of Nursing, University of Leeds, Leeds

Tim Kilner BN RGN PGCE DipIMC RCSEd
Lecturer in Emergency Nursing,
University of Birmingham, Birmingham

Lindsey Lorkin RN RSCN DipHealthStudies
Senior Sister/Paediatric Adviser, Paediatric A&E,
King's College Hospital, London

Janet Marsden MSc BSc(Hons) RGN OND MIMgt
Senior Lecturer,
Manchester Metropolitan University, Manchester

Barbara Neades BN RGN RMN PGCE(FE) RNT
Lecturer, Department of Adult Nursing,
Napier University, Edinburgh

Mike Paynter RGN REMT
Charge Nurse, Accident and Emergency Services,
Bristol Royal Infirmary, Bristol

Stewart Piper   MSc(HealthEd) PGDE RGN
Senior Lecturer,
Homerton College, Cambridge,
School of Health Studies

Lynne Poucher   BHSc
Senior Nurse, Continuing Professional Development,
North East Lincolnshire NHS Trust

Marion Richardson   BD(Hons) RGN DipN(Lond) CertEd
Senior Lecturer, Department of Post-registration Nursing,
University of Hertfordshire

Elspeth Richie   RMN RGN
Surgical Services Manager, Monklands Hospital,
Lanarkshire Acute Hospitals Trust, Airdrie

Karen L. Sanders   MA RGN RNT
Senior Lecturer,
South Bank University, London

Anita Tyler   BN RGN RSCN
Emergency Nurse Practitioner,
Emergency Unit, University Hospital of Wales

Jamie Walthall   RGN DipN(Lond)
Senior Charge Nurse,
Royal Berkshire Hospital A&E Department, Reading

Barbara Warncken   MA BSc(Hons) RN RMN
Senior Lecturer, A&E Nursing/ENB199 Programme Leader,
Anglia Polytechnic University

Andrew Whitfield   MSc BSc(Hons) CertEd(FE) RN
Senior Lecturer (Nursing and Paramedic Sciences),
University of Hertfordshire, Hatfield

Rosemary Wilkinson   RGN OND RNT CertEd
Adviser in Nursing Practice,
Royal College of Nursing

Grant Williams   BSc(Hons) DipN(Lond) RGN RNT
Lecturer Practitioner, Emergency Unit,
University Hospital of Wales, Cardiff

Cherine Woolwich   BSc(Hons) DipNP(RCN) RGN ONC
Nurse Practitioner, Primary Health Care,
Colville Health Centre, Ladbroke Grove, London

Bob Wright   HonMSc RGN RMN
Clinical Nurse Specialist — Crisis Care,
Accident and Emergency,
Leeds General Infirmary, Leeds

Ann P. Young   BA MBA RGN RNT
Head of Strategic and International Management,
East London Business School, University of East London,
London

Preface

In the last decade, emergency care has been transformed from being a Cinderella service to one that is increasingly seen as an environment representing the best of innovation and new ways of working. Nurses working in emergency care have found that their knowledge, skills and practice are increasingly valued – patients are now likely to be diagnosed, treated and discharged by an emergency nurse without seeing a doctor.

Accident and Emergency: Theory into Practice was conceived several years ago, when the editors realised that existing books did not meet the comprehensive and changing needs of nurses working in emergency care settings in the UK. The vibrancy and energy of emergency care, and the changes occurring within it, were not reflected in the texts available. By drawing together experts from practice, education, management and research, this book seeks to redress this imbalance.

Following the Introduction, *Accident and Emergency: Theory into Practice* is organised into eight parts: Trauma Management; Trauma Care; Psychological Dimensions; Life Continuum; Physiology for A&E Practice; Emergency Care; Practice Issues in A&E; and Professional Issues in A&E. It is worth briefly identifying a number of the innovative approaches adopted in this text.

While it might be expected that trauma organisation and management would feature prominently and at length in this book, as can be seen in Parts 1 and 2, the inclusion of Psychological Dimensions as early as Part 3, is intended to highlight the editors' belief that the psychological care of the patient and his or her relatives plays a critical rather than supplementary role in delivering a quality emergency service. Part 4, the Life Continuum, is a novel approach to this subject. The authors concentrate on the developmental changes and attendant clinical conditions that are most prevalent across different parts of the life span, and the editors hope that readers will find this a useful approach for quickly accessing information about patients in their care.

Part 5 reflects the growing importance of understanding physiology, pain management and anaesthesia, highlighting the sophistication and expected depth of knowledge now required by nurses in clinical practice. Detailed consideration is also given to wound care. The range of emergencies discussed at length in Part 6 includes medical, surgical and ophthalmic conditions, to name but a few. Parts 7 and 8 consider some of the important practice and professional debates currently being held in the field of emergency care and, hopefully, will both contribute to and generate discussion for some time to come.

Those who have been in emergency nursing for some time occasionally comment that it has turned full circle. Whereas once emergency nurses would, for instance, suture patients to relieve the pressure on overworked junior doctors on busy Saturday nights, a long period of professional inertia seemed to occur where every nursing action appeared to need a supporting certificate. Now, with the growth of nurse practitioners and advancing practice, emergency nurses are, as suggested above, developing an ever widening repertoire of skills and activities. There is one key difference between emergency nursing now and in years gone by; in the past nurses taking on roles that were previously undertaken by medical colleagues did so surreptitiously, often when there was no-one else around. Now, nursing practice is increasingly recognised for its comprehensive, patient-orientated approach to care. On the other hand, a common thread linking today's practice with that of the past is the recognition that good, knowledgeable emergency nurses give good quality care.

Emergency nurses have always spoken up for patients at a time when they are at their most vulnerable and when there is often no one else to speak up for them. It is this that is the hallmark of good care and is the difference between technical skill and compassionate concern. This book is imbued with a philosophy that recognises that combining technical skill and compassionate concern enables emergency nurses to become confident, knowledgeable practitioners. In essence, this book is for those who wish to blend the best of the art and science of our discipline.

As emergency nursing grows in scope, recognition and confidence, so too must it avoid the complacency of believing it has 'arrived'. In reality, emergency nursing is a journey without end, ever striving to deliver better patient-centred care. *Accident and Emergency: Theory into Practice* is a text that can be used as a guide on that journey.

Brian Dolan and Lynda Holt
Stratford upon Avon, 1999

Introduction: Nursing in Accident and Emergency

Gary Jones

- The coming of casualty
- From casualty to accident and emergency
- Patient attendance
- A&E nursing today
- Models of nursing
- The nurse/patient relationship
- Patient assessment
- Waiting times
- Clinical practice
- Towards a Faculty of Emergency Nursing
- Conclusion

Accident and emergency (A&E) nursing is dynamic, complex and progressive. It is about providing an immediate nursing response to meet the full spectrum of human need. To understand A&E nursing, and indeed A&E nurses themselves, it is necessary to review the history of the speciality, to consider patient attendance and to show how changing attitudes influence the service provided. In addition, this chapter will consider key reports which have shaped the organisation and delivery of A&E care and trends will be identified.

The Coming of Casualty

Like the A&E service itself, A&E nursing has developed from the casualty departments of the old voluntary hospitals and workhouses. In England, until the time of the dissolution of the monasteries in the Middle Ages, medicine, nursing and welfare were traditionally in the hands of the church. Between then and the 18th century there was no urge to build hospitals for the sick or to establish nursing orders. The main reason for this apparent lack of interest was that no more effective care could be given in a hospital than could be given at home by relatives and friends.

As medicine developed and a new spirit of philanthropy emerged, the initiative for founding charity hospitals became a reality. By 1825, 154 charity hospitals had been built in England (Baly 1973). These hospitals, which became the voluntary hospitals in the 19th century, received funding from public subscription. Admission was often by a ticket system and the employer made a contribution to the hospital for his employees. Within these voluntary hospitals, the outpatients department provided care for casual attenders. This service, which was often provided free of charge, allowed doctors to select patients who were 'interesting' and were of use to their developing speciality. Nurses resembled domestic workers and were few in number.

Although the outpatient service provided for both the patient's as well as the doctor's needs, it was unpopular with the newly emerging general practitioner (GP). The GPs felt the outpatient system was unfair competition, and many patients with primary health care problems attended the outpatients department rather than seeking health care from them. Because of these complaints, it was agreed that a patient should only be seen at hospital if referred by a GP; however, this system could be bypassed in an emergency. The 'casualty' could be seen as a casual attender in the newly established casualty departments.

From Casualty to Accident and Emergency

Casualty comes from the word 'casual'. Although not an inspiring term, it is still in use today despite the introduction of the term 'accident and emergency' nearly 40 years ago. The Platt Report (Standing Medical Advisory Committee 1962) recommended the change of title in a deliberate attempt to discourage casual attenders and recommended that casualty departments should change in function. Primary care to casual attenders, it suggested, should be secondary to the provision of a 24-hour A&E service. The major

responsibility was to provide care for serious accidents, and medical and surgical emergencies. The report further recommended that this new service should be appropriately staffed and equipped and a named consultant identified.

Nursing in these new-look A&E departments went through the same evolution as nursing in general. Gradually, as nurses worked in the speciality, they began to develop knowledge and skills beyond their general training. In 1972, the Accident & Emergency Nursing Forum (now an association) was established within the Royal College of Nursing (RCN). In 1975, the Accident & Emergency Nursing Course was developed. This course, run by the Board of Clinical Nursing Studies, is still available in England as the ENB course 199. More recently, a Health Services Accrediation working group (1997) has developed agreed service principles for an A&E service which stress quality standards of care (Box I.1).

Patient Attendance

Although the Platt Report (Standing Medical Advisory Committee 1962) identified that the major responsibility of the A&E department should be to provide

---

Box I.1 – *Service principles for an accident and emergency service*

A first class service that will always deliver to the highest standards
- Patients are entitled to the highest possible standards from their A&E department
- Minor injuries units are expected to provide the same level of relevant standards as A&E services and contemporary standards of best practice
- Pre-hospital care will be constantly developed to provide a system that meets the highest expectations and contemporary standards of best practice
- Every A&E department will be organised to receive patients of all types and severity and should always be open
- Clinical audit shall be developed to ensure the professional assessment of clinical treatment and the effectiveness and efficiency of services
- Staff shall be appropriately trained, qualified and experienced, with staffing levels that reflect the work patterns of the department

A service that is part of hospital–wide provision
- Hospitals with an A&E department will give priority to emergency cases over non–urgent cases for admission
- Where possible, acute management of a single episode of care will be managed on one hospital site
- Appropriate hospital facilities must be on site to support the A&E department
- Treatment shall be coordinated with other specialities and integrated to form a single service

A service that puts patients first
- Service provision will ensure equity for all sections of the population, not least in respect of access to services
- The service should be provided in a manner which is sympathetic to the individual's privacy, dignity and religious and cultural beliefs
- Patients and, where appropriate, relatives, friends or significant others (with the patient's consent) will be kept informed of clinical progress and prognosis
- Where the consent of a patient is required for treatment or participation in research, patients will be given the choice of whether to participate, with the potential benefits and any possible attendant risks clearly explained

care for serious emergencies, it also recognised that the secondary or subsidiary function was still to provide care for casual attenders. Perhaps because of this, the public's perception of the A&E service did not change, and consequently, today the public continue to use the service for both emergency and primary health care needs.

The National Audit Office (1992a,b) and Audit Commission (1996) reports highlighted the continued increase in new attenders. In England, there was an increase from 9.2 million patients in 1979 to 11.2 million in 1990/91. By 1995, this figure had risen to 15 million per year (Audit Commission 1996). In Scotland, in the 10 years from 1982 to 1992 there was an increase of 230 000 new patient attenders (National Audit Office 1992b). The reports identified that patients attend A&E departments with a wide variety and range of illnesses and injuries. Only a small proportion, less than 0.5%, are seriously ill or severely injured (Audit Commission 1996).

Chambers and Johnson (1986) indicated that while factors such as age, sex, social class, geographical location and availability of GP services are likely to influence attendance, their effects are largely unknown. Walsh (1990a), in his study of 2000 adults aged 16–60, found attendance to be predominantly from the young male group. He also noted a correlation between lower socioeconomic status and attendance. Travelling distance to the department was another major factor which influenced A&E attendance.

The primary care research project at King's College Hospital (Department of General Practice and Primary Care/Department of Accident & Emergency Medicine 1991) found that the most common reason patients gave for attending the A&E department was a problem with access to their GP, and nearly one-third of patients considered that their problem was not appropriate to general practice.

Appropriateness of attendance

Over the last 30 years, the appropriateness of attendance to an A&E department has been debated both formally and informally, with many departments actively seeking to discourage patients who, in the opinion of the staff, are 'inappropriate attenders'. Calnan (1984) interviewed patients in their own homes following an A&E attendance: 62% had made no attempt to contact their general practitioner, and of those who did, a third were unsuccessful. The study concluded that most people who go directly to hospital do so because of the circumstances in which they find themselves. Geographical location, peer pressure and

perceived urgency of the condition were all factors in the decision.

Walsh (1990b), using a medical definition of 'appropriate attendance', found that of those patients in his study who were allocated one of the two categories 'appropriate' or 'inappropriate', 27.5% were considered inappropriate. He also found that the majority of the patients considered inappropriate were suffering from non-traumatic conditions and were much more likely to require medication. While recognising that the term 'inappropriate attender' is not acceptable, it is important to differentiate between those patients who attend the A&E department suffering with a primary health care problem and those who are suffering with an A&E problem. A patient suffering with a primary health care problem requires the expertise of the GP and a nurse with skills in primary care. The A&E patient requires care that can only be given by A&E medical and nursing specialists. The issue of primary care in A&E is discussed in detail in Chapter 32.

A&E Nursing Today

A&E nursing and the role of the A&E nurse have been influenced, and in many instances directed, by patient attendance. It is somewhat ironic that the casualty departments of the pre-1962 era were developed because of pressure from GPs, yet now a number of patients attend the A&E department as a direct result of GP mistrust or of not being included on a GP list (Walsh 1990b). In addition, as a result of the Platt Report (Standing Medical Advisory Committee 1962), which rightly identified the seriously ill or injured as the first priority, many A&E nurses were, and still are, drawn into the appropriate/inappropriate attender debate.

In an attempt to identify and clarify the current position of A&E nursing, the RCN A&E Nursing Association (1994) set out its beliefs with regard to where A&E nursing is today. The Association believes the patient must be the main focus of attention and that care must be provided within a collegiate relationship between health care professionals. The Association (1994) sees the A&E department as the interface between primary and secondary care and believes the service should be seen as part of the community and not simply as a department within a hospital. It believes that certain aspects of the current service, such as minor injury and emergency primary health care, can be provided by nurse-run clinics within the community. The care of patients suffering from life-threatening or potentially life-threatening problems is the first priority and all other problems identified by the patient, nurse, family or others are then considered. Care should always be provided with the overall objective of health promotion.

The A&E nurse is seen as the leader in the initiation and coordination of patient care. She acts as a focus for the coordination and delivery of multidisciplinary care and delivers that care in partnership with the patient and significant others. Put in its most simplest terms, A&E nursing is all about the three rights: the *right* patient receiving the *right* care at the *right* time. What it means in reality is the A&E nurse providing a complex service to the patient.

The RCN A&E Association (1994) recognises the difference between the nurse working in the A&E department and the A&E specialist nursing practitioner. An A&E specialist nursing practitioner is responsible for providing immediate nursing care to people who have undifferentiated and undiagnosed problems. She accepts, without prior warning, any person of any age requiring health care, with problems originating from social, psychological, physical, spiritual or cultural factors, and she is the key decision-maker in selecting and deciding upon the priorities for care. Further, the A&E specialist nursing practitioner prescribes and initiates appropriate interventions, monitors, refers or discharges. The A&E specialist nursing practitioner also takes autonomous decisions with, or on behalf of, the patient, and acts as advocate to maximise health potential and promote continuity of care. To achieve this, the nurse must have an appropriate education and competency must be continually assessed.

Pamela Kidd (Assistant Professor, University of Kentucky, USA), in her address to the International A&E conference in New South Wales in 1993, argued that A&E nurses look beyond the physiological and anatomical problems to the complexities of the patient's needs and to the reason behind the accident or problem. They look at the social and environmental factors and the ongoing care of the patient. The A&E nurse realises that her care is not isolated but is the beginning of what can be a very lengthy process for the patient, relatives and friends.

Models of Nursing

A model of nursing is simply a framework that provides a structure to nursing care. Numerous models of nursing are available and the debate continues as to which one, if any, is suitable not only for A&E but also for nursing practice generally. Chalmers (1990) defines a model of nursing as a set of formulated ideas about the practice of nursing in which the nature of people is central. She argues that nursing models provide a much needed alternative knowledge base from which nurses can practise in an informed way.

Melia (1990) opposes this view and considers that not only has the development and use of nursing models not had a positive influence upon nursing practice, but that this trend has served to limit the development of nursing. She considers it is a phase that nursing is going through which has had little effect on patient care. Kenny (1993) believes that while nursing models are relevant to the nursing profession, they have not always been seen as relevant to individual nurses and consumers of health care. He argues that nurses still need a set of explicit concepts to guide their practice; however, instead of being seen as a restrictive straightjacket, models should inform and assist nurses.

Ali (1990) introduced three distinct models to nurses working in an A&E department, over a 12-week period. These models were Orem (1980), Roper and the Human Needs model (Roper *et al.* 1983). Ali found that Orem and Roper were less suitable than the Human Needs model and that the department's philosophy could be placed easily within the human needs framework. She also found that by using a model of nursing within the A&E setting, it helped to develop the relationships between A&E nurses and their patients and relatives. It provided the foundation for quick, concise and accurate patient assessment and made joint care planning and evaluation possible.

Walsh (1985) argues that any profession must have well established theoretical foundations and that a model of nursing provides this for accident and emergency. Walsh believes that the model used in A&E should be based on the concept of self-care and favours Orem as a model that should be considered. He believes that Orem's (1980) view of nursing, moving from a wholly compensatory phase to a partly compensatory phase and on to a final educational developmental stage, is appropriate for A&E. He suggests that Orem (1980) encourages nurses to anticipate potential problems and to include the family circumstances in care planning and that, by providing a concise and relevant assessment model from which a care plan can be derived, nurses will avoid the sort of pitfalls that are all too familiar in A&E.

Jones' (1990) care structure is based on a process of care which allows the nurse to return to looking at the patient and acting on the basis of professional judgement. The process comprises a model of nursing, a triage system, a problem-oriented approach encompassing assessment, problem identification, goals, intervention and evaluation, and the necessary documentation. Jones (1990) believes that practice-based models are more acceptable to A&E nurses and

Box I.2 – *The value of a model of nursing in A&E*

- It provides a structure to nursing care
- It provides a framework for holistic care
- It makes the patient a person
- It allows for social as well as physical problems to be addressed
- It provides health promotion and environmental safety opportunities
- It develops a partnership between the nursing staff and the patient and relatives
- It is the foundation for quick, concise and accurate patient assessment, intervention and evaluation
- It allows for joint care planning
- It provides for an organised and structured documentation system
- It ensures that all staff are moving in the same direction
- It prevents aspects of care being missed

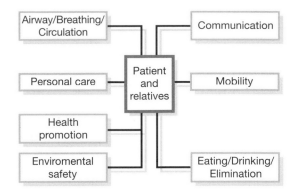

Figure I.1 – *Components of Life Model*

Box I.3 – *The four universal goals for A&E nurses*

- To establish a partnership with the patient/relatives
- To achieve a level of independence in the patient appropriate to his condition or injury and by so doing, assist him to restore health and maintain quality of life
- To enable the individual to avoid ill-health or injury through self-care, health education and environmental safety
- To ensure that the patient receives optimum effectiveness from medically prescribed treatment

that such models can provide the framework for organised nursing assessment, planning, intervention and evaluation. He believes it is impossible to ignore the medical model, as a great deal of nursing care is based around restoring normal anatomical and physiological activity, but argues that a nursing model provides a better framework for holistic care (Box I.2). His Components of Life model (Jones 1990) is based on an analysis of practice and represents what actually exists. The Components of Life model is not conceived from an idea in the same way as a theory-based model, but takes into account more than one model of nursing; nevertheless, he believes it is a model in its own right.

One of the major features of the Components of Life model is the simplicity of its use. The seven identified components can be easily memorised and lend themselves to simple documentation (Fig. I.1). Working through each component, the nurse is able to build up a picture of the patient's problems and intervene in a logical manner. The communication component encourages the nurse to assess the patient's consciousness level, human behavioural state and physiological senses and to identify any complaint of pain. This component also links up with one of the model's four universal goals (Box I.3), which is the establishment of a partnership with the patient and the relatives and friends.

The Nurse/Patient Relationship

Communication and the establishment of a partnership with the patient and significant others are essential parts of A&E nursing care. Unless a partnership is formed, it will be difficult for the individual to appreciate the process of care and the need for self-care guidance. *The Patient's Charter* (Department of Health 1991a) identifies a named, qualified nurse to be responsible for the patient's nursing care. In addition, one of the national charter standards requires the nurse to wear a name badge. Both of these charter standards are designed to create a better partnership between the patient/significant other and the nurse.

The development of the named nurse standard has presented some problems within the A&E department. These problems have mainly stemmed from the confusion between methods of delivering care and the purpose of the named nurse standard. Crinson (1995) notes that many of the principles underpinning *The Patient's Charter* (Department of Health 1991a) and *The Health of the Nation* (Department of Health 1992) had support among senior nursing staff, but these organ-isational developments have had less impact on the quality of care in A&E than intended, essentially because of a failure to provide sufficient resourcing. Jones (1993b) indicates that the named nurse in A&E is the nurse allocated to a patient and that this can be achieved irrespective of the method used to deliver care. If primary nursing is the method used within the A&E department, then the primary nurse and the named nurse are one and the same. If team nursing is in use then either the team leader or other nurses within the team can be identified as the named nurse. With patient allocation, a given number of patients can be allocated to each named nurse. The number of patients will vary depending on the patients' dependency.

The triage nurse may be the most appropriate person to be the named nurse for patients arriving and waiting to be seen by the doctor or nurse practitioner. While it is appreciated that continuity is important, it is also unrealistic in many departments for the same nurse to follow the patient through all stages of care. When a change of named nurse does occur, the patient as well as the relative/friends must be informed. While both the patient and the nurse have a joint responsibility for establishing the partnership, it is the nurse who has the prime responsibility for achieving a good working relationship with the patient. The nurse must attempt to prevent her own attitude or prejudices damaging the establishment of the partnership, and thereby causing a breakdown in communication. Stockbridge (1993) states that if the nurse has negative perceptions of the patient, her own non-verbal communication will cause the patient to behave in such a way that the nurse's perceptions are confirmed. The patient may be labelled as difficult.

Wright (1991) identifies that most complaints from relatives of sudden death victims involve basic com-munication skills. Many patients complain of doctors not sitting down, not using eye contact and only spending a brief period of time with them. Listening and having the ability to react appropriately to the patient's problems require the nurse to have a working knowledge of social, psychological, physical, spiritual and cultural factors that can cause problems with communication and with the development of a partner-ship. The nurse must understand that altered body image, mental health, drugs, alcohol and many other factors will often create barriers to good communication.

Anxiety-provoking factors, such as fear of the unknown, personal arrangements, possible com-plications and treatments, can also lead to poor communication (Walsh 1993). Wright (1986) indicates

that due to the breakdown in the individual's coping mechanisms, the nurse may no longer be seen as a person who can help, but rather an obstacle preventing that individual getting what he wants. Through formal A&E nursing education, the nurse may learn to overcome many of these problems and develop skills to ensure that the nurse/patient relationship is maintained.

Patient Assessment

The Patient's Charter (Department of Health 1991a) indicates that patients will be seen immediately and their need for treatment assessed. This standard caused much debate, primarily because of the word 'immediate' and the government's insistence that waiting time from arrival to assessment had to be monitored and national league tables produced.

Nursing assessment occurs in various phases throughout the patient's stay. On arrival, and irrespective of the mode of arrival, the patient must receive an initial nursing assessment. While this standard was achieved for ambulance patients, many departments had difficulty in complying with this standard for walking patients. Departmental design, nurse staffing levels and the intensity of the initial nursing assessment were all factors that had to be addressed. As 24-hour initial assessment costs each department a minimum of £90 000/year, or between 10 and 15% of the total nursing budget, it is essential that it is done well (Audit Commission 1996). Following a major study on behalf of the Patient's Charter Unit (Jones 1995), several consultation documents were published, and in October 1997 the Initial Assessment standard was modified. The current standard, which had to be fully implemented by April 1998, is as follows:

> *If you go to an Accident & Emergency Department needing immediate treatment you will be cared for at once. Otherwise you will be assessed by a doctor or trained nurse within 15 minutes of arrival. Following assessment you will be given a priority category which will be communicated to you. This priority will determine the urgency with which you will be treated.*

By providing a much more logical time-frame to the standard, initial assessment can once again become an essential part of a full triage process and provide the quality of service that patients require.

Initial, or primary, assessment identifies the chief complaint, determines the effectiveness of the airway, breathing and circulation, and confirms the patient's conscious state. The chief complaint and the patient's general condition determine the priority for medical/nursing care. The initial nursing assessment should be brief but must ensure patient safety. A recorded chief complaint of an arm injury without a record of assessing the distal pulse is unacceptable.

Once the priority for medical or nursing intervention has been determined (triage), a secondary nursing assessment should be conducted. This secondary assessment can be conducted either by the same nurse or by the nurse who will continue to care for the patient, i.e. the named nurse. Secondary assessment should only be conducted by the nurse who performed the initial assessment if this does not create a delay for newly arriving patients. Triage is discussed in detail in Chapter 34.

The completed nursing assessment should identify the patient's actual and potential problems, which both the patient and a relative/friend may encounter. Wilkinson (1991) highlighted the plight of an 85-year-old lady and her husband when admitted to an A&E department. The lady, incontinent and suffering from a fractured neck of femur, lay on a trolley for 6 hours. During this time she did not receive pressure area care and later developed a sacral sore. Wilkinson asked:

If we cannot give care such as this woman needed, when she needed it, what can we do? What is the point of 'high tech' medicine if the essentials somehow get forgotten or neglected along the way? How can a six-hour wait in an accident and emergency department be justified? Is this an indicator of a 'high-quality service'?

Waiting Times

Another of the local *Patient's Charter* standards that directly affects the A&E department is waiting times after the need for treatment has been assessed. While the causes of long waiting times are complex and no two departments have exactly the same set of problems, many factors are within their control. For instance, re-attendance rates vary from less than 1% to over 54%. The Audit Commission (1996) suggests ways in which re-attendances can be reduced (Box I.4).

Emergency nurse practitioners are often introduced in the belief that waiting times will be instantly reduced. Waiting times are a constant source of irritation to patients and staff alike. Introducing nurse practitioners may reduce the waiting times, but whether they are present or not, Dolan (1998) argues, patients have a right to be kept informed about what is going on. While a nurse practitioner service can

> **Box I.4 –** *Ways to reduce planned A&E attendances*
>
> ■ Ensuring more patients are seen by experienced A&E doctors the first time they attend. Uncertainty by junior doctors about diagnosis or treatment can lead to more investigations and more return visits
>
> ■ Requiring SHOs to consult a middle or senior grade doctor, if one is present in the department, before booking clinical appointments for patients
>
> ■ Ensuring all re-attenders are seen by a senior doctor or nurse
>
> ■ Asking GPs or practice nurses to assess the quality and outcomes of treatment provided rather than arranging return A&E attendances for these to be monitored
>
> ■ Improving knowledge of facilities offered by GP practices, e.g. for removal of sutures and renewal of dressings, both through personal contact and by making a directory available
>
> ■ Periodic audit of reasons for re-attendance to ensure that all are justified clinically or by the need to assess outcomes and the quality of care. This audit may require better information systems
>
> ■ Agreeing protocols with other specialities for deciding who should be seen in which clinics
>
> ■ Discontinuing minor operations which could be performed more appropriately elsewhere

reduce overall waiting times, for some patients their individual overall time in the department may increase because of the service provided. Many emergency nurse practitioners identify the need for health education and safety awareness instruction and thereby increase the overall time the patient spends in the department. The emphasis must be on improved care rather than the conveyer belt approach. Nurse practitioners are considered in detail in Chapter 35.

Clinical Practice

Clinical practice, while being patient-driven, is also directly affected by national, regional and local initiatives. Several national documents published in recent years are having, and will continue to have, dramatic effects on the way nursing is carried out (Clinical Standards Advisory Group 1995, Audit Commission 1996). *A Vision for the Future* (Department of Health 1993) provides, as its title suggests, a vision for nursing and a framework for action. Providing the reader with five key areas and 12 targets, it indicates that the participation of nurses will improve the general health and life expectancy of the whole population. This statement, coming so closely after the publication of *The Health of the Nation* (Department of Health 1992), encourages A&E nurses to develop the health promotion and accident prevention aspects of their role.

Challenging the Boundaries (RCN A&E Association 1994) has set out the role, boundaries and targets for the future. The strategy, in line with the UKCC's proposals for post-registration education and practice (PREP) (UKCC 1991), identifies the specialist nurse and recognises that some patients may require services other than medical intervention. It proposes the development of an advanced level of practice which offers direct access to clients seeking health care.

Sudden death

About 1 in 400 A&E patients either die while in A&E or are brought in dead. Recommendations put forward by the British Association of Accident & Emergency Medicine and The Royal College of Nursing (1995) to the Chief Nursing Officer and Chief Medical Officer at the Department of Health aim to improve the care of the relatives and friends of sudden death victims. As well as providing guidance on the design of sitting rooms and visiting rooms, the recommendations also explore methods of educating staff and supporting relatives during this crucial time. Dealing with sudden death in A&E is described in detail in Chapter 13.

Children

Nationally, one-quarter of all A&E patients are under 16. The Children Act (Department of Health 1989) and the work of the RCN Children in A&E Special Interest Group have had major effects on the way children are cared for in the A&E environment. The Clinical Standards Advisory Group (1995) has stated that every hospital with an A&E department should have on-site paediatricians and the Department of Health (1991b) has set a target that each A&E department seeing children should have at least one registered sick children's nurse on duty 24 hours a day. More departments are now employing registered sick children's nurses and many departments have, by creating children's areas, responded to the needs of the child. (See Part 4, 'Life continuum'.)

Trauma care

The nurse's role in the care of the trauma patient has grown considerably. Scott (1990) recognised that in the front line of an A&E department, the ability to perform the tasks needed to save life when time is of the essence is as essential for nurses as it is for ambulance personnel and doctors. The publication of the Royal College of Surgeons of England's (1988) *Report on the Management of Patients with Major Injuries* stimulated interest in the care of trauma patients. Within 2 years of its publication, two trauma nursing courses had been established within the UK. Both courses were developed by nurses for nurses. The Advanced Trauma Nursing Course is provided jointly by the Royal College of Nursing and the Royal College of Surgeons of England. The Trauma Nursing Core Course is a bought package from the United States and is provided by the RCN A&E Nursing Association. By 1997, the TNCC courses had trained over 1000 trauma nurse providers.

There is a long-standing recommendation that hospitals should have a trauma team (Campling *et al.* 1989). Paynter (1993) believes that the philosophy of trauma nursing is spreading and indicates that as more A&E trauma trained nurses return to their individual departments, the procedure for assessing and managing critically injured patients is improving. (See Part 1, 'Trauma Management' and Part 2, 'Trauma Care'.)

Towards a Faculty of Emergency Nursing

In recent years, there has been a tendency to develop generic 'critical care' courses. In some ways, these detract from the speciality of A&E nursing and fail to recognise the uniqueness and diversity of A&E practice (Crouch & Jones 1997). It is the belief of the A&E Nursing Association Steering Group that a radical change is required in the preparation and career development of A&E nurses to meet the changing health needs of the nation and the evolving role of nursing practice. To achieve this, a proposal to form a Faculty of Emergency Nursing has been developed. Although trends within the speciality have influenced this proposal, a number of external trends in nursing have contributed to the thinking behind it. These include the:

■ increasing moves to the deregulation of professional groups
■ shift of accreditation from central government bodies to professional bodies
■ greater emphasis on multidisciplinary training and collaboration
■ local determination of educational needs for nursing

- continued debate over generic, specialist and advanced practice
- confusion over basic competency levels in nursing practice.

Box I.5 outlines the aims of the proposed faculty.

Box I.5 – *Aims of the Faculty of Emergency Nursing*

The Faculty would aim to develop:
- A national education framework to facilitate career development at all levels in the speciality
- A programme to recognise specialist practice and advanced practitioners in the speciality
- A number of clinical research posts at regional level for specialists in the field of A&E nursing.

An authoritative body that would:
- Establish national standards of clinical competency through the monitoring and accreditation of education
- Seek funding, commission and coordinate national A&E research
- Coordinate and provide a structure for the educational activities by the RCN A&E Nursing Association
- Act as an advisory group, to statutory bodies, on issues pertaining to A&E service and appointments to senior nursing posts
- Assess and validate training posts for the faculty.

The purpose of the Faculty would be to produce the 'gold standard' for education and development of A&E nurses. The standard would be promoted throughout the UK to ensure that each A&E nurse has the opportunity to advance his or her career in a structured way. The faculty proposal has gained the full support of the Royal College of Nursing and the RCN A&E Nursing Association and it is hoped that the Faculty will provide the opportunity to advance the speciality and provide a career structure for A&E nursing.

Conclusion

From the development of the casualty service in the 19th century to today's modern A&E departments, the nurse has always been an essential and influential member of the multidisciplinary team. It was A&E nurses who developed the RCN A&E forum, who created the A&E course, and who pioneered the developments of nurse triage, the emergency nurse practitioner, bereavement care, trauma nursing and nurse-run minor injury units. It is A&E nurses who continue to develop the service despite some of the current difficulties and the ongoing debate about how, when and where emergency care should be provided.

With increased patient attendance and the extra demands placed on the A&E nurse from the patient, statutory bodies and government departments, stress is inevitable. Stress invokes tension and anxiety (Walsh & Dolan 1999), and there is a need for more awareness and openness regarding stress within A&E nursing. Many things contribute to stress in the A&E unit, and the result of unrelieved stress and emotional burn-out is often multifactorial (Wilson 1991).

So what of the future for A&E nurses? Well, there are numerous developments to be taken forward: the faculty of emergency nursing, trauma care, primary health care, health promotion and accident prevention, to name but a few. *The New NHS* white paper (Department of Health 1997) also offers nurses opportunities to further enhance their role, through their involvement, for instance, in NHS Direct, a 24-hour telephone advice line which may lead to reductions in the numbers of patients attending A&E because it is inappropriate for their clinical needs.

A&E nurses need strong leadership at departmental level. All departments should have clinical nurse managers who will take the speciality forward into the next century. Research and clinical practice must go hand in hand. Care must be properly evaluated and practice changed where necessary. A&E nurse managers should be part of an A&E provider unit dealing directly with the purchasers of health care. Jones' (1993a) vision for the A&E nurse is both in the community setting and in the A&E department, a partnership the *New NHS* white paper implicitly supports (Department of Health 1997). The development of the A&E nurse specialist, providing a range of services to patients from advanced trauma care to direct access to those suffering with a minor injury – and moving between community minor injury units and the A&E department, is seen as the way forward.

In an 'activity scoping exercise' undertaken for the Department of Health, Jones (1997) reported a range of initiatives, such as fast-tracking patients with fractured neck of femur to the wards, enhanced pathways for children with asthma and following trauma, 24-hour bed management systems, emergency community psychiatric liaison teams, trauma courses, etc. He believes that what is emerging is not a doctor substitute but a new type of practitioner who legitimately is providing a service that is new.

A&E nurses have a great future ahead, but must never forget that however much we strive to develop the role of the A&E nurse, however much we push to move the boundaries of our practice forward, it must never be at the expense of patient care. Any change must always be for the good of the patient and his relatives and friends. Wilson (1991) stated, that:

...when we take away all the high-tech equipment, human beings are still there with all their needs, some *fulfilled, some not. Nursing, in essence, requires human to human contact and if we cannot provide such contact, then nursing is a myth, a game and a drain on the financial and moral structure of society.*

A&E nurses must never forget that (see also Kitson 1999).

References

Ali L (1990) Models in accident and emergency. *Nursing Standard*, **5**(3), 33–35.

Audit Commission (1996) *By Accident or Design: Improving A&E services in England and Wales*. London: HMSO.

Baly M (1973) *Nursing and Social Change*. Heinemann: London.

British Association of Accident & Emergency Medicine and Royal College of Nursing (1994) Bereavement care in A&E departments. *Report to Chief Medical and Nursing Officers*. London: RCN.

Calnan M (1984) The junctions of the hospital emergency departments: a study of patient demand. *Journal of Emergency Medicine*, **2**, 57–63.

Campling EA, Devlin HB, Hoile RW, Lunn JN (1989) *The Report of the National Confidential Enquiry into Perioperative Deaths*. London: Royal College of Surgeons of England.

Chalmers H (1990) Nursing models: enhancing or inhibiting practice? *Nursing Standard*, **5**(11), 34–35.

Chambers J, Johnson K (1986) Predicting demand for A&E services. *Community Medicine*, **8**(2), 93–103.

Clinical Standards Advisory Group (1995) *Urgent and Emergency Admissions to Hospital*. London: HMSO.

Crinson I (1995) Impact of *The Patient's Charter* on A&E departments. *British Journal of Nursing*, **4**(21), 1280–1287.

Crouch R, Jones G (1997) Towards a faculty of A&E nursing: planning for the future. *Emergency Nurse*, **5**(6), 12–15.

Department of General Practice and Primary Care/Department of Accident & Emergency Medicine (1991) *Providing for Primary Care: Progress in A&E*. King's College School of Medicine and Dentistry: London.

Department of Health (1989) The Children Act, London: HMSO.

Department of Health (1991a) *The Patient's Charter*. London: HMSO.

Department of Health (1991b) *Welfare of Children and Young People in Hospital*. London: HMSO.

Department of Health (1992) *The Health of the Nation. A Strategy for Health in England*. London: HMSO.

Department of Health (1993) *A Vision for the Future*. London: HMSO.

Department of Health (1995) *The Patient's Charter and You*. London: HMSO.

Department of Health (1997) *The New NHS: Modern, Dependable*. London: The Stationary Office.

Dolan B (1998) Waiting times (Editorial). *Emergency Nurse*, **6**(4), 1.

Health Services Accreditation (1997) *Standards for Accident & Emergency Services*. Battle: Health Services Accreditation.

Jones G (1990) *Accident & Emergency Nursing: A Structured Approach*. London: Faber & Faber.

Jones G (1993a) A&E nursing: all change ahead. *Emergency Nurse*, **1**(1), 7–8.

Jones G (1993b) The patient's charter in the accident & emergency department. *Accident & Emergency Nursing*. **1**, 211–218.

Jones G (1995) *The Value of Initial Assessment within the Accident & Emergency Department and The most Effective Way of Achieving this Activity*. London: Patient's Charter Unit, NHS Executive.

Jones G (1997) *Accident & Emergency: A Scoping Report*. London, Department of Health.

Kenny T (1993) Nursing models fail in practice. *British Journal of Nursing*, **1**(22), 133–135.

Kitson A (1999) The essence of nursing. *Nursing Standard*, **13**(23), 42–46.

McKee C (1990) Accident and emergency services in the United Kingdom: the past, present, and future. *The Journal of Emergency Surgery and Intensive Care*, **13**(4), 257–263.

Melia K (1990) Nursing models: enhancing or inhibiting practice? *Nursing Standard*, **5**(11), 36–39.

National Audit Office (1992a) *NHS Accident & Emergency Departments in England*. London: HMSO.

National Audit Office (1992b) *NHS Accident & Emergency Departments in Scotland*. London: HMSO.

Orem D (1980) *Nursing: Concepts of Practice*, 2nd edn. New York: McGraw Hill.

Paynter M (1993) Trauma support: revolution in care. *Emergency Nurse*, **1**(2), 7–9.

Roper N, Logan W, Tierney A (eds) (1983) *Using a Model for Nursing*. Edinburgh: Churchill Livingstone.

Royal College of Nursing A&E Association (1994) *Challenging the Boundaries*. London: RCN.

Royal College of Nursing and British Association of Accident & Emergency Medicine. (1995) *Bereavement Care in A&E Departments*. London: RCN.

Royal College of Surgeons of England (1988) *Report of the Working Party on the Management of Patients with Major Injuries*. London: Royal College of Surgeons of England.

Scott S (1990) Nurses in the front line. *Nursing Standard*, **4**(27), 50.

Standing Medical Advisory Committee (1962) *Accident & Emergency Services*, (Platt report). London: HMSO.

Stockbridge J (1993) Parasuicide: does discussing it help? *Emergency Nurse*, **1**(2), 19–21.

UKCC (1991) *The Report of the Post Registration Education and Practice Project*. London: UKCC.

Walsh M (1985) *Accident & Emergency Nursing: A New Approach*. London: Heinemann.

Walsh M (1990a) Why do people go to the A&E? *Nursing Standard*, **5**(7), 24–28.

Walsh M (1990b) Patient's choice: GP or A&E department? *Nursing Standard*, **5**(10), 28–31.

Walsh M (1993) Pain and anxiety in A&E attenders. *Nursing Standard*, **7**(26), 40–42.

Walsh M, Dolan B (1999) Emergency nurses and their perceptions of caring. *Emergency Nurse*, **7**(4), 24–31

Wilkinson R (1991) No care, no excuses. *Nursing Standard*, **5**(49), 44.

Wilson G (1991) Technology and stress. *Nursing*, **4**(32), 31–34.

Wright B (1986) *Caring in Crisis*. Edinburgh: Churchill Livingstone.

Wright B (1991) *Sudden Death*. Edinburgh: Churchill Livingstone.

Part 1

Trauma Management

1. Pre-hospital Care   15
2. Trauma Life Support   25
3. Major Incident Planning   33

Chapter 1

Pre–hospital Care

Tim Kilner

■ Introduction
■ Major incidents
■ Equipping the mobile team
■ Inadequate training and experience
■ Defining the role of the mobile medical and nursing team
■ Non-major incidents
■ Delivery of care
■ Patient assessment
■ Unique role played by nurses in providing pre-hospital care
■ Conclusion

Introduction

There is considerable debate regarding the role for nurses in the provision of pre-hospital care as part of hospital-based mobile teams (Carley *et al.* 1998, Kilner 1998, Mathews 1998). The simple response is that nurses, like any other health care provider, should only engage in activity in the pre-hospital setting if it will be of clear benefit to patient care and, in addition, to those services already provided.

To achieve this, guidelines for call-out must be established and the role of the team and its members must be clearly defined. Additionally, activity must be supported through education, training, rehearsal and operational experience. Failure to do so will result in ill-equipped, poorly trained, undisciplined teams working in an environment in which there is no place for them. With appropriate preparation, it is possible for the A&E nurse to contribute to and improve the quality of care patients receive from the scene of the incident to their transfer to the A&E department. This chapter will address these issues in relation to the role of the nurse as part of a medical and nursing team providing pre-hospital care at both major incidents and single/small multiple casualty incidents.

Care of the ill and injured is often perceived as beginning when the patient passes over the threshold of the A&E department. This is far from the reality of the situation, as care provided by the ambulance service at the scene of the accident and *en route* to hospital has become increasingly sophisticated. Although much of the hands-on care is provided by the ambulance service, there are occasions where the team needs to be broadened to include other health care professionals, in order to provide optimum care for the patient. The concept of pre-hospital care is based upon the team approach, with the involvement of a range of health care providers and members of the statutory emergency services. This chapter will examine the role of the A&E nurse in the provision of pre-hospital care in the context of the multidisciplinary team.

In exploring this role, it is important to define the philosophy of pre-hospital care from a medical and nursing perspective. Pre-hospital care, in this context, may be viewed as the provision of specific, skilled, medical and nursing intervention for the ill or injured individual at the scene of the incident. However, these interventions should encompass more than just physical care; as Eaton (1993) suggests, 'it [pre-hospital care] extends beyond the preservation of life to the prevention of complications and the relief of suffering'. Definitive care for both the injured and acutely ill, realistically, can only be carried out in hospital. Therefore, pre-hospital care must not be an attempt to take the A&E department to the patient, but to provide interventions to stabilise the patient's condition prior to and during evacuation to hospital. There is no place for definitive care in the pre-hospital environment.

In reality, contemporary pre-hospital care in the UK is far from ideal. As Donald Trunkey (1983) observed: 'In general, trauma care is frequently, disorganised and has an unacceptable outcome. Pre-hospital care of the accident victim is sub optimal.' In many cases little has changed since then in terms of medical and nursing intervention at the accident site. The contemporary problems in pre-hospital care often emerge when the ambulance service requests the attendance of a medical and nursing team from the local A&E department at the scene of an accident or major incident. As a consequence of this type of request being such a rarity, the team members have no clearly defined role or function, they are poorly trained and inadequately equipped for work outside the A&E department. Most importantly they will have little or no operational experience in the pre-hospital setting.

Such requests made by the ambulance service are usually in response to difficult situations, for example in the event of a prolonged entrapment of a multiply injured individual where access to the patient is problematic. Thus the least experienced are requested to deal with the most complex situations. This is a reflection of a common phenomenon seen in hospital. Consider, for example, the experienced nurse who encounters difficulty in placing a nasogastric tube and calls the junior doctor – the doctor may in fact have considerably less experience in this procedure.

Major Incidents

Following the declaration of a major incident, the ambulance service will alert the receiving hospital and will 'request the attendance of a mobile medical/nursing team, where the initial reports suggest that this is desirable' (Regional Ambulance Officers Group 1990). Unfortunately, the report offers no indication of the circumstances which would make the attendance of such a team desirable. This lack of clarity is manifest in the way many such teams have an ill-defined role and purpose at the site of a major incident.

Guidelines on major incident planning in the NHS, issued jointly by the Department of Health/NHS task group, offer little help in clarifying the situation. They provide no indication of the purpose of these teams other than that they will 'report to the Medical Incident Officer at the Ambulance Control Point to receive instructions' (NHS Management Executive 1990). This problem is exacerbated by the 'it won't happen to us' syndrome, which results in poorly formulated plans and ill-prepared team members. Although the perspective may be disputed, it may be clearly tested in two ways. Firstly, colleagues who may be requested to be team members could be asked to define their role at the scene of a major incident. The second strategy is to examine the department's own major incident plan for a clear definition of the purpose of the mobile medical/nursing team. Are colleagues aware of their role as team members, is there a clear statement of purpose in the plan and do perceptions match it?

The confusion that results from this lack of clarity was graphically illustrated in an account of the experience of the medical and nursing team at the scene of the Regent's Park bombing in 1982. An ill-prepared team who did not know the protocols or the contents of the equipment bags were dispatched to the scene of the incident, where they waited for more than half an hour before returning to the hospital along with a second team who were also not required, having not treated any patients (Fletcher 1986).

An ill-defined role is a fundamental problem in the operation of a hospital-based team at the site of a major incident, although it is not a problem in isolation. Confusion often arises as to which hospital should provide the medical/nursing team, often resulting in too many teams arriving at the site of the incident, adding to the chaos. Recent experience has shown that many of these teams are dispatched to the scene too late to be of any practical benefit, and when they do arrive they are inappropriately equipped and inadequately trained for work in the pre-hospital environment (New 1992). Resourcing the team often results in the hospital being depleted of key, experienced personnel at a time when their expertise is in greatest demand. If several hospitals provide teams then each hospital is depleted of key resources, whilst at the same time the incident becomes congested with personnel who are not required and who therefore become an additional liability (see also Ch. 3).

Which hospital should provide the mobile medical and nursing team?

Salt (1989) supports the commonly held belief that the mobile medical and nursing team should be provided by a local supporting hospital and not the hospital designated as the receiving hospital, so that the receiving hospital is not depleted of its key personnel. Although this principle is sound and works in theory, it is somewhat divorced from reality. The King's Fund report on the health-related services' response to a series of major incidents in London (New 1992) stated that: 'In practice, the first receiving hospital to be notified that a major incident has been declared will send out a medical team. Often, other receiving hospitals will do the same.'

Guidelines on emergency planning in the NHS suggest that when selecting staff to make up the team, 'care must be taken not to deplete staff required in the A&E department or elsewhere in the hospital who will be needed to provide care for gravely injured patients arriving at the hospital' (NHS Management Executive 1990). If experienced staff from the A&E department form the team, then the department will be depleted of the very people who are needed, while non-A&E staff may not be skilled in triage and care of the poly-traumatised patient. It could be argued that unless problems of training and operational experience are addressed then neither group is appropriate.

Deployment of the team is often delayed, principally for logistical reasons, such as assembly of the team, collection of the equipment and availability of transport for the team. Transport is a particular problem as most ambulances and their staff will be committed to patient care and transport and it may be some time before a vehicle is made available to transport the team.

Equipping the Mobile Team

Most A&E departments have a supply of clothing and equipment to be used by the mobile team in the event of a major incident (Kilner 1995). Often equipment, at best, is packed in inappropriate bags or, at worst, in cases or boxes (Peter & Taylor 1994). Frequently, staff are unfamiliar with the contents of the bags/boxes, where specific equipment is kept and how specific equipment is operated. It is critical, therefore, for potential team members to know the contents of the bags and where to find specific equipment.

Protective clothing is often inappropriate in terms of either design or size. Team members arriving at an incident without the correct safety wear will be prevented from entering the incident site, on the

---

Box 1.1 – *Essential equipment for mobile teams (Hodgetts & Miles 1996)*

- Carbon fibre helmet with chin strap and visor. Helmet should be green in colour with 'nurse' or 'doctor' in white lettering on each side

- Ear defenders – for team members and the patient

- Fire-retardent suit – designed to offer some protection to the wearer should a fire occur, but not designed to allow the wearer to enter a fire

- Warm underclothing – essential during cold weather, especially if the incident is likely to be protracted

- High-visibility jacket – with designation clearly marked front and back. Jacket to have green shoulder and fluorescent lower section with reflective bands

- Heavy duty gloves

- Latex gloves

- Oil- and acid-resistant boots. Wellington boots are not appropriate for the demands of pre-hospital care; they are cold, limit movement and are prone to having liquids poured into them

Additional essential equipment

- Personal identification and money

- Notebook – ideally plasticised with water-resistant pen

- Action card

---

grounds of health and safety. Protective clothing which must be included is outlined in Box 1.1.

Inadequate Training and Experience

It has been recognised for some time that a team of hospital doctors and nurses who are untrained and inexperienced in pre-hospital care is of little practical benefit at the scene of a major incident (Savage 1979). It is not possible to address the issue of training until the purpose of the medical and nursing team has been determined. Devising a training package for a team whose purpose remains nebulous is a seriously flawed approach. There is the potential risk that the team members will acquire skills they do not need at the expense of being unskilled in areas of practice which are essential at the site of a major incident. At the root of many of these problems is the lack of a clearly defined role. This is the focus through which many of these problems may be addressed.

Defining the Role of the Mobile Medical and Nursing Team

Deployment of a medical and nursing team must clearly benefit patient care at the site of the incident. If no clear benefit can be identified then the team should remain at the hospital where they will have a positive impact on patient care. The team should therefore have clear aims and objectives, which should be clearly identified in the local major incident plan as well as being familiar to all potential team members (Flynn 1997).

A team of two doctors and two nurses is going to have little impact on direct hands-on care amongst the wreckage. Firstly, four people will only be able to treat a relatively small number of casualties and it is likely that they will attempt to treat the first casualties they encounter regardless of need. Thus members of a medical and nursing team may find themselves at the scene treating patients with non-life-threatening injuries while patients with potentially treatable, life-threatening injuries are being ignored. In addition, the team members will find themselves working in an environment which is hostile and alien to them, having implications for their safety, efficacy and efficiency.

The management of medical and nursing resources at the scene is the responsibility of the medical and nursing incident officer(s) (MIO/NIO). Most of the initial treatment at the incident site should be carried out by the ambulance service personnel, under the direction of the ambulance incident officer (AIO), who are trained, experienced and capable of working in this environment. Furthermore, since the advent of paramedic training, hands-on care may be provided with a relatively high degree of sophistication.

The Function of the Mobile Team

Close to the accident site, but outside the inner cordon surrounding the actual incident site, a casualty clearing point will be established. This is the interface between the incident site and the chain of evacuation. It is at this point that the mobile team may be of most use.

Casualties will initially be treated by ambulance personnel prior to evacuation to the casualty clearing point. At the casualty clearing station the mobile team will triage the casualties for transport, identifying those patients who should be dispatched to hospital immediately and those who may wait a short time. The team may also become involved in stabilising patients

awaiting transportation to hospital. A further role the team may play is in the confirmation of death, thus preventing resources being deployed where they will be of no practical benefit. It is important that, if life has been declared extinct, the body should be clearly labelled to that effect, as it is not uncommon for a doctor to be requested to see the same casualty several times by different rescuers.

Triage at a Major Incident

In a mass casualty situation, there is a serious risk of prioritising casualties without regard for need. Thus triage for transport is essential so that the greatest benefit is achieved for the greatest number. It is important to stress that triage at the scene of a major incident is philosophically different from triage occurring on a day-to-day basis in the A&E department. As numbers of casualties will outstrip resources, triage includes a category not used routinely in hospital – dead/expectant. 'Dead' is self-explanatory; 'expectant' refers to those casualties whose injuries are so severe that they are expected to die in the absence of involved care. These patients are those who would receive the care of the hospital trauma team at the A&E department under normal circumstances. If the team become involved in treating these people, however, a greater number of others may die because of being denied simple life-saving interventions. This form of triage is often difficult for nurses and doctors to accept, but the aim is to do the greatest good for the greatest number.

Triage for initial treatment must be rapid, using a simple method of assessment (Box 1.2).

Box 1.2 – *Triage sieve (Hodgetts et al. 1995)*

This is carried out to rapidly determine priorities for treatment and is initially carried out at the incident site.

■ *Is the patient able to walk?*
  Yes → **Delayed**
  No → Go to next stage

■ *Check breathing. Is it present?*
  No → Open the airway (breathing now present?)
    Yes → **Immediate**
    No → **Dead**
  Yes → Check rate
      \> 30 or < 10/min → **Immediate**
      10–30/min   → Go to check circulation

■ *Check circulation* (capillary refill time (CRT) or pulse)
  CRT > 2 s or pulse > 120/min → **Immediate**
  CRT < 2 s or pulse < 120/min → **Urgent**

Triage for transport

After initial treatment in situ and in the casualty clearing station, patients must be prioritised for transport to hospital. Some patients who receive a high priority for treatment may receive a lower priority for transportation. For example, an unconscious person with a simple airway obstruction would receive 'immediate priority' for treatment; however, once the airway problem is resolved they would become a lower priority than a patient with time-critical hypovolaemia.

Triage for transport employs the triage sort system, which is somewhat less crude than the triage sieve. The triage sort requires the measurement of the Glasgow Coma Score, respiratory rate and systolic blood pressure (Box 1.3).

Box 1.3 – *Triage sort (Hodgetts et al. 1995)*	
Parameters within each category are allocated a coded value between 0 and 4.	
■ Patients with a score of 12 receive 'delayed priority'	
■ Patients with a score of 11 receive 'urgent priority'	
■ The remainder receive 'immediate priority'	
Glasgow Coma Score	*Coded value*
13–15	4
9–12	3
6–8	2
4–5	1
3	0
Respiratory rate	*Coded value*
10–29	4
>29	3
6–9	2
1–5	1
0	0
Systolic blood pressure	*Coded value*
≥ 90	4
76–89	3
50–75	2
1–49	1
0	0
Total of coded values	
Priority	*Coded value total*
Immediate	1–10
Urgent	11
Delayed	12

Training

Training must enable the team members to function safely, effectively and efficiently at the scene of a major incident. The team members must know the roles of other team players as well as the command structure. They must be skilled in rapid assessment, triage and stabilisation of the injured, but most importantly they must be disciplined in the discharge of their role. Making unilateral decisions without considering the implications for the whole team inevitably leads to chaos.

Formal training for those who will potentially be asked to attend the scene of a major incident is available through the British Association for Immediate Care (BASICS), who provide a course on the medical management of major incidents. Rehearsal may be important in the training cycle, by testing out procedures, skills and teamwork; however, rehearsals are carried out infrequently because of expense and the logistics of arranging a full-scale major incident exercise. Although parts of the plan may be rehearsed on a small scale at a reduced cost, they may have less impact than a full-scale rehearsal. The largest single benefit of this type of exercise is experience gained in working as part of a large multidisciplinary team.

Non-Major Incidents

At the request of the ambulance service, the hospital may provide a medical and nursing team to attend an incident where there is either one or a small number of casualties. These incidents usually involve entrapment of the casualty (or casualties) where removal to hospital is delayed and where interventions may be required which fall outside the skills or protocols of the paramedics.

The teams provided by the hospital fall into two distinct groups; the team arranged on an ad hoc basis, as described in the section on major incidents; and the established team who attend incidents on a regular basis, colloquially called 'flying squads'.

There are potential difficulties in the operation of these teams, which differ slightly from the teams deployed at a major incident. It is essential that, prior to deployment of a team, there is a clear indication that the team's intervention will be of benefit to the patient. One may well argue that additional resources at the scene of the accident will naturally enhance patient care. However, this is not strictly true as there is a risk that the team may attempt to provide definitive care at the roadside, delaying transfer to hospital. Once release of the casualty has been effected and immediate management of early life-threatening conditions has been initiated, the patient should be transported to hospital. This is essential if mortality and morbidity are to be reduced in those patients with time-critical injuries.

One of the major contributory factors to this potential delay in transfer to hospital is the lack of understanding of the concept of pre-hospital care. Pre-hospital is the provision of skilled care at the roadside and en route to hospital. It is not an attempt to take the A&E department to the patient. Definitive care can only be carried out in the hospital setting, and pre-hospital care should aim to facilitate the removal of the stabilised patient to hospital at the earliest and most appropriate opportunity.

Expeditious removal to hospital of the poly-traumatised patient is based upon the notion of the 'golden hour', the maximum time it should take from injury to definitive care. The golden hour does not belong to the pre-hospital providers, nor does it belong to the A&E department; it belongs to the patient (Porter, personal communication 1994). Ideally, on-scene treatment of the patient should last no longer than 10 minutes, the 'platinum 10 minutes'. This may be somewhat compromised if the patient is trapped, and in such circumstances the delay should be reduced to an absolute minimum.

Difficulties may be experienced by medical and nursing staff, when working in the pre-hospital environment, in adapting to the subtle changes in their respective roles. This is illustrated in the situation where the hospital team focuses upon the medical and nursing care of the individual to the exclusion of everything else, rather than considering the scene in its broadest context. For example, the patient may have had her airway secured, been provided with high-flow oxygen, had intravenous volume replacement, be connected to monitoring equipment, and had her fractures immobilised and her wounds dressed. During this time, however, the fire service may have been prevented from continuing the rescue and the ambulance service may have been deployed fetching and carrying equipment. The result is that the patient will have received medical and nursing care but is still trapped and no nearer to being transported to hospital.

This lack of understanding of teamwork in its broadest sense is largely explained by a lack of operational experience of the team and is therefore less likely to be a problem where the team is used frequently, as opposed to those teams that are rarely mobilised. Many of these problems may be addressed through multidisciplinary training in both theory and practice, the practical element being reinforced through supervised operational experience. This means that a less experienced, not necessarily junior, member of staff is mentored by an experienced colleague, during 'live' call-outs.

Formal training

Historically, formal training in pre-hospital care for both doctors and nurses, if it existed at all, was based upon in-house training schemes and informal discussion with colleagues. Wood & Davies (1994) note that the situation has changed in recent years with the advent of the Pre-hospital Trauma Life Support Course (PHTLS) and the Pre-hospital Emergency Care Course (PHEC). Both courses are open to doctors, nurses and ambulance service paramedics, thus promoting multidisciplinary dialogue. There may be scope to train with the local emergency services as part of ongoing in-service training (Noone & Goncalves 1997). The opportunity to train collectively offers a greater dimension of realism than does training in isolation.

Delivery of Care

Safety

The delivery of care in the pre-hospital environment is fraught with hazards, some of which are common to many areas of practice and others of which are unique to the pre-hospital environment. Those hazards to which the nurse is exposed on a day-to-day basis in the A&E department are likely to be recognised and appropriate precautions taken. In the pre-hospital environment, these precautions may not always be taken. For example, when caring for a multiply injured person in the A&E department, few nurses would consider not wearing gloves, yet at the scene of the accident gloves may not be worn because they become torn on the wreckage or when carrying equipment, or may not be easily accessible. Similarly, gloves are not always replaced when they do become torn.

On arrival at the scene of the incident, the team must liaise with the senior officers from the emergency services and take expert advice regarding specific hazards. Accident scenes are intrinsically hazardous; the rescuer is at risk from a whole range of potential or actual hazards, such as wreckage, chemicals, electricity, moving vehicles and the weather. In addition, when moving about accident sites, the nurse should beware of jagged metal edges, glass, extrication equipment, rubble and blood (Gwinnutt et al. 1996) In a highly stressed situation, it is easy to lose sight of hazards in an eagerness to be of assistance. For instance, when arriving at the scene of an accident on the motorway it is easy to step out of an ambulance or police car into a 'live' traffic lane. High-visibility fluorescent jackets offer the nurse no protection in such circumstances, and in fact may lull nurses into a false sense of security. Those who work in the pre-hospital environment need to develop a sixth sense, having a heightened awareness of the environment which surrounds them. As the nurse becomes 'streetwise', he may react to these hazards in an intuitive way.

The personal safety of the rescuers is paramount, and this question of safety extends beyond the duration of the incident, particularly in respect of psychological safety. By the very nature of the work, the nurse who attends the serious incident is exposed to sights which would be psychologically disturbing to anyone who witnessed them. In order to reduce the risks of developing long-term psychological symptomatology, all rescuers should be able to access debriefing sessions on request (Kilner 1996).

Patient Assessment

Assessment of the patient at the scene of an incident relies heavily on basic clinical assessment skills, rather than the more sophisticated methods employed in hospital. It is a pointless exercise to attempt to auscultate the chest at the side of a motorway as the fire service are cutting the car apart, as is attempting to listen to a blood pressure in the same circumstances. It is almost impossible to see central cyanosis at 4 a.m. in the rain at the side of railway track. A high index of suspicion based upon the mechanism of injury is an invaluable assessment tool.

Technological aids are not always helpful; for example, a pulse oximeter is of little use if the patient is cold and peripherally shut down. If the patient is attached to a number of monitors, as well as the oxygen and bags of intravenous fluid, it becomes quite difficult to remove them without one or more of the appendages snagging. The assessment must be based on identifying the problems the patient is likely to have (reading the wreckage) and then identifying or excluding them. Assessment at the scene should be based upon the primary survey, with the secondary survey being carried out, if possible, en route to hospital. Transport to hospital should not be delayed in order to carry out the secondary survey.

Airway with cervical spine control

The rationale and techniques for airway management and cervical spine control in the trauma patient are well documented (American College of Surgeons 1997, Driscoll et al. 1993). A large proportion of the literature explores these techniques in the context of the A&E department. What is important for the pre-hospital provider, however, is how these principles are applied in the pre-hospital environment.

Reduced levels of consciousness with positional airway obstruction are common and require urgent attention (Gwinnutt et al. 1996). When managing the airway, as with much of the practice of pre-hospital care, the nurse needs to have thought two or three steps ahead. It is extremely frustrating to have gained access to a small space to treat the patient, armed with a size three oropharyngeal airway, only to find that the patient needs a size four. This lack of preplanning could be disastrous to patient outcome, e.g. if the patient vomits during an airway intervention and the suction equipment has not been requested as routine.

Similarly, it is frustrating for medical staff to have successfully intubated the patient but still be unable to inflate the cuff as no syringe is available, with the patient aspirating in the interim. These problems are less likely to occur in the A&E department where equipment is readily available and staff are familiar with its whereabouts. Members of the team should be skilled in a range of airway management techniques, and it is important that these skills have been practised in a range of scenarios. The team member is likely to experience difficulty if faced with an unconscious person with a compromised airway who is trapped upside down, when he has learned the jaw thrust manoeuvre on supine patients.

In the A&E department, the cervical spine is immobilised with a semi-rigid collar, sand bags and tape, whereas in the pre-hospital environment, immobilisation is often provided by the rescuer's hands. It may not be possible to apply a collar because of space restrictions and while the patient is trapped it will not be possible to use sandbags and tape.

With the advent of extrication devices, used in conjunction with a cervical collar, protection may be offered to the cervical, thoracic and lumbar spine. The extrication devices (such as the Russel Extrication Device, RED™, or the Kendrick Extrication Device, KED™) are short, moulded, rigid boards which are placed along the spine and strapped to the patient. The device may be inserted from above, or from the side depending on the space available. The use of this equipment requires some skill, which the hospital team needs to acquire. Failing this, the ambulance staff who are trained in its use and who work with the equipment on a daily basis are well placed to carry out this procedure. Many ambulance services are now using long spinal boards as a means of extrication as well as providing spinal immobilisation during transport. Again, the medical/nursing team should be familiar with the equipment and skilled in its use. This is best achieved through training with staff from the ambulance service.

If an extrication device or long spinal board is not used, it is important that the patient's head is not taped to a conventional ambulance trolley. It is extremely difficult to turn the patient quickly and in a controlled manner, should they vomit en route to hospital, while they are taped to the trolley.

Breathing and ventilation

As Driscoll et al. (1993) suggest, all trauma patients need a high concentration of inspired oxygen. This is an important feature of the pre-hospital management of the patient, and the team members should be alerted to a number of safety issues. Firstly, high-flow oxygen used in a confined space may result in an oxygen-rich atmosphere which presents a potential fire hazard. Fire service personnel should be made aware of this as it may have implications for the techniques they use to extricate the patient. Secondly, there is a potential explosion and fire risk if oxygen therapy equipment comes into contact with grease. This hazard is limited in the hospital setting, but is significantly increased at the scene of an accident.

The environment may present the team with difficulties in performing certain procedures. For instance, it may be difficult to identify the surface anatomy required to site a needle for a needle thorocentesis, because of the position of the patient. This may change priorities in terms of the speed of extrication. Should the extrication be slow with greater control, or should it be rapid with less control, in order to undertake a life-saving procedure?

Circulation

One of the major ongoing debates in trauma management is which intravenous fluid should be used for volume replacement – crystalloid or colloid? The controversy of this debate has been fuelled by emerging schools of thought which dispute the benefits of volume replacement in the pre-hospital delivery (Deakin 1994). These debates are likely to continue for some time in relation to both the hospital and pre-hospital management of trauma patients. It may be further complicated by factors which relate specifically to the pre-hospital environment. In providing pre-hospital care, consideration must be given to the shelf-life of equipment, which is likely to be an important factor for those teams who are called out less frequently. Synthetic colloids such as Gelofusine are more expensive than crystalloids, but they do have a longer shelf-life.

Storage and transport of the equipment may also influence the choice of fluid carried. Colloid should be replaced one for one, i.e. the replaced volume is equal to the estimated volume of fluid the patient has lost. Crystalloid is replaced at a rate of three to one, i.e. the replaced volume is three times the estimated volume lost. Therefore, if crystalloid is to be used, the team must carry greater volumes of intravenous fluid.

The environment may complicate volume replacement in the pre-hospital setting. Intravenous fluids rapidly cool when working outside in the winter months. The temperature of the fluid falls prior to and during administration to the patient. Much of the heat is lost as the fluid flows along the giving set tubing. Fluids may be cold before dispatch to the scene if they are stored in cupboards in draughty corridors or in store huts. Colloid solutions are prone to gelling in cold weather, thus preventing them from being administered to the patient. Rapid infusion of cold fluid may have a catastrophic effect on the physiology traumatised patient, yet currently available equipment designed for warming fluid and maintaining its temperature in the pre-hospital setting is suboptimal.

Although volume replacement for the trauma patient is supported by ATLS training, this practice may be of little benefit to the patient in the pre-hospital setting. It may even be the case that volume replacement in the pre-hospital setting could increase mortality (Deakin & Hicks 1994), thus making the difficulties discussed above largely academic.

Disability

Neurological assessment may be conducted in the form of the mini-neurological assessment (ATLS), based upon the AVPU acronym:

- **A** – **a**lert
- **V** – responds to **v**erbal stimuli
- **P** – responds to **p**ainful stimuli
- **U** – **u**nresponsive.

Exposure and environmental control

Exposure of the patient should be sufficient to conduct the primary survey, while being conscious of the patient's dignity in such a vulnerable position. It is also essential to be aware of the effects the environment is having on the patient. The carer may have warm, waterproof clothing, but the patient will not be so well prepared. Protection of the patient from the elements is vital, yet it is often forgotten, partly because it assumes a relative low priority (Advanced Life Support Group 1995). Hypothermia has both physiological and psychological implications for the patient and should be avoided if at all possible.

Transport

Most of the patients to whom the hospital team are called out will have time-critical injuries. They should therefore be transported by the most appropriate means, to the most appropriate hospital, being that which has the facilities on site to provide the patient with definitive care. This is not necessarily the closest hospital with an A&E department or the hospital which is the team's base. There is no place to 'stay and play' in the pre-hospital environment. Once extricated, there is little, if any, reason to delay transport to hospital.

Unique Role Played by Nurses in Providing Pre-Hospital Care

Some of the skills which nurses refine in the A&E department are transferable into the pre-hospital arena and of these skills many form the uniqueness of the nurse's role in this environment. The nurse may be a skilled communicator who is able to establish a rapport with the patient early into the incident and follow this through into the hospital phase of care. This may have a significant impact on the psychological well-being of the patient, especially as the nurse has already established a degree of credibility, through having been there at the scene and therefore knowing what it was like. This continuity is more than a familiar face, although this is important; rather, it is reassurance for the patient through a relationship based upon security and trust.

The psychological support is not undertaken in isolation, as the nurse is able to assimilate information from the scene in order to support the patient and gain her cooperation. The nurse may become the interface between the patient and the rescue team, interpreting events for the patient and protecting him or her from a barrage of repetitive questions. The nurse is able to provide the rescue team with vital information that the patient is unable to verbalise, e.g. if the patient winces in pain when a particular activity is undertaken.

A nurse is well placed to act as the patient's advocate, which is an acknowledged skill of nurses and is less likely to be taken on by other team members. The nurse may also be skilled in caring for distressed relatives who may be at scene and who may accompany the patient to the hospital. Again, establishing and sustaining a rapport with the relatives will enhance the quality of care those relatives receive.

Conclusion

Nurses can make a valuable contribution to the delivery of pre-hospital care as part of a multidisciplinary team. Yet, with a few exceptions, the service which is currently provided is suboptimal. Optimal care may be achieved through effective planning, multi-agency training and education, research, operational experience and adequate funding, with standards developed and agreed at a national level.

Failure to address these issues will result in the continuation of a fragmented service of dubious quality, which ultimately may result in the demise of nursing input in the provision of pre-hospital care.

References

American College of Surgeons (Committee on Trauma) (1997) *Advanced Trauma Life Support Programme*. Illinois: American College of Surgeons.

Advanced Life Support Group (1995) *Major Incident Medical Management and Support: the Practical Approach*. London: BMJ Publishing Group.

Carley S, Stadthagen A, Cabrera Esquenazi A *et al.* (1998) Pre-hospital forum – nurses in pre-hospital care. *Pre-hospital Immediate Care*, **1**, 144–151.

Deakin CD, Hicks IR (1994) AB or ABC: prehospital fluid management in major trauma. *Journal of Accident and Emergency Medicine*, **11**, 154–157.

Driscoll PA, Gwinnutt CL, LeDuc Jimmerson C, Goodall O (1993) *Trauma Resuscitation: the Team Approach*. Basingstoke: Macmillan.

Eaton CJ (1993) *Essentials of Immediate Medical Care*. Edinburgh: Churchill Livingstone.

Fletcher V (1986) When the music stopped. *Nursing Times*, **30**(4), 30–32.

Flynn R (1997) *Sitting in the Hot Seat: Leaders and Teams for Critical Incident Management*. Chichester: John Wiley.

Gwinnutt CL, Wilson AW, Driscoll P (1996) Prehospital care. In: Skinner D, Driscoll P, Earlam R, eds. *ABC of Trauma*, 2nd edn. London: BMJ Publishing Group.

Hodgetts T, McNeil I, Cooke M (1995) *The Pre-hospital Emergency Management Master*. London: BMJ Publishing Group.

Hodgetts T, Miles S (1996) Major incidents. In: Skinner D, Driscoll P, Earlam R, eds. *ABC of Trauma* 2nd edn. London: BMJ Publishing Group.

Kilner T (1995) Equipping the pre-hospital care team. *Emergency Nurse* **3**(4),16–19.

Kilner T (1996) Psychological aspects of pre-hospital care. *Emergency Nurse*, **4**(2), 16–18.

Kilner T (1998) Pre-hospital forum – nurses in pre-hospital care (letter). *Pre-hospital Immediate Care*, **2**(2), 116.

Mathews J (1998) Pre-hospital forum – nurses in pre-hospital care (letter). *Pre-hospital Immediate Care*, **2**(2), 115–116.

NHS Management Executive (1990) *Emergency Planning in the NHS: Health Service Arrangements for Dealing with Major Incidents.* London: NHS Management Executive.

New B (1992) *Too Many Cooks? The Response of the Health Related Services to Major Incidents in London.* London: Kings Fund Institute.

Noone P, Goncalves D (1997) A flying start. *Emergency Nurse,* **4**(4), 4–5.

Peter L, Taylor C (1994) Rucksacks for flying squads. *Emergency Nurse* **2**(2), 4–5.

Regional Ambulance Officers Group (1990) *Ambulance Service Operational Arrangements – Civil Emergencies.* London: Regional Officers Group.

Salt P (1989) The mobile team. In: Walsh M, ed. *Disasters: Current Planning and Recent Experience.* London: Edward Arnold.

Savage (1979) *Disasters: Hospital Planning.* Oxford: Pergamon Press.

Trunkey DD (1983) Trauma. *Scientific American*, **249**, 28–35.

Wood I, Davies S (1994) Beyond the department's doors: prehospital emergency care. *Accident and Emergency Nursing,* **2**(3), 149–154.

Chapter 2

Trauma Life Support

Lisa Hadfield-Law

- Introduction
- Preparation
- Primary survey
- Secondary survey
- Trauma in children
- Definitive care
- Conclusion

Introduction

The last decade has seen significant changes in how patients with major injuries are managed. However, trauma continues to be a leading cause of death in people under 40 years of age in developed countries and is the third commonest cause of death at all ages (Robertson & Redmond 1994). In the UK this translates to 25 000 fatalities as a direct result of trauma, with 500 000 sustaining major injury per annum. The estimated fiscal cost for one individual who dies as the result of a road traffic accident is over £800 000 and, in total, accidents consume approximately 1% of the gross national product, some £5000 million annually in the UK (Robertson & Redmond 1994). Conversely, Underhill & Finlayson (1989) found that trauma deaths account for fewer than two deaths per 10 000 new attendees to A&E departments. It places into context the health economics of care and the resultant responsibilities placed on A&E staff to play their part in ensuring patients receive the best quality care possible.

The multiply injured patient presents a great challenge to the A&E or trauma team. Failure to recognise and correctly treat traumatic injuries promptly will have a detrimental effect on early and delayed mortality and morbidity (Royal College of Surgeons 1988). A careful and thorough assessment must be made as quickly as possible, supported by life-saving interventions. A trauma team may comprise an informal group of individuals who care for the multiply injured patient, or a more formal resuscitation team identified as the 'trauma team' (Driscoll & Vincent 1992). All team members should be appropriately prepared to care for the trauma patient in a systematic manner (Hadfield 1993a). The A&E nurse is part of this team.

Within the team, nurses have diverse roles to fulfil. These include: (Hadfield 1993a):

- assessment and resuscitation
- communication

- evaluation
- documentation
- planning
- debriefing
- advocacy.

A widely adopted management plan for trauma victims is the Advanced Trauma Life Support (ATLS) system (American College of Surgeons 1997) which follows a sequence that prioritises care with the objective of minimising mortality and morbidity. Initial assessment comprises:

- preparation
- primary survey
- resuscitation
- secondary survey
- continuous monitoring and evaluation
- definitive care.

This chapter will follow the sequence of events; in reality, however, many activities occur simultaneously and involve a number of team members.

In the multiply injured patient, resuscitation of physical condition takes immediate priority, but it is important that psychological needs are not overlooked. In practice, this often falls to one member of the team. Despite this, all health professionals involved should be careful not to cause further emotional or spiritual distress to patients (Edwards 1995).

Preparation

In many instances, the ambulance service alerts the A&E department to the impending arrival of a multiply injured patient. This allows time for the most appropriate preparations for receipt of the patient. The size and mix of the team of staff will depend on the level of resources available to each unit and will vary widely around the country. Some will comprise a junior A&E nurse and doctor, while others will have specialist nursing and medical support available 24 hours a day. Irrespective of the level of staffing, a systematic approach to care should apply on every occasion and it should be constantly monitored to maintain its optimum effectiveness and efficiency (Sexton 1997). Each team member should have a clear role and pre-designated responsibilities.

A safe and appropriate environment is essential. This requires careful preparation. All team members who have direct patient contact must use protective clothing. This should include goggles, gloves and aprons to protect against contamination from patient's body fluids. Universal precautions should be taken with *all* trauma patients (Fuller 1993). Such patients

also need protection from nosocomial infection and death due to sepsis. The use of lead aprons for all staff involved means that care can continue while X-rays are taken, without undue risk to staff. The treatment area should be kept warm to reduce the risk of hypothermia in the trauma patient (Kosmos 1995). It should also be spacious enough for team members to work safely and simultaneously.

Primary Survey

Each patient should have an initial physical examination to identify and prioritise potentially life-threatening injuries (Paynter 1993). This should take place immediately and systematically using an ABC approach:

- Airway with cervical spine control
- Breathing and ventilation
- Circulation with haemorrhage control
- Disability: neurological status
- Exposure/environmental control.

The primary survey and resuscitation aspects of initial assessment are completed together. Jutzi-Kosmos (1995) claims the primary survey can be completed within 30 seconds by an experienced trauma nurse.

Airway with cervical spine control

To prevent secondary cervical spine injury, the patient should be approached from an angle at which he can see the assessor without moving his head. A simple statement which requires a response can then be made, e.g. 'How are you Mr Smith?' or 'Hello, what's your name?' If the patient is able to speak, two important assumptions can be made. Firstly, the airway is clear, and secondly the patient's brain is being perfused with blood. Even if a patient's airway *sounds* clear, the assessor should not move onto the next stage without physically checking the airway for potential problems by looking for foreign bodies or damage to the mouth and neck.

Simultaneous cervical spine precautions must be taken from the outset (Tippett 1993). Any trauma patient, particularly with injuries above the clavicle or those with an altered conscious level, should be considered to have a cervical spine injury until proven otherwise. Manual immobilisation of the head and neck should be followed as soon as possible by the application of a semi-rigid collar and specifically designed immobilisers firmly in place. This is the minimum intervention in terms of acceptable precautions. Specifically designed boards for complete spinal immobilisation are most effective. For those patients who are unable to remain still and who are thrashing around on the trolley, a semi-rigid collar can be applied until the patient is calm enough to tolerate further measures.

If the patient does not respond to a simple question, airway obstruction should be assumed and measures should be taken to relieve this immediately. The most common reason for obstruction in the unconscious patient is partial or complete occlusion of the oropharynx by the tongue. Saliva, vomit and blood may exacerbate the problem. Interventions should begin with the simplest, progressing to the more complex if necessary. A chin lift or jaw thrust should pull collapsed soft tissues out of the airway. Any debris or foreign bodies must be physically removed. Suction can be very effective, using a tonsil tip/rigid (Yankeur) sucker.

For those patients who vomit profusely and unexpectedly, airway and cervical spine control can be difficult. Mechanical suction apparatus, including a Yankeur sucker, must always be available for use *immediately*, so that the patient can be tipped, head downwards, on the trolley and his airway cleared, minimising the risk of aspiration of gastric contents.

More active airway intervention may be required for those who are unable to maintain their own airway. A nasopharyngeal airway will ensure patency in the conscious patient, without causing a gag reflex. This may be particularly useful for those with a fluctuating conscious level. For the unconscious patient, an oropharyngeal (guedal) airway may be helpful; however, its use increases the risk of vomiting.

Many multiply injured patients need emergency endotracheal (ET) intubation early on in their management. This procedure carries with it certain risks, particularly in the trauma patient. Cervical spine immobilisation must be maintained throughout intubation, making the procedure more complex. The patient is often shocked, can have a damaged airway, and frequently has a full stomach. ET intubation in inexperienced hands can be fraught with danger. Ideally, it should be performed by someone with appropriate trauma and anaesthetic skills.

If oral or nasal intubation fails to secure an airway in the patient with obstruction, within 60 seconds, and the patient cannot be ventilated with a bag–valve–mask system owing to facial fractures, the nurse should prepare for an emergency cricothyroidotomy. Several periods of apnoea caused by repeated attempts at intubation can result in dangerous levels of hypoxia for the patient. A needle cricothyroidotomy can establish a temporary airway swiftly, but will need to be followed by a surgical cricothyroidotomy or a tracheostomy within 30–45 minutes. After any intervention, the patency of the airway should be rechecked.

Breathing

A patent airway does not automatically mean that the patient is able to breathe properly. The patient's chest should be watched carefully, for the rise and fall of the chest wall. The assessor should listen for breath sounds and feel for exhaled breath. If the patient is not breathing or is breathing inadequately, then mechanical ventilation using a bag–valve–mask system (Ambu bag) with high-flow oxygen should be instituted. This is usually more effective when performed by two people, one to seal the airway and one to squeeze the Ambu bag.

Efficiency of breathing should be established by observing for rate and depth, cyanosis, use of accessory muscles, tracheal shift from the midline, engorged neck veins, any sucking chest wounds, and, of great importance, any change in conscious level. Pulse oximetry is a valuable monitor, as peripheral oxygen saturation is a good measure of breathing efficiency. All trauma patients should receive high-flow oxygen (American College of Surgeons 1997). Its purpose is to reduce further strain on the heart and it can be achieved by administering oxygen at 15 l/min through a clear mask with a reservoir bag attached. A concentration of approximately 95% arterial saturation will result.

Any life-threatening condition encountered during the assessment of breathing should be corrected immediately. These include:

■ airway obstruction
■ tension pneumothorax
■ open pneumothorax (sucking chest wound)
■ massive haemothorax
■ flail chest
■ cardiac tamponade.

Sucking chest wounds should be covered. A needle thoracentesis may be required in the event of a tension pneumothorax. A large flail segment with pulmonary contusion or a massive haemothorax should be treated straight away. If the patient is unable to maintain adequate ventilation unassisted, endotracheal intubation may be required, with mechanical ventilation. Equipment for inserting a chest drain should be prepared following a needle thoracentesis. After any manoeuvre is used to correct inadequate ventilation, breathing should always be rechecked.

Circulation with haemorrhage control

Assessment of the patient's circulatory status should be made by measuring the quality and rate of the pulse and the level of consciousness. If the patient does not have a pulse, external cardiac massage should be commenced. It may be appropriate to prepare for open thoracentesis, pericardiocentesis or needle thoracentesis if cardiac tamponade or tension pneumothorax is suspected.

Any external bleeding should be controlled by direct pressure or by elevation, as there is little point in trying to replace fluid if no attempt is being made to conserve it. Tourniquets should not be used, as the tissue damage incurred can be irreversible. By checking the skin of the patient, other indicators of circulatory status may be available, e.g. colour, warmth, sweating and capillary refill. Every trauma patient should be presumed hypovolaemic until proved otherwise. Erring on the side of caution may prevent some of the unnecessary deaths and disability which occur.

At least two short, wide-bore cannulae must be inserted (14–16 gauge) with an initial fluid bolus of 2 L of warmed Hartmann's solution given through a blood giving set. It is important to remember that the rate of intravenous (I.V.) infusion is not determined by the size of the vein, but by the internal diameter of the cannula, and is inversely affected by its length. At this time a blood sample can be taken for grouping and cross-matching of at least six units, and full blood count and urea and electrolyte baselines should be taken. Women of child-bearing years should have a pregnancy test (Smith 1996).

The two peripheral I.V. lines should be started in upper extremities if not contraindicated. Lines should not be placed in injured extremities if they can be avoided. If difficulties arise with insertion, or more lines are required, venous cut-downs should be performed.

Restoration of adequate circulating blood volume and oxygen-carrying capacity is essential. Fluid best suited to the trauma patient remains controversial. As crystalloids are cheaper than colloids, and are more effective in restoring intravascular volume (Schierhout & Roberts 1998), Hartmann's solution is a good option. It is important to remember that for every millilitre of estimated blood volume lost, 3 ml of crystalloid should replace it (Kosmos 1995). Crystalloids cannot enhance oxygen-carrying capacity, and therefore the fluid of choice is blood, which should be transfused as soon as possible, if the patient does not respond to a rapid infusion of 3 L of crystalloid solution.

Ideally, blood should be typed and cross-matched, but this can result in an unacceptable delay. If so, type-specific blood can be used. Risk of reaction is relatively low. In dire emergencies, O-negative blood can be used and should be stored in small quantities in the A&E department for such cases. Patient blood samples should be taken early as infusion of large quantities of O-negative blood can cause difficulties with grouping and cross-matching later. Monitoring the patient's fluid intake and output is a vital part of the A&E nurse's role. Knowing precisely how much and what kind of fluid the patient has received is essential in determining subsequent intravenous fluid management.

ECG monitoring provides circulatory information from the heart rate and rhythm. It also provides an indicator of hypoxia, hypoperfusion and hypothermia in the form of ectopic beats, aberrant conduction and bradycardia. Electromechanical dissociation (EMD) is suggestive of profound hypovolaemia, cardiac tamponade or tension pneumothorax and has a poor prognosis unless the underlying cause can be determined and treated (Belson 1993).

Application of a pneumatic anti-shock garment (PASG) is controversial (Mattox *et al.* 1986) and is rarely used in the trauma situation in the UK. Initially it was thought that the PASG increased blood pressure (BP) by causing an autotransfusion effect of 1–1.5 L of blood from the lower extremities back to the systemic circulation (Kemmer 1984). Other evidence indicates, however, that only around 200 ml is actually shunted back (Frumkin 1985). The rise in BP is much more likely to be due to an increase in peripheral vascular resistance in the lower extremities. Contraindications for the use of PASG include left ventricular failure, pulmonary oedema, CNS injury or an intrathoracic injury (Driscoll *et al.* 1994). It is very important, therefore, that the patient is continuously monitored while the suit is in place.

Disability: neurological status

A simple and rapid assessment of neurological status should take place during the primary survey. A mnemonic using the acronym AVPU is used along with pupil size and reaction. An accurate impression of conscious level can be surmised by eliciting the best eye opening response to stimulus:

- A – **A**lert
- V – responds to **V**erbal stimuli
- P – responds to **P**ainful stimuli
- U – **U**nresponsive.

A decreased level of consciousness should alert the

assessor to four possibilities (Pre-Hospital Trauma Life Support Committee 1994)

■ decreased cerebral oxygenation (hypoxia and hypoperfusion)
■ central nervous system injury
■ drug or alcohol overdose
■ metabolic derangement (diabetes, seizure, cardiac arrest).

A full Glasgow Coma Score is completed at this stage. Although this score is considered by some to be a crude measure of level of consciousness, a sequence of readings will tend to show fairly subtle changes quickly.

Exposure/environmental control

At the end of the primary survey, every item of clothing must be removed without risking any further damage to the patient (American College of Surgeons 1997). It is prudent at this point to log roll the patient so that the back, which comprises 50% of the body, can be fully examined. Failure to assess the back of the patient can mean that the assessor misses a life-threatening injury.

Trauma patients are at great risk from hypothermia. Many have been exposed to low temperatures outside. Wet conditions, wind and blood loss contribute further to a drop in core temperature. Hypothermia increases the morbidity and mortality of the trauma patient and must be prevented and reversed. Secondary hypothermia should be prevented from occurring in the resuscitation room. Various measures can be used, including:

■ warm blankets over the patient from a warming cabinet, radiator or microwave
■ i.v., blood and lavage fluids warmed to 39°C (Hadfield 1993b)
■ adequate environmental temperature in resuscitation area
■ specifically designed warming plate suspended over patient trolley
■ controlled exposure of the patient (Kosmos 1995)
■ external warming device, e.g. Behr Hugger.

Full history

A comprehensive history surrounding the patient and event will ensure a quicker idea of the status of the patient. Ambulance crews, paramedics, witnesses and relatives are an invaluable source of information. If the patient is conscious, he may possibly hold the most relevant information (Box 2.1).

Box 2.1 – *Ample history (American College of Surgeons 1997)*

■ Allergies

■ Medications – current

■ Past illnesses/medical history
 – respiratory disease
 – cardiovascular disease
 – endocrine disease
 – neurological disease
 – splenectomy
 – other
 – tetanus immunisation
 – previous/current infectious disease
 – female – date of last menstrual period

■ Last meal/drink

■ Events preceding injury
 – height/weight
 – place of incident

Details regarding the mechanism of injury can indicate the site and seriousness of many potential injuries. This can save a great deal of time, which may be a life saver for the patient (Halpern 1989). Following blunt trauma, patients should have two X rays as part of the primary survey:

■ chest
■ pelvis.

These are the only X-rays which are required to identify life-threatening injuries. Any other X-rays required can be taken during the secondary survey.

Pain relief can be overlooked during the activity of resuscitation, but it is an essential part of good patient care. Intravenous opiates work well, although intramuscular routes are only appropriate for less acute situations. Entonox can provide useful pain relief during the early stages, but should be avoided if there is the possibility of a pneumothorax.

Secondary Survey

The primary survey and resuscitation must be completed before the secondary survey begins. If, at the end of the primary survey, the patient's condition remains unstable, each step should be repeated until stability is achieved. During the secondary survey less obvious injuries, which may pose a latent threat to life, should be detected.

At this stage a full set of observations should be taken, including:

- temperature – rectal or tympanic membrane (Hadfield 1993c)
- pulse – radial, femoral or carotid
- respirations
- blood pressure
- Glasgow Coma Score.

All these parameters will provide the assessor with a much clearer idea of the state of the patient. Early signs of shock may be detected if a rise in pulse and respirations and diastolic blood pressure are noted. These should be repeated every 5 minutes initially, preferably by the same person, to avoid assessor variability.

Trauma patients are vulnerable to the effects of pressure on their skin, and every effort should be made to prevent any unnecessary risk. Patients who arrive in A&E on a spine board should be transferred from it as soon as is safe (Cooke 1998).

Head and face

The patient should be asked about any pain he may be experiencing and examined for evidence of injury to the bones or soft tissue, mouth or eyes. Otorrhoea or rhinorrhoea should be noted. The 'halo test' should be performed on any drainage from the ear, nose or mouth, to check for the presence of cerebrospinal fluid following basilar skull fracture. To do this, a drop of the fluid is placed on a paper towel; if it contains cerebrospinal fluid, as it disperses, it will become lighter towards the edges.

Neck

Cervical spine immobilisation should be maintained at all times. If immobilising devices must be removed, then manual in-line immobilisation should be substituted (Sing 1998). While maintaining careful cervical spine immobilisation, the neck should be examined for any obvious injury to the bones or soft tissues. Any evidence of damage should lead the assessor to be concerned about airway obstruction. The assessor should check for tracheal deviation or distended neck veins which may indicate a missed tension pneumothorax or cardiac tamponade.

Chest

The patient should be asked about pain or dyspnoea. Any sign of obvious injury should be noted, e.g. sucking chest wounds, surface/penetrating trauma, paradoxical movements, subcutaneous emphysema, bruising or crepitus over the ribs. Life-saving interventions should already have been performed for open chest wounds or a tension pneumothorax.

It is important to remember that every patient has a posterior chest, which should already have been examined during the log roll at the end of the primary survey. A 12-lead ECG will determine dysrhythmias and may indicate cardiac contusion. This is demonstrated by elevation of the ST-segment of the affected area, atrial fibrillation or an unexplained tachycardia.

Abdomen

An assessment of pain should be made, providing the patient is conscious. The abdomen should be examined for any obvious injury, distension, rigidity, guarding, contusions, scars and bowel sounds. Such an examination should be careful and thorough, as bleeding into the abdomen from damaged organs is frequently the cause of life-threatening hypovolaemia. The most important aspect of the abdominal assessment is to determine whether the patient requires surgery or not.

A urinary catheter attached to a urometer should be inserted, providing no contraindications exist, such as blood at the urinary meatus, scrotal haematoma or a high riding prostate, which would indicate urethral damage. A urometer will ensure that accurate hourly measurements of urine output can be taken. If urethral catheterisation is contraindicated due to urethral damage, a suprapubic catheter should be inserted by a suitably skilled team member. A urinary output of >50 ml/h is a good indicator of satisfactory tissue perfusion (Mills *et al.* 1995).

A nasogastric tube should be inserted to decompress the stomach, thereby helping to avoid regurgitation. This can be caused by a paralytic ileus or air in the stomach as the result of assisted manual ventilation. A gastric tube may also signify blood in the gastric contents. A nasogastric tube should not be inserted if a cribriform plate fracture is suspected, in case it is inadvertently passed into the cranial cavity. In this event, the tube can be inserted orally.

A naso- or orogastric tube and a urinary catheter should always be inserted before diagnostic peritoneal lavage (DPL) is performed. Such measures will ensure that abdominal and pelvic organs are less likely to be damaged during the procedure. DPL is a quick diagnostic procedure to determine intra-abdominal bleeding. It is indicated when results of physical examination are equivocal or the patient is unable to participate in the assessment. It should always be performed by, or in the presence of, the surgeon who will be acting upon any positive findings.

Pelvis and genitalia

Patients should be asked about pain and whether they have an urge to pass urine. Male patients should be examined for bruising, blood at the urinary meatus, priapism and oedema. The presence of femoral pulses should be ascertained. If a rectal examination was not performed when the patient was log rolled at the end of the primary survey, it should be carried out now. The assessor should look for blood in the rectum, which may indicate damage to the gut or pelvis. A high riding prostate may be indicative of urethral injury, and loss of sphincter tone is often associated with spinal injury. Bony fragments may also be felt, indicating pelvic damage.

A vaginal examination should be performed in women, to look for blood and lacerations resulting from either direct damage or pelvic fractures. The pelvic ring should not be 'rocked' by applying heavy manual pressure to the iliac crests, but should be carefully examined to investigate for lack of continuity. 'Rocking' can be extremely painful and causes further damage and bleeding.

Extremities

Both arms and legs should be examined. Each should be assessed for:

- pain
- pallor
- pulse
- paraesthesia
- paralysis
- cold
- perspiration
- instability
- crepitus.

Any injuries should be realigned or splinted. Every time this is done, the limb must be reassessed. Any open wounds should be covered with a sterile dressing. If at any time during the secondary survey a patient's condition deteriorates, returning to the primary survey with institution or reinstitution of resuscitative measures is essential.

Trauma in Children

Trauma is a major cause of death in children. Many of the principles for managing children are exactly the same as for adults, but it is essential that team members with paediatric experience are available. The priorities for assessment and management are identical (Jorden 1994). The only differences lie in certain aspects of their anatomy, physiology and emotional development. With children it can be difficult for the inexperienced to recognise early problems.

The small size and shape of the child tend to mean that from the mechanism of injury, different patterns of injury result, and there is an increased chance of multiple injuries with the same force. Bones are flexible, which mean they tend to bend, and the structures underneath can be damaged. The high ratio between body surface area and volume puts children at higher risk of hypothermia due to loss of heat through the skin. Children have not had the experience to develop the emotional coping strategies of adults. Particular attention should be paid to psychological considerations. If at all possible, someone known to the child is almost always a helpful support in the trauma room and should be given the opportunity to stay throughout the resuscitation.

Definitive Care

Once the trauma patient has been assessed using the ABCDE approach, has been successfully resuscitated and has undergone a head to toe assessment to find all injuries, the patient can be moved on to the next stage of care. Definitive care may be provided in the operating theatre, intensive care unit, trauma ward or another hospital. Serious injuries are treated and definitive plans for the comprehensive care of the patient are made. It is essential the patient is in the best condition possible to undergo transfer either intra-hospital or inter-hospital. Many of the areas and routes are limited, in terms of facilities, should the patient's condition deteriorate, and therefore the team should be as confident as possible about the stability of the situation. Nevertheless, appropriate items of resuscitation equipment should accompany the patient, along with suitably skilled staff.

Copies of the comprehensive records and reports, which must be kept up to date, should accompany the patient wherever he is transferred. While a resuscitation is in progress, it is tempting to leave documentation until afterwards. Unless there are very few members of the team present, someone should be made responsible for recording all assessments, interventions, evaluations and plans. Preprinted trauma sheets can be very useful on these occasions, both to save time and to act as an aide memoire. Fully comprehensive notes regarding all details of the patient contribute significantly to the optimal standards of communication supporting the patient, which are vital to good care, not to mention medicolegal and audit purposes.

Family members and significant others should be

kept carefully informed of the proceedings. The distress experienced by this group of people during resuscitation can be far longer lasting than that experienced by the patient. If possible, someone should be allocated to liaise between the resuscitation room and relatives. Although the nurse may be the ideal person, chaplains, social workers or staff from other areas of the hospital can often assume this role. Relatives can provide important information, and they should be included in the efforts to provide optimal patient care. Inviting relatives into the trauma room appears to be appropriate in some instances (Barratt & Wallis 1998, RCN and BAEM 1995).

Conclusion

Good trauma care relies heavily on a multidisciplinary approach. Not all trauma team members give 'hands-on' care, but each department and speciality has a valuable part to play. Successful initial assessment using a systematic approach *every* time, by every team member, will ensure that injuries are not missed. This gives the trauma patient the best possible chance of a complete and speedy recovery.

A great deal of progress has been made over the last decade, but there still remains a great deal to do. In the past, trauma patients have died as the result of relatively simple problems like hypovolaemia and hypoxia. Many of us are now aware of ways to prevent such deaths. However, it is essential that all those who come into contact with trauma patients have the necessary skills and knowledge. Investment in training of this nature is a small price to pay for a reduction in trauma deaths.

References

American College of Surgeons (Committee on Trauma) (1997) *Advanced Trauma Life Support Programme*. Illinois: American College of Surgeons.

Barratt F, Wallis DN (1998) Relatives in the resuscitation room: their point of view. *Journal of Accident and Emergency Medicine* **15**, 109.

Belson L (1993) ACLS: cardiac care for the Nineties. *Emergency Nurse* **1**(1), 9–12.

Cooke MW (1998) Use of the spinal board within the accident and emergency department. *Journal of Accident and Emergency Medicine* **15**, 108–109.

Driscoll PA, Vincent CA (1992) Organising an efficient trauma team. *Injury* **23**(2), 107–110.

Driscoll PA, Gwinnutt C, Brook S (1994) Extremity trauma. In: Discoll P, Gwinnntt CL, LeOne Jimmerson C, Goodall O, eds. *Trauma Resuscitation: the Team Approach* London: Macmillan.

Edwards B (1995) Management of spiritual distress. *Emergency Nurse* **3**(2), 23–25.

Frumkin K (1985) The pneumatic antishock garment. In Robert JR, Hedges JR, eds. *Clinical Procedures in Emergency Medicine.* Philadelphia: WB Saunders.

Fuller A (1993) Spillages of blood and body fluids in accident and emergency departments. *Accident and Emergency Nursing* **1**(2), 98–103.

Hadfield L (1993a) Preparation for the nurse as part of the trauma team. *Accident and Emergency Nursing* **1**(3), 154–160.

Hadfield L (1993b) Review of the level one fluid warmer. *Accident and Emergency Nursing* **1**(1), 58–59.

Hadfield L (1993c) Review of tympanic membrane thermometry. *Accident and Emergency Nursing* **2**(1), 57.

Halpern JS (1989) Mechanisms and patterns of trauma. *Journal of Emergency Nursing* **15**(5), 380–388.

Jorden RC (1994) Evaluation and stabilisation of the multiply injured traumatised patient. In: Barkin RM, Rosen P, eds. *Emergency Paediatrics: A Guide to Ambulatory Care*, 4th edn. St Louis: Mosby.

Jutzi-Kosmos C (1995) Assessment of multiple trauma and thoracic trauma. In: Kitt S, Selfridge-Thomas J, Proehl JA, Kaiser J, eds. *Emergency Nursing – a Physiological and Clinical Perspective* Philadelphia: WB Saunders.

Kemmer DL (1984) Antishock trousers. *American Family Physician* **30**, 163–166.

Kosmos CA (1995) Multiple trauma In: Kitt S, Selfridge-Thomas J, Proehl JA, Kaiser J, eds. *Emergency Nursing – a Physiological and Clinical Perspective* 2nd edn. Philadelphia: WB Saunders.

Mattox KL, Bickell WH, Pepe PE, Manglesdorff AD (1986) Prospective randomised evaluation of antishock MAST in post-traumatic hypotension. *Journal of Trauma* **26**, 779–786.

Mills K, Morton R, Page G (1995) *Colour Atlas and Text of Emergencies.* London: Mosby-Wolfe.

Paynter M (1993) Trauma support: revolution in care. *Emergency Nurse* **1**(2), 7–9.

Pre-Hospital Trauma Life Support Committee (1994) *PHTLS: Basic and Advanced Pre-hospital Trauma Life Support.* St Louis: Mosby Lifeline.

Robertson C, Redmond AD (1994) *The Management of Major Trauma* 2nd edn. Oxford: Oxford University Press.

Royal College of Nursing (RCN) and British Association for Accident and Emergency Medicine (BAEM) (1995) *Bereavement Care in Accident and Emergency.* London: RCN.

Royal College of Surgeons of England (1988) *Report of the Working Party on the Management of Patients with Major Injuries.* London: Royal College of Surgeons of England.

Schierhout G, Roberts I (1998) Fluid resuscitation with colloid or crystalloid solutions in critically ill patients. *British Medical Journal* **316**(7136), 961–964.

Sexton J (1997) Trauma epidemiology and team management. *Emergency Nurse* **5**(1), 14–16.

Sing RF (1998) Letter to the Editor. *The Journal of Trauma* **44**(2), 417.

Smith S (1996) Care of the pregnant woman in A&E. *Emergency Nurse* **4**(2), 7–9.

Tippett J (1993) Spinal immobilisation of the multiply injured patient. *Accident and Emergency Nursing* **1**(1), 25–33.

Underhill TJ, Finlayson BJ (1989) A review of trauma deaths in an accident and emergency department. *Archives of Emergency Medicine* **6**, 90–96.

Chapter 3

Major Incident Planning

Andrew Whitfield & Tim Kilner

- Introduction
- Definition
- Planning
- Exercise and training
- The hospital's response to a major incident alert
- Medicolegal issues
- Aftermath
- Conclusion

Introduction

In recent years, the United Kingdom has witnessed a number of major incidents, many of which have become household names: Hillsborough, King's Cross, Kegworth, Bradford Football Stadium, The Herald of Free Enterprise, Clapham. From a local perspective, however, the threat of a major incident occurring in the UK is often viewed as remote and the perception of individuals or communities who are affected by a specific incident is very low (Kreps 1992). Consequently, major incident management often attracts a low priority in relation to more immediately pressing issues of the health service. Additionally, emergency planning and exercising are often viewed as being time-consuming, disruptive and expensive (Rushing 1990).

By their very nature, major incidents are unpredictable, the only certainty being that at some time, somewhere, the unexpected will happen. But when it does, the health services must be able to respond rapidly, mobilising additional human and material resources. Procedures must also be in place to make the most efficient use of those resources in the given circumstances. Achieving this requires the health services to be proactive in the planning of emergency management measures, thus reducing the need for reactive management in an extremely stressful situation. The A&E department provides the focus for the hospital's patient care activity during the response to an incident.

This chapter discusses the role of the health services in contingency planning and service provision for major incidents. Consideration will be given to hospital-based activity, both in general terms and specifically in relation to A&E services. The on-scene response to a major incident is considered in Chapter 1.

Definition

In England, the NHS Executive, in its document *Emergency Planning in the NHS: Health Services*

Arrangements for Dealing with Major Incidents (HSE 1996a, b), states that a major incident arises when

> *... any occurrence presents a serious threat to the health of the community, disruption to the service, or causes (or is likely to cause) such numbers of casualties as to require special arrangements by the health service.*

This definition is the basis for the health service's major incident planning and response. Guidance for emergency planning in the NHS was provided by Health Circular (HMSO 1990). This guidance was subsequently replaced by HSG(93)24 and the handbook was updated in relation to reception and dispersal of military casualties evacuated to the UK in 1994 by EL(94)28, and in relation to protective clothing by a new chapter in the handbook in 1994. A revised handbook of guidance with the same title as the original was produced and circulated in 1996 by the Emergency Planning Coordination Unit of the NHS Executive (HSE 1996a,b) to replace the majority of the chapters in the original handbook. Guidance was also offered in Wales (WHC(93)69; Welsh Office 1993), Scotland (SHHD/DGM(1990)73; Scottish Office 1990) and Northern Ireland (HSS EMP 1/93; Health and Personal Social Services Northern Ireland 1993) prior to the revised publication of HSE (1996a,b).

A major incident may be declared by any of the emergency services or any hospital that considers that the criteria for such an incident have been fulfilled. Major incidents do not make equal demands upon all services. For example, a civil disturbance at a sports event may have limited implications for the fire service, while making a great demand on other services; similarly, a large chemical warehouse fire in an isolated area may make greater demands on the fire service than on other services. However, all incidents are dynamic and present the potential for demands to change.

Consequently, all emergency services should respond accordingly with the appropriate predetermined responses, which may initially only require the service to activate the standby mode. All incidents, where the scale and magnitude are questionable, should be regarded as serious in the first instance, even if the criteria for a major incident have not been met. Often, seemingly innocuous events can, if not dealt with speedily and efficiently, develop into major incidents.

Planning

The very nature of major incidents brings together diverse groups of professionals in large numbers, each group having distinct roles and responsibilities. When faced with the complexities of a major incident, it is unrealistic to expect such a large multidisciplinary team to function in an effective and coordinated manner without detailed prior planning. Yet major incident planning in most district general hospitals does not attain a high priority. In terms of actual numbers of major incidents, the UK has relatively little experience, which inevitably results in the 'it won't happen to me' factor – unfortunately it sometimes does.

Several sound reasons for emergency planning in general can be identified which are applicable to the health service (see Box 3.1).

Box 3.1 – *Reasons for emergency planning*

■ It reduces uncertainty and softens the impact that the unusual circumstances produced by a major incident may have

■ It reduces thinking time during an incident – it may be too late to plan at the time of an incident

■ It promotes a systematic, orderly and effective approach to circumstances which might otherwise result in arbitrary, chaotic and ineffective responses

■ It helps to contain and control the incident by attempting to ensure that appropriate actions take place by utilising determined procedures, understood responsibilities, designated authority, accepted accountability and trained personnel

■ To formulate an aide-memoire, or checklist, of actions prior to when they may need to be taken (action cards detailing individuals' responsibility and preventing information overload; individuals are provided only with information that is relevant to them)

■ It maximises the preservation of life and the utilisation of personnel and resources to this end

■ It maximises the protection of personnel and the organisation

■ It is an educational activity which enables and encourages practitioners to maintain an up-to-date knowledge base regarding their role and responsibility in a major incident

■ It is a requirement of the Department of Health

The primary guidance for major incident planning in the NHS is contained within HSE (1996a,b). The overall aim of this guidance is to ensure that the health care services, i.e. health authorities, hospitals, ambulance services and family health service authorities, are prepared for 'an effective response to any major incident' (HSE 1996a,b).

The documents describe what government requires of regional and district health authorities, health boards and, consequently, hospitals and A&E departments, and outlines the general principles that ought to be adopted when planning for emergencies in the NHS. Major incident management in the NHS embraces an 'all hazards' approach to planning, i.e. all reasonable planning measures are taken to enhance response capabilities to deal with any major incident that may result in an abnormal casualty situation or pose a threat to normal services. NHS major incident planning seeks to provide a 'seamless' cover using this all hazards approach, but maintaining an in-built flexibility to take into account all incidents of any scale or duration. This 'all hazards' and 'all risks' approach to hospital major incident planning can be supported by the fact that, regardless of the nature of a major incident, hospitals fulfil several basic functions that will remain constant. These functions are (Hindman 1990):

- the receiving and triage of casualties
- the treatment of casualties
- the integration of casualties into the hospital facilities
- the allocation of personnel and resources.

To fulfil the functions of emergency management, several common elements should be considered (see Box 3.2).

Box 3.2 – *Functions of emergency management planning (Nudell & Antokol, 1998)*

- Assessing risk
- Deciding policies
- Producing an emergency plan
- Identifying, gathering and utilising resources
- Selecting an emergency management team
- Locating an emergency management centre
- Equipping an emergency management centre
- Training personnel for response to an emergency
- Testing emergency plans
- Dealing with victims and their relatives
- Dealing with the media
- Dealing with affected staff
- Continuing the normal functions of the organisation
- Returning to normality

The hospital major incident plan will also need to include:

- The allocation of an area which can be used as a temporary mortuary should the number of casualties who die after admission or who are dead on arrival exceed the established mortuary facilities available.
- Accommodation for a hospital information centre, where internal collation of casualty information will be centred.
- Facilities for the police documentation team, who will be responsible for the identification of casualties and who will supply information to the police's casualty bureau. The police will also act on behalf of HM coroner in the event of casualties resulting from the major incident dying before arrival and after admission to hospital. The documentation team will require office facilities, preferably with a dedicated telephone and fax line. Equipment and documentation may be stored at the hospital or at a local police station depending upon local arrangements.
- Facilities for an ambulance liaison officer who will be responsible for the supervision of ambulance service activity and liaison with the hospital. The ambulance liaison officer will also supply any mobile communications equipment needed for use of ambulance service staff at the hospital and for communication between the scene and the hospital.

All such designated areas involved in the major incident response should be clearly identified and signposted for both staff and others needing to make use of their facilities.

Some incidents may involve the clash of opposing factions, e.g. civil disturbance or sporting events. It is prudent for the ambulance service to dispatch each faction to a different receiving hospital to prevent a continuance of the incident within the hospital! If this is not possible, it is wise for the A&E department to attempt to separate opposing groups into different treatment areas. If the hospital has a specific risk of becoming involved with such an occurrence, such as a sports stadium within its catchment area, arrangements to deal with this potential problem should be considered in its operational plans (Martin 1999).

Responsibility for planning

Within the NHS a number of bodies have responsibility for hospital major incident planning:

- Health authorities (HAs)
- Health emergency planning officer (HEPO)
- NHS ambulance service trusts
- 'Listed' hospitals (NHS trusts).

Regional HAs are charged with the responsibility of ensuring that comprehensive major incidents plans are in place within each district HA. Arrangements for dealing with major incidents are secured through contractual arrangements between purchasing authorities and provider units (directly managed units and NHS trusts) specifying the role, services and training that each unit is to perform. NHS Executive regional offices must monitor these contracts to ensure they provide a seamless cover within and between regions. They must also ensure that there is a health emergency planning officer in post at regional level to advise upon, coordinate and monitor these plans.

The NHS Executive regional office is also required to maintain a list of hospitals with A&E departments that are adequately equipped to receive casualties on a 24-hour basis and provide, when required, a medical incident officer and a mobile medical and nursing team. These hospitals are known as 'listed' hospitals. District HAs are charged with ensuring that comprehensive planning provision exists to safeguard all of the residents of their district and to cover any 'at risk' sites or installations within their district by ensuring that all listed hospitals and ambulance services have comprehensive, coherent and up-to-date plans that are regularly reviewed and exercised. All listed hospitals are required to have in place a plan for dealing with major incidents, known as a 'hospital major incident plan' (HMIP). The HMIP forms part of the district HA's plan

The ultimate responsibility for the compilation of the HMIP and for the hospital's major incident response lies with the chief executive. However, due to the complexity and multidisciplinary nature of emergency management and the need for rapid decision-making, a small and cohesive core 'hospital coordination team' is needed. This team commonly includes the senior manager, (usually the chief executive or senior duty manager), the senior medical officer (usually the senior consultant, consultant or senior registrar in A&E or the other most senior medical officer in the hospital) and the senior nurse manager in A&E (or other most senior nurse manager). Other valuable additions to this team may include the bed manager and a public relations manager. Each team member is likely to have deputies or liaison officers who will ensure that the strategies formulated by the coordination team are successfully translated into tactics, and objectives are met by personnel involved in the major incident response.

Exercise and Training

Major incident exercises

Major incident exercises fall broadly into three main categories:

- large-scale exercises involving all emergency services role-playing a simulated incident with simulated casualties
- small-scale exercises involving a single hospital, a department in the hospital or the mobile team
- table-top exercises, where a fictitious incident is created and the major incident plan is worked through on paper or using table-top models.

Large-scale exercises serve a number of purposes: enabling major incident plans to be tested; allowing the rehearsal of practical skills in realistic environments; and working alongside other services, establishing working relationships with individuals and organisations likely to be involved in a true response. However, large exercises do not allow detailed scrutiny of any one aspect of the plan; rather, there is a superficial overview of the plan as a whole. Large-scale exercises should be as realistic as possible in all respects and be based upon the more likely incidents that may occur locally, to gain full benefit from testing the emergency response and making the experience as meaningful as possible.

The timing of an exercise is also of importance. If possible, it is preferable not to advise personnel exactly when the exercise will take place, as forewarning inevitably will create a false state of preparation and readiness which will not truly reflect the response to a 'real' incident. However, there is a need to ensure that exercises do not unduly disrupt the normal functioning of the service, so an acceptable compromise must be reached when planning and informing staff of exercises. The organisation and enactment of full or 'live' exercises are expensive in terms of time, personnel and resources, and these factors make exercises of considerable financial cost. Combining exercises with other services and agencies, many of which also have statutory requirements to exercise, can cut costs. It may be that in some circumstances other forms of exercise, which may be more cost-effective and appropriate in meeting response and training needs, should also be considered.

Small-scale exercises allow part of the plan to be examined in detail, utilising skill and task-specific activities, but do not always highlight problems which may occur when influenced by the activity of other departments or organisations. *Table-top exercises* allow a greater range of activities to be scrutinised in detail, but are largely theoretical and may not highlight logistical problems or poor skill levels resulting from inadequate training.

Given that each method has limitations, there is a case for exercise and training to make use of a combination of these techniques and not to be reliant upon on one method. The freedom for hospitals to decide upon the method of testing their major incident plan is constrained, in terms of minimum requirements, by government. The Department of Health requires that provisions are made to exercise and test major incident plans in the health service, that full-scale practical exercising of a HMIP should take place not less than every 2 years and that this exercise should involve:

- full implementation of the HMIP
- implementation of the plan in conjunction with a joint emergency services major incident exercise
- deployment of a medical incident officer and a mobile medical team
- receipt of simulated casualties into the hospital during the exercise.

In addition to these requirements, the hospital should carry out an internal communications/call-in exercise at least every 6 months and exercise communications systems between themselves and the ambulance service at regular intervals. Exercising of plans also provides an opportunity to review procedures and make amendments in the light of lessons learned from testing implementation. Lack of practice in implementing the plan allows deficits, inconsistencies and errors to go undetected until a major incident occurs.

Training

The NHS Executive (HSE 1996a,b) highlights the need for training of members of mobile teams and incident officers. Members of mobile teams should be proficient in the delivery of emergency care and systematic approaches to trauma care, such as that suggested by ATLS. Specific training courses which may prove of use to medical and nursing staff involved in a response at the site of an incident include the Immediate Medical Care course, Pre-hospital Trauma Life Support and Pre-hospital Emergency Care, as well as the Major Incident Management and Support course for incident officers. While the Department of Health offers no guidance for the training of individuals who will be required to deal with the major incident within the hospital and the A&E department, staff would find the Advanced Trauma Nursing course and the Trauma Nursing Core course of benefit to them, as well as observing on the ATLS course. In addition, training in the use of emergency radio communications equipment will be necessary. However, it is questionable whether any of these courses will truly prepare nurses or doctors to function to their optimum clinically or managerially in a major incident.

The courses available at the present time do not adequately prepare personnel to function in the hostile and hazardous environment of an incident scene. This is one of the factors that has brought into question the desirability, or need, to have hospital doctors and nurses at the scene of a major incident. With the increase in the numbers and skills of ambulance service 'paramedics' (Mackay *et al*. 1997), the role for mobile medical teams may, in most cases, become redundant and the majority of major incidents in the future will be manageable without the need for hospital-based medical/nursing support (New 1992). This issue is considered further in Chapter 1 on pre-hospital care.

The Hospital's Response to a Major Incident Alert

A&E department

The ambulance service will alert the most appropriate listed hospital(s) and these hospitals will then be referred to as the 'receiving' hospitals. This is the most likely route for the major incident plan being activated; however, due consideration must be given to the possibility of a major incident occurring and casualties bringing themselves or being brought to the A&E department, possibly in large numbers, without the involvement of the ambulance service. In such circumstances, the hospital will have the responsibility for declaring a major incident. Consequently, the hospital must have a mechanism to activate the HMIP and to inform ambulance control appropriately.

Alerting stage

The HMIP should clearly state the actions to be taken by the person receiving such a call to initiate major incident responses. The nature of the alert message from the ambulance service, whether the receiving hospital is the first to be alerted or whether it will act in a supporting role, and the nature of the incident will all affect the response from the hospital. The information recorded by the person receiving the initial and subsequent calls from the ambulance service is extremely important and the HMIP should ensure that those who receive such calls have clear guidelines for their role and responsibilities (see Box 3.3). The recognised alerting messages to receiving hospitals (HSE 1996a,b) are as follows:

- **Major incident – standby**, which may be rescinded by
- **Major incident – cancelled**
- **Major incident – declared – activate plan** which may be rescinded at the conclusion of the incident by
- **Major incident – casualty evacuation complete**, or
- **Major incident – stand down**.

Box 3.3 – *Information to be recorded from the ambulance service in the event of major incident*

- Type and location of the incident

- Type and estimated number of casualties (if known)

- Names of other receiving/supporting hospitals

- Whether a medical incident officer is required (usually from the first receiving hospital to be alerted)

- Whether a mobile medical and nursing team is required

- Request for a general and intensive care (or other speciality) bed state

'Standby' provides a warning that an incident may occur, e.g. warning of an improvised explosive device, that an incident has the potential of developing into a major incident, or that a declared major incident is progressing in a manner that may require the response of further hospitals. The 'major incident – declared – activate plan' alert may be the first alert that the hospital receives or may follow a standby alert. This alert indicates that a major incident has occurred and that the hospital should activate its HMIP and thereby make preparations for the receipt, treatment and absorption of casualties into the hospital.

During this stage of the incident, relevant nursing and medical staff will be contacted and deployed to activity pre-determined by individual action cards. If additional nursing staff are required by the A&E department, then an appropriately designated person should initiate a 'call-in' procedure. Other involved areas in the hospital will also activate similar procedures, which may also involve the use of personnel from voluntary organisations. It is often advisable to call in staff rostered for the next shift, but one in the department, as this allows for an already rostered fresh shift to come in to relieve those involved in the initial response and allows the present and called-in shifts an opportunity to rest. This is not always possible as the bulk of the current shift may be rostered for the shift after next, e.g. today's late shift staff are tomorrow's early shift staff.

It may also be advisable to distinguish A&E nurses and doctors from other staff deployed to the department from elsewhere by the use of identifying tabards. If possible, additional staff deployed into A&E should have A&E or critical care experience and should not be utilised in treatment teams without the presence of at least one experienced A&E nurse. Nurses from other areas can play useful roles in dealing with minor injuries and in transferring casualties from the treatment areas to admission wards.

Receipt of casualties

Within A&E, all of the patients in the department at the time of the major incident alert should have the situation explained to them and their conditions reassessed. Those awaiting treatment or with minor injuries should be given any appropriate first aid treatment and advised to go home, attend their local community hospital or see their GP. More seriously injured or ill patients should be rapidly stabilised and transferred to a ward.

It should be borne in mind that during a major incident A&E may still receive casualties who have not been involved in the incident, especially if they make their own way to the department. It may be prudent to make facilities available to treat such casualties and to ensure their details and documentation do not become included with those of the major incident casualties. The department should prepare facilities for the reception and treatment of casualties according to their priority for treatment. This commonly involves the utilisation of appropriately identified areas, adjacent to A&E if possible, for the collection and treatment of low-priority casualties. In most hospitals, a ward is also cleared of patients, by discharges and internal or external transfers, for receiving major incident victims. This is often an A&E admissions ward or an 'observation' ward. Within the A&E department and other areas identified for casualty reception and treatment, appropriate types and amounts of equipment should be prepared. To enable this essential equipment to be rapidly available for use, stocks should be held in an easily accessible place within the department and planning with the central sterile supply department, pharmacy and other departments should enable additional supplies to be quickly procured to replenish the stocks held in A&E, such as chest drain packs and controlled analgesic drugs.

Each casualty should receive a uniquely numbered identification bracelet and set of records. As immediate identification of the casualty may be difficult and time-consuming, this unique number will accompany her throughout the hospital system. The triage labels used at the incident scene should also be uniquely numbered and, if it is practical to use this number within the hospital as well, tracking of the casualty will be assisted. A stock of casualty documentation for major incidents should also be stored in the A&E department and can be incorporated into a casualty treatment pack (see also Ch. 1).

In the A&E department, arrangements should be made to receive and treat casualties with appropriate priority. On arrival at the hospital all casualties should be re-triaged, documented and directed to an appropriate treatment area. Triage should be carried out by a triage team consisting of an experienced A&E doctor and nurse. If separate entrances have been designated for minor and other categories, due to the geography of the hospital, two triage teams may be needed. Each casualty will be assigned a triage category and a unique identification number – preferably the same as on the triage label from the scene. Further identification and documentation of casualties will take place as their condition allows and will be carried out by members of the police documentation team and hospital administrative staff. Information regarding the numbers and identities of casualties will be compiled by the police documentation team and relayed at regular intervals to the police's casualty bureau, where it will be combined with information from the scene, rest centres, mortuary and other sources, such as transport companies' passenger lists.

Treatment of casualties

Treatment may be facilitated by organising available staff into 'treatment teams'. A treatment team can consist of two doctors and two nurses. At least one of the nurses should be an A&E nurse. Each 'immediate priority' casualty will require one treatment team for her care in the department. However, one team should be able to manage the care of two or three urgent priority casualties and the area designated for delayed priority ('minor') casualties should be manageable using two teams. The medical and nursing staff in A&E should aim to treat, stabilise and transfer immediate and urgent casualties out of the initial treatment areas as rapidly as possible, to allow treatment of the maximum numbers of casualties. However, in reality, the number of immediate and urgent casualties that a hospital will be able to accept will be limited by the number of intensive care, high-dependency care and operating theatre spaces available.

While casualties in the minor area may be initially regarded as having a low priority, their conditions may change. It is therefore important that at least some of the nurses allocated to this area are suitably experienced and are able to re-triage casualties into higher categories when required and arrange for their transfer to a more appropriate treatment area as necessary, especially as areas designated for the treatment of minor injuries may be geographically separated from the main A&E treatment areas, such as an outpatients department.

Transfer teams will also be required to transfer critically ill patients from the treatment area to critical care areas or to the operating theatres. These teams may consist of a doctor and a nurse, preferably both with critical care experience, and preferably two porters, as medical and nursing staff are needed for patient care and should not be pushing trolleys. The transfer of non-critical casualties to their admission destination can be facilitated by a nurse and a porter. In order that there is continuity of care for casualties and of record-keeping and handover, it may prove useful for one nurse to remain with the casualties in immediate and urgent categories during their stay in the A&E department. However, the practicality of this arrangement will depend upon the number of casualties involved and the number of nurses available. It may be that this role should be fulfilled by a nurse drafted into the department from elsewhere in the hospital. During a mass casualty incident the knowledge and skills of the A&E nurse are at a premium and if their numbers are limited then they are probably best utilised in the care of critical casualties and in a resource and organisation of care role, making use of other hospital nurses drafted into the department.

Chemical/radioactive contamination

Any casualties who are contaminated by either chemical or radioactive materials should be decontaminated appropriately, and A&E staff should be protected from contamination by using appropriate protective clothing. All A&E departments should have a designated area for decontamination procedures and a dedicated entrance for such cases. Coordination of the response to chemical and nuclear incidents does not lie with the health service.

County emergency planning officers (CEPOs) will have prepared operational plans for 'off-site' incidents and will be familiar with 'on-site' plans drawn up by chemical site operators. The health service's response should be planned in consultation with the CEPO. In the case of unforeseen nuclear accidents, the national arrangements for dealing with incidents involving radioactivity, the NAIR scheme, exists and is coordinated by the police and identifies sources of expert advice, resources and action. Expert advice should be followed regarding the treatment of those who are likely to have been exposed to or contaminated by radioactive material.

Arrangements also exist for the planning and response to an emergency involving a civil nuclear installation and hospitals with such an installation in or adjacent to their location should be familiar with these arrangements. In all of these incidents, close liaison with the scene, the police, the fire and rescue service, NAIR advisors, site operators and local authorities' emergency planning officers is necessary.

Chemical and radiation incidents present particular difficulties and require specific incident plans. Discussion of this issue is beyond the scope of this chapter, but guidance is provided in Chapter 9 of HC(90)25 and Handbook of Guidance Volume 2 (HSE 1996a,b), respectively.

Hospital response

Alerting stage

The hospital switchboard and A&E department should initiate a telephone/paging 'cascading' system to alert personnel and departments to notify further personnel and to activate their planned responses to the particular alert status.

A cascading system of alert reduces the pressure on the main switchboard, but relies upon each person being aware of whom they should contact. The major incident control team will be alerted during this stage and will assemble and commence internal management of the incident response from an identified hospital control centre. The control centre should:

■ have sufficient communications hardware and software available within it to facilitate efficient internal and external communications
■ provide as stress-free a working environment as possible
■ be large enough for meetings of the coordination team with other managers and agencies
■ be located in an area where interruptions will be kept to a minimum.

The alerting stage and the subsequent actions of personnel should be preplanned to be largely automatic without the need for management or the major-incident control team, and should result in the preparation of the hospital to receive casualties and the dispatch, if requested, of a medical incident officer/mobile medical and nursing team to the incident scene. This can be facilitated by the use of clear and detailed 'action cards'.

If the hospital is to receive casualties, it is also likely that routine operating lists will be suspended and as many intensive care and high-dependency spaces as possible made free. In addition, it may be thought necessary to clear as many beds as possible in other wards by means of early discharges and by transferring patients to other, unaffected hospitals – the use of the voluntary aid societies and their vehicles may be indicated for this task.

Restriction of access

Maintaining security, controlling access to the hospital and the containment of casualties, relatives and the media in specified areas of the hospital are vital tasks essential to the effectiveness of the hospital's response. Full security and containment arrangements must be in place as soon as possible after the hospital has received notification to activate its HMIP.

If possible, access to all involved areas should be limited to one entrance and egress to one exit. All other entrances should be locked or closed by security personnel. Only those staff with appropriate identification should be allowed into the hospital, the A&E department and associated treatment and collection points. Major incidents cause a convergence of individuals and groups on the hospital, focusing upon the A&E department. Well-meaning and interested hospital and non-hospital nursing and medical staff, various volunteers and voluntary groups will cause a disrupted and confused response and their access must be prevented.

It is advisable that hospital staff do not leave their own departments or come to the hospital until they are requested to do so via the recognised communication channels. A decision will also have to be made whether or not to use non-requested, non-hospital medical, nursing and other volunteers who offer their services. The potential legal ramifications of using possibly unqualified impostors and/or the possibility of negligence claims resulting from their practices may well outweigh any useful function that they may be able to perform.

The media

The media, who who will no doubt have gathered at the hospital, should be provided with regular and accurate press releases. The media are under pressure during a major incident to meet deadlines and if they do not receive adequate and appropriate information they may set about seeking it out for themselves. The needs of the media should be addressed in ways which will not compromise the emergency response of the hospital and its staff or the confidentiality of casualties and relatives. Only designated members of staff, who preferably have been prepared for this role, should address the media and only statements prepared in consultation with the appropriate emergency services and approved by the hospital's major incident coordination team should be released. Any access to casualties and staff should be very carefully controlled, with ground rules being agreed and consent obtained before any interviews take place.

Medicolegal Issues

During the response to a major incident in the hospital or at the scene, nurses must consider a number of legal and professional issues. Major incident scenes are considered to be 'scenes of crime' until proven otherwise and consideration must be given to the preservation of forensic evidence. Such evidence, e.g. clothing, debris, etc., may leave the scene with casualties and, as a result, be present in the A&E department and other areas of the hospital. Every effort should be made to collect and preserve this evidence in collaboration with the police. Of course, in all circumstances, preservation of life takes priority over the preservation of evidence.

Criminal investigations and prosecutions, civil actions, official inquiries and inquests are all possible following a major incident. Some of the staff involved in the management of the incident are likely to be required to provide statements and/or give evidence. It should also be remembered that all documentation completed during the incident can be used not only as a source of evidence to explain what happened, but possibly also to suggest negligence.

Although staff are working under considerable pressure at the time of an incident, all documentation should be adequate, clear and accurate. Nurses should consider that the pressures of a major incident do not remove their professional accountability for practice, and they may well be asked to justify the actions that they took, both inside and outside of the A&E department, at a later date (Montague 1996). Staff should also be aware that the HMIP, including any action cards, is a written document and, as such, essentially becomes an approved policy document of the organisation and provides standards and descriptions of expected activities against which the actions of staff may be judged by any investigation, whether internal or external (see also Ch. 39).

Aftermath

During and in the aftermath of a major incident, it is important to recognise that both casualties and staff may be psychologically and/or spiritually affected by events that are outside the normal range of experience. As a consequence they may be at risk of developing post-trauma stress reactions and doubting long-held beliefs.

Hospital major incident plans must include arrangements to provide casualties, relatives and staff with appropriate psychological and spiritual support during and after the event. Psychological support may be provided by appropriately trained personnel from the mental health professions or other statutory or voluntary bodies. Religious representatives from the major groupings should also be available, as well as a contact list of representatives from a broad range of spiritual beliefs so that individual needs may be met as far as is possible. Both psychological and spiritual support should be available from the outset and throughout the incident. Follow-up services such as psychological debriefing should also be made available to all of those involved as part of the HMIP (Whitfield 1994).

Conclusion

Major incidents are rare, but they do happen. In this eventuality, many factors cannot be controlled, such as the type and location of the incident or the time of day. What can be controlled are the degree and quality of the preparation, in terms of planning, testing and training, that has taken place prior to the event. Excessive and unnecessary decision-making during a major incident is of little help in mounting the most effective response.

Further reading

Advanced Life Support Group (1995) *Major Incident Medical Management and Support: the Practical Approach.* London: BMJ Publishing.

Dethick L (1999) Managing major incidents: a dynamic educational initiative. *Emergency Nurse,* **7**(1), 21–25.

Dethick L, Hicks P (1999) Risk management in major incident and emergency planning. *Emergency Nurse,* **7**(2), 10–15.

Dethick L, Man D (1999) Declaring a major incident. *Emergency Nurse,* **7**(3), 21–24.

Dethick L (1999) Co-ordinating major incident trauma care: international responses. *Emergency Nurse,* **7**(4), 8–12.

Flynn R (1997) *Sitting in the Hot Seat: Leaders and Teams for Critical Incident Management.* Chichester: John Wiley.

Montague A (1996) *Legal Problems in Emergency Medicine.* Oxford: Oxford University Press.

Parker D, Handmer J (eds) (1992) *Hazard Management and Emergency Planning Perspectives on Britain.* London: James and James Science Publishers.

Thornly F (1990) Major disasters: an ambulance service view. *Injury* **21**(1), 34–36.

Wardrope J, Hockey MS, Crosby AC (1990) The hospital response to the Hillsborough tragedy. *Injury,* **21**(1), 53–54.

Walsh M (1989) *Disasters Current Planning and Recent Experience.* London: Edward Arnold.

References

Health and Personal Social Services Northern Ireland (1993) Emergency planning for health and personal social services in Northern Ireland. *Circular HSS EMP 1/93*. Belfast: HMSO.

Hindman D (1990) Nurse educator planning a disaster drill: checklist for success. *Journal of Emergency Nursing*, **16**(4), 298–299.

HMSO (1990) Emergency planning in the NHS: health services arrangements for dealing with major incidents. *HC(90)25*. London: HMSO.

HSE (1996a) *Emergency Planning in the NHS: Health Services Arrangements for Dealing with Major Incidents*, vol. 1. London: Department of Health.

HSE (1996b) *Emergency Planning in the NHS: Health Services Arrangements for Dealing with Major Incidents*, vol. 2. London: Department of Health.

Kreps G (1992) Foundations and principles of emergency planning. In Parker D, Handmer J, eds. *Hazard Management and Emergency Planning: Perspectives on Britain*. London: James and James Science Publishers.

Mackay CA, Burke DP, Bowden DF (1997) Effect of paramedic scene times on patient outcomes. *Pre-hospital Immediate Care*, **1**(1), 4–7.

Martin G (1999) Drumcree. *Emergency Nurse*, **6**(10): 8–12

Montague A (1996) *Legal Problems in Emergency Medicine*. Oxford: Oxford University Press.

New B (1992) *Too many cooks? The Response of the Health-related Services to Major Incidents in London*. London: King's Fund Institute.

Nudell M, Antokol C (1988) *The Handbook for Effective Emergency and Crisis Management*. Massachusetts: Lexington Books.

Rushing D (1990) Disaster preparedness: a serious responsibility (guest editorial). *Journal of Emergency Nursing*, **16**(4), 234.

Scottish Office, National Health Service in Scotland (1990) Emergency planning guidance to the National Health Service in Scotland. *Circular SHHD/DGM (1993) 73*. Edinburgh: HMSO.

Welsh Office (1993) Emergency planning in the NHS Wales: health service arrangements for dealing with major incidents. *Circular WHC (93) 69*. Cardiff: HMSO.

Whitfield A (1994) Critical incident stress debriefing. *Emergency Nurse*, **2**(3), 6–9.

Part 2

Trauma Care

4. Head Injuries 45
5. Skeletal Injuries 67
6. Spinal Injuries 109
7. Thoracic Injuries 119
8. Abdominal Injuries 137
9. Facial Injuries 147
10. Burns 159

Chapter 4

Head Injuries

Deborah Dawson & Karen Sanders

- Introduction
- Anatomy and physiology
- Physiology of raised intracranial pressure (ICP)
- Classification of head injuries
- Assessment of head injury
- Management of serious injury
- Transfer to a specialist neurosurgical unit
- Brain stem death
- Management of minor injury
- Conclusion

Introduction

Caring for patients with head injuries accounts for about 10% of an A&E department's workload (Bullock & Teasdale 1996) and this type of injury is the commonest cause of traumatic death in young adults (Chandler & Cummins 1995). Approximately 300/100 000 of the population per year require hospitalisation; of these, 9/100 000 die, about 5000 patients per year in Britain (Lindsey *et al.* 1991). Many of these deaths are inevitable, but around 7% are preventable (Royal College of Surgeons of England 1988).

There are many causes of head injuries: occupational-related accidents, sporting accidents, falls, assaults and road traffic accidents (RTAs). Although only 25% of head injuries are due to RTAs, 60% of deaths result from this cause, with half of the deaths occurring before the patient has reached hospital (Lindsey *et al* 1991). There is an increased incidence of head injuries in young males and many are associated with alcohol. Age is a significant factor in determining outcome, especially in patients who become deeply unconscious: mortality is 19% in patients aged 20, but 71% in those aged 60 and over (Hickey 1992).

A good understanding of the anatomy and physiology of the brain and its related structures is vital in caring for patients with head injuries. It allows the A&E nurse to relate mechanisms of injury to the classification of brain injury and to plan care appropriate to the physiological processes occurring at a particular stage post-injury. A structured approach to the care of head-injured patients, such as the system advocated by Advanced Trauma Life Support (ATLS; American College of Surgeons 1997), provides a mechanism for assessment and immediate management and minimises the risk of secondary brain injury.

This chapter will outline relevant anatomy and physiology and examine brain injury, before discussing assessment and management of patients. The chapter will also offer guidance on preventing secondary brain injury and give indications for transfer to specialist units.

Anatomy and Physiology

To fully understand the importance of the mechanisms of injury, and the management needed, it is imperative that A&E nurses are aware of both the anatomy of the skull and brain and the physiological processes that maintain homeostasis.

The skull

The skull is a rigid bony cavity composed of 29 individual bones, the eight bones of the cranium, 14 facial bones, the six ossicles of the ear and the hyoid bone. To ensure maximum protection, strength and support, bony capsules surround the brain, the eyes, the nasal passages and the inner ear; and bony buttresses extend upwards from the teeth through the facial bones. To relieve the potential weight, the skull is made lighter by the paranasal sinuses, which also give resonance to the voice.

The cranium is one of the strongest structures in the body and provides the bony protection for the brain. It is composed of the parietal (2 no.), occipital, frontal, temporal (2 no.), sphenoid and ethmoid bones. Figure 4.1 shows an exploded view of the cranial skull, however the bones are fused along main sutures, the saggital, coronal, lambdoidal and squamosal. The facial bones form the framework for the nasal and oral cavities and include the zygomatic bones (2 no.), palatine bones (2 no.), mandible, maxilla (2 no.), lacrimal bones (2 no.), nasal bones (2 no.), vomer and the inferior nasal concha (2 no.) (see Fig. 4.2).

Figure 4.3 shows the irregular internal surfaces of the skull. These irregular surfaces account for injury to the brain as it moves within the skull under acceleration/deceleration forces.

The meninges

The brain and the spinal cord are encased by three layers of membrane – the dura mater, the arachnoid mater and the pia mater – known collectively as the meninges (see Fig. 4.4).

The dura mater

The dura mater consists of two layers: the outer layer is the periosteal layer of the skull which terminates at the foramen magnum, and the inner layer is a strong, thick membrane that is continuous with the spinal dura mater. There is only a potential space between the two dura, except at the falx cerebri, which divides the left and right hemispheres of the cerebrum; the tentorium cerebelli, which divides the cerebrum and cerebellum; the falx cerebelli, which divides the lateral

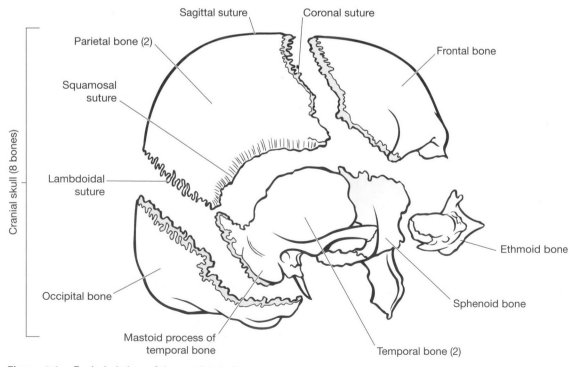

Figure 4.1 – *Exploded view of the cranial skull.*

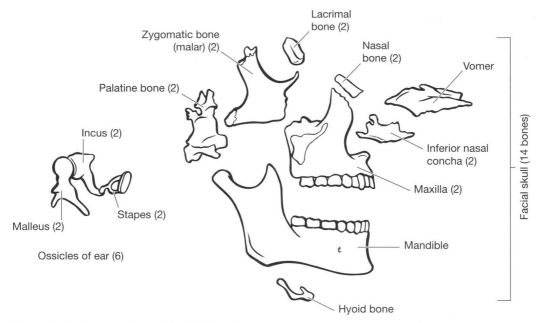

Figure 4.2 – *Exploded view of the facial skull.*

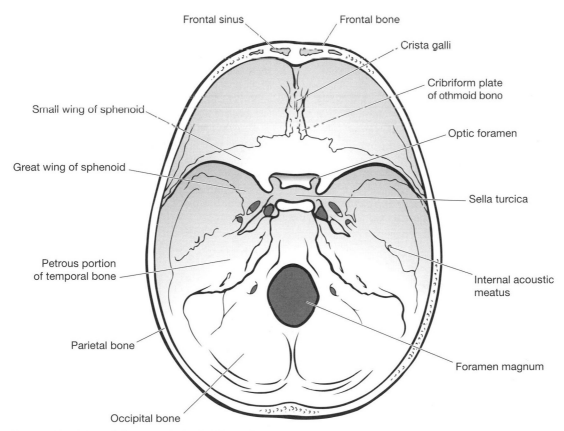

Figure 4.3 – *View of the base of the skull from above.*

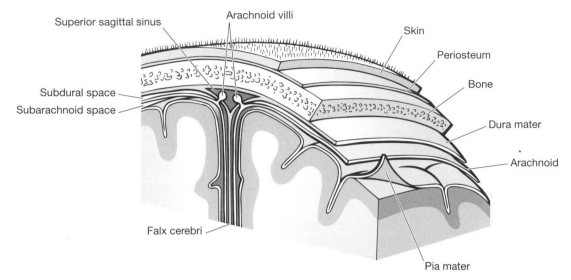

Figure 4.4 – *The cranial meninges.*

lobes of the cerebellum; and the diaphragm sellae, creating a roof for the sella turcica (which houses the pituitary gland). These compartments provide support and protection for the brain and form the sinuses which drain venous blood from the brain.

The arachnoid mater

The arachnoid mater is fine serous membrane that loosely covers the brain. There is a potential space between this and the inner dura mater, known as the subdural space. Between the arachnoid mater and the pia mater is an actual space, known as the sub-arachnoid space, which contains the arachnoid villi, cerebrospinal fluid (CSF) and small blood vessels.

The pia mater

The pia mater follows the convolutions and is attached to the surface of the brain. It consists of fine connective tissue, housing the majority of the blood supply to the brain.

The ventricles and cerebrospinal fluid

Within the brain there are four connected cavities called ventricles, which contain cerebrospinal fluid (CSF). These are the left and right lateral ventricles, the third ventricle and the fourth ventricle. The lateral ventricles lie in the cerebral hemispheres, the third in the diencephalon and the fourth in the brain stem. The lateral ventricles are connected to the third ventricle by the interventricular foramen, sometimes known as the foramen of Munro, and the third ventricle is connected to the fourth by the cerebral aqueduct,

sometimes known as the aqueduct of Sylvius (see Fig. 4.5).

CSF is a clear, colourless fluid composed of water, some protein, oxygen, carbon dioxide, sodium, potassium, chloride and glucose. Its purpose is to protect the brain from injury by providing a cushioning effect. The major source of CSF is from the secretions of the choroid plexus, found in the ventricles. The choroid plexus produce approximately 500 ml of CSF daily, however the average adult brain only holds between 125 and 150 ml. CSF is renewed and replaced approximately three times daily, being reabsorbed through the arachnoid villi, which drain into the superior saggital sinus, when the CSF pressure exceeds the venous pressure. Normal CSF pressure is 60–180 mmH$_2$O in the lumbar puncture position (lateral recumbant) and 200–350 mmH$_2$O in the sitting position.

The brain

The brain consists of three main areas:

- the cerebrum
- the cerebellum
- the brain stem.

The major structures within these divisions are summarized in Box 4.1.

The cerebrum

The cerebrum consists of two cerebral hemispheres, which are partially separated by the longitudinal fissure and connected at the bottom by the corpus

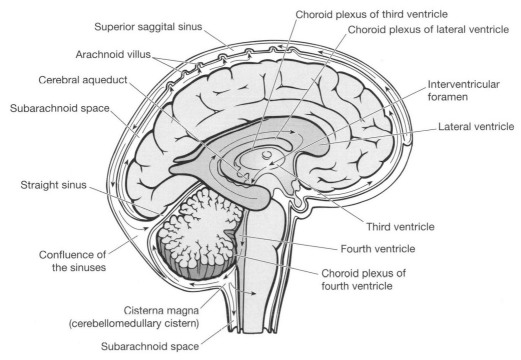

Figure 4.5 – *Ventricles of the brain and circulatory path of cerebrospinal fluid through the cranial pathways.*

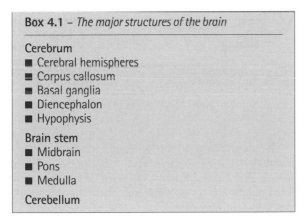

Box 4.1 – *The major structures of the brain*

Cerebrum
- Cerebral hemispheres
- Corpus callosum
- Basal ganglia
- Diencephalon
- Hypophysis

Brain stem
- Midbrain
- Pons
- Medulla

Cerebellum

The surface area of the brain, the cerebral cortex (grey matter), is much increased by the presence of gyri and sulci (see Fig. 4.6), resulting in a 3:1 proportion of grey to white matter. Below the cortex is the white matter. The cerebral hemispheres are composed of four lobes, the frontal, parietal, temporal and occipital lobes. Box 4.2 summarizes the main functions of these lobes.

The diencephalon is located deep into the cerebrum and consists of the thalamus, hypothalamus, subthalamus and epithalamus. It connects the midbrain to the cerebral hemispheres. The hypothalamus includes several important structures, such as the optic chiasma, the point at which the two optic tracts cross, and the stalk of the pituitary gland (hypophysis).

Cerebellum

The cerebellum is situated behind the pons and attached to the midbrain, pons and medulla by three paired cerebellar peduncles. It consists of three main parts:

- the cortex
- the white matter, which forms the connecting pathways for impulses joining the cerebellum with other parts of the central nervous system
- four pairs of deep cerebellar nuclei.

callosum. It is generally accepted that one hemisphere (usually the left) is more highly developed than the other. The left side of the brain has been shown to control the right side of the body, spoken and written language, scientific reasoning and numerical skills, whereas the right side is more concerned with emotion and artistic and creative skills. However, at birth, the hemispheres are of equal ability and very early injury to one side or another usually results in skills being acquired by the opposite side of the brain. Each cerebral hemisphere has an area of grey matter called the basal ganglia, which assists in the motor control of fine body movements.

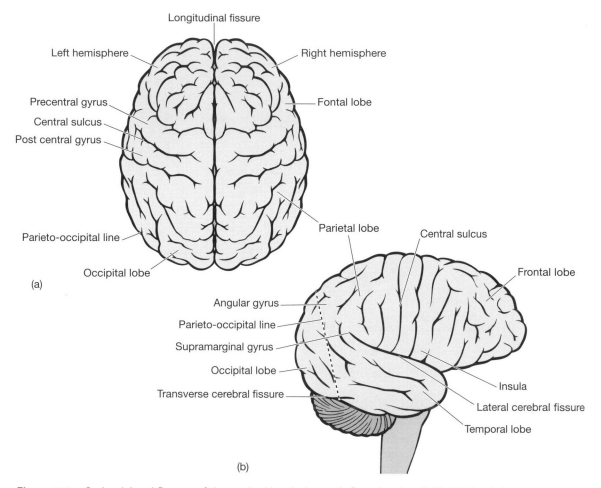

Figure 4.6 – *Gyri, sulci and fissures of the cerebral hemispheres. A: Superior view. B: Right lateral view.*

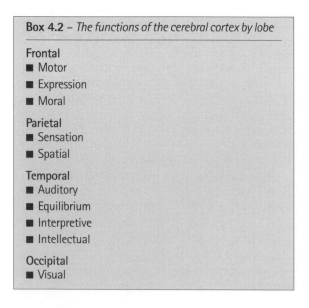

Box 4.2 – *The functions of the cerebral cortex by lobe*

Frontal
■ Motor
■ Expression
■ Moral

Parietal
■ Sensation
■ Spatial

Temporal
■ Auditory
■ Equilibrium
■ Interpretive
■ Intellectual

Occipital
■ Visual

The cerebellum is the processing centre for co-ordination of muscular movements, balance, precision, timing and body positions. It does not initiate any movements and is not involved with the conscious perception of sensations.

Brain stem

The brain stem is the connection between the brain and the spinal cord, and is continuous with the diencephalon above and the spinal cord below. Within the brain stem are ascending and descending path-ways between the spinal cord and parts of the brain. All cranial nerves, except the olfactory (I) and optic (II), emerge from the brain stem (see Fig. 4.7). It is formed from three main structures: the midbrain, pons and medulla.

The midbrain connects the pons and the cerebellum to the cerebrum. It is involved with visual reflexes, the movement of the eyes, focusing and the dilation of the

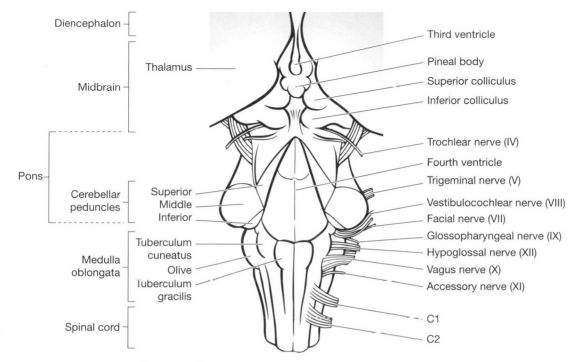

Figure 4.7 – *Brain stem (dorsal view).*

pupils. Contained within the midbrain and upper pons is the reticular activating system, which is responsible for the 'awake' state. The pons is located between the midbrain and the medulla and serves as a relay station from the medulla to higher structures in the brain. It is involved with the control of respiratory function. The lowermost portion of the brain stem is the medulla, which connects the pons and the spinal cord. The point of decussation of the pyramidal tract occurs within the medulla. The vital centres associated with autonomic reflex activity are present in its deeper structure. These are the cardiac, respiratory and vasomotor centres and the reflex centres of coughing, swallowing, vomiting and sneezing.

Cerebral circulation

The brain is supplied with blood by four major arteries: two internal carotid arteries, which supply most of the cerebrum and both eyes; and two vertebral arteries, which supply the cerebellum, brain stem and the posterior part of the cerebrum. Before the blood enters the cerebrum it passes through the circle of Willis, which is a circular shunt at the base of the brain consisting of the posterior cerebral, the posterior communicating, the internal carotids, the anterior cerebral and the anterior communicating arteries (see Figs 4.8 and 4.9). These vessels are frequently anomalous, however they allow for an adequate blood supply to all the brain, even if one or more is ineffective.

The venous drainage from the brain does not follow a similar pathway (Fig. 4.10). Cerebral veins empty into large venous sinuses located in the folds of the dura mater. Bridging veins connect the brain and the dural sinuses and are often the cause of subdural haematomas. These sinuses empty into the internal jugular veins, which sit on either side of the neck and return the blood to the heart via the brachiocephalic veins.

The brain, especially the grey matter, has an extensive capillary bed, requiring approximately 15–20% of the total resting cardiac output, about 750 ml/min. Glucose, required for metabolism in the brain, requires about 20% of the total oxygen consumed in the body for its oxidation. Blood flow to specific areas of the brain correlates directly with the metabolism of the cerebral tissue.

Physiology of Raised Intracranial Pressure (ICP)

Intracranial pressure (ICP) represents the pressure exerted by the cerebrospinal fluid (CSF) within the ventricles of the brain (Hickey 1992). The exact

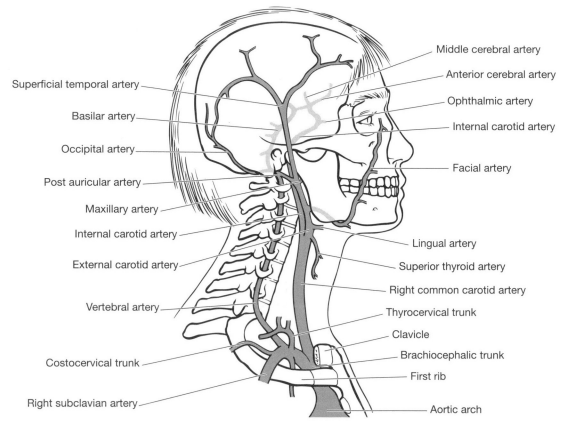

Figure 4.8 – *Major arteries of the head and neck.*

pressure varies in different areas of the brain. Its normal range is 0–15 mmHg when measured from the foramen of Munro. Intracranial pressure also varies with activities like coughing or sneezing.

The ICP is fundamental in maintaining adequate brain function. This is because the brain lies in the skull which is a rigid compartment. This compartment is filled with non-compressible contents, i.e. brain matter (80%), intravascular blood (10%) and cerebrospinal fluid (10%). In the healthy brain these components maintain a fairly constant volume, therefore creating equilibrium therein. The Monro–Kellie hypothesis states that if one component increases, another must decrease to maintain the dynamic equilibrium. If this does not occur, intracranial pressure will rise (Hickey 1992). In the healthy brain dynamic equilibrium is maintained by a number of compensatory mechanisms in order to maintain a stable cerebral blood flow. These include:

■ increasing CSF absorption
■ decreasing CSF production
■ shunting of CSF to the spinal subarachnoid space
■ vasoconstriction – reducing cerebral blood flow.

Maintenance of the dynamic equilibrium in the brain is further aided by autoregulation. Autoregulation is initiated by cerebral perfusion pressure (CPP), which is calculated by subtracting ICP from the systemic mean arterial pressure (MAP):

CPP = MAP – ICP

Autoregulation is necessary to maintain cerebral blood flow. If MAP falls and ICP increases, there is a risk that cerebral perfusion pressure will fall to too low a value to maintain adequate cerebral blood flow. This can result in hypoxia and cerebral ischaemia, causing secondary brain injury. If autoregulation is occurring, the CPP should be maintained between 80 and 100 mmHg. Autoregulation fails below 60 mmHg or above 160 mmHg. It is important to maintain an adequate but not elevated blood pressure in trauma patients to allow autoregulation to occur.

Chemoregulation is triggered by changes in extracellular pH and metabolic by-products. It is also triggered by changes in P_{CO_2} or a dramatic reduction in P_{O_2} (see Fig. 4.11). In the head-injured patient, maintaining adequate oxygenation is vital, because allowing the P_{CO_2} to rise initiates chemoregulation,

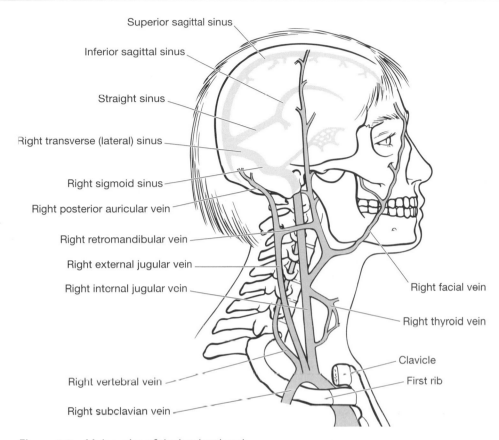

Figure 4.9 – *Major veins of the head and neck.*

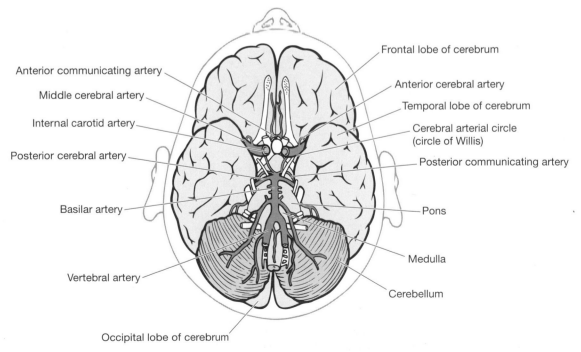

Figure 4.10 – *Cerebral circulation.*

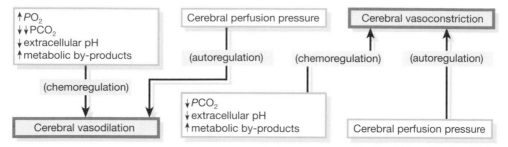

Figure 4.11 – *Chemoregulation of the brain.*

which in turn increases ICP, because it increases overall brain mass. Cerebral vasoconstriction reduces brain mass, and it is for this reason that some ventilated head-injured patients are hyperventilated, as this reduces $P\text{CO}_2$ and activates chemoregulation, thus inducing vasoconstriction which helps to reduce ICP. Hyperventilation is not a definitive treatment for raised ICP – it is used to buy time until the cause is treated.

Following brain injury, if autoregulation is impaired, cerebral perfusion falls as ICP rises, usually as a result of traumatic cerebral oedema. This causes a reduction in cerebral blood flow and can result in cerebral ischaemia. If the patient is poorly ventilated, for whatever reason, cerebral vasodilation further increases ICP. It is raised ICP or reduced CPP which is responsible for most secondary brain injury. The mechanisms which maintain ICP in the healthy brain can compensate for rises in ICP initially, but will fail as ICP reaches 15–20 mmHg. From then on, small increases in brain mass, blood volume or CSF have a profound effect on ICP.

Classification of Head Injuries

Head injuries can be classified under three anatomical sites: the scalp, the skull and the brain. Patients often present with a combination of injuries.

Scalp injuries

There are four types of injury to the scalp:

■ *abrasion* – minor injury that may cause a small amount of bleeding
■ *contusion* – no break in the skin, but causing bruising to the scalp that may cause blood to leak into the subcutaneous layer
■ *laceration* – a cut or tear of the skin and sub-cutaneous fascia that tends to bleed profusely
■ *subgaleal haematoma* – a haematoma below the galea, a tough layer of tissue under the sub-

cutaneous fascia and before the skull. The veins here empty into the venous sinus, and thus any infection can spread easily to the brain, despite the skull remaining intact.

Abrasions may not require any treatment, but ice applied to the area may reduce any haematoma formation (Hickey 1992). Lacerations can bleed extensively, however bleeding from the scalp alone is unlikely to cause shock in the adult patient. In small children, a scalp laceration may be sufficient to cause hypovolaemia. Scalp lesions should be explored under local anaesthetic for foreign bodies or skull fracture, with an X-ray examination if there is any doubt in diagnosis, and any wound should be sutured or glued according to depth and position. There is controversy surrounding the treatment of subgaleal haematomas, due to the risks of infection; therefore some doctors argue that it is best to evacuate the haematoma, while others suggest that it is best to let it reabsorb. If the scalp injuries are only part of other injuries, it is important they are documented to allow further investigation at a more appropriate time. They may need to be cleaned and dressed or temporarily sutured.

The skull

Skull fractures are classified into four groups:

Linear. These are the most common types of injury. They usually result from low-velocity direct force. They are usually diagnosed from skull X-ray and need no specific treatment. If the patient has no neurological deficit, he can be discharged with family/ friends after a period of observation (Sheehy 1992).

Depressed skull fractures may be very evident clinically, but will require X-ray examination to discover the full extent of the damage. They are managed according to their severity and whether there are any accompanying injuries.If there are no other injuries requiring surgical management, they may not be surgically elevated, due to the risks of infection. However, if there is debris disturbing the brain tissue then surgery will be required.

Basal fractures are diagnosed clinically as they are difficult to detect on X-ray. Signs include CSF leakage from the nose (rhinorrhoea) or ears (otorrhoea). If this is suspected, fluid should be tested both for glucose and using the 'halo test'. In the halo test, a small amount of fluid is placed on blotting paper; if CSF is present it will separate from blood and form a yellow ring around the outside of the blood. Patients with a base of skull fracture may also have bruising behind the ears (Battle's signs) and around the eyes ('raccoon eyes'). Patients with no neurological deficit are usually prescribed antibiotics, because this type of fracture poses a high risk of infection to the brain. The patient can be discharged home with adult companions. Where other injuries or neurological deficits exist, the patient should be admitted. If gastric decompression is indicated, an orogastric tube should be used, as nasogastric insertion carries a risk of introducing infection to the cranium.

Comminuted fractures. These are detected on X-ray: the skull is broken into multiple fragments. These patients should be closely observed and any neurological deficits managed appropriately. Surgical intervention is sometimes required to remove fragments or elevate bone, and a cranioplasty may be performed once any cerebral oedema has subsided.

The brain

Brain injuries are usually categorised into either focal or diffuse injuries. Focal injuries cause direct damage to the area of the brain injured. Mechanisms of injury are usually blunt trauma and acceleration/deceleration injury. They are generally space-occupying lesions and are liable to cause secondary brain injury if not detected early. The exact type and location of injury are diagnosed by CT scan, but early focal (e.g. pupillary changes), lateralising (e.g. paresis) and localising (e.g. speech loss) signs should highlight the type of brain injury. Focal injuries include contusions and haemorrhage (see Fig. 4.12).

Contusion

This is the most common type of brain injury. Cerebral contusions are bruises of the surface of the brain, most commonly the frontal and temporal lobes, are diagnosed by computed tomography (CT) scan. Bleeding may occur into contusions, and it is this bleeding that would cause an early decrease in the conscious level (Lindsey *et al.* 1991). Nausea, vomiting and visual disturbance are also common signs. The brain will swell around the sites of contusion, and if the

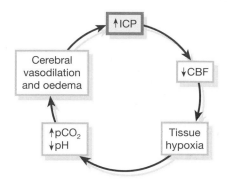

Figure 4.12 – *Cycle of progressive brain swelling.*

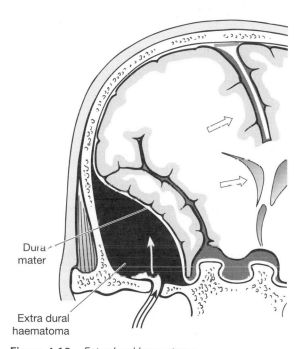

Figure 4.13 – *Extradural haematoma.*

contusions are large or widespread, the swelling may cause the ICP to rise, raising the mortality rate for this type of injury to 45% (Hudak & Gallo 1994). Lacerations are tears of the cortical surface and occur in similar locations to contusions.

Haemorrhage

There are four types of traumatic bleed: extradural (EDH), subdural (SDH), intracerebral (ICH) and subarachnoid (SAH). Subarachnoid bleeds are usually not traumatic in origin; however, they may be seen on CT scan following trauma. This is for one of two reasons – either the patient has suffered a SAH prior to an incident (possibly the cause of the incident;

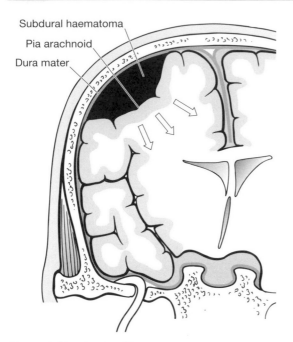

Subdural haematoma
Pia arachnoid
Dura mater

Figure 4.14 – *Subdural haematoma.*

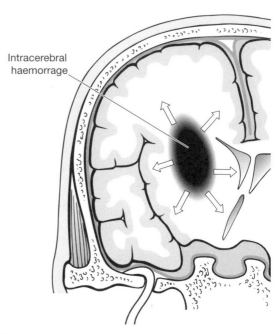

Intracerebral
haemorrage

Figure 4.15 – *Intracerebral haematoma.*

Sakas *et al.* 1995), or the vessels in the subarachnoid space have been damaged by shearing forces.

Extradural haematomas are situated between the periosteum and the dura mater (see Fig. 4.13). They are usually caused by a laceration to the middle meningeal artery or vein or, less commonly, the dural venous sinus, following a blow to the temporal–parietal region. EDHs make up 16% of all haematomas (Lindsey *et al.* 1991), and in 85% of patients the EDH will be accompanied by a skull fracture (Hudak & Gallo 1994).

Patients with EDHs present with a history of transient loss of consciousness. If the EDH is not diagnosed they will then be lucid for a period of time (hours to days) dependent on the rate of the bleed. They will then rapidly lose consciousness and deteriorate very quickly. A common presentation is the patient who falls, gets up after a short period of time, then goes home to bed; the next morning his family or friends are unable to rouse him and he is brought to A&E. Surgical treatment is required to evacuate the haematoma and ligate the damaged blood vessel. Early signs of deterioration are irritation and headache, and later signs are seizures, ipsilateral pupil dilation, reduced level of consciousness and contralateral hemiplegia (Sherman 1990). Relatives or friends of these patients require a great deal of reassurance, as they often feel responsible for not bringing the patient to hospital earlier.

Subdural haematomas are situated between the dura mater and arachnoid mater and make up 22% of all haematomas (Lindsey *et al.* 1991) (see Fig. 4.14). SDHs are caused by the rupture of bridging veins from the cortical surfaces to the venous sinuses. They can be seen in isolation, but more commonly are associated with cerebral contusions and intracerebral haematomas (this group comprises 54% of all haematomas).

Subdural haematomas are classified into acute, subacute and chronic: acute refers to symptoms which manifest before 48 h post-injury; subacute to those manifesting between 48 h and 2 weeks; and chronic to those manifesting after 2 weeks. Subacute and chronic SDHs are often seen in the elderly and in alcoholics. Both groups can suffer regular falls and have a degree of cerebral atrophy which puts strain on the bridging veins. Acute SDHs are associated with major cerebral trauma. The onset of symptoms such as headache, drowsiness, slow cerebration and confusion is slower than in EDHs, but often associated with other injuries, and therefore the symptoms can become confused within a general head injury picture. Small SDHs may be treated conservatively, as they will reabsorb over time. Larger SDHs will require evacuation, due to the secondary damage they will cause.

Intracerebral haematomas are found deep within the brain parenchyma. As mentioned before, they are related to contusions and are therefore usually found

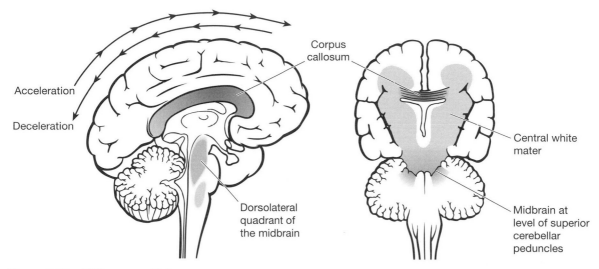

Figure 4.16 – *Diffuse axonal injury.*

in the frontal and parietal lobes. Other causes include penetrating/missile injuries and shearing of blood vessels deep within the brain following acceleration/deceleration injuries. They are caused by bleeding within the substance of the brain (see Fig. 4.15). Symptoms include headache, contralateral hemiplegia, ipsilateral dilated/fixed pupil and deteriorating level of consciousness, progressing to deep coma (Glasgow Coma Score < 8).

Treatment tends to be conservative, due to the associated injuries and the difficulty in evacuating a haematoma that is situated so deeply within the brain. Not surprisingly, mortality is high within this group of patients.

Diffuse injury

These injuries account for 35% of deaths from head injury and 50% of hospital admissions. Diffuse injuries occur throughout the brain matter rather than to a specific area. They result in generalised dysfunction. Diffuse injuries range from concussion, with no residual damage, to diffuse axonal injury and persistant vegetative state.

Concussion. This is a transient form of diffuse injury which occurs following blunt trauma. It causes a temporary neuronal dysfunction because of transient ischaemia or neurol depolarisation. This manifests as a headache, dizziness, inability to concentrate, disorientation, irritability and nausea. Concussion can occur with or without memory loss. Concussion is graded in line with the severity of symptoms (see Box 4.3).

Recovery is usually rapid, but if neurological symptoms persist, a CT scan should be performed to rule

Box 4.3 – *Grading concussion*	
Grade I	No loss of consciousness, transient confusion and rapid return to normal function
Grade II	Confusion and mild amnesia
Grade III	Profound confusion with pre- and post-traumatic amnesia
Grade IV	Loss of consciousness, variable confusion, amnesia

out more severe injuries. Skull X-ray should only be performed if the mechanism of injury or existing clinical findings are suggestive of a skull fracture. Most patients with concussion can be discharged with an accompanying adult. If there has been a loss of consciousness greater than 10 minutes, the patient should be admitted for observation even if he appears fully recovered. Some patients will have symptoms, such as headache, fatigue, inability to concentrate, irritability and anxiety, persisting for several months (Jackson 1995).

Acute axonal injury. This is usually the result of an acute rotation/deceleration injury, typically following a road traffic accident (Fig. 4.16). The patient usually becomes unconscious rapidly after injury, due to the shearing injury to the brain. Mortality is high in this patient group, and those who do survive usually have severe neurological dysfunction. Initially, a CT scan may show little abnormality, but gradually with repeated scans, many small diffuse haemorrhagic areas will begin to appear commonly in the corpus callosum, midbrain and pons; accompanied by generalised cerebral oedema.

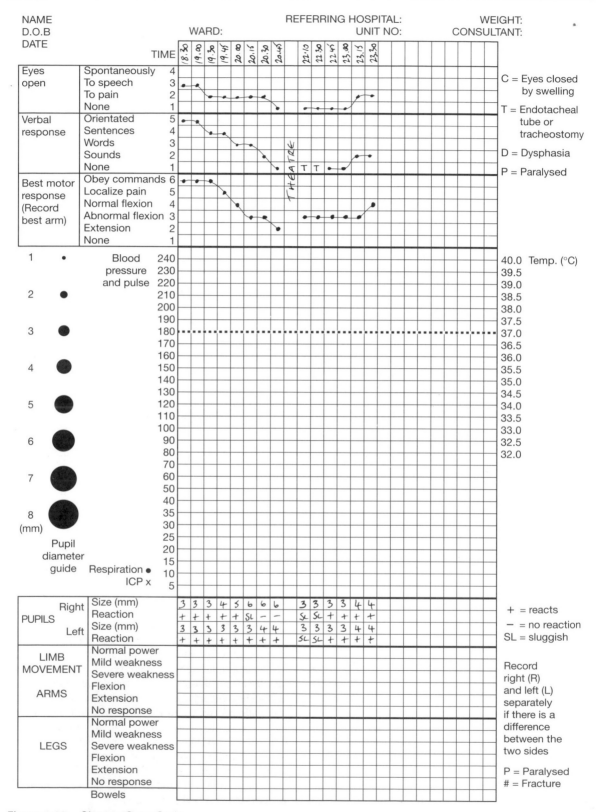

Figure 4.17 – *Glasgow Coma Scale.*

Patients with diffuse axonal injury may also develop autonomic dysfunction, such as excessive sweating, hyperpyrexia and hypertension, due to the common area of haemorrhage being in the corpus callosum, midbrain and pons. Severe cerebral oedema usually accompanies such injuries. Management revolves around maximising cerebral perfusion and preventing secondary brain injury (see below).

Hypoxic injury

This occurs if the brain is deprived of oxygen, e.g., following cardiac arrest, obstructed airway, cervical spine injury and prolonged epileptic-type seizures. The severity of hypoxic injury varies with the time span of hypoxia, ranging from mild cognitive disorder to death. As brain tissue becomes hypoxic, it also becomes oedematous, which compounds the injury by causing cerebral oedema.

Assessment of Head Injury

History

As with all patients, accurate history-taking gives vital clues to the type and potential severity of the head injury (Shah 1999) (see Box 4.4). This may have to be obtained from a witness or paramedic. Even if the history is obtained from the patient, it should be corroborated by a witness/relative if possible.

Box 4.4 – *History-taking in head injury*

- Mechanism of injury
- Time elapsed
- Period of loss of consciousness
- Any pre/post-traumatic amnesia
- Condition since injury, such as nausea, vomiting, confusion, visual disturbance, lethargy or dizziness

---

Physical assessment

If the mechanism of injury or the patient's presenting condition suggests potentially severe injuries, an ATLS approach to assessment should be adopted (Gentleman *et al.* 1993) (see also Ch. 2). Full neurological assessment forms part of the secondary survey, as should thorough examination of the scalp for lacerations, haematomas or evidence of a depressed skull fracture. Neurological assessment should include vital signs:

- blood pressure
- pulse
- respiration
- temperature.

As well as providing a baseline for assessing the patient's progress, vital signs give important information about potential secondary brain injury, e.g. respiration rate and hypoxia. The Glasgow Coma Score (GCS), developed by Teasdale & Jennett (1974), provides an objective, standardised and easily interpreted tool for neurological assessment without relying on subjective terminology such as 'stupor', 'semi-coma' and 'deep coma' (see Box 4.5). The GCS records what you see, measuring arousal, awareness and activity, by assessing eye opening, verbal response and motor ability. Each activity is allocated a score, therefore enabling objectivity, ease of recording and comparison between recordings. It also provides useful information for patient outcome prediction. The score ranges from 15 (fully conscious) to 3 (no response).

As a stimulus is applied, it is good practice to commence with light pressure and then increase to elicit a response. When assessing motor function, always record the best arm; there is no need to record left and right differences as the GCS is not aiming to measure focal deficit; this should be completed in the limb assessment. There is no reason to measure leg response as this may be measuring a spinal rather than a brain-initiated response.

When recording the GCS it is important to record the individual scores as well as the total score (i.e. E2, V3, M4: GCS=9), the motor response being the most reflective for determining prognosis. The GCS may be misleading in patients who have a high cervical injury, or brain stem lesion, and in those who are hypoxic, haemodynamically shocked, fitting or post-ictal. These patients may be unable to move their limbs or may show no responses at all. It is important to attempt to assess the spinal patient using facial movements, being aware of the possibility of a combined head and neck injury. Patients who show no response should be re-evaluated following correction of any shock or hypoxia.

A limb assessment is useful to assess for focal damage; however, although it is usual for a hemiparesis or hemiplegia to occur on the contralateral side to the lesion, it may occur on the ipsilateral side. This is due to indentation of the contralateral cerebral peduncle and is known as a false localising. Spontaneous movements are observed for equality. If there is little or no spontaneous movement, then painful stimuli must be applied to each limb in turn, comparing the result. It is most appropriate to complete this while assessing the motor component of the GCS.

Pupils are assessed for their reaction to light, size and shape, and cranial nerves II (optic) and III (oculomotor). Each pupil needs to be assessed and

Box 4.5 – *The Glasgow Coma Score*

Eye opening

4 – *Spontaneously*: when the patient's eyes open without stimulation of any sort

3 – *To speech*: when the patient's eyes open to verbal stimulation which may need to be repeated, but no physical stimulation is required

2 – *To pain*: when the patient' eyes open either to vigorous shaking or following the application of a painful stimulus

1 – *None*: when the patient's eyes do not open even with persistent verbal or adequate painful stimuli

Verbal response

5 – *Orientated*: when the patient is able to tell the assessor with complete accuracy the date, where he is and who he is

4 – *Sentences*: when the patient is not orientated, but formulates a full sentence or sentences; these may be inappropriate

3 – *Words*: when the response from the patient is restricted to words which are comprehensible, but may be inappropriate

2 – *Sounds*: when the patient makes sound that are not recognisable as words

1 – *None*: when no sound is made by the patient in response to either verbal or painful stimuli

(If the patient is dysphasic, then the letter 'D' should be put in the none column. If the patient is intubated then the letter 'T' should be put in the none column.)

Motor response

6 – *Obeys commands*: when the patient follows simple instructions, such as 'hold up your arms' or 'squeeze and release my hands'

5 – *Localising*: when the patient raises his hands, at least to chin level, in response to a stimulus applied above that level

4 – *Normal flexion*: when the patient's arms bend at the elbow in response to a painful stimulus, without rotation at the wrist.

3 – *Abnormal flexion*: when the patient's arms bend at the elbow, the forearm rotates and the wrist is flexed, in response to a painful stimulus

2 – *Extension*: when the patient's arm straightens at the elbow and rotates towards the body, while the wrist flexes, in response to a painful stimulus

1 – *None*: when there is no response following the application of a deeply painful stimulus

(If the patient is receiving medicines to maintain muscle paralysis, record the letter 'P in the none column.)

recorded individually. Pupils are measured in millimeters, the normal range being 2–6 mm in diameter. They are normally round in shape and abnormalities are described as ovoid, keyhole or irregular (Hickey 1992). A bright light is shone into the side of each eye to assess the pupils' reaction to light. This should produce a brisk constriction in both pupils, the consensual light reaction. Herniation of the medial temporal lobe through the tentorium directly damages the oculomotor (IIIrd) nerve, resulting in dilation of the pupil and an impaired reaction to light. The pupil dilates on the side of the lesion. Neurological observations should be recorded on an observation or trauma chart.

Patients with head injuries can be classified into three groups depending on their GCS:

■ A score of 13–15 is indicative of a *minor head injury*. In some patients, a one point drop in their GCS can be alcohol- or drug-induced. This necessitates extra vigilance from nursing staff as subtle changes in the patient's cognition or conscious level may be masked by alcohol and/or drugs.

■ A GCS of 9–12 suggests a *moderate head injury*, or a more serious injury evolving. Any changes in the patient's condition should be closely monitored.

■ A *severe head injury* is classified by a GCS of 8 or less. These patients are potentially at risk of secondary brain injury, and their GCS and vital signs should be monitored at frequent intervals.

When assessing vital signs in conjunction with GCS, it is important to remember the following:

■ Hypotension is only of neurological origin in end-stage brain injury or spinal shock. Other causes of hypotension, such as hypovolaemia, should be investigated.

■ Cushing's triad (hypertension, bradycardia and bradypnoea) indicates a life-threatening rise in ICP.

■ Pyrexia with hypertension may indicate autonomic dysfunction.

Generally, in the assessment of head injury, skull X-ray is not necessary. In unconscious patients with a history of significant head injury, CT scanning is more useful. Skull X-ray should only be considered if there is marked bruising or significant laceration of the scalp, CSF or blood oozing from the nose or ear, a suspected penetrating injury or abnormal neurology in a conscious patient (Bullock & Teasdale 1996). CT scanning should be considered if:

■ GCS <15 with a skull fracture
■ abnormal neurology and skull fracture
■ seizure and skull fracture

- GCS <15 for longer than 8 h
- a decreasing GCS with normal BP and P_{O_2}
- persistent vomiting with no other obvious cause.

Management of Serious Head Injury

Management of serious head injury in A&E revolves largely around preventing or limiting secondary brain injury while the patient awaits definitive treatment such as surgery. Secondary brain injury should be suspected if the patient's consciousness level alters. Causes of secondary brain injury are shown in Box 4.6.

> **Box 4.6** – *Causes of secondary brain injury*
>
> - Hyperpyrexia
> - Cerebral ischaemia
> - Cerebral oedema
> - Raised intracranial pressure
> - Infection
> - Metabolic disorder
> - Evolving intracranial bleed
> - Hypotension

Airway/breathing

Management should follow the sequence laid down by ATLS (American College of Surgeons 1997). Airway management is paramount in preventing hypoxia and therefore secondary brain injury. Airway patency can be threatened by oedema/debris following injury, loss of gag reflex and vomiting. If a clear airway cannot be maintained with simple aids, such as a Guedel or oropharyngeal airway then intubation should be performed. Suctioning should be kept to a minimum as it raises ICP. Cervical spine immobilisation should be maintained unless neck injury has been excluded.

The neurophysiology of breathing is complex and involves several areas of the brain. Following head injury the normal pattern of breathing is easily disrupted, leading to hypoxia. As good oxygenation is imperative, head-injured patients should be given oxygen via a face mask and reservoir bag: if bradypnoeic this should, be assisted by mechanical ventilation. It is important to maintain adequate oxygenation, as a rise in P_{CO_2} levels initiates autoregulation, causing cerebral vasodilation and a rise in ICP. If unchecked, this can lead to secondary brain injury. Induced hyperventilation is used to reduce P_{CO_2} levels, but this

> **Box 4.7** – *Indications for intubation*
>
> - An absent gag reflex in an unconscious head-injured patient
> - For airway protection from bleeding or vomit
> - If adequate ventilation cannot be maintained, i.e. P_{O_2} < 10 kPa on maximal O_2 via mask*
> - Hypoventilation causing a P_{CO_2} > 6 kPa*
> - Hyperventilation causing a P_{CO_2} < 3.5 kPa*
> - Flail chest injury*
> - To facilitate interhospital transfer in a patient with a GCS < 8
>
> *Indicates need for mechanical ventilation.

should be discussed with a neurosurgeon first (Bullock & Teasdale 1996). Indications for intubation with or without mechanical ventilation are listed in Box 4.7.

If urgent intubation is indicated, it should be assumed that the patient has a full stomach, and cricoid pressure should be applied to prevent vomiting or gastric regurgitation. In adults, this should be maintained until the cuff of the ET tube is inflated, creating a secure airway. Short-acting sedatives and muscle relaxants should always be used for intubation, to minimise the impact on neurological observations. Hypoxia is a major cause of cerebral ischaemia and care should always be taken to maintain adequate oxygenation levels by monitoring respiratory effort closely with arterial blood gases (ABGs) and O_2 saturation measurement and intervening with supportive therapy at an early stage.

Circulation

Hypotension is rarely of neurological origin. It usually results from systemic hypovolaemia following multiple trauma. Causes of hypotension should be identified and fluid resuscitation is imperative to prevent a drop in cerebral ischaemia and secondary brain injury. Hypertension is a late sign of pending brain injury. Arterial blood pressure increases in an attempt to maintain the perfusion pressure in the brain. In the late stages of head injury, hypertension occurs with bradycardia and bradypnoea. This is referred to as Cushing's triad. The aim of this is to maintain cerebral perfusion pressure, but it is a late sign which often precedes death. The decreases in respiration and heart rate are due to pressure on the medulla.

Raised intracranial pressure

Uncontrolled elevation in ICP is the most common cause of mortality and secondary brain injury in the head-injured patient. This is because it alters tissue perfusion, causing cerebral ischaemia. It is therefore important to ensure that signs of raised ICP are noted and treated early. Disorientation, irritation, headache, seizures, nausea and vomiting are all possible indicators of raised ICP, and later signs include deterioration in the GCS, limb and pupil changes and finally alteration in the vital signs (Cushing's triad).

Hypercapnia can cause secondary brain injury which results from either inadequate ventilation or a response to hypermetabolism following trauma. High Pco_2 levels result from cerebral vasodilation in an attempt to increase oxygenation. This increases cerebral blood flow and, therefore, intracranial pressure. Hyperventilation is controversial (Harrahill 1997), but is the most common treatment for inducing vasoconstriction, and reduces Pco_2 and thus intracranial pressure. Arterial blood gas analysis should be frequently recorded in patients being artificially hyperventilated/ventilated.

Fluid management is crucial to ensuring adequate maintenance of ICP. As previously stated, patients should have adequate fluid resuscitation to ensure they are normotensive; however, it is common to restrict crystalloid input to 70% of normal. Osmotic diuretics, such as 20% Mannitol, with or without frusemide, should be administered to reduce cerebral oedema. All patients should have close observation of their fluid input and output. For this reason, and to reduce discomfort, patients receiving Mannitol should have a urinary catheter inserted. If possible, the patient should be positioned with the head raised to 30° (following clearance of the cervical spine) and the neck should be in neutral alignment, to maximise venous drainage.

Seizures

Seizures will increase metabolic activity in the brain, which in turn may raise the intracranial pressure. If seizure activity is continuous, i.e. status epilepticus or serial fitting, severe cerebral oedema may occur. Patients having seizures should be protected from harm, but if they are not in any danger then they should not be handled. The seizure should be observed for origin, sequence of events and time of start/finish. This information should be clearly recorded in the patient's notes.

Seizures may require muscle relaxant and/or anticonvulsant drugs to be brought under control.

Both the post-ictal state and medication may alter the neurological observations, so extra vigilance is required. Regular GCSs should be completed until the pre-seizure state is regained.

Transfer to a Specialist Neurosurgical Unit

The most common reason for interhospital transfer in the head-injured patient is the need for surgical intervention, such as evacuation of heamatoma or treatment of a depressed skull fracture. Less than 1% of all head injuries are treated in specialist units (Bullock & Teasdale 1996). Once the decision to transfer has been made, it is imperative that the patient is adequately resuscitated and stable prior to transfer. Patients should have i.v. access and fluid replacement before leaving.

The neck should be fully examined to identify or exclude cervical injury (see also Ch. 6). Chest or abdominal injuries (Chs 7 and 8) should be treated if potentially life-threatening and fractures splinted where appropriate (see Ch. 5). Airway management is a major cause for concern during transfer; unconscious patients, those who are vomiting or those whose condition appears to be deteriorating (GCS ≤8) should be intubated prior to transfer (Munro & Laycock 1993). Patients who are intubated should also be sedated whether or not they were previously conscious (Gentleman *et al.* 1993).

Any patient being transferred should have a suitably qualified medical and nurse escort (NHSE 1996). During transfer, the patient should be carefully observed and ECG, oxygen saturation levels and blood pressure should be monitored continuously (Parkins 1998). If the patient is not sedated, pupil size and reaction and GCS should be recorded. All documentation and results of clinical investigations, such as CT, should accompany the patient (Jones 1993).

Brain Stem Death

The diagnosis of brain stem death is usually made in the intensive care unit; however, in rare cases this may occur in the A&E department. Initially, certain preconditions must be fulfilled, as follows:

- There is a known cause of irremediable structural brain damage.
- The patient must have normal electrolyte levels, normal glucose levels and a normal acid–base balance.

- The patient must have no CNS depressant drugs or neuromuscular blocking drugs on board and must be normothermic.

Having satisfied the preconditions a number of tests are performed. The following results confirm brain stem death:

- The pupils are fixed and dilated, not responding to sharp changes in the intensity of light.
- There is no corneal reflex.
- There are no vestibulor-ocular reflexes.
- There is no motor response.
- There is no gag or cough reflex.
- There is no respiratory effort, despite allowing the $P\text{CO}_2$ to rise above the threshold for stimulus of respiration.

Two senior doctors must perform these tests on two occasions. This condition alone limits the probability of the full testing occurring in A&E; however, some or all of the tests may be performed, either to complete a clinical picture or to reach an endpoint in an inevitable situation. This is a very difficult situation to manage, even in the intensive care unit, when the nurse may be familiar with the patient's family and friends.

Management of Minor Head Injury

The majority of patients treated in A&E with head injury will have a 'minor' head injury. Some 92% of these patients will have normal neurology (Klauber 1993) and the majority will be discharged home. A thorough assessment of the patient's condition should be performed, which should include pulse, respirations, blood pressure, pupil size and reaction, and the patient's GCS. Although only 1% of head-injured patients have skull fractures (Ramrakha & Moore 1997), there are certain circumstances where a skull X-ray is appropriate (see Box 4.8).

Box 4.8 – *Indications for skull X-ray*

- Suspected penetrating injury
- Decreased consciousness (if GCS below 8/15, CT is indicated)
- Altered neurology
- CSF from nose or ear
- Significant scalp bruising or swelling
- Difficulty in clinical examination, where mechanism of injury is suggestive of fracture

---

The key to managing minor head injury is giving adequate information and advice to the patient and his carer. The patient should be advised to rest quietly and should be discouraged from taking part in strenuous activities and from undertaking long periods of VDU work or watching TV, which will exacerbate any headache. Simple analgesia should be suggested, such as paracetamol, which should be sufficient to alleviate headaches without masking other signs of deterioration. The patient should be discouraged from taking alcohol until symptoms have subsided. Written advice should always be given to the patient/carer to reinforce any verbal information (Box 4.9). (see also Ch. 36).

Box 4.9 – *Typical head injury advice sheet*

- General advice about observing a patient every 2 hours; ensure he wakes easily and is orientated when awake. Ensure the patient is able to move all limbs

- You should return to hospital if any of the following occur:
  - persistent vomiting
  - confusion
  - excessive sleeping; difficulty in rousing patient
  - severe headache
  - double vision
  - limb weakness
  - convulsions or 'passing out'
  - discharge of blood/fluid from nose/ears

- You should not drink alcohol until all symptoms have subsided

- The name and telephone of the hospital should be included

When discussing the outcomes of a minor head injury, it is important that the A&E nurse explains post-concussion type symptoms to the patient. Approximately one-third of patients with head injuries who are discharged from A&E have persistent symptoms for longer than 6 months. This is due to mild diffuse axonal injury. The majority of these patients will have been knocked out for a short time and may have other mild neurological signs. As there is no treatment for mild diffuse axonal injury, and recovery is usually spontaneous, reassurance and psychological support are vital to the patient's recovery. Symptoms are shown in Box 4.10. Head-injured patients should be discharged into the care of a responsible adult. Not all patients with minor head injury are appropriate for discharge (see Box 4.11).

Box 4.10 – *Symptoms of mild diffuse axonal injury*

- Headache
- Fatigue
- Irritability
- Poor concentration
- Dizziness
- Poor balance
- Depression

Box 4.11 – *Indications for hospital admission*

- Decreased consciousness
- Neurological deficit
- Severe headache and persistent vomiting
- Confusion
- Intoxification rendering clinical assessment unreliable
- Coexisting conditions such as clotting disorders
- Social circumstances making discharge unwise

Conclusion

Head trauma can have a devastating effect on a person's life and some mortality and morbidity are inevitable. The A&E nurse is fundamental to keeping morbidity to a minimum by being vigilant and preventing secondary brain injury. The majority of head-injured patients treated in A&E have minor injuries; however, these can have an enormous impact on the lives of the patient and his carer. The information and psychological support given in A&E are vital to facilitate recovery.

Further reading

Johnson BP (1995) One family's experience with head injury: a phenomenological study. *Journal of Neuroscience Nursing* **27**(2), 113–118.

Thompson RF (1993) *The Brain: a Neuroscience Primer*, 2nd edn. New York: WH Freeman.

Thomson R, Gray J, Madhok R, Mordue A, Mendelow AD (1994) Effect of guidelines on management of head injury on record keeping and decision making in accident and emergency departments. *Quality in Health Care* **3**(2), 86–91.

References

American College of Surgeons (Committee on Trauma) (1997) *Advanced Trauma Life Support Programme*. Illinois: American College of Surgeons.

Bullock R, Teasdale G (1996) Head injuries. In: Skinner D, Driscoll R, Earlam R, eds. *ABC of Trauma*, 2nd edn. London: BMJ Publishing Group.

Carola R, Harley JP, Noback CR (1990) *Human Anatomy and Physiology*. Booton: McGraw-Hill.

Chandler CL, Cummins B (1995) Initial assessment and management of the severely head-injured patient. *British Journal of Hospital Medicine*. **53**(3), 102–108.

Dadley L (1998) Trauma scoring in A&E. *Emergency Nurse*, **6**(7), 15–17.

Gentleman D, Dearden M, Midgley S, MacLean D (1993) Guidelines for resuscitation and transfer of patients with serious head injury. *British Medical Journal* **6903**, 347–352.

Harrahill M (1997) Management of severe head injury: new document provides guidelines. *Journal of Emergency Nursing* **23**(3), 282–283.

Hickey JV (1992) *The Clinical Practice of Neurological and Neurosurgical Nursing*, 3rd edn. Philadelphia: JB Lippincott.

Hudak CM, Gallo BM (1994) *Critical Care Nursing*, 6th edn. Philadelphia: JB Lippincott.

Jackson S (1995) Not so minor head injuries? *Emergency Nurse* **3**(1), 19–22.

Jones H (1993) Safe transfer. *Nursing Times*, **89**(41), 31–33.

Klauber K (1993) Rehabilitation of the trauma patient: In Neff JA, Kidd PS, eds. *Trauma Nursing: the Art and Science*, St Louis: Mosby Year Book.

Lindsey KW, Bone I, Callander R (1991) *Neurology and Neurosurgery Illustrated*, 2nd edn. Edinburgh: Churchill Livingstone.

Munro HM, Laycock JRD (1993) Inter-hospital transfer. *British Journal of Intensive Care*, **16**, 210–214.

NHSE (1996) *Admission to and Discharge from Intensive and High Dependency Care*. London: Department of Health.

Parkins DR (1998) Transportation of the injured: head injuries. *Pre-hospital Immediate Care*, **2**, 25–26.

Ramrakha P, Moore K (1997) *Oxford Handbook of Acute Medicine*. Oxford: Oxford University Press.

Royal College of Surgeons of England (1988) *Report of the Working Party on the Management of Patients with Major Injuries*. London: Royal College of Surgeons of England.

Sakas DE, Dias LS, Beale D (1995) Subarachniod haemorrhage presenting as a head injury. *British Medical Journal* **310**, 1186–1187.

Shah S (1999) Neurological assessment. *Nursing Standard*, **13**(22), 49–56

Sheehy S (1992) *Emergency Nursing Practice and Principles*, 3rd edn. St Louis: Mosby Year Book.

Sherman DW (1990) Managing an acute head injury. *Nursing* **20**(4), 47–51.

Teasdale G, Jennett B (1974) Assessment of coma and impaired consciousness: a practical scale. *The Lancet* **2**(7872), 81–84.

Chapter 5

Skeletal Injuries

Lynda Holt

- Introduction
- Anatomy and physiology
- Pelvic injury
- Hip injury
- Limb injury
- Femoral fractures
- Lower leg injury
- Ankle fractures
- Foot fractures
- Injury to the shoulder
- Upper arm injury
- Elbow injury
- Forearm injury
- The wrist
- The hand
- Soft tissue injuries
- Conclusion

Introduction

Skeletal and soft tissue injuries range in severity from life- or limb-threatening to self-limiting minor injuries. International research has demonstrated that patients with musculoskeletal injuries represent approximately 25% of the A&E workload. It is imperative for A&E nurses to be able to assess musculoskeletal injury and identify life- or limb-threatening trauma, some of which may not seem devastating at first glance.

This chapter will provide the underpinning anatomy and physiology of the musculoskeletal system, before looking at areas such as pelvis, neck of femur and limb injuries. Each of these will be examined in detail, principles of assessment and management will be discussed, and particular problems related to specific injuries will be identified.

Anatomy and Physiology

In order to appreciate the impact of injury, it is useful for the A&E nurse to have a thorough understanding of the make-up and purpose of the human skeleton (Fig. 5.1) and skeletal muscle. The skeleton comprises two parts with specific functions:

- *the axial skeleton*, consisting of the skull, vertebral column, ribs and sternum – supports and protects vital organs
- *the appendicular skeleton*, consisting of the shoulder girdle, pelvic girdle and limbs – provides shape and facilitates movement.

Bone is a form of connective tissue comprising three major components:

- organic matrix of collagen – creates tensile strength
- mineral matrix of calcium and phosphate – creates rigidity and strength
- bone cells, including osteoblasts, osteoclast, osteocytes and fibroblasts.

Compact cortical bone, which is found on outer parts of all bone, forms the shaft of long bones and

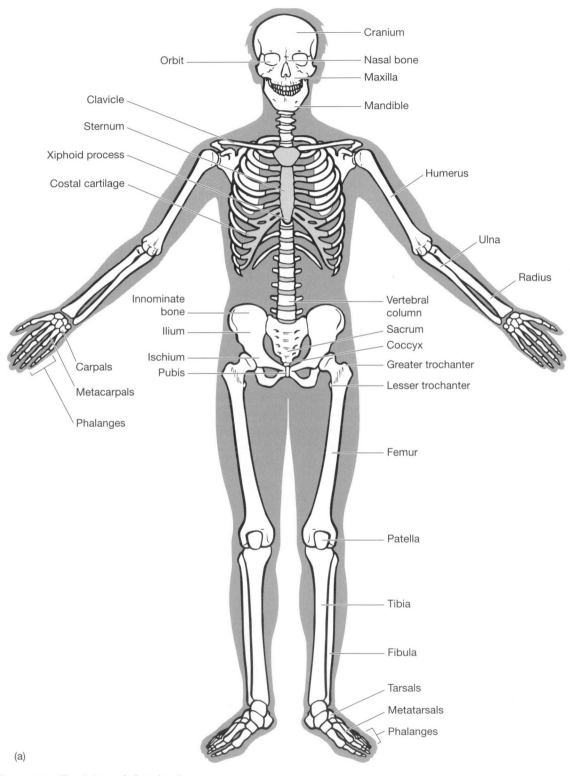

Figure 5.1 – *The skeleton. A: Anterior view.*

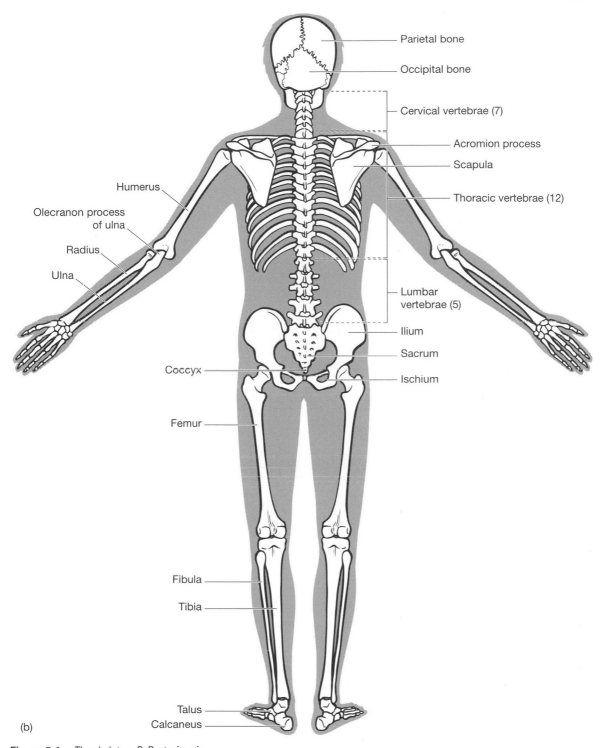

Parietal bone

Occipital bone

Cervical vertebrae (7)

Acromion process

Scapula

Thoracic vertebrae (12)

Humerus

Olecranon process
of ulna

Radius

Ulna

Lumbar
vertebrae (5)

Ilium

Sacrum

Coccyx

Ischium

Femur

Fibula

Tibia

Talus

Calcaneus

(b)

Figure 5.1 – *The skeleton. B: Posterior view.*

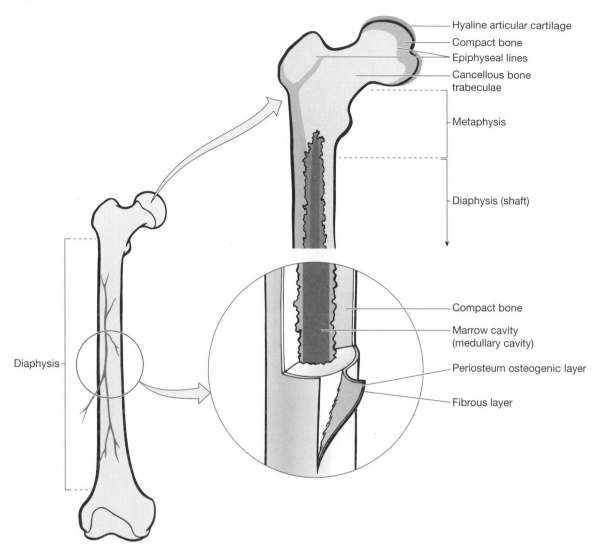

Figure 5.2 – *Cross-section of bone.*

encloses marrow cavities (see Fig. 5.2). Compact bone contains Haversian canals with osteocytes which facilitate the exchange of nutrients and waste. Cancellous bone (trabeculae) is organised in a lattice system and contains fewer Haversian canals. Red and fatty bone marrow fills the cavities in the lattice. Cancellous bone is found at the ends of the long bone and in the vertebrae and flat bones.

The periosteum is a fibrous tissue layer covering bone, but not cartilage or synovial joints. It transmits blood vessels and nerve fibres. The periosteum also provides attachments for ligaments and muscles. Beneath this layer are osteoblasts which aid bone growth and, as a result, the periosteum does not attach

to the bone surface until adulthood when growth is complete. Because of abundant nerve supply, the periosteum is responsible for bone pain. Damage to periosteum or pressure on it from tumours or trauma can cause severe pain.

Bone cells

Osteoblasts. These are present on all bone surfaces and form a uniform layer. Their purpose is the synthesis and secretion of collagen and protein, and they promote calcification during rapid phases of this process.

Osteocytes. These form from osteoblasts trapped

in matrix. The exact function of these cells is not known, but they appear to act as a pump, controlling calcium release in response to hormones.

Osteoclasts. These are found near bone surfaces and are responsible for reabsorption of bone. They are very mobile and are found in great numbers where bone is undergoing erosion. Their activity is controlled by a number of hormones including parathyroid and thyroxin.

Joints

Joints are the area of contact between bone and bone, or bone and cartilage. They are classified by the type of movement they permit.

Fibrous joints permit no movement at all, e.g., skull joints. Fibrous connective tissues merges into the periosteum of each bone.

Cartilaginous joints permit limited movement because of flexible cartilage between bones. The symphyses have cartilage pads, or discs, between bones, e.g. symphysis pubis or intervertebral joints. Complex ligament arrangements stabilise these cartilage pads to limit movement and facilitate recoil. Synchondroses are cartilage joints which ossify in adulthood and prevent movement, e.g. epiphysis of long bone.

Synovial joints form most of the body's joints. They are further classified by the type and range of movement they allow (see Table 5.1). All synovial joints have a number of similar structured features. They are enclosed in a capsule which is lined with synovial membrane, which secretes synovial fluid. Bone ends are not in direct contact and are covered by hyaline cartilage. The fibrous capsule is held in place by a number of ligaments.

Muscular system

Muscle tissue is formed to convert chemical energy into mechanical contraction, creating movement. Movements are generated both at joints and in soft tissue. Muscles also assist in maintaining body posture and muscular activity is associated with maintaining body heat.

Muscles are made up of bundles of fibres (fasciculi). The length of these fibres relates to the range of movement the muscle performs; that is, the longer the fibre, the greater is the range of movement. The number of fibres relates to the strength of the muscle. Muscles are attached to the periosteum by tendons. There are two points of attachment, the origin of which remains fixed during contraction while the insertion moves. Skeletal muscles have a rich blood supply which increases dramatically during exercise.

Table 5.1 – *Classification of synovial joints*

Type of joint	Site	Range of movement
Hinge	Elbow Fingers Ankle Toes	Flexion Extension
Pivot	Vertebral column	Rotation
Gliding	Shoulder girdle Vertebral column	Limited motion in several directions
Ball and socket	Hip Shoulder	Extensive range of movement: Flexion Extension Rotation
Saddle	Hand Base of thumb	Flexion Extension Abduction Adduction Opposition
Ellipson	Wrist Hand Foot	Flexion Extension Abduction Adduction Opposition

Tendons

Tendons are made up of fibrous connective tissue carrying parallel bundles of collagen fibres. This gives greater flexibility but prevents stretching when under pressure, such as in muscle contraction. They act like a spring, allowing the transition of movement from muscle to bone. Tendons have a sparse blood supply which inhibits healing if damaged.

Ligaments

Ligaments are made up of collagen and elastin bundles. They are attached to bone and are responsible for maintaining joint stability. Stretching or tearing of ligaments results in painful, swollen and, in severe cases, unstable joints.

Pelvic Injury

Anatomy and physiology

The pelvis is designed to provide structure, strength for weight-bearing, and protection of internal organs. It houses the rectum, bladder and, in women, the reproductive organs. The pelvis forms a ring, comprising the sacrum and two innominate bones, each made up of an ilium, pubic bone and ischium (see Fig. 5.3).

The bones are supported by strong ligaments at the sacroiliac joint, and cartilaginous joint at the symphysis pubis. The innominate bones do not fuse until around 16–18 years of age, and in children are supported by cartilage. The pelvis has a rich blood supply from the internal and external iliac arteries.

Mechanism of injury

Major trauma to the pelvic girdle is relatively uncommon and accounts for approximately 3% of all skeletal injuries; however, the mortality associated with major pelvic fractures ranges from 4 to 50% (Monsell & Ross 1998, Muir *et al.*, 1996). Most pelvic fractures are caused by motorcycle accidents, accidents involving pedestrians, direct crush injuries or falls from a height (American College of Surgeons 1997).

Fracture patterns

In adults, isolated pelvic fractures rarely occur. This is because of the strength and ligamentous stretch of the pelvic ring. If significant force is applied, two or more breaks in the pelvic ring are likely to occur. The pelvis has predictable areas of strength and weakness, and therefore, in adults, potential patterns of fractures are easy to predict. In children, the increased elasticity of the pelvis prior to fusion of the innominate bones makes isolated fractures far more likely.

Lateral compression fractures (graded I, II, III) are caused by a side impact, usually to motorcyclists or pedestrians in collision with vehicles. A compression fracture of the pubic bone or rami is combined with compression fracture on the side of impact (see Fig. 5.4A). With greater force of impact, the iliac wing on the side of the impact will also break; this is a grade II injury (Fig. 5.4B). A grade III injury also involves the opposite side to the impact (Fig. 5.4C).

Anteroposterior compression fractures (graded I, II, III) are caused by direct pressure or crushing and result in the pelvis opening outwards from wings rather like a book. The result is fracturing of the pubis or rami together with sacroiliac distribution. In grade I injuries, the symphysis is separated by less that 2 cm (see Fig. 5.5A); in grade II injuries the sacrospinous

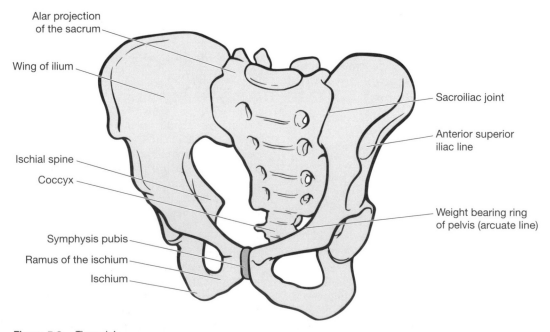

Figure 5.3 – *The pelvis.*

Alar projection of the sacrum
Wing of ilium
Ischial spine
Coccyx
Symphysis pubis
Ramus of the ischium
Ischium
Sacroiliac joint
Anterior superior iliac line
Weight bearing ring of pelvis (arcuate line)

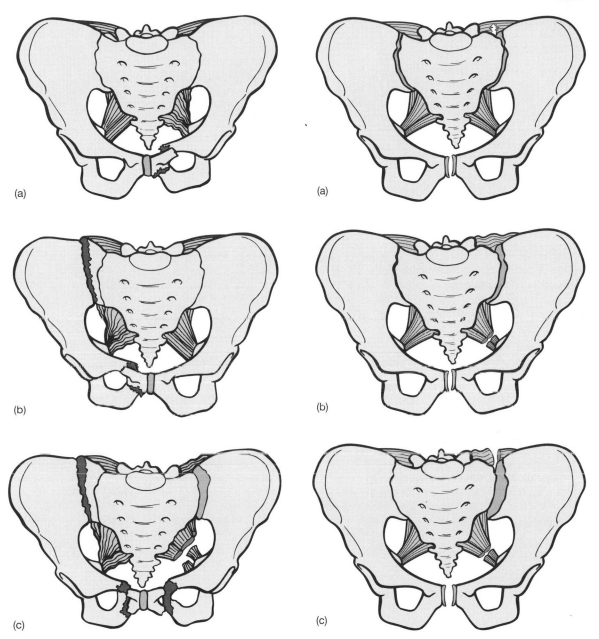

(a)

(b)

(c)

(a)

(b)

(c)

Figure 5.4 – *Lateral compression (LC) fractures of the pelvis. (a): Grade I. (b): Grade II. (c): Grade III.*

Figure 5.5 – *Anteroposterior compression (APC) fractures of the pelvis. (a): Grade I. (b): Grade II. (c): Grade III.*

and sacrotuberous ligaments rupture (Fig. 5.5B); and in grade III injuries the iliolumbar ligament can rupture (Fig. 5.5C). This type of pelvic fracture has double the mortality rate of the lateral compression injuries.

Vertical shearing force fractures result from falls or from knees hitting a car dashboard with great speed. The pattern of injury is similar to antero-posterior compression, but with vertical displacement (see Fig. 5.6). With combined mechanical forces, such as being run over by a motor vehicle, a combination of the above fracture patterns may occur simultaneously.

Patterns of single fracture injury to the pelvis include:

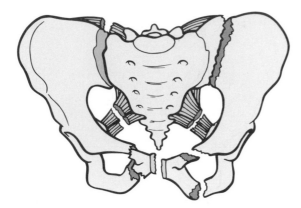

Figure 5.6 – *Pelvic ring fracture.*

- *acetabulum* – these are not common in isolation, but can occur with direct force to the leg, driving the head of the femur into the acetabulum
- *sacrum* – again these are uncommon in isolation, but can result from a backward fall or falls from a height
- *coccyx* – this is often fractured by falls onto the buttocks, particularly in women where the coccyx is more prominent
- *single pubic ramus* – these appear to be common in elderly patients following falls; however, evidence suggests that they usually occur with other pelvic injuries that are not initially detected
- *avulsion fractures* – these occur in young athletes, where excessive muscle strain can avulse growth cartilage on the apophyseal plates
- *iliac wing fractures* – these injuries commonly result from direct trauma and should always be considered in conjunction with intra-abdominal injury.

Assessment of pelvic ring injury

Fractures involving the pelvic ring carry potentially life-threatening complications of haemorrhage if not rapidly identified and treated. Mechanisms of injury should give some clues as to a potential pelvic fracture. The assessing nurse should carry out a primary assessment following the ABCDE approach laid out in ATLS guidelines (American College of Surgeons 1997). A patient with a pelvic ring fracture will have severe pelvic pain and progressive flank, perianal or scrotal swelling and bruising. Disruption of the pelvic ring can also be identified by differences in leg length and external rotation of a leg without an associated limb fracture.

Mechanical instability of the pelvis can be tested by manual manipulation or compression of the pelvis. This should be carried out once by an experienced

clinician. It is a very painful procedure for the patient and carries the risk of exacerbating haemorrhage. When the clinician manipulates the pelvis, pressure should be applied gently to the iliac crest. If the pelvis has rotated, the clinician will be able to close the ring by gently pushing the iliac crests together. Diagnosis can be confirmed by X-ray. Most patients with a pelvic ring fracture will have moderate to severe hypotension. Abdominal/pelvic X-rays will aid diagnosis.

Assessment should also include examination of groins, perineal area and genitalia. Femoral pulses should be checked on both sides. Absent pulses are indicative of damage to the external iliac artery and surgery is required to preserve the limb of the affected side. Decreased pulse pressure should be closely monitored, as it may be indicative of a worsening systemic condition or damage to the iliac artery. The perineum should be inspected for laceration and bleeding. Prophylactic antibiotics should be prescribed for wounds because of the high infection risk from faecal flora (Ruiz 1995).

In men, testicles should be examined, as a swollen testicle is indicative of testicular rupture requiring surgical decompression. The penis should be examined for blood at the meatus, suggestive of urethral damage. In women, the vulva should be examined, and the vagina and urethral meatus inspected for blood. In male and female patients where there is no evidence of urethral injury, a urinary catheter should be inserted. If urethral injury is likely then suprapubic catheterisation should be considered for bladder decompression. A rectal examination should be performed to test sphincter tone – a reduction in tone is suggestive of a sacral fracture. Frank blood is usually indicative of a rectal tear and surgical intervention is necessary. In men, the position of the prostate should be established as a high, boggy prostate indicates a urethral transection.

Management of pelvic ring fractures

Pelvic fracture is a potentially life-threatening injury because of significant haemorrhage. Initial management focuses on volume replacement, stabilisation of fractures and, therefore, the rate of haemorrhage and pain control. Fluid replacement should follow ATLS guidelines with a rapid infusion of warmed crystalloid fluid, ideally Ringer's lactate (American College of Surgeons 1997). This is because Ringer's solution closely resembles the electrolyte content of plasma and therefore provides transient intravascular expansion followed by interstitial and intracellular replacement. Normal saline can be used, but large amounts are not recommended because it can induce hypercholaemic acidosis. After an initial 2 L, or 20 ml/kg in children, blood or colloid solutions should be commenced. The patient's haemodynamic condition should be continuously monitored during this period.

Haemorrhage control relies on fracture stabilisation. This can be achieved in a number of ways. The use of a pneumatic anti-shock garment (PASG) serves a dual purpose of haemorrhage and pain control. It provides mechanical stabilisation of the fractures and external counter-pressure. Circulation to extremities should be regularly checked. Decompression of the PASG should take place in a controlled environment, at a pace which does not exacerbate haemodynamic instability. Usually this takes place in the operating theatre. If a PASG is not available, longitudinal skin traction can be used (American College of Surgeons 1997). Early external fixation provides definitive haemorrhage control. Pain control is initiated by fracture immobilisation, but inhaled analgesia, such as Entonox in the conscious patient, and i.v. opiates are also necessary.

Uncomplicated, isolated pelvic fractures not involving the pelvic ring should be assessed in a similar manner. The management of these injuries is usually conservative. Patients usually require hospital admission for initial bed rest, pain control and rehabilitation support. Most of these fracture injuries have an uncomplicated recovery pattern. Acetabular fractures, however, have a high morbidity. They are caused by extreme force, commonly road traffic accidents (RTAs), where the knees hit the dashboard at speed. Long-term prognosis is improved by surgical intervention (Snyder 1998).

Hip Injury

Anatomy and physiology

The femoral head and neck lie within the joint capsule of the hip joint. The head of the femur moves within the acetabulum. This is supported by three ligaments: iliofemoral, ischiofemoral and pubofemoral. Blood supply to the head of the femur is largely from the profunda femoris artery, which has circumflex branches around the neck of femur, off which smaller branches supply the head. This pattern of blood supply is particularly vulnerable to disruption from impacted fractures – hence the high risk of vascular necrosis with neck of femur fractures. The periosteum is very thin or non-existent around the neck of femur, therefore making it very susceptible to fractures. This susceptibility increases with age, particularly for women where osteoporosis has further weakened bone strength.

Classification of fractures

Neck of femur

Garden's classification of neck of femur (NOF) fractures has been used for over 30 years (Garden 1964). He highlighted four stages of fracture (Fig. 5.7):

Stage I represents impacted fractures. The trabeculae and cortex are pushed into the femoral head. This is considered a stable fracture as the inferior cortex usually remains intact. This type of fracture is not very susceptible to avascular necrosis and therefore operative treatment usually entails

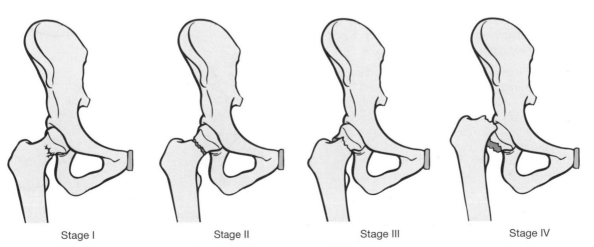

Stage I   Stage II   Stage III   Stage IV

Figure 5.7 – *Garden's classification of femoral neck fractures: stages I–IV.*

pinning rather than prosthetic replacement of the femoral head. Union rates are good and morbidity is low following this treatment (Ruiz 1995).

Stage II. These are non-displaced fractures across the femoral neck. Because there is no impaction, the fracture is unstable, but as there is no displacement the risk of avascular necrosis is low. These injuries are therefore fixed with screws.

Stage III. These are displaced fractures, with the femoral head abducted in relation to the pelvis. Fragments of the fracture are in contact with each other. Disruption of the blood supply is common and for this reason operative repair usually involves the insertion of a prosthesis to replace the femoral head.

Stage IV. Similar to stage III fractures, these are displaced, but the femoral head is adducted in relation to the pelvis, fracture fragments are completely separated and avascular necrosis is likely. In most cases, prosthetic replacement of the femoral head is the treatment of choice in younger patients; however, attempts may be made to reduce and internally fixate the fracture. This prevents degeneration of the acetabulum caused over time by a prosthesis.

Intertrochanteric fractures

Although these have specific differences from NOF fractures, the assessment of injury and initial A&E management are similar. In terms of anatomy, the main difference is in bone density, as periosteum is present over the trochanters, although osteoporosis has a detrimental effect in women. In younger people and older men these fractures are far less common than NOF fractures. These injuries are not affected by avascular necrosis as the circumflex arterial branches of the NOF are not damaged. Because of the periosteum, the risk of non-union is also lower.

Several fracture classifications are used and all have slight variations from each other. To provide a general idea of fracture classification, Kyle *et al* (1979) described four types of injury (see Fig. 5.8):

- *Type I* – stable, undisplaced intertrochanteric fracture, requiring simple internal fixation.
- *Type II* – stable but displaced with fragmentation of the lesser trochanter; these are internally fixed.
- *Type III* – unstable fractures of the greater trochanter with posteromedial comminuted bone and deformity. These are fixed, but if a stable reduction cannot be achieved because of the amount of comminuted bone, osteotomy to the base of greater trochanter may be performed.
- *Type IV* – these have the components of type III fractures, but also have subtrochanteric fractures. Internal fixation is attempted using screws and sliding plates.

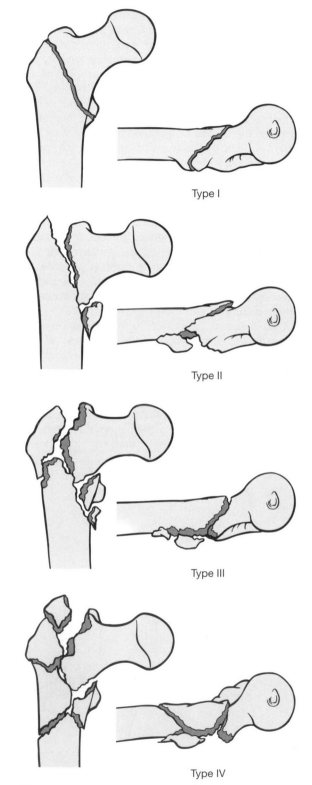

Type I

Type II

Type III

Type IV

Figure 5.8 – *Kyle's classification of intertrochanteric fractures.*

In children, NOF or intertrochanteric fractures are uncommon and are caused by severe force. Internal fixation is not the treatment of choice because of growth patterns. Children are treated with bed rest and traction.

Assessment of patients with hip injury

These patients are usually elderly, predominantly women and commonly attend A&E following a fall (Audit Commission 1996). Although these injuries are rarely immediately life-threatening, attributed mortality is as high as 20% (Ruiz 1995). The patient usually complains of groin pain, and pain through the thigh to the knee. Pain is worsened by any movement and the majority of patients will have been unable to weight-bear since injury. In most NOF and intertrochanteric fractures, the injured limb will be externally rotated, and is shortened if displacement exists at the fracture site. Neurovascular integrity should be checked distally to the fracture, although damage of this type is extremely uncommon. The patient's haemodynamic status should be regularly observed, particularly with intertrochanteric fractures where blood loss from surrounding tissues is higher than NOF fractures. The patient's general health should be discussed and pre-existing medical conditions and medication established. It is also necessary to establish the cause of the fall to rule out medical reasons. The patient's hydration and nutritional status should be assessed, as should skin integrity and risk level for pressure sores (Wickham 1997a).

Initial management

In most instances, these fractures can be broadly diagnosed clinically. X-rays provide supplementary information which is necessary for ongoing management. As a result, patients with clinically diagnosed fractures should receive appropriate analgesia, such as morphine sulphate, prior to X-ray. Hydration at an early stage reduces mortality, and therefore i.v. fluids should be commenced, particularly for patients with intertrochanteric fractures where blood loss is greater. Regular observations should be undertaken to ensure haemodynamic stability is maintained, and the patient is neither dehydrated nor becomes overloaded by fluid replacements. Many hospitals have fast-track policies to get patients into a ward bed and off hard A&E trolleys (Audit Commission 1996). If tissue viability is to be maintained, this together with regular pressure area care is vital (Wickham 1997b). If the patient's general condition prohibits internal repair of the fracture, skin traction should be applied at the earliest opportunity.

Hip dislocation

The majority of hip dislocations occur in people with total hip replacements or femoral head replacements. Hip dislocations in patients who have not had previous hip surgery are uncommon and demand a great deal of force. Posterior dislocation is commonly caused by high-impact RTAs where the patient's knee hits the dashboard. Posterior dislocation accounts for about 90% of non-prosthetic dislocations. The patient will present in severe pain, with an internally rotated, flexed leg. Anterior dislocation is much less frequent and results from a fall from a height where the patient lands on an extended leg. This type of injury can be confused with a fractured NOF in elderly patients, and therefore careful history-taking and limb assessment are vital.

In both anterior and posterior dislocations, early limb relocation is essential. Closed reduction should be performed, provided associated fractures of the femoral head have been excluded. Therefore, management priorities in A&E involve pain relief, X-ray and relocation of the hip joint under sedation. Once the hip is relocated, the patient should be admitted for traction. If relocation attempts are unsuccessful with sedation in A&E, then urgent transfer to theatre for closed or open reduction under general anaesthetic is appropriate.

Limb injury

Anatomy and physiology

Limbs form part of the appendicular skeleton and are vital for movement. Both arms and legs comprise long bones, with complex joints and bone systems in the hands and feet. Limb injuries treated in A&E fall into two categories: fractures and soft tissue injury.

Classification of fractures

A break or fracture of the bone occurs when it is no longer able to absorb the mechanical energy placed on it. This usually results from trauma (Hinchliff et al. 1996). Fractures are classified into the following groups (see Fig. 5.9):

- *Simple* – this is a closed fracture; therefore the skin is intact and the fracture is undisplaced. These can be further categorised by the direction in which the fracture travels:
  — transverse: across the bone
  — oblique: at an angle to the length of the bone
  — spiral: encircle the bone in a spiral around its diameter
  — linear: runs parallel to the axis of the bone.

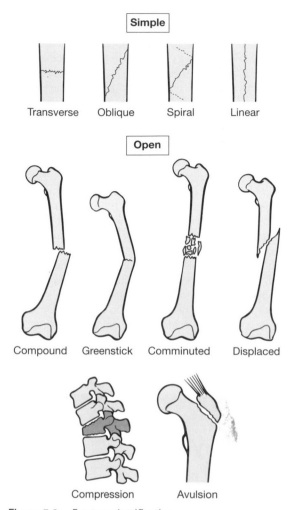

Figure 5.9 – *Fracture classification.*

- *Compound* – an open fracture where bone has punctured skin. These can exist with any of the above types of fracture. It is also possible for fracture fragments to puncture blood vessels, nerves and organs.
- *Greenstick* – these occur in children and are incomplete fractures, like a bend which disrupts the bone cortex but does not pass right through
- *Comminuted* – fragmented fracture with two or more pieces.
- *Displaced* – bone ends are completely separated at the fracture site.
- *Compression* – adjacent bones are compacted.
- *Avulsion* – bone ends or condyles pulled off when the ligaments remain intact under extreme force.

Fracture healing follows a specific pattern. It has three main phases: inflammatory, reparative and remodelling. The inflammatory phase lasts approxi-

mately 72 hours. Initially a homeostatic response to the physiological damage to bone, tissue and blood vessels occurs. Basically, a dot is formed in which the fibrin networks collect debris, blood and marrow cells. Capillary network increases over 24 hours and neutrophils invade the area. In the following 48 hours, phagocytosis takes place. In the reparative stage, chondroblasts and osteoblasts proliferate. The chondroblasts unite fracture ends in a fibrous tissue called callus which begins to calcify after 14 days. Osteoblasts create the trabeculae of cancellous bone and osteoclasts destroy dead bone. Remodelling takes several months; osteoblasts and osteoclasts restore bone shape, replacing cancellous with compact bone (see Fig. 5.10).

Assessment of limb injury

Following ATLS principles, assessment of extremity injury should take place after only the primary survey is completed and more serious injuries are dealt with. The assessment has three stages

- identification and intervention in life-threatening haemorrhage (primary survey)
- identification and intervention in limb-threatening haemorrhage (secondary survey)
- identification and management of other limb injuries.

Assessment should follow a set pattern regardless of how severe or trivial an injury may appear. The assessing nurse should establish the history, perform an examination and, if appropriate, refer the patient for X-ray. When assessing the history, the nurse should establish a number of factors (see Box 5.1). Mechanism of injury should include what happened, the direction and magnitude of force, and how long the patient was exposed to the force. When determining symptoms, the nurse should establish pain, loss of function and perceived swelling. The nurse should also enquire about the duration of symptoms and whether they are worsening or improving. Past

Box 5.1 – *Establishing history of musculoskeletal injury*

- Mechanism of injury
- Symptoms
- Duration
- Pain
- Previous relevant injury, illness, medication

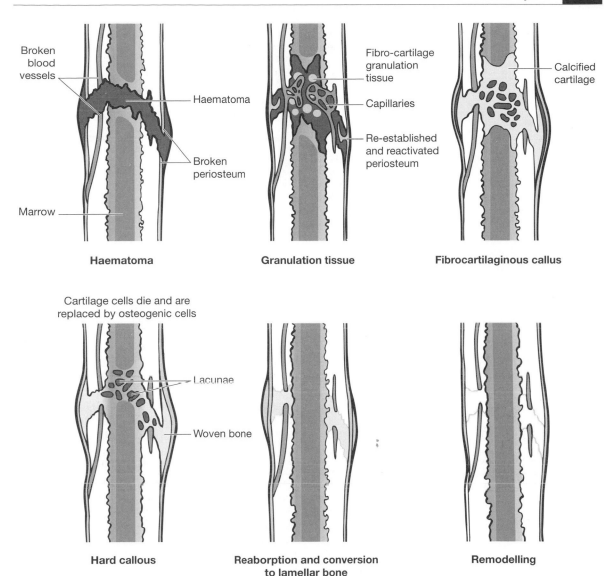

Figure 5.10 – *Bone healing process.*

history should include pre-existing injuries to that limb, medical conditions which affect the musculo-skeletal system or bone density and factors which would influence recovery.

Examination

Examination should follow a specific pattern, starting from the joint above, moving through the site of the injury, and finally checking neurovascular function distal to the injury. Principles of examination are shown in Box 5.2. Examination starts from the joint above the injury site both to assess function and limits

of injury and to gain the patient's cooperation and confidence. The examination should also include assessment of pain, and factors influencing it, such as movement, pressure and guarding (Mooney 1991).

If a patient presents with a mechanism of injury or the clinical examination is suggestive of a fracture then X-ray should be requested. X-rays should not, however, be performed for purely medicolegal reasons (Ward 1999).

Femoral Fractures

The femur is the longest, strongest human bone. It is

Box 5.2 – *Principles of examination*

Look
- Colour
- Perfusion
- Deformity
- Swelling
- Wounds
- Bruising
- Compare with opposite limb

Feel
- Palpate from joint above injury
- Identify tender spots
- Note areas of reduced sensation
- Note obvious crepitus – *never* test for crepitus because of the pain it causes
- Assess distal pulses and capillary refill
- Test temperature of the limb
- Test sensation distal to wound

Move
- Assess active movement
- Assess passive movement
- Test resistance to establish muscle injury

Function
- Observe how patient uses limb
- Observe walking/weight-bearing for lower limbs

Box 5.3 – *Assessment of femoral fracture*

- Severe pain in thigh
- Reduced leg movement – unable to weight-bear
- Deformity – shortening because of muscle spasm and external rotation in proximal fractures
- Swelling in surrounding tissue due to soft tissue damage and bleeding
- Crepitus – possibility of damage to popliteal nerves and blood vessels. Check distal circulation and sensation

surrounded by muscles and is fed by the profunda femoris artery. The shaft of femur also has a good collateral blood supply in the periosteum. Most of the bleeding associated with femoral fracture is due to rupture of small branches of the profunda femoris artery. The femur only fractures under great force and the most common cause of injury is RTA, particularly motorcycle accidents (Crimmins & Ruiz 1995).

Assessment

Fractures of the femur fall into three anatomical categories: proximal, midshaft and distal. Examination findings are shown in Box 5.3. The patient should be carefully assessed for signs of hypovolaemia as blood loss from a shaft of femur fracture can be 2–3 units. Although isolated femoral fractures rarely cause significant shock, fractures occurring with other traumatic injury do contribute to significant hypovolaemia. Observation should therefore be vigilant and X-ray will confirm diagnosis.

Management priorities

Two main management priorities exist in A&E: preventing secondary damage and pain control. Preventing secondary damage includes managing blood loss by initiating i.v. fluid replacement. Reduction in blood loss and significant pain reduction can be achieved by correct application of an appropriate traction splint, such as a Haire splint or a Thomas splint. These stabilise the fracture until definitive repair can take place. In doing this, the extent of the trauma to surrounding soft tissue is minimised. Pain is reduced because bone ends are immobilised. Distal and proximal pulses, capillary refill and sensation should be rechecked after splint application. If the fracture is open, broad-spectrum antibiotics should be given and the patient's tetanus status checked. The wound should be covered with a wet dressing. Povidone-iodine soaks are commonly used because of the devastating effects of infection (see also Ch. 23). Intravenous analgesia should also be given. Fractured femurs take about 8–16 weeks to heal in an adult and 6–12 weeks in a child. Definitive treatment is usually internal fixation for an adult which means they can usually be walking within 2 weeks post-surgery. Surgery is not recommended for children because of growth and speed of repair; therefore traction is recommended for older children, and plastering with hip spica for toddlers and small children.

Supracondylar fractures of the femur are assessed in the same way as shaft fractures. The mechanisms of injury are similar, with pain usually localised to the knee. These fractures do not cause the same extent of blood loss as shaft fractures and are repaired by either long leg casting or surgery.

Lower leg injury

The principles of assessment are common to all limb

injuries and have been highlighted earlier in the chapter. This section describes specific advice, identifying common mechanisms of injury, assessment findings and initial management.

Fractures and dislocations

Patellar fractures occur following a direct blow or fall onto the knee. Indirect twisting injury can also result in a fracture as the patella is ripped apart by the quadriceps muscles. The patient presents with pain, swelling and a knee effusion. As a result, range of movement is restricted, particularly full extension. Usually, patellar fractures can be repaired by long leg cylindrical casting for 4–6 weeks. Surgical intervention is necessary for open fractures; those fractures where fragmentation of the patella leaves gaps greater than 4 mm; and longitudinal fractures.

Patellar dislocation results from a direct blow to the medial aspect of the knee, common in football or similar contact sports. The knee locks and remains in a flexed position. On examination, obvious lateral deformity is present with medial tenderness and pain on attempted movement. Haemarthrosis rapidly occurs, causing generalised swelling of the knee. Treatment seeks to relocate the patella. This is usually straightforward and achieved by extension of the knee. It is painful because of muscle spasm and therefore analgesia and muscle relaxants should be used. A supportive long leg bandage should then be applied, or a long leg cast

Tibial plateau fractures

Tibial plateau injury commonly occurs from pedestrian/car accidents, usually at lower speeds where the car bumper hits the standing pedestrian. Fractures also occur as a result of a fall from a height, causing compression of the plateau. Patients usually present with pain over the fracture site and inability to weight-bear. Swelling varies considerably, with haemathrosis sometimes present. Conservative treatment with long leg casting is less common than internal fixation because of the morbidity risk of long immobilisation, particularly in older patients (Harris & Haller 1995).

Tibial shaft fractures

Mechanisms of injury are varied. The tibia has little muscular protection, so fractures from direct blows are common. Torsional or indirect forces are also common causes of fracture, particularly in children. Similar mechanisms cause tibial and fibular fracture, although much more force is needed to break both bones. Direct trauma tends to cause transverse or comminuted fractures, and indirect trauma causes oblique and spiral fractures. The patient presents with localised pain and is usually unable to weight-bear. Surrounding soft tissue damage varies from a haematoma, causing swelling, to an open wound caused by fracture ends. Treatment for tibial fractures varies: children with greenstick fractures need casting for 6 weeks; in adults, displaced fractures may need internal fixation. Open fractures warrant prophylactic antibiotics and tetanus prophylaxis if not covered (Beales 1997). The risk of compartment syndrome is high, and therefore admission for 24 hours' observation and limb elevation should be considered in very swollen proximal tibial fractures.

Fibular fractures

Isolated fibular fractures are not common and usually occur in conjunction with tibial fractures. Isolated fibular fractures usually occur as a result of direct trauma to the lateral aspect of the calf. Distal fibular/malleolar fractures occur with excessive rotational forces. They are discussed in more detail under ankle injury below. Stress fractures of the fibula are relatively common in runners (Adams 1989). The patient will complain of pain over the fracture site, with radiation along the length of the fibula on palpation. Because the fibula is not a weight-bearing bone, the patient may be walking with discomfort. Swelling is usually minimal. Depending on the degree of pain, isolated fractures are treated by either plaster cast or compression bandage.

Tibial and fibular fractures

Combined tibial and fibular fractures are fairly common in contact sports, such as football. In injuries where indirect force causes the fracture, the tibia and fibula may be fractured in different places. Commonly, the tibial shaft fractures at the distal third, and because of a twisting mechanism the fibula fractures at the proximal end. This reinforces the need to assess from the joint above to the joint below the injury. If injury is caused by direct force and both bones are fractured at the same level, the leg will appear unstable and flexible at the fracture site. It is important that temporary immobilisation occurs as soon as possible, both to reduce pain and to prevent further soft tissue damage. These fractures will need surgical fixation.

Ankle Fractures

Most ankle injuries seen in A&E are soft tissue

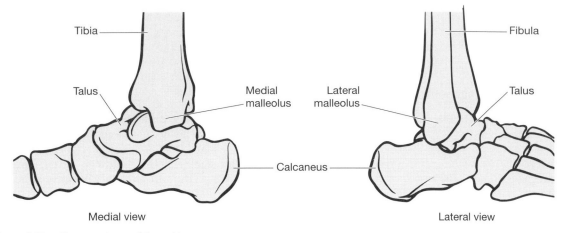

Medial view   Lateral view

Figure 5.11 – *Bone anatomy of the ankle.*

injuries (Wilkerson 1992). Patients with fractures risk significant morbidity if these are not identified and treated early. The ankle joint is made up of three bones – the tibia, fibula and talus – and three collateral ligaments – the lateral, medial and interosseous. These ligaments stabilise the ankle joint; the lateral ligament allows for some inversion of the joint, whereas the medial and interosseous have less stretch (see Fig. 5.11 and Box 5.4).

Isolated lateral malleolus fractures can occur following inversion injury. Patients present with swelling and bony tenderness on the lateral aspect of the ankle and are usually unable to weight-bear (Whelan 1997). Most isolated fractures are either a chip or avulsion fracture with ligament injury. These can be treated by a below-knee weight-bearing cast. Some fractures above the joint line or comminuted fractures may warrant surgical intervention. Isolated medial malleolar fractures are less common and usually result from a direct blow or eversion and, occasionally, inversion injury. The patient presents with pain over the medial aspect, swelling and limited range of movement. Usually, the patient will be non-weight-bearing (Wyatt *et al.* 1999). Simple avulsion fractures can be managed by below-knee casting. Fractures into the joint space should be referred for specialist opinion as internal fixation may be necessary (see Fig. 5.12).

Bimalleolar fractures involve two of the lateral, medial and posterior malleoli, usually the lateral and medial. The patient presents with a history of inversion or eversion injury and will have bilateral bony tenderness and swelling, with or without deformity, and will be non-weight-bearing. These are unstable fractures with a significant risk of ankle dislocation.

Box 5.4 – *Lange–Hansen classification of ankle injury (After Mayeda 1992.)*

Supination – adduction (inversion injury)
Stage I   Fracture of lateral malleolus at joint level or below, or tear of lateral collateral ligament
Stage II   As above with fracture of medial malleolus

Supination – lateral rotation
Stage I   Rupture of anterior tibiofibular ligament
Stage II   As above with spiral fracture of distal fibula
Stage III As above with posterior tibiofibular ligament disruption with/without avulsion fracture of posterior malleolus
Stage IV   As above with medial malleolar fracture

Pronation – abduction
Stage I   Transverse fracture of medial malleolus or deltoid ligament tear
Stage II   As above with posterior and anterior tibiofibular ligament disruption with/without avulsion fracture of posterior malleolus
Stage III As above with fracture of distal fibula at ankle joint level

Pronation – lateral rotation
Stage I   Transverse fracture of medial malleolus or tear or deltoid ligament
Stage II   As above with disruption of anterior tibiofibular ligament and interosseous membrane
Stage III As above with fracture of distal bone 6 cm or greater above joint
Stage IV   As above with posterior tibiofibular ligament disruption with/without avulsion fracture of posterior malleolus

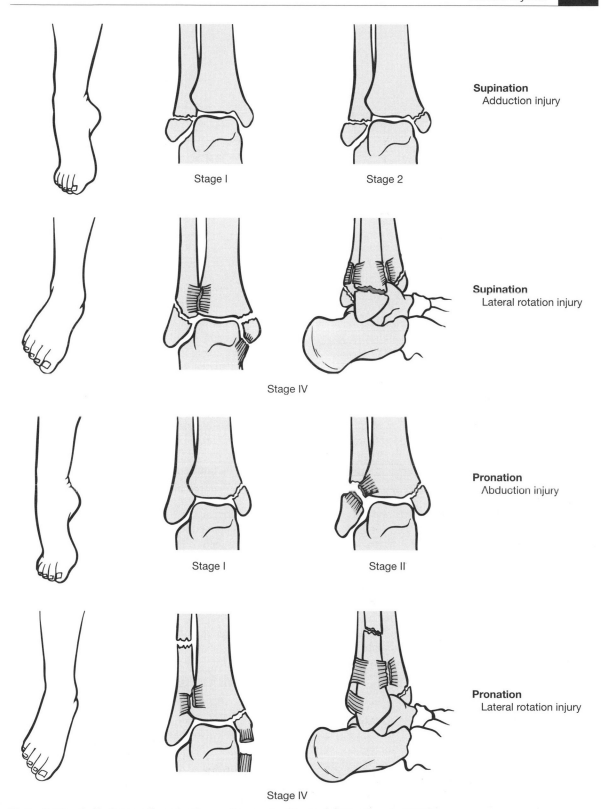

Stage I

Stage 2

Supination
Adduction injury

Stage IV

Supination
Lateral rotation injury

Stage I

Stage II

Pronation
Abduction injury

Stage IV

Pronation
Lateral rotation injury

Figure 5.12 – *Ankle fracture (based on Lange-Hansen classification). (After Mayeda 1992.)*

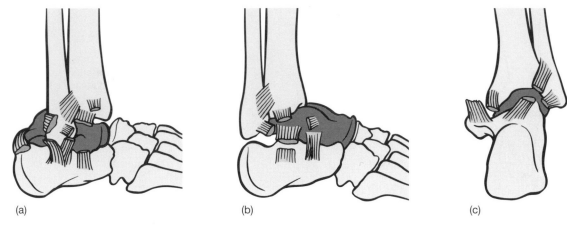

Figure 5.13 – *Ankle dislocations. (a): Posterior. (b): Anterior. (c): Lateral.*

The ankle should be temporarily immobilised, adequate pain relief should be given and hospital admission facilitated. Restoration of function requires accurate medial malleolus reduction and joint space alignment (Mayeda 1992). Lateral malleolar reduction is desirable but less crucial. This is usually achieved by open reduction and fixation in theatre, but can be achieved by closed methods if surgery is contraindicated.

Trimalleolar fractures involve the posterior malleolus as well and are usually combined with ankle dislocation. They are caused by falls or, most commonly, tripping, e.g. off a kerb. Management priorities are limb realignment (see discussion of dislocations below) and subsequent internal fixation, using the same principles as for bimalleolar fractures.

Ankle dislocation

Ankle dislocation occurs in one of three directions: posterior, anterior and lateral (see Fig. 5.13). Stability of the ankle is normally maintained by tight articulation of the talus with the tibia and fibula. Because of the amount of force needed, isolated ankle dislocation is extremely rare (Greenbaum & Papp 1992). It is usually associated with malleolar fractures and ligament rupture. Common causes of dislocation are sports injuries, direct force or RTA (Harris 1995). Complicated dislocations associated with multiple ankle fractures are most common in osteoporotic women (Purvis 1982).

The ankle will be oedematous, the joint locked, with the distal tibia prominent under stretched skin. Management priorities in A&E are to preserve neurovascular integrity. If there appears to be neurovascular compromise, the ankle dislocation should be reduced urgently, without waiting for X-rays. If neurovascular integrity appears intact, X-rays can be obtained, but the foot should remain supported to prevent further injury. Reduction should be carried out swiftly after X-ray. Nitrous oxide is a useful initial pain relief, for its therapeutic effects of analgesia, increasing oxygen intake and for its distraction potential, i.e. by getting the patient to concentrate on breathing. While dislocation is being reduced, the patient should have adequate intravenous analgesia and muscle relaxant. The patient's cardiac and respiratory function should be monitored during this procedure.

Ankle reduction is a two person job. It is achieved by flexing the patient's knee to reduce tension on the Achilles tendon. One carer supports the lower leg while the other applies downward traction to the foot and force is applied in the opposite direction to that of the original injury. When reduction is completed, neurovascular integrity should be rechecked, by checking for pedal pulse, capillary refill and sensation. The ankle should then be immobilised in an above-knee plaster case which is either bivalved or guttered, because of the degree of swelling associated with fracture manipulation. Most patients need internal fixation of associated fractures.

Foot Fractures

The foot is divided into three anatomical areas (see Fig. 5.14). It is considered vital for balance, movement and as a shock absorber for movement.

The hindfoot

The talus supports the body weight and forces above by allowing movement at the ankle joint and between

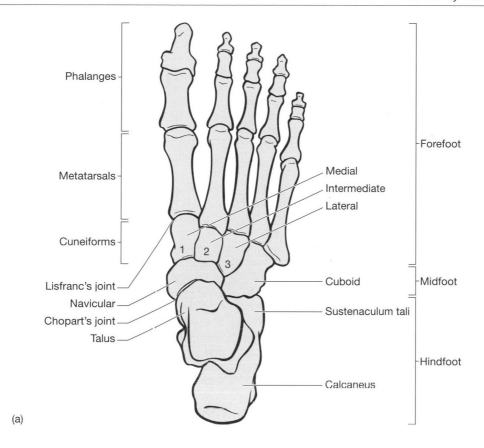

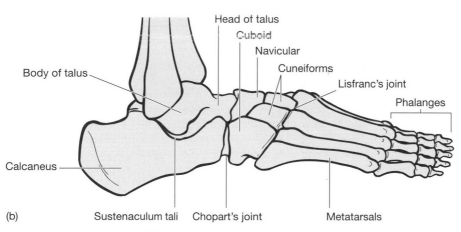

Figure 5.14 – *The right foot. (a): Dorsal view. (b): Lateral view.*

the calcaneus and midfoot. It is well secured by ligaments surrounding the ankle joint and therefore fracture is uncommon (Harris 1995). This risk of fracture complication is high because 60% of the surface is covered by articular cartilage and vascular supply is low, creating a significant threat of avascular necrosis. It is usually injured as a result of falls,

landing on the heel or forefoot, causing fractures through the body or neck of the talus. Fractures to the neck of the talus also result from head-on RTAs where the driver's foot is pressed against compressed floors or pedals, causing extreme dorsiflexion.

The patient will present with ankle pain, there may be visible disruption to normal ankle anatomy and swelling is common. Fractures to the talar neck are usually treated by below-knee casting, but if any displacement cannot be reduced, open reduction is necessary. Fractures to the talar body frequently require internal fixation. Fractures of the talar head are extremely uncommon and management varies with the extent of the injury and associated injuries. Specialist orthopaedic advice should be sought for specific management.

The calcaneus

This is the largest bone of the foot and it absorbs the body's weight when standing or moving. The calcaneus is a relatively hollow bone consisting of an outer thin cortical shell filled with cancellous bone. As a result, it fractures when subjected to vertical forces such as falling from a height. There is an associated crush fracture of the lumbar spine in about 10% of cases resulting from a fall. The Achilles tendon attaches to the tuberosity and can cause an avulsion fracture when damaged. Fractures resulting from a fall are most common in men between 30 and 50 years old (Clisham & Berlin 1981), whereas avulsion fractures are more common in women showing signs of osteoporosis.

The patient presents with pain over the rear of the foot and both sides of the heel. Swelling is usually present and patients are usually unable to weight-bear on their heel. Calcaneal fractures are categorised into two groups: those involving the subtalar joint and those which do not, i.e. extra-articular fractures. The outcome for patients with extra-articular fractures is considerably better than those involving the subtalar joint. Extra-articular fractures are managed conservatively with compression and elevation in the first instance. After swelling has subsided, the injury is immobilised in a cast. The majority of fractures do involve the subtalar joint and the prognosis for these patients is poor. About 50% have some long-term problems from the injury (Mayeda 1992), including restricted movement, pain and subtalar arthritis. Most are treated with internal fixation.

The midfoot

This region includes the navicular, cuboid, cuneiform and metatarsal bones. The midfoot provides foot flexibility. Fractures to this area are uncommon and result from direct force, such as crush injuries. Transverse dislocation of the forefoot result from direct force. Patients present with localised tenderness and swelling. These injuries heal well and can usually be treated with below-knee non-weight-bearing casts.

There are two exceptions to this: the first relates to avulsion fractures of the navicular, which occur as a result of eversion injury. If 20% or more of the articular surface is avulsed, the fracture should be internally fixed. If less than 20% is avulsed, a below-knee cast should be adequate. The second exception is the Lisfranc dislocation, which occurs when the forefoot is dislocated across the metatarsal joints. This is an extremely rare condition, occurring in one in 55 000 cases (Mayeda 1992). Neurovascular compromise is common, partly because the force necessary to cause dislocation also causes extensive soft tissue damage, resulting in oedema and vascular compromise. The patient presents with moderate to severe midfoot pain and large amounts of swelling which can hinder diagnosis. There is usually a shortening of the foot length, compared with the uninjured foot, and the injured foot will have transverse broadening.

Patients with Lisfranc dislocation will not be able to stand on their toes. Treatment of this injury revolves around rapid reduction of the dislocation and cast immobilisation, because the risk of circulation compromise and subsequent necrosis is so high. If a base of second metatarsal fracture coexists, an accurate reduction may not be possible, or will prove unstable. In such cases, internal fixation should be considered. Hospital admission is usually necessary during the initial days post-injury, whatever the method of reduction.

The forefoot

The forefoot consists of the five metatarsal bones and the phalanges.

Metatarsal fractures

The metatarsals are susceptible to fractures because of their length. The mechanisms of fracture varies; the second and third metatarsals are relatively fixed and therefore susceptible to stress fractures. The first, fourth and fifth metatarsals are more mobile. Fractures are caused by direct blows to the foot, e.g. a heavy object falling across the foot.

Twisting injury can also result in fractures, particularly of the second to fourth metatarsals. The patient presents with swelling over the foot, localised pain and inability to weight-bear. Reduction of swelling is imperative as skin necrosis and neurovascular compromise can occur. Elevation of the foot is essential. Most fractures can be managed by immobilisation in a short leg cast.

Fifth metatarsal fracture is one of the most common foot injuries (Rockwood & Green 1975). It usually results from an inversion injury causing sudden

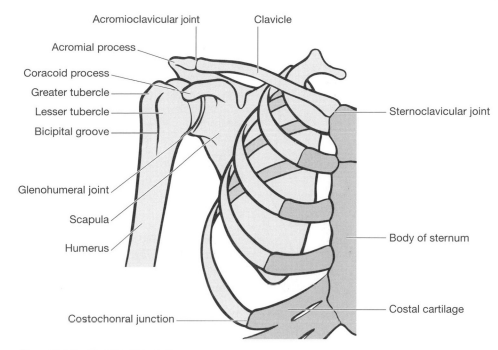

Acromioclavicular joint

Acromial process

Coracoid process

Greater tubercle

Lesser tubercle

Bicipital groove

Glenohumeral joint

Scapula

Humerus

Costochonral junction

Clavicle

Sternoclavicular joint

Body of sternum

Costal cartilage

Figure 5.15 – *The shoulder girdle.*

contraction of the peroneus brevis muscle. The tendons joining this muscle with the base of the fifth metatarsal can cause an avulsion fracture. The management of fifth metatarsal fractures is either neighbour (or buddy) strapping and crutches or a below-knee cast, depending on the patient's pain. Occasionally, displaced fractures require internal fixation.

First metatarsal fractures warrant special consideration because of the weight-bearing capacity of the first metatarsal and its contribution to balance and stability. If the metatarsal head has been displaced in plantar rotation, the patient will have trouble with weight-bearing and with the 'push-off' mechanism in walking. Many of these fractures can be reduced in A&E with adequate analgesia, and then immobilised in a cast. If reduction cannot be achieved in this manner, internal fixation should be considered.

Phalangeal fractures

These result from stubbing injury or from dropping heavy objects on toes. The patient presents with pain, swelling and often bruising or a subungal haematoma. The clinical symptoms can make fracture diagnosis difficult and often X-rays do not offer much assistance (Mayeda 1992). If angulation or deformity of the toe exists, then X-rays are more helpful. Most fractures can be managed by neighbour strapping and elevation. Obviously angulated fractures should be reduced

using a digital block, then the toe neighbour strapped. Big toe fractures needing reduction may warrant immobilisation in a cast with toe support.

Injury to the Shoulder

The shoulder girdle consists of three bones: the scapula, the clavicle and the humerus (see Fig. 5.15). The shoulder attaches the arms to the axial skeleton.

Scapular fractures

The scapula is situated above and lateral to the posterior thorax. It is well protected from injury by thick muscle and extreme force is necessary to fracture it. Injury commonly results from high-speed RTAs, crush injury or falls. Occasionally, a scapular fracture occurs as a result of electric shock, when both scapulae are fractured (Dumas & Walker 1992). Fractured scapulae most frequently occur in young men (McGuinness & Denton 1989) because of the force needed to cause fractures and associated injuries such as pneumothorax, chest wall injury or related shoulder girdle injuries.

Anatomically, scapular fractures fall into three categories (Fig. 5.16):

■ *type I fractures* involve the body and spine of the scapula

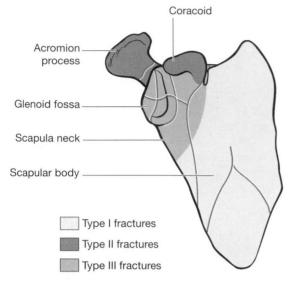

Type I fractures
Type II fractures
Type III fractures

Figure 5.16 – *Classification of scapular fractures.*

Table 5.2 – *Classification of clavicular fractures*

Type	Mechanism of injury	Frequency (% of all clavicular fractures)
Proximal third	Direct blow to anterior chest	5%
Mid-third	Indirect force to lateral aspect of shoulder	80%
Distal third	Direct blow to top of shoulder	15%

- *type II fractures* involve the acromion or coracoid process
- *type III fractures* involve the scapular neck and glenoid fossa.

Type I fractures to the scapula are difficult to palpate because of thick muscle and pain. An adducted shoulder and the mechanism of injury should suggest possible fracture, which can be confirmed on X-ray (Knapton 1999). Treatment is usually conservative and involves pain relief and simple immobilisation using a broad arm sling bandage on the injured side. Controversy exists over the benefits versus risks of plating scapular body fractures. It has been suggested that fractures in young patients where extensive displacement exists are best treated by plating (Nordqvist & Petersson 1992). In contrast, a high complication rate has been identified following surgical management of fractures (Schmidt *et al.* 1992).

Type II acromion and coracoid process fractures occur from direct trauma and are similar in that patients have pain over the site of injury and adduction of the shoulder. They differ in that acromion fractures cause pain on elbow flexing, while in coracoid fractures the patient actively flexes the elbow as a form of pain relief. Both types are usually managed conservatively unless concurrent shoulder girdle injury exists, such as dislocation or clavicular fracture. Type III fractures of the neck or glenoid fossa result from lateral to medial rotation of the humeral head. The patient presents with pain around the humeral head and shoulder adduction, and is usually supporting an injured arm. Treatment involves immobilisation of the arm on the injured side, however difficulty in regaining full range of movement following this injury is high.

Clavicular fractures

The clavicle provides anterior support for the shoulder. It is a slightly S-shaped bone which articulates laterally with the acromion process and medially with the sternum. The clavicle gives definition to body shape as well as providing protection for the subclavian neurovascular bundle. Calvicular fractures most commonly occur from direct contact or, less often, due to a fall onto an outstretched hand. In children it is the most commonly fractured bone (Newman 1988). Clavicular fractures are divided into three groups: proximal third fracture, mid-clavicular fracture and distal fractures (see Table 5.2).

Common presenting symptoms include pain over the fracture site, crepitus and sometimes a palpable deformity. The patient is usually supporting the arm of the injured side. In midclavicular fractures, deformity is common. The patient presents with a downward shoulder stump, sometimes rotated inward and forward. This is because of gravitational forces and the pectoralis major. The proximal fragment is displaced upward. Because of the location of the neurovascular bundles and the great blood vessels, a careful assessment of neurovascular function of the arm on the injured side must be carried out. Management of clavicular fracture is usually conservative. Immobilisation with a simple sling is as effective as other less comfortable methods and is therefore the treatment of choice. Displaced fractures of the distal third usually require surgical repair because of the risk of nonunion (Rockward & Green 1975). Complications frequently include malunion, regardless of the support mechanism used; however, evidence suggests that this malunion is of little functional or cosmetic consequence (Newman 1988).

Shoulder dislocation

The glenohumeral joint is the most commonly dislocated major joint, accounting for 50% of A&E attendances with dislocation (Simon *et al.* 1987). The wide range of movement carried out at the shoulder, and its lack of bony stability, predisposes the joint to dislocation. Two main patient groups can be identified: men between the ages of 20 and 30, and women over 60 (Kroner *at al.* 1989). Glenohumeral joint dislocation can be categorised into four groups: anterior (>90% of dislocations), posterior (<5%), inferior (<1%) and superior (<1%).

Anterior dislocation

Anterior dislocations occur following a fall onto an outstretched hand where the arm is extended and externally rotated. They can also be caused by direct trauma to the posteriolateral aspect of the shoulder.

The patient presents in extreme pain, usually holding the injured arm in abduction and external rotation (Genge Jagmin 1995). On examination, the shoulder will be obviously deformed when compared with the uninjured side. It will have a square appearance and the acromial process will be prominent (see Fig. 5.17). Assessment should include a detailed examination of neurovascular function (Box 5.5).

Before shoulder dislocation is treated, humeral fracture should be excluded on X-ray. Fractures of the humeral head or neck prohibit early reduction of dislocation in A&E and orthopaedic opinion should always be sought. If no fracture exists, reduction of shoulder dislocation should be carried out as soon as

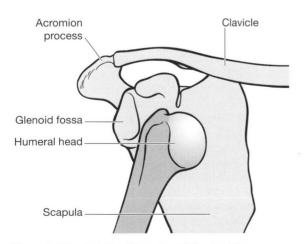

Figure 5.17 – *Anterior dislocation of the shoulder.*

Acromion process

Clavicle

Glenoid fossa

Humeral head

Scapula

> **Box 5.5** – *Assessment of neurovascular function following shoulder injury*
>
> Posterior cord of brachial plexus – test for wrist extension
>
> Axillary nerve damage – test for sensation over lateral aspect of upper arm
>
> Axillary artery damage – test for brachial pulse

possible. Prompt reduction is always necessary as the procedure becomes more difficult as time passes and the dislocation may prove irreducible (Mills *et al.* 1995), partly because muscle spasm increases with the length of time the joint is dislocated. Early relocation is also vital in maintaining the integrity of the humeral head. Because the scapular neck is harder than the humeral head, a compression fracture occurs, causing long-term deformity to the humeral head. (Hill–Sachs deformity), which leads to recurrent dislocation. This is thought to occur in between 11 and 50% of patients with anterior dislocation (Tullos *et al.* 1984).

Four types of anterior dislocation exist, classified by the exact position of the humeral head. Management is broadly the same. Successful reduction of shoulder dislocation depends on overcoming muscle spasm. This is achieved by intravenous administration of muscle relaxant, such as midazolam, together with appropriate analgesia, usually opiates. The mechanics of shoulder reduction are achieved by traction or leverage, or a combination of both.

Traction methods include lying the patient on her front with the injured arm over the side of the trolley and hanging a 5–7 kg weight, depending on the patient's muscularity, on the affected arm. Over 20–30 minutes this reduces muscle spasm by gently elongating muscles, pulling the humeral head off the scapular and allowing the rotator cuff muscles to relocate it in the glenoid fossa. This method is thought to be less painful than some more aggressive relocations and the risk of complication is low (Quaday 1995). The most commonly used and safest method of reduction is a two-person traction/counter-traction approach. One person applies longitudinal traction to the injured arm, reducing muscle spasm, while the other person applies counter-traction by wrapping a sheet around the patient's chest and under the axilla of the injured side and then pulling towards the patient's ear on the unaffected side. This helps to disengage the humeral head from the scapula. The arm should then be adducted and immobilised.

Traditional traction/counter-traction methods of putting a foot in the patient's armpit and then pulling on the arm is not recommended because of its high association with neurovascular injury and lower success rate than other methods (Quaday 1995). Leverage techniques involve some traction to lift the humeral head off the scapula, but then lever it back into place. These methods are fast, but increase the risk of injury to the glenoid rim or humeral shaft. The external rotation method of reduction is the least traumatic. It works by slowly adducting the injured arm and then flexing the elbow to 90°. The elbow is then held in place while the forearm is externally rotated by its own weight and gravity, not by force. This allows the smallest profile of the humeral head to be relocated into the glenoid fossa. The traditional method of leverage is Kocher's technique. This involves a three-step external/internal rotation manoeuvre which is both painful for the patient and dangerous because of the high risk of vascular tearing, rotator cuff injury and humeral fracture (Riebel & McCabe 1991). If reduction cannot be achieved, orthopaedic referral should be made for manipulation under general anaesthetic.

Whatever method of reduction is used, it is important that neurovascular integrity is rechecked, and an X-ray taken to check position. The affected arm should be immobilised to prevent redislocation. The arm should be adducted and internally rotated. To prevent shoulder stiffness, the patient should be advised to extend the elbow and rotate the arm to a neutral position several times a day. In older patients, the risk of joint stiffness is greater, and therefore it is usual to remobilise the arm sooner than in younger people. Patients over 40 should not be immobilised for longer than 3 weeks. The redislocation is higher in younger people, and therefore those patients under 40 years of age are immobilised for up to 6 weeks.

Posterior dislocation

The anatomy of the shoulder girdle makes posterior dislocation difficult because the glenoid fossa is positioned posteriorly to the humeral head. The angle of the scapula helps to buttress this structure. When dislocation occurs, the humeral head sits behind the glenoid and usually below the acromion (see Fig. 5.18).

Posterior dislocation is caused by a fall onto an outstretched hand where the arm is flexed and internally rotated. Posterior dislocation also occurs following significant electric shock, epileptic seizures and, occasionally, from direct force to the anterior aspect of the shoulder. The patient will have severe pain and will present holding the arm in internal rotation, supported in a sling type position. There is usually a loss of definition of the anterior shoulder and

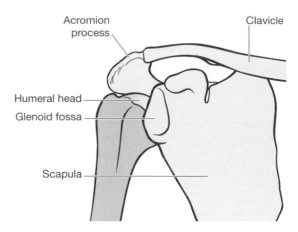

Figure 5.18 – *Posterior dislocation of the shoulder.*

a prominent acromial and coracoid process, with the humeral head sometimes palpable posteriorly. The patient is unable to lift the arm above 90° and cannot externally rotate.

Diagnosis should be made from the mechanism of injury and patient presentation as anteroposterior X-rays are inconclusive and up to 50% of posterior dislocations are missed initially (Quadray 1995). Lateral and axillary X-ray views will confirm diagnosis. Neurovascular injury is less common with posterior dislocation because the major structures lie anterior to the joint and are thus protected. Although closed reduction with muscle relaxant and analgesia may be attempted, orthopaedic consultation should determine this.

Because of the strong anterior muscle mass, reduction in A&E is usually only recommended for elderly or frail patients and reduction under general anaesthetic is generally required. If attempts at reduction are made in A&E, the process involves slow in-line traction, while maintaining internal rotation, with gentle pressure on the humeral head to lift it off the glenoid. If reduction is attempted, neurovascular integrity should be checked afterwards and X-rays performed. The affected arm should be immobilised but not internally rotated. For this reason, shoulder spicas are often used to create slight external rotation (Brown 1992). Immobilisation should not exceed four weeks.

Upper Arm Injury

The humerus is surrounded by strong muscle compartments – anteriorly the biceps and posteriorly the triceps. The neurovascular bundle lies on the medial border of the biceps and contains the brachial artery, the brachial vein and the medial and ulnar nerves. The radial nerve runs posteriorly until it reaches the distal humerus, where it travels laterally until it is anterior to the humerus. The muscle design of the upper arm is appropriate for pulling or hanging activities.

Humeral fractures are common in two main patient groups:

- women aged between 56 and 65 years, usually with osteoporosis – fractures occur as a result of a fall and occasionally direct force; injury is usually to the proximal humerus, neck or shaft.
- young men aged between 16 and 24 years – mechanisms of injury include RTAs (transverse humeral fractures), falls from a significant height (oblique or spiral fractures) and stress fractures from throwing actions.

The patient will present with localised pain, or shoulder pain in fractures of the humeral neck. The upper arm is usually swollen and may have obvious shortening with normal movement at the point of fracture. Very careful neurovascular assessment is necessary, especially with distal third fractures. Circulation should be assessed at the brachial pulse, radial pulse and along the ulnar artery. Capillary refill of the fingertips and hand should also be assessed. Sensory and motor function should be checked in line with radial, ulnar and median nerve activity.

The muscle masses help to splint humeral fractures, and gravity helps with lengthening and aligning the bone. However, this is a very painful option for the patient, and non-union is common. Although exact alignment is not vital because the shoulder's mobility can compensate, four basic steps to fracture management should be followed:

- traction to restore length and align fragment
- any angulation should be reduced
- initial immobilisation for pain control and healing
- encourage mobilisation of shoulder and elbow to prevent loss of function.

A number of immobilisation methods exist. Open reduction with internal fixation is one option, usually performed for open or severely comminuted fractures and in patients with multiple fractures where conservative management would delay overall recovery and mobility. Hanging casts and U-slabs have been used for many years as a method of immobilising the upper arm. As well as being extremely uncomfortable and restrictive for patients, these casts can cause posterior angulation of the fracture (Ciernick *et al.* 1991). Slings are commonly used, but these offer little immobilisation or pain control. The treatment of choice appears to be an interlocking upper arm brace with forearm support. These have 95% excellent functional rotation and 85% minimal shortening of the limb (Zagorski *et al.* 1988).

Elbow Injury

The elbow joint consists of the distal humerus, radius, ulna and olecranon (see Fig. 5.19). The distal humerus forms two columns; the lateral and medial epicondyles

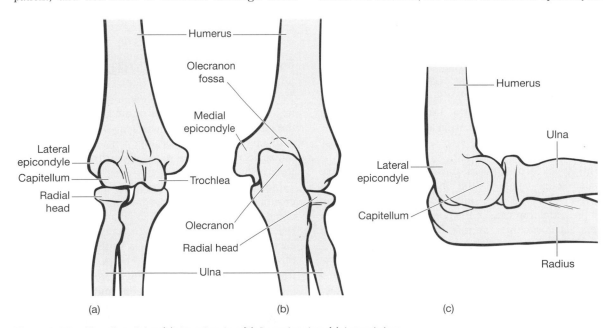

Figure 5.19 – *The elbow joint. (a): Anterior view. (b): Posterior view. (c): Lateral view.*

form the proximal part of these columns and are significant for their muscle attachments facilitating wrist movement. The wrist extensors originate from the lateral epicondyle, and flexors from the medial epicondyle. The trochlea articulates with the olecranon to allow flexion/extension at the elbow, and the capitellum allows pronation and supination of the forearm by articulation with the radial head. The radial nerve travels around the humerus to the anterior of the lateral epicondyle, and supplies the wrist and finger extensors. Because of its proximity to the distal humerus, it is very susceptible to injury. The medial nerve travels anterior to the humerus with the brachial artery. It provides sensation to the thumb and index finger and coarse hand movement, like grip. If damaged above the elbow, the index finger cannot be flexed (Ochsner's test). If damaged in the forearm, the interphalangeal thumb joint cannot be flexed if the base of the thumb is held to immobilise it.

The ulnar nerve crosses behind the medial epicondyle and is therefore susceptible to damage when elbow injury occurs. It supplies the flexor muscles and intrinsic hand nerves. Sensation to the ulnar side of the hand is also provided by the ulnar nerve. The brachial artery travels down the anterior of the humerus and crosses the elbow with the median nerve. This is the major blood supply to the hand and forearm and compromise of this supply following injury can result in Volkmann's ischaemia. This is muscle wasting of the hand and forearm which leads to contracture.

Supracondylar fractures

These are distal humerus fractures, proximal to the epicondyles. They are the most common fracture in children accounting for 60% of childhood fractures (Nicholson & Driscoll 1995). Supracondylar fractures are categorised into two groups depending on mechanism of injury: extension and flexion fractures.

Extension fractures

This type of fracture is caused by a fall onto an outstretched hand with the elbow locked in extension (see Fig. 5.20). This results in posterior displacement of the distal fragment of the humerus, and puts neurovascular structures at risk because of the jagged proximal humerus which becomes anteriorly angulated. This injury is most common in those under 15 years of age, because the tensile strength of the ligaments and joint capsule is greater than bone, and therefore fracture occurs. In adults, the reverse is true and dislocation of the elbow joint is more common (Magnusson 1992).

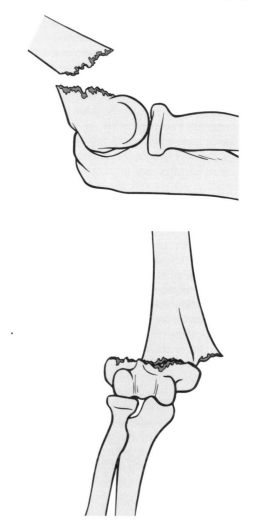

Figure 5.20 – *Supracondylar extension fracture.*

The patient will present holding the arm partially flexed. There is usually severe pain and swelling above the elbow. A thorough assessment should be made of neurovascular and motor function, as injury to the radial nerve occurs in about 8% of patients (Tsai & Ruiz 1995) (see Table 5.3).

Management depends on clinical findings. If circulatory compromise exists then immediate reduction should be considered in A&E. This carries significant risk of neurovascular damage and should only be carried out in limb-threatening situations (St Claire-Strange 1982). In most cases prompt reduction of the fracture should be carried out in theatre. In undisplaced fractures, a plaster backslab can be applied, and provided neurovascular integrity is maintained the patient can be discharged with limb care advice and fracture clinic follow-up.

Table 5.3 – *Assessing neurological function following elbow injury*

Nerve	Position	Motor function	Sensory function
Radial	Spirals humerus to anterior of lateral epicondyle	Wrist and finger extensor muscles – test for wrist drop on elbow flexion and forearm pronation	Snuff box area and dorsal aspect of thumb – test for sensation
Median	Anterior to humerus	Coarse hand movement, e.g. grip Test location of injury – above elbow there will be inability to flex index finger; below elbow there will be inability to flex thumb	Thumb and index finger – test for sensation
Ulna	Posterior to medial epicondyle	Flexor muscles of wrist and fingers and intrinsic muscles of the hand – damage can present as claw-like hand	Palmar and dorsal aspects of ulnar half of hand

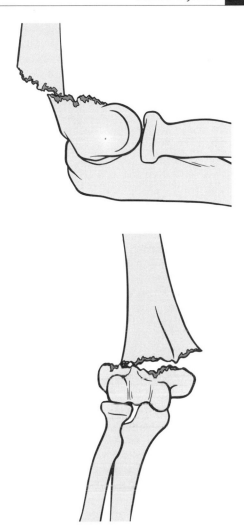

Figure 5.21 – *Supracondylar flexion fracture.*

Flexion fractures

These are less common than extension and fractures comprise approximately 2–4% of the total number of supracondylar fractures (Tsai & Ruiz 1995). They are caused by direct force to a flexed elbow, from a fall or a blow (see Fig. 5.21). The patient will have significant pain around the site and will be supporting the injured arm in a flexed position, but the olecranon prominence will be decreased. There may be a prominent proximal fragment of the humerus anteriorly, and these injuries are commonly seen in open fractures. Although nerve damage is less likely with flexion fractures, the ulnar nerve is at risk because of fracture displacement. Vascular injury is uncommon. If only minimal displacement exists, the fracture can be treated by closed reduction and an above-elbow back-slab in flexion. Fractures with significant displacement or open injuries should have open reduction and internal fixation of the fracture.

Elbow dislocation

Although elbow dislocation is not uncommon in adults, considerable force is needed to cause dislocation. As a result, a 1 in 3 likelihood of an associated fracture exists. The most common type of dislocation is posterior, where the coronoid process slips back and lies in the olecranon fossa, or jams into the distal humerus. The joint capsule is damaged and collateral ligaments are torn.

The patient will have pain, the arm will be supported in mid-flexion and the limb will appear shortened. The olecranon is prominent. Careful neurovascular examination is necessary. Management involves urgent relocation for both pain control and neurovascular integrity. This is achieved with good muscle relaxants and adequate analgesia followed by a traction/counter-traction approach where one carer applies sustained traction distally from the wrist followed by flexion with posterior pressure. When the reduction is completed, range of movement should be checked to rule out a mechanical blockage, neurovascular integrity should be rechecked, and then the arm should be immobilised in at least 90% flexion. Medial, lateral and anterior dislocations can also occur, but less commonly. Management of these should be led by the orthopaedic team.

Radial head fractures

In this type of fracture the radial head becomes compressed upwards against the capitellum following a fall onto an outstretched hand. It is an important feature in elbow flexion/extension and forearm rotation. The patient will present with localised pain, which is worse with passive rotation of the forearm. For management purposes, fractures are classified into three types (see Table 5.4).

Forearm Injury

The forearm consists of two long bones: the radius and ulna. They run essentially parallel, although the ulna is straight and the radius bows laterally to allow supination and pronation. The radius and ulna articulate with each other at both ends and are held together by the elbow and wrist joints and their ligaments. The radiocarpal joint connects the radius and the articular disc of the ulna with the carpal bones. This allows palmar and dorsiflexion of the wrist and abduction of the ulna. The union and alignment of the radius and ulna are vital to the function of the forearm and wrist.

Table 5.4 – *Classification and management of radial head fractures*

Type	Description	Management
I	Undisplaced	Sling with early mobilisation
II	Marginal fracture with displacement	Joint aspiration if necessary Sling and early mobilisation
III	Comminuted fracture	Treatment options vary from internal fixation to partial or total extension of the radial head

Fracture of both radius and ulna

This occurs following a direct blow, fall or RTA involving significant force or longitudinal compression. Displacement of fractures is common because of the force needed to break both bones. Injury commonly occurs where the mid- and distal thirds merge because there is less muscle protection. These fractures are easy to diagnose as the patient presents with severe pain and marked deformity, sometimes with abnormal movement of the forearm, which mainly depends on the degree of deformity. If there is no angulation or displacement, a long arm Plaster of Paris (POP) slab with 90° flexion of the elbow is applied. Usually open reduction with internal fixation is required because displacement is common. If good reduction is not achieved and maintained, non-union of the bones or union with loss of function will occur.

Ulnar fractures

Ulnar shaft fractures are caused by direct force to the arm, commonly when it is raised to protect the face from injury. The patient presents with pain over the area, and swelling and deformity if the fracture is displaced. Management depends on the degree of displacement. Fractures with more than 50% displacement or 10% of angulation should be internally fixed as they carry a significant risk of non-union (Dymond 1984). Fractures with less displacement/angulation can be treated in a long arm POP cast with the elbow in 90° flexion and the forearm in a neutral position. Non-displaced fractures initially treated by immobilisation respond well to early remobilisation at about 10 days post-injury.

Proximal ulnar fractures rarely occur independently and are associated with radial head dislocation. This is called a Monteggia fracture. Several classifications of these fractures exist, usually defined by the position of the radial head (Carr 1995). The patient presents with localised pain, and depending on the position of the radial head, it may be palpable and shortening of the forearm may also be noted. The patient will resist any movement of the elbow. Management usually involves open reduction and internal fixation in adults, as non-union and persistent dislocation of the radial head are common. A closed reduction under general anaesthetic can usually be achieved in children, as slight radial angulation of the ulna will not restrict movement. In adults, about 95% have some morbidity following this injury (Oveson *et al.* 1990), i.e. non-union, loss of reduction and infection. Radial nerve paralysis can also occur as a result of compression from the displaced radial head. This causes weak wrist and hand extensors.

Fractures of the radius

Proximal third fractures are rare because of the muscular support attached to the forearm. When they do occur, these fractures are usually caused by direct force to the forearm. The patient usually has pain around the fracture site and pain on longitudinal compression of the radius. Deformity is not as easy to detect as in other forearm fractures because of the amount of soft tissue surrounding the proximal radius. Associated ulnar injury is common because of the force needed to fracture the radius at this level.

The shape of the radius must be maintained to restore function. In proximal third fractures this is complicated by the force exerted by the supinator and biceps brachii muscles, creating supination and displacement of the proximal fragment. The pronator teres muscle causes pronation of the distal fragment which compounds deformity. This deforming process can occur within a POP cast, and therefore if fractures occur proximal to the point of pronator teres insertion in the mid-third of the radius, internal fixation of the fracture is recommended. Fractures in the proximal fifth of the radius are unsuitable for internal fixation because orthopaedic metalwork/hardware cannot be accommodated. These fractures should be treated in a long arm cast with 90° elbow flexion and forearm supination to minimise muscle forces and maintain reduction. The outcome of closed reduction is better in children than in adults.

Distal third shaft fractures also occur because of direct force, but are more common because of the lack

Table 5.5 – *Deforming forces in Galeazzi fractures*

Mechanism	Deformity
Gravity	Subluxation or dislocation of radioulnar joint Angulation of radial fracture
Pronator quadratus	Rotation of distal fragment in a proximal and volar direction
Brachioradialis	Shortening because of distal fragment rotation
Thumb abductors and extensors	Compounds shortening

of soft tissue protection. Isolated fractures are less common than more complicated injury (Goldberg *et al.* 1992). Dislocation of the radioulnar joint is usually concomitant with fractures around the midshaft and distal shaft junction. This is called a Galeazzi fracture. Pain is the primary diagnostic feature. Tissue swelling may obscure deformity, but shortening is sometimes apparent. The deforming forces, shown in Table 5.5, make closed reduction less successful than open reduction with internal fixation.

The Wrist

Anatomically, the wrist is an area which contains multiple joints connected by ligaments. It extends from the distal radius and ulna to the distal carpal bones (see Fig. 5.22). Injury to the wrist usually

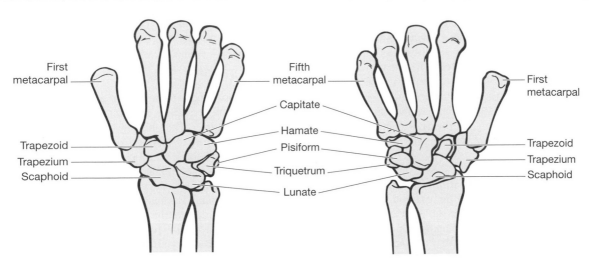

Figure 5.22 – *The wrist.*

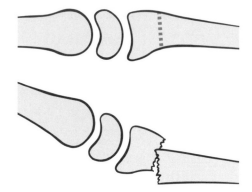

Figure 5.23 – *Colles' fracture.*

results from a fall onto an outstretched hand, which causes hyperextension of the hand and force to be exerted on the volar aspect of the radius causing fracture. Injury pattern varies with age, gender and the amount of force involved.

Distal radius fractures

The distal radius is a common site of injury in adults. Fractures of this area are broadly grouped into three categories depending on the displacement of the distal radius and ulna. The most common of these is the Colles' fracture (see Fig. 5.23). This describes a distal radius fracture with dorsal displacement of the distal fragment. This causes a loss of the usual volar tilt and pronation of the distal fragment over the proximal fragment. An associated ulnar styloid fracture is present in 60% of cases (Cooney *et al.* 1991). The injury is most prevalent in women over 50, particularly those with signs of osteoporosis. Colle's fractures are easy to identify at triage as the patient presents with classic dinner-fork deformity of the wrist because of dorsal displacement and loss of volar angulation.

The patient usually has significant swelling around the fracture site and localised pain. Nerve involvement is not uncommon and paraesthesia may be present in areas served by the median or ulnar nerve. Severe swelling can cause vascular compromise and compartment syndrome. Neurovascular function should therefore be carefully checked on assessment. Management priorities involve restoration of anatomical alignment, in particular the degree of volar tilt, and the exact restoration of a neutral radioulnar joint if good function of the wrist is to be restored. Fractures with minimal displacement with no shortening and maintenance of volar tilt are managed in a forearm POP back-slab or split cast with the hand pronated and ulnar deviation, and flexion at the wrist (Brown 1996).

Most displaced fractures can be managed by closed

reduction in A&E. To facilitate this, adequate analgesia is required. Debate persists as to which method of anaesthesia is most appropriate, and various methods are discussed in Chapter 25. Bier's block is often favoured by orthopaedic staff, but demands skilled operators, not A&E SHOs unfamiliar with the equipment. Haematoma block carries the risk of subsequent tissue toxicity from the lignocaine/lidocaine used, and has been criticised for providing inadequate anaesthesia to complete the reduction (Cooney *et al.* 1991). Despite this, haematoma block is commonly used and is successful in the treatment of elderly women. As a general rule, haematoma block is not suitable for Colles' fracture reduction in younger patients, particularly men with greater muscle spasm creating resistance to reduction. An accurate reduction is vital for restoration of full function in younger patients, and therefore multiple attempts at manipulation are sometimes needed. This is more easily facilitated under Bier's block.

The reduction involves a traction/counter-traction approach, with the first person applying longitudinal traction through the hand to lengthen the radius, while the other applies counter-traction through the forearm until disimpaction of the distal fragment can be felt. Then the first person applies pressure to the top of the distal fragment to reduce it. Again, volar movement will be felt and visible deformity should be resolved. The wrist should be immediately immobilised in a POP slab with ulnar deviation and wrist flexion. Post-reduction X-rays should be obtained to establish the degree of volar tilt, length and neutral radioulnar joint position. If this cannot be achieved by closed manipulation, open reduction and internal fixation should be considered. In complicated or severely comminuted injuries, open reduction and internal fixation should be considered and closed manipulation not attempted in A&E.

Smith's fractures

In both anatomical presentation and mechanism of injury, a Smith's fracture represents the opposite of a Colles' fracture. The distal radius is displaced proximally and the distal fragment is volar to the radial shaft. There are three classifications depending on the direction of the fracture (see Figure 5.24).

The mechanism of injury is an impact on the distal aspect of the hand. Because significant force is needed to cause this fracture, the cause is usually an RTA or cyclist going over the handlebars. Smith's fractures are most common in young men. The patient presents with severe pain, obvious volar deformity of the wrist, making the hand appear anteriorly displaced, and

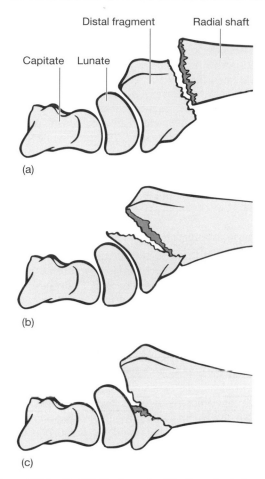

Capitate Lunate Distal fragment Radial shaft

(a)

(b)

(c)

Figure 5.24 – *Smith's fracture: classification of anterior displacement. (a): Type I–transverse fracture. (b): Type II–oblique fracture from proximal volar surface through dorsal particular surface. (c): Type III–oblique fracture with joint space involvement (same as Barton fracture-dislocation).*

often swelling to the dorsal aspect of the wrist. Neurological compromise to median and ulnar nerves is possible with significant deformity, as is vascular compromise. Careful triage will highlight these complications.

Type I fractures can usually be treated in A&E. Closed manipulation involves restoring length and dorsal alignment of the radius. This can be achieved using Bier's block anaesthesia and manual traction. Once deformity is corrected, the arm should be immobilised in an above-arm split POP cast with the forearm in a supinated position. Type II and type III fractures are unstable injuries, and to ensure maximum functional recovery, orthopaedic advice should

also be sought. Open reduction with internal fixation is usually required.

Carpal fractures

The carpal bones form two rows (see Fig. 5.22). The proximal row consists of the scaphoid, lunate, triquetrum and pisiform bones. The scaphoid has a bridging position with the distal row which consists of the trapezium, capitate and hamate bones. These bones are supported by three strands of ligaments stemming from the radial styloid. The radial and ulnar arteries provide vascular supply, and the radial, ulnar and median nerves provide neurological function.

Fractures of the carpal bones are less common than other wrist injuries (Collier 1995), but are often associated with ligament injury, creating an unstable wrist joint. Long-term disability is not uncommon in missed fractures. Assessment of wrist injury should focus on the mechanism of injury, force involved and exact site of impact as well as the age of the patient, as wrist anatomy and relative strengths change with age.

Scaphoid fracture

Because of its unique position in relation to the radius and both rows of carpal bones, the scaphoid is the most commonly fractured carpal bone. It occurs in both adults and children, most often between early teens and mid-life. The scaphoid is an oblong bone divided into four anatomical areas (see Fig. 5.25).

The scaphoid has a good vascular supply to the middle and distal areas, but the proximal pole has no dedicated blood supply. This results in a high incidence of vascular necrosis if fracture union is not rapidly achieved (Gumucio 1989). Scaphoid fractures are usually classified as stable or unstable according to Herbert & Fisher (1984), and time taken to union differs with the fracture location (Box 5.6). Stable fractures are incomplete or completely undisplaced, heal rapidly and are treated with immobilisation. An

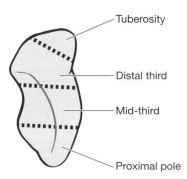

Figure 5.25 – *The scaphoid bone.*

Tuberosity, Distal third, Mid-third, Proximal pole

Box 5.6 – *Herbert's classification of scaphoid fractures*

Type A (stable)
A1   Crack fractures
A2   Tubercle fractures

Type B (unstable)
B1   Distal third
B2   Waist
B3   Proximal pole
B4   Carpal dislocation
B5   Comminuted

unstable fracture has been defined as displacement of the fracture by 1 mm or more on X-ray.

The most common mechanism of injury is a fall onto an outstretched hand. Externally, there is little visible evidence of a fracture, although swelling can sometimes be present. The patient will have generalised pain, which is worse on wrist movement, particularly gripping actions. On examination, the patient will have specific tenderness in the anatomical snuff box. She may also have longitudinal pressure on the thumb and index finger, and pain on dorsiflexion of the wrist. Because of the location of pain and lack of external signs, patients often delay A&E attendance as they do not automatically relate symptoms with a broken bone.

X-ray findings can be misleading as up to 20% of patients with scaphoid fracture have normal initial X-rays (Collier 1995). For this reason, diagnosis should be based on clinical findings, specifically mechanism of injury and localised tenderness in the anatomical snuffbox. Although management of scaphoid fractures can be controversial (Dyson 1997), a general consensus exists that all fractures, whether clinical or radiological, should be immobilised as failure to do this can result in delayed or non-union healing or avascular necrosis. A POP cast or splint which incorporates the forearm and thumb, with the wrist in slight volar flexion, should be used. Complicated fractures should be referred to the orthopaedic team because of the risk of avascular necrosis. Some fractures are internally fixed at an early stage to prevent non-union and to ensure good functional recovery. Fractures not initially visible on X-ray will be apparent about 10 days post-injury (Chin *et al.* 1992).

Lunate fracture

The lunate is in the middle of the proximal carpal row and rests in the lunate fossa of the radius. Injury of the lunate bone is relatively uncommon because it is protected by the lunate fossa. When fracture does occur it is usually due to a fall onto an outstretched hand, where force is taken through the heel of the hand. The patient presents with mid-dorsal pain and wrist weakness; however, swelling is uncommon. As a result, A&E attendance is sometimes days or weeks after the initial injury.

Radiological evidence of fracture is not always obvious, therefore clinical diagnosis is necessary based on location of pain and mechanism of injury. Non-displaced fractures should be treated in a forearm POP cast, with orthopaedic follow-up. Displaced fractures are prone to avascular necrosis and non-union, with a potential for secondary osteoarthritis. For this reason, patients should be referred to the orthopaedic team for possible internal fixation.

Triquetrum fractures

The triquetrum is the second most commonly fractured carpal bone. Such fractures often occur with other carpal fractures or perilunate dislocation (Botte & Gelberman 1987). Isolated injury is less common and usually minor. Triquetrum fractures are usually caused by hyperextension injury of significant force. The patient usually complains of pain over the dorso-ulnar area of the wrist. Management involves a short arm POP cast or splint for 3–6 weeks in the case of isolated injury or referral to the orthopaedic team where the fracture is associated with other wrist injuries. Other carpal fractures generally occur as part of a more complicated hand or wrist injury, and demand specialist orthopaedic input after initial diagnosis in A&E.

Perilunate and lunate dislocation

These dislocations occur as a result of disruption to the lesser arc of ligaments. They can be graded into four groups depending on the degree of disruption (see Box 5.7). They are caused by extreme hyper-

Box 5.7 – *Stages of perilunate disruption and midcarpal dislocation (After, Mayfield 1984.)*

■ **Stage 1: scapholunate instability**–due to torn radioscaphoid and scapholunate interosseous ligaments with/without scaphoid fracture

■ **Stage 2: dorsal perilunate dislocation**–capitate dislocates dorsally from lunate at the midcarpal joint

■ **Stage 3: disruption of lunate and triquetrum**–occurs with avulsion fracture of triquetrum with/without scaphoid or capitate fracture

■ **Stage 4: volar dislocation of lunate**

extension, such as a motorcycle accident or fall from a height. Because of the force needed to cause perilunate and/or lunate dislocation, concurrent injury is common. The patient presents with extreme pain and a fork-type deformity, and is usually unable to hold the fingers in a flexed position. Nerve disruption is not uncommon, so paraesthesia may also be present. Fractures and severe ligament disruption are usual with these injuries, which should always be managed by the orthopaedic team and often require open reduction when associated with fractures.

The Hand

The hand is a complex structure whose skeletal outline is shown in Figure 5.26. The back of the hand is referred to as the dorsal aspect and the palm of the hand the volar aspect. The intricate mechanisms of hand movement are particularly vulnerable to injury because of its environmental exposure and functional purpose. Hand function relies on intact muscle and tendon structures and sensory motor connection to the central nervous system, as well as adequate circulation. The treatment of any hand injury revolves firstly around restoring function and secondly around appearance. Anatomy will be considered in greater detail where relevant to specific injuries.

Thumb injury

The flexor surface of the thumb is perpendicular to that of the fingers and has a saddle joint which allows 45° of rotation. The range of thumb movements include flexion/extension, adduction/abduction and opposition. It provides both strength and grip.

First metacarpal fractures

These are treated differently from other metacarpal fractures because of the degree of functional restoration needed.

Metacarpal shaft fractures

These usually occur in the proximal half of the bone and are often associated with adduction of the distal

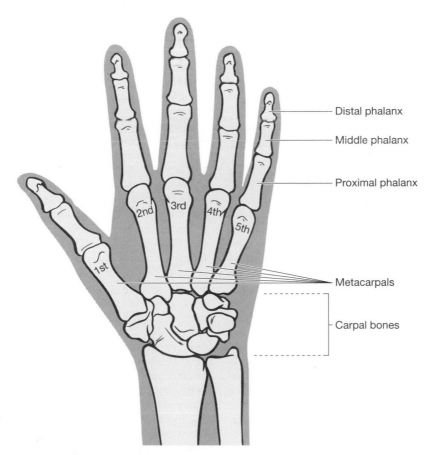

Figure 5.26 – *Anatomy of the hand.*

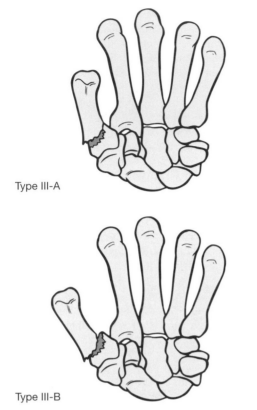

Type III-A

Type III-B

Figure 5.27 – *Extra-articular fracture to the base of the first metacarpal.*

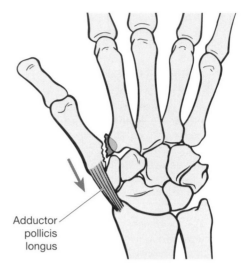

Adductor pollicis longus

Figure 5.28 – *Intra-articular fracture to the base of the first metacarpal (Bennett's fracture).*

segment. Management usually involves longitudinal traction and POP cast incorporating the thumb. Early orthopaedic follow-up is advisable.

Base of metacarpal fractures

These are usually more complicated and result from flexion injuries, commonly from clenched fists. They can be classified as intra-articular fractures, such as Bennett's fractures, or extra-articular transverse or oblique fractures. Extra-articular fractures are the most common fracture types. The fracture occurs within the joint capsule but does not involve the articular surface of the joint (see Fig. 5.27). These injuries are usually managed by closed reduction and POP cast incorporating the thumb. In order to retain good function, it is important not to hyperextend the thumb at the metacarpophalangeal joint. Some oblique fractures may remain unstable with closed reduction and plaster immobilisation alone, and therefore orthopaedic referral for percutaneous pinning is necessary.

Intra-articular fractures can be divided into two groups: the more common *Bennett's fracture* and

Rolando's fracture. The Bennett's fracture is categorised by the displacement of the metacarpal shaft while the palmar articular fragment retains its correct anatomical location as shown in Figure 5.28. The mechanism of injury is similar to that of an extra-articular fracture, with interpersonal fracas being a common cause of injury. The patient has limited movement of the base of the thumb with pain and swelling around the area. Effective emergency management is essential to prevent degenerative post-traumatic arthritis and to restore adequate range of movement.

The injury is considered unstable because of the adductor pollicis longus tendon, which is attached to the base of the first metacarpal. Its tensile strength prevents union of fracture without the aid of percutaneous pins or orthopaedic reduction and internal fixation.

Rolando's fracture is similar to a Bennett's fracture, but in addition to the palmar articular fragment remaining in place, the dorsal fragment displaces from the base, creating a Y-shaped or more severely comminuted base of metacarpal fracture. Mechanism of injury and patient presentation are similar to those of a Bennett's fracture, but the prognosis is poor as functional integrity is difficult to restore with orthopaedic reduction and internal fixation or closed reduction and immobilisation. Persistent pain and degenerative arthritis are common. Phalangeal fractures of the thumb are generally managed in the same manner as fingers and are discussed later in this chapter, (p. 100).

Second to fifth metacarpal fractures

The metacarpals are anatomically sectioned into base, shaft, neck and head. Unlike other long bones, the base is at the proximal point and the head at the distal end.

Base of metacarpal fractures (II–IV)

The patient presents with a history of a fall onto an outstretched hand or punch injury. The fractures are often associated with carpal fractures and second and third metacarpal base fractures often have intra-articular involvement, but this causes little or no disability because of the relative immobility of the first and third carpometacarpal (CMC) joint. As a result, treatment focuses on maintaining patient comfort. A removable splint is the treatment of choice. Fractures of the fourth and fifth metacarpal bases are usually associated with CMC dislocation. Fourth metacarpal base fractures can usually be managed in A&E with closed reduction and splinting followed up by the orthopaedic team. Fifth metacarpal base fractures will usually require pinning because of displacement.

Good fracture alignment is necessary to retain normal mobility of the CMC joint. When splinting hand injuries, it is vital that metacarpophalangeal joints are immobilised in at least 70° of flexion to prevent shortening of the collateral ligaments. If these ligaments contract during immobilisation, the patient is left with considerable disability because of joint stiffness.

Shaft of metacarpal fracture

These are caused by a number of mechanisms of injury (see Table 5.6). Principles of management revolve around correction of any rotation, angulation and shortening of the finger to ensure functional recovery. Even a small degree of rotation can cause problems with flexion of the metacarpophalangeal joint. Effective closed reduction and immobilisation are usually achievable in A&E unless severe swelling or open fractures exist. If rotation cannot be corrected with manipulation, the patient should be referred for percutaneous pinning or orthopaedic reduction and internal fixation.

Table 5.6 – *Metacarpal shaft fractures*

Type	Cause
Transverse	Direct blow
Oblique	Torque force
Comminuted	Crush injury/gunshot wound

Metacarpal neck fractures

Second and third metacarpal neck fractures often need wiring to correct angulation in order to restore functional mobility, and therefore orthopaedic opinion should be sought. The fourth metacarpal is more mobile and neck fractures will heal without functional deficit even if volar angulation at the metacarpal neck exists. Any rotation in these fractures must be corrected to prevent functional deficit.

Fifth metacarpal neck fracture (Boxer's fracture). This is one of the most common hand injuries treated in the A&E department and usually results from a punch injury. Management of these fractures is controversial, but there is a consensus that any rotational injury needs manipulation and either splinting or wiring. Volar angulation can, however, be treated in a number of ways, ranging from orthopaedic reduction and internal fixation to no treatment and early mobilisation (Ford *et al.* 1989)

Clinical trials (Rusnak 1995) have found that no treatment at all or supportive splinting which facilitates mobilisation has quicker functional repair, with minimal cosmetic deformity in the majority of cases. Where closed reduction is carried out, maintaining that reduction is difficult without causing further damage to the function of the hand. This is because 70° of flexion at the metacarpophalangeal joint is necessary to prevent contractures, but this position will not provide the three-point fixation needed to stabilise the metacarpal neck.

If the patient is exceptionally concerned about the cosmetic result and the possible loss of knuckle definition, then surgical fixation should be considered; however recovery is significantly slower with this method. Whatever method is used, the patient should have adequate follow-up from a hand surgeon to ensure the fullest functional potential is achieved. Metacarpal head fractures should be managed conservatively unless they are displaced or comminuted, when an orthopaedic opinion should be sought.

Fracture of phalanges

As with other hand fractures, the key management priority is to maintain good function by correcting rotation.

Soft Tissue Injuries

Soft tissue injuries are commonly treated in A&E and are usually considered 'minor' in nature by A&E staff. The impact on the patient, however, is far from minor; loss of normal function in the short term is common, usually because of pain. If soft tissue injuries are not detected and treated properly, long-term or recurrent problems can occur. Soft tissue injury (STI) is the all-encompassing term given to injury to muscles, ligaments, tendons and skin. As a result, the diagnosis of a STI has a number of possible causative factors. The common ones are described below.

Sprains

These are injuries to the fibres of ligaments supporting a joint. This results from abnormal movement of the joint which causes stretching and tearing of the ligament. The degree of this varies from some fibrous tearing to total disruption of the ligament complex supporting a joint (see Table 5.7).

The patient will present with mechanisms of injury and symptoms similar to those with fractures. The joint has often been subjected to forces in opposite or abnormal directions, creating joint stress. The patient will usually describe a sudden onset of acute pain, and often describe hearing a 'snap' at the time of injury. Many patients are convinced this means they have broken their limb and the nurse must therefore be careful to assess the injury thoroughly and provide the appropriate reassurance (Whelan 1997). Although specific injury management can vary, common principles of sprain management apply:

Rest. Most acute sprains benefit from a 48-hour period of rest, with minimal use.

Ice. As well as being a useful first aid measure, ice packs, or wrapped crushed ice, help to decrease both pain and swelling. The patient should be advised to apply the ice for 10–15 minutes every 2–3 hours for the first 12 hours post-injury.

Compression. Elastic tubular bandages or strapping provide support for the injury and help to reduce swelling. Tubular bandage should be removed by the patient at night to prevent oedema distal to the injury. In severe sprains, POP casts may be more appropriate for specific injuries.

Elevation. Together with ice packs and rest, elevation of the injured part helps to reduce the accumulation of blood and lymph in tissues surrounding the injury, which in turn reduces both pain and healing time. This is particularly important for distal limb injuries, such as those of the hand, foot or ankle.

Strains

These are injuries to muscles and tendons. They occur after forced stretching or sudden violent contraction. As with sprains, the severity of strain injury is classified by the extent of damage (Table 5.8).

Treatment of strains is similar to that of sprains. Management of first-degree strains involves rest, ice,

Table 5.7 – *Classification of sprains*

	Physiology	Clinical signs
First degree	Minor tearing of ligament fibres with mild haemorrhage	Minimal swelling Tenderness over ligaments – worse with motion, stressing the ligaments
Second degree	Partial tear with moderate haemorrhage and reduced active motion	Significant pain – worse with passive movement and swelling Injuries prone to recurrence and can cause joint instability
Third degree	Complete rupture of ligament; moderate haemorrhage with significant loss of function	Less painful with significant swelling and abnormal motion of joint on active/passive movement Usually need surgical repair if joint instability exists.

Table 5.8 – *Classification of strains*

	Physiology	Clinical signs
First degree	Minor tearing of muscle/tendon unit	Spasm, swelling and localised pain
Second degree	More severe pain but incomplete tearing of fibres	Muscle spasm, swelling, localised pain and loss of strength
Third degree	The muscle or tendon is completely disrupted with separation of muscle from tendon, tendon from muscle or tendon from bone	Palpable defect is often present Muscle spasm, pain, swelling and loss of function.

compression and elevation as described under 'sprains' above. Second-degree injuries may require immobilisation, depending on the site affected, and usually take longer to heal. Third-degree injuries should be immobilised and the patient referred for early orthopaedic consultation at the fracture/STI clinic. Some injuries benefit from surgical repair, but many require simple immobilisation. Many factors influence this decision: the site of injury, as well as the age, activity level and occupation of the patient.

Tendinitis

This is an inflammatory condition usually caused by overuse. Less commonly it is caused by direct trauma. The patient complains of pain at the point where the tendon attaches to bone. Pain is worse on movement and function is sometimes restricted. Occasionally, palpable crepitus exists. Common sites include the rotator cuff of the shoulder, the insertion of hand extensors to the humeral epicondyle (tennis elbow), the radial aspect of the wrist (De Querrain's tenosynovitis) and the Achilles tendon. Management involves rest and non-specific anti-inflammatories (NSAIDs).

Bursitis

This is inflammation of the bursa. The bursa is a sac of synovial fluid situated between muscle, tendon and bony prominences to facilitate movement. Bursitis can result from friction between the bursa and musculoskeletal tissue, direct trauma or infection. It results in inflammation and oedema, which causes sac engorgement, and the area becomes painful.

This condition is most common in middle age (Genge Jagmin 1995). The patient usually presents to A&E with a swelling at 2–3 days post-injury or strain. Pain can increase gradually over this time or may be of sudden onset. It is usually worse on movement and radiates distally from the site of bursitis. The area will appear classically inflamed with erythema and swelling and will be hot to the touch. Areas commonly affected include the knee, elbow and big toe (gout bursitis). If infection is suspected, e.g. following a puncture wound, or if the patient has pyrexia, the bursa should be aspirated and the aspirate sent to the laboratory for culture. Otherwise, the injured area should be managed conservatively with rest and NSAIDs.

Haematoma

This is a collection of blood resulting from vascular injury within the soft tissues, bone or muscle. It is a result of direct or blunt trauma. Large haematomas not only threaten homeostasis, due to loss of circulatory volume, but are also a potential host for infection. As a result, surgical drainage and antibiotic therapy may be necessary. Smaller haematomas can be treated with compression bandages, ice as described above, and elevation.

Contusions

These usually result from direct trauma, which results in localised pain, swelling and bruising. Most are self-limiting and symptoms are relieved by ice treatment, analgesia and early mobilisation.

Specific soft tissue injuries

There are a number of soft tissue injuries that are so commonly treated in A&E departments that they warrant individual discussion within this chapter.

Knee injury

The knee gives support and flexibility to body movement. Ligaments and musculotendinous structures maintain its stability. Because of its load-bearing task, the knee is very susceptible to injury, particularly during sporting activities like rugby and football. Medial injuries tend to be the most common; lateral injuries, however, are often more disabling (Mayeda 1992). The mechanism of injury gives a strong indication of the likely structural damage, so accurate history-taking is vital (see Table 5.9).

Table 5.9 – *Mechanisms of knee injury*

Force	Cause	Injury
Hyperextension Forced flexion	Running/sudden deceleration, e.g. from rugby tackles	Tearing of anterior cruciate ligament
Twisting or flexed knee injury	Direct or blunt trauma	Meniscal injury
Valgus stress with external rotation	Skiing	Medial collateral ligament injury
Varus stress internal rotation	Skiing in snowplough position	Lateral collateral ligament
Direct force	Fall, hitting dashboard in RTA	Posterior cruciate ligament

Examination of the knee should be carried out with the patient lying on a trolley. The nurse should look at both knees to detect subtle differences. Bruising, swelling or redness are all signs of soft tissue injury. Swelling is frequently caused by haemarthrosis if it has a rapid onset; this could be the result of ligament/meniscus tear or a fracture of the tibial plateau and is therefore an indication for X-ray. Aspiration should be carried out in strict aseptic conditions, both for symptom relief and for diagnostic purposes. If the aspirate contains fat globules then a fracture is present. All patients with a rapid-onset haemarthrosis have significant knee trauma and should be referred for orthopaedic follow-up. Swelling can occur gradually and usually represents a reactionary effusion. These are also aspirated for symptom relief if large or restrictive.

The nurse should carefully assess knee movement, as this will give clues as to what ligamentous damage exists. Most ligament injuries can be healed with the treatment described above for sprains. Because of the load-bearing nature of the knee tendon, ruptures are often associated with fractures and frequently need surgical repair. For this reason, patients with total ruptures should be referred to the orthopaedic team.

Achilles tendon rupture

This is a common tennis and badminton injury, associated with sudden jumping movements with a heavy landing. The patient complains of a sudden sharp pain at the back of the ankle, not dissimilar to a direct blow. Swelling is present in some cases, as is bruising, but often it is simply pain and the mechanism of injury which initially indicate Achilles tendon rupture. The calf squeeze test (Simmonds' test) is useful in confirming diagnosis. The patient kneels backwards over a chair or lies face down on a trolley with the ankles over the end. When the calf is squeezed, plantarflexion of the ankle should occur unless the Achilles tendon is ruptured. All of these patients should be referred for orthopaedic follow-up.

Most are initially managed in long leg equinous plaster, with the ankle in plantarflexion. Some patients benefit from surgical repair, particularly young athletic people. Patient outcomes appear similar whether or not open repair is performed (Mayeda 1992). Achilles tendinitis should not be confused with partial rupture. Tendinitis is caused by overuse or sudden change in activity such as dancing or running. The patient will have localised pain, swelling and crepitus over the tendon. The range of movement will be normal but painful. The patient should be treated with rest and NSAIDs.

Ankle sprain

Large numbers of patients with ankle injuries are treated in A&E, and one of the priorities for A&E nurses lies with identifying serious or potentially limb-threatening injury. Assessment for all ankle injuries should be systematic and thorough, although the majority will turn out to be straightforward sprains. Assessment should include mechanism of injury, the most common being an inversion injury causing damage to the anterior talofibular ligaments. This results from slipping off kerbs or twisting the ankle in a manner where the sole of the foot turns inwards.

Eversion injury is less common, but is more likely to be associated with an avulsion fracture and causes damage to the deltoid ligament; it is characterised by an injury where the sole of the foot turns outwards. Patients will often have heard a 'snap' or 'crack' at the time of injury which they will probably associate with a broken bone. The nurse needs to provide reassurance as well as a thorough assessment, particularly when an X-ray is not clinically indicated. The patient with an ankle sprain usually has pain at the site of injury, swelling over that area and reduced mobility because of pain. Examination usually identifies the area immediately below the respective malleolus to be the most severe point of pain, as opposed to a fracture where pain is worse over the bony prominence. To reduce unnecessary X-rays a set of criteria called the 'Ottowa ankle rules' have been developed (Stiell *et al.* 1992). These provide the criteria within which patients with ankle injury should be X-rayed (see Box 5.8).

Management involves initial rest with compression bandaging, intermittent ice therapy and support. Recovery usually takes 2–4 weeks, however most long-term problems stem from prolonged immobilisation. For this reason, patients should be encouraged to exercise the ankle gently and resume activity after 1–2 weeks as pain and swelling permit.

Rotator cuff injury

The varied mobility of the shoulder joint makes it sus-

Box 5.8 – *Ottawa ankle rules*

- Patients with tenderness over bony prominences of malleolus or posterior tenderness

- Pain up proximal fibula

- Specific tenderness of calcaneus, navicular or base of fifth metatarsal

- Unable to weight-bear immediately post-injury or in A&E

Table 5.10 – *The rotator cuff muscles*

Muscle	Action
Infraspinatus	External rotation
Teres minor	External rotation
Subscapularis	Internal rotation
Supraspinatus	Internal rotation

ceptible to injury. Shoulder stability is maintained by the rotator cuff. It comprises a sheath of muscles listed in Table 5.10. Degenerative conditions such as rheumatoid arthritis are not uncommon and increase the likelihood of injury. Acute injury includes tearing or tendinitis. The supraspinatus is the most commonly injured area; this results from falls with hyperextension or hyperabduction of the shoulder. Rest and analgesia comprise the management of choice, and most patients benefit from orthopaedic follow-up, as recurrent injury is not uncommon.

Rotator cuff tendinitis is usually a chronic condition, but a patient may present to A&E following an acute exacerbation. Unlike a rotator cuff tear, the patient will describe a gradually worsening discomfort, inability to sleep and decreased range of movement. NSAIDs and rest are the treatment of choice.

Thumb sprain

Stability and function of the thumb rely on the ulnar collateral ligament (UCL). Injury to the UCL is caused by hyperextension of the thumb from ball games or a fall, or by hyperabduction, usually from falling while moving, such as during skiing. If the history is suggestive of a UCL injury and the patient has pain in that area, then an X-ray should be performed to exclude a thumb fracture before joint stability is formally tested. If no fracture is present, the joint should be examined with the thumb in flexion and extension to determine stability. If UCL rupture is suspected, the patient should be referred to the orthopaedic team, as open surgical repair is often beneficial. If an uncomplicated sprain exists then elastoplast strapping in the form of a thumb spica will provide the compression and rest the joint to enable the sprain to heal.

Mallet finger

This is caused by a direct blow to the end of the finger or more commonly occurs as a result of forced flexion of the distal interphalangeal (DIP) joint. It is caused by rupture or avulsion of the extensor tendon. If an avulsion fracture of the distal phalanx is present, healing is usually more rapid than a tendon rupture.

The patient presents in A&E with pain and a deformed finger and is unable to actively extend the fingertip distal to the DIP joint. Management involves splinting the finger to below the DIP joint in slight hyperextension. Patient education and cooperation are vital to the success of this treatment. The splint is usually plastic and needs to be removed frequently to clean the finger and prevent skin damage. It is important, however, that hyperextension of the DIP joint is maintained during this time. The patient should therefore be taught to apply and remove the splint while supporting fingertip on a firm surface.

Compartment syndrome

Compartment syndrome is essentially an increased tissue pressure with a closed space. If this pressure is allowed to rise and stay high, it causes permanent damage to the soft tissue structures and nerves within that compartment. The limbs contain compartments, so injuries where swelling occurs have the potential to cause compartment syndrome. The forearm contains dorsal and volar compartments, and the lower leg is divided into four compartments: lateral, anterior, superficial posterior and deep posterior. In addition to internal tissue swelling, constricting dressings or plaster of Paris, which is too tight, can cause compartment syndrome. This is one reason why casts on new injuries tend to be either split or bivalved or back-slabs are applied.

Tissue pressure rises for a number of reasons, and often the primary injury is not in itself devastating. Any injury with the potential for haemorrhage or tissue swelling can result in compartment syndrome. There is no correlation between fractures and severity and tissue pressure. If pressure rises there is an increased volume in that area. There are two main causes:

■ bleeding into the compartment, perhaps following a fracture or rupture of small vessels, will result in clot formation and increased compartmental pressure
■ muscle swelling – this usually occurs after a period of ischaemia, e.g. following vascular damage.

During the ischaemic period, fluid leaks into tissues through damaged capillaries and membranes. When blood supply is restored, however, this situation continues because of capillary damage. This results in muscle oedema. This is why compartment syndrome is so common after major burn injury or as a follow-up to major crush injuries. Increased tissue pressure leads to hypoperfusion of the structure within the affected compartment. Tissue perfusion rises, restricting venous return and causing reduced blood flow in major vessels; therefore the patient will have no tangible change in systemic blood pressure and pulses in the affected compartment will remain palpable. Tissue ischaemia can cause irreversible muscle and nerve damage unless nurses are familiar with the physiology of compartment syndrome and do not rely solely on traditional determinants, such as major pulses, to assume all is well.

The patient will complain of severe pain, which is incompatible with the severity of the injury, and often in response to analgesia. Pain may also occur away from the site of the primary injury. Symptoms are usually worse on movement or manual compression of the compartment. The patient often complains of numbness of the extremities distal to the compartment because of neurological compression. Motor function may also be impaired.

If any restrictive splints or dressings are in place these should be removed and the limb elevated in an attempt to reduce swelling. If conservative treatment fails to restore sensation and relieve pain, fasciotomy will be necessary within the first few hours to prevent long-term damage. In all patients susceptible to compartment syndrome, early involvement of the orthopaedic team is essential. Specialist tissue pressure monitoring gives an accurate portrait of how the patient is responding to conservative management and and an indication of how quickly to intervene with fasciotomies.

Conclusion

Musculoskeletal injury is one of the most common types of presentation to A&E departments. As this chapter has highlighted, it is imperative for A&E nurses to be able to assess musculoskeletal injury and identify life- or limb-threatening trauma, some of which may not seem devastating at first glance. An understanding of the underpinning anatomy and pathophysiology of the musculoskeletal system has been provided in order to inform clinical decision-making and meet the needs of the individual patient and avoid long-term, preventable disability. In doing so, the A&E nurse may be assured of delivering quality care to this vulnerable group of patients.

References

Adams I (1989) Sports injuries. In: Rutherford W, Illingworth R, Marsden A, Nelson P, Redmond A, Wilson D, eds. *Accident and Emergency Medicine*. Edinburgh: Churchill Livingstone.

American College of Surgeons (1997) *Advanced Trauma Life Support*. Chicago: American College of Surgeons.

Audit Commission (1996) *United they Stand*. London: The Stationary Office.

Beales J (1997) Tetanus immunisation: Implications in A&E. *Emergency Nurse*, **5**(5), 21–23.

Botte MJ, Gelberman RH (1987) Fractures of the carpus, excluding the scaphoid. *Hand Clinic*, **3**, 149–161.

Brown AFT (1996) *Accident & Emergency Diagnosis and Management*. Oxford: Butterworth-Heinemann.

Brown DE (1992) Shoulder Injuries. *Primary Care*, **19**, 265–281.

Carr M (1995) Forearm injuries. In: Ruiz E, Cicero JJ, eds. *Emergency Management of Skeletal Fractures*. St Louis: Mosby.

Chin HW, Propp PA, Orban DJ (1992) Forearm and wrist. In: Rosen P, Barkin RM, Braen GR *et al.*, eds. *Emergency Medicine: Concepts and Clinical Practice*, 3rd edn. St Louis; Mosby Year Book.

Ciernick IF, Meier L, Hollinger A (1991) Humeral mobility after treatment with a hanging cast. *Journal of Trauma*, **31**, 230–233.

Clisham MW, Berlin SJ (1981) The diagnosis and conservative treatment of calcaneal fractures – a review. *Journal of Foot Surgery*, **20**(1), 28.

Collier R (1995) The wrist. In: Ruiz E, Cicero JJ, eds. *Emergency Management of Skeletal Fractures*. St Louis: Mosby.

Cooney WP, Linscheid RL, Dobyns JH (1991) Fractures and dislocations of the wrist. In: Rockward CA *et al.*, eds. *Fractures in Adults*. Philadelphia, JB Lippincott, vol. 1.

Crimmins TJ, Ruiz E (1995) Shaft fractures of the femur. In: Ruiz E, Cicero JJ, eds. *Emergency Management of Skeletal Fractures*. St Louis: Mosby.

Dumas JL, Walker N (1992) Bilateral scapular fracture secondary to electric shock. *Archives of Orthopaedic Trauma Surgery*, **111**, 287–288.

Dymond IW (1984) The treatment of isolated fractures of the distal ulna. *Journal of Bone Joint Surgery*, **66**, 408–410.

Dyson S (1997) The diagnosis and treatment of scaphoid fractures in A&E. *Emergency Nurse*, **5**(6), 23–25.

Ford DJ, Ali MS, Steel WM (1989) Fractures of the 5th metacarpal neck – is reduction or immobilisation necessary? *Journal of Hand Surgery*, **14B**(2), 165–167.

Garden RS (1964) Stability and union in subcapital fractures of the femur. *Journal of Bone Joint Surgery*, **46-B**, 630.

Genge Jagmin M (1995) Musculoskeletal injuries. In: Kitt S, Selfridge-Thomas J, Proehl JA, Kaiser J, eds. *Emergency Nursing: a Physiologic and Clinical Perspective*, 2nd edn. Philadelphia: Saunders.

Goldberg HD, Young JWR, Reiner BI (1992) Double injuries of the forearm: a common occurrence. *Radiology*, **185**, 223–227.

Greenbaum MA, Papp GR (1992) Ankle dislocation without fracture – an unusual case. *Journal of Foot Surgery*, **31**, 238–240.

Gumucio CA (1989) Management of scaphoid fractures – a review and update. *South African Medical Journal*, **82**, 1377–1388.

Harris CR (1995) Ankle injuries. In: Ruiz E, Cicero JJ, eds. *Emergency Management of Skeletal Fractures*. St Louis: Mosby.

Harris CR, Haller PR (1995) The tibia and fibula. In: Ruiz E, Cicero JJ, eds. *Emergency Management of Skeletal Fractures*. St Louis: Mosby.

Herbert T, Fisher W (1984) Management of the fractured scaphoid using a new bone score. *Journal of Bone and Joint Surgery*, **71-A**(6), 938, 941.

Hinchliff S, Montague S, Watson R (1996) *Physiology for Nursing Practice*, 2nd edn. London: Baillière Tindall.

Knapton P (1999) Shoulder injury: a case study. *Emergency Nurse*, **6**(10), 25–28.

Kroner K, Lind T, Jenson J (1989) The epidemiology of shoulder dislocation. *Archives of Orthopaedic Trauma & Surgery*, **108**, 288.

Kyle RF, Gustilo RB, Premer RF (1979) Analysis of 622 intertrochanteric hip fractures: a retrospective and prospective study. *Journal of Bone Joint Surgery*, **61**, 216.

McGuinness M, Denton JR (1989) Fractures of the scapula: a retrospective study of 40 fractured scapula. *Journal of Trauma*, **29**, 1485–1493.

Magnusson AR (1992) Humerus and Elbow. In: Rosen P, Barkin RM, Braen GR *et al.*, eds. *Emergency Medicine: Concepts and Clinical Practice*, 3rd edn. St Louis: Mosby Year Book.

Mayeda DV (1992) Ankle and foot. In: Rosen P, Barkin RM, Braen GR *et al.*, eds. *Emergency Medicine: Concepts and Clinical Practice*, 3rd edn. St Louis, Mosby Year Book.

Mayfield JK (1984) Patterns of injury to carpal ligaments. *Clinical Orthopaedics*, **187**, 36–42.

Mills K, Morton R, Page G (1995) *Color Atlas and Text of Emergencies*, 2nd edn. London: Mosby-Wolfe.

Monsell FP, Ross ERS (1998) Pelvic injuries. In: Driscoll P, Skinner D, eds. *Trauma Care: Beyond the Resuscitation Room*. London: BMJ Books.

Mooney N (1991) Pain management in the orthopedic patient. *Nursing Clinics of North America*, **26**, 73–87.

Muir L, Boot D, Gorman DS, Teanby DN (1996) Epidemiology of pelvic fractures in the Mersey region. *Injury*, **27**, 199–204.

Newman AP (1988) Fractures of the shoulder. *Topics in Emergency Medicine*, **10**(3), 65.

Nicholson DA, Driscoll PA (1995) Elbow. In: Nicholson DA, Driscoll PA, eds. *ABC of Emergency Radiology*. London: BMJ Publishing Group.

Nordqvist A, Petersson C (1992) Fracture of the body, neck or spine of the scapula: a long-term follow up study. *Clinical Orthopaedics*, **283**, 139–144.

Oveson O, Brok KE, Arreskov J *et al.* (1990) Monteggia lesions in children and adults: an analysis of aetiology and long-term results of treatment. *Orthopedics*, **13**, 529–534.

Purvis GD (1982) Displaced, unstable ankle fractures: classification, incidence and management of a consecutive series. *Clinical Orthopaedics*, **165**, 91.

Quaday K (1995) Shoulder Injuries. In: Ruiz E, Cicero JJ, eds. *Emergency Management of Skeletal Fractures*. St Louis: Mosby.

Riebel GD, McCabe JB (1991) Anterior shoulder dislocation: a review of reduction techniques. *American Journal of Emergency Medicine*, **9**(3), 180–188.

Rockward CA, Green DP (1975) *Fractures*. Philadelphia: JB Lippincott.

Ruiz E (1995) Pelvic, sacral and acetabular fractures. In: Ruiz E, Cicero JJ, eds. *Emergency Management of Skeletal Fractures*. St Louis: Mosby.

Rusnak RA (1995) Examination of the hand and management of finger-tip injuries. In: Ruiz E, Cicero JJ, eds. *Emergency Management of Skeletal Fractures*. St Louis: Mosby.

St Claire-Strange FG (1982) Entrapment of median nerve after dislocation of the elbow. *Journal of Bone and Joint Surgery*, **64B**, 224.

Schmidt M, Armbrecht A, Havermann D (1992) Results of surgical management of scapula fractures. 78th annual meeting of the Swiss Society of Accident Surgery and Occupational Diseases. *Z-Unfallchir Versicherungsmed*, **85**, 186–188.

Simon RR, Koenigsknect SJ, Stevens C (1987) *Emergency Orthopedics: the Extremities*, 2nd edn. Conneticut: Appleton & Lange.

Snyder PE (1998) Fractures. In: Maher AB, Salmond SW, Pellino TA, eds. *Orthopaedic Nursing*, 2nd edn. Philadelphia: WB Saunders.

Stiell IG, Greenberg GH, McKnight RD, Nair RC, McDowell I, Worthington JR 1992. A study to develop clinical decision rules for the use of radiography in acute ankle injuries. *Annals of Emergency Medicine*, **21**(4), 384–390.

Tsai AK, Ruiz E (1995) The elbow joint. In: Ruiz E, Cicero JJ, eds. *Emergency Management of Skeletal Fractures*. St Louis: Mosby.

Tullos HG, Bennett JG, Braly WG (1984) Acute shoulder dislocations: factors influencing diagnosis and treatment. In: *The American Academy of Orthopaedic Surgeons Instructors Course Lectures*. St Louis, Mosby, vol. 33.

Ward W (1999) Key issues in nurse requested X-rays. *Emergency Nurse*, **6**(9), 19–23.

Whelan L (1997) Ankle injury: a case study. *Emergency Nurse*, **5**(7), 24–27.

Wickham N (1997a) Pressure area care in A&E: part one. *Emergency Nurse*, **5**(3), 26–31.

Wickham N (1997b) Pressure area care in A&E: Part Two. *Emergency Nurse*, **5**(4), 25–29.

Wilkerson CA (1992) Ankle injury in athletes. *Primary Care*, **19**, 377–392.

Wyatt JP, Illingworth RN, Clancy MJ, Munro P, Robertson CE (1999) *Oxford Handbook of Accident & Emergency Medicine*. Oxford: Oxford University Press.

Zagorski JB, Latta LL, Zych GA *et al.* (1988) Diaphyseal fractures of the humerus: treatment with prefabricated braces. *Journal of Bone and Joint Surgery*, **70A**, 607–610.

Chapter 6

Spinal Injuries

Mike Paynter

- Introduction
- Anatomy and physiology
- Pathophysiology
- History-taking
- Examination
- Cervical spine fractures
- Thoracolumbar spine fractures
- Spinal cord injury
- Conclusion

Introduction

At present the annual incidence of spinal cord injury in the UK is about 10–15 per million of the population. The majority of patients with spinal cord injury are male, usually below the age of 40, with a quarter of all cord-injured patients being below the age of 20 (Perez-Avila 1986). Many of these patients are left with permanent disabilities. The overall physical, emotional and financial consequences of disability are devastating for those injured, and for their families and friends.

Although the effect of the initial injury is irreversible, the spine and spinal cord are at further risk from secondary insult either by accidental ill-handling at the accident scene or by subsequent poor management in the A&E department. This chapter explores the identification and management of spinal cord injuries in A&E.

Anatomy and Physiology

The vertebral column is a series of stacked bones that support the head and trunk and provide the bony encasement for the spinal cord. It comprises 33 vertebrae – seven cervical, 12 thoracic, five lumbar, five fused sacral and usually four rudimentary coccygeal vertebrae. With the exception of the atlas (C1) and the axis (C2), all vertebrae are anatomically alike but differ in size and function (see Fig. 6.1).

The human vertebral column enables people to assume an upright position. It provides a base of muscle attachments, protects the spinal cord and vital organs in the thorax, and allows for body movements to occur. Intervertebral cartilaginous discs provide cushioning and shock absorption between vertebral segments.

The spinal cord lies protected within the spinal canal, which is a hollow tunnel extending the length of the vertebral column. The spinal cord descends from the medulla oblongata near the atlas to the level of the second lumbar vertebra. The spinal cord is nearly

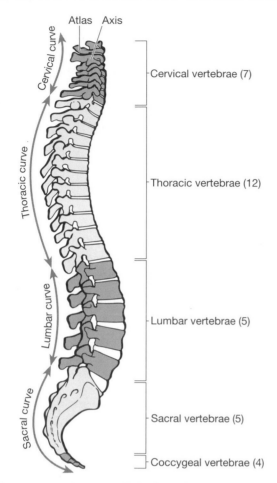

Figure 6.1 – *Anatomy of spinal vertebrae.*

circular in section and about 1 cm in diameter, with two enlargements. On cross-section, the spinal cord has a grey matter, appearing in the form of the letter H. The grey matter consists of nerve cells that act as relay stations for nerve impulses transmitted up and down the spinal cord. White matter surrounds the grey matter and contains longitudinal myelinated fibres organised in tracts or bundles to carry information to and from the brain. Ascending tracts are sensory, and descending tracts are motor (Jaworski & Wirtz 1995).

Pathophysiology

Vertebral column injury, with or without neurologic deficits, must always be sought and excluded in a patient with multiple trauma. Any injury above the clavicle should prompt a search for a cervical spine (c-spine) injury. Approximately 15% of patients sustaining such an injury will have an actual (c-spine) injury. Approximately 55% of spinal injuries occur in the

cervical region, 15% in the thoracic region, 15% at the thoracolumbar junction, and 15% in the lumbosacral area. Approximately 5% of patients have an associated spinal injury, while 25% of spinal injury patients have at least a mild head injury (American College of Surgeons 1997).

The majority of spinal cord injuries are closed. The specific mechanisms of injury that cause spinal trauma are (Pre-Hospital Trauma Life Support Committee 1994):

■ excessive flexion or hyperextension
■ axial loading or compression-type injuries
■ hyperrotation, sudden or excessive lateral bending
■ distraction
■ a combination of any of the above.

The most common type of injury mechanism is excessive flexion. This usually occurs following road traffic accidents (RTAs) when the patient's head strikes the steering wheel or windscreen and the spine is forced into hyperflexion with the chin thrown forward to the chest. Rupture of the posterior ligaments results in forward dislocation of the spine (see Fig. 6.2).

Axial loading or compression-type injuries can occur when the head strikes an object and the weight of the still moving body bears against the now stationary head, such as when the head of an unrestrained car passenger is flung into the windscreen or during a dive into shallow water. Vertebral bodies are wedged and compressed, and the burst vertebral fragments enter the spinal canal, piercing the cord (Jaworski & Wirtz 1995) (see Fig. 6.3).

Rotational injuries (e.g. Fig. 6.4) can result from a number of causes. Disruption of the entire ligamentous structure, fracture and fracture-dislocation of spinal facets may occur. Flexion-rotation injuries are highly unstable fractures.

Distraction, or over-elongation of the spine, occurs when one part of the spine is stable and the rest is in longitudinal motion. This 'pulling apart' of the spine can easily cause stretching and tearing of the cord. It is a common mechanism of injury in children's playground accidents and in hangings (Pre-Hospital Trauma Life Support Committee 1994).

Table 6.1 outlines the categories of movement that may result in spinal cord injury.

History–taking

The importance of obtaining the patient's history and establishing the mechanism of injury cannot be over-emphasised. Obtaining an accurate history represents 90% of the diagnosis (American College of Surgeons 1997). A fully documented pre-hospital history should

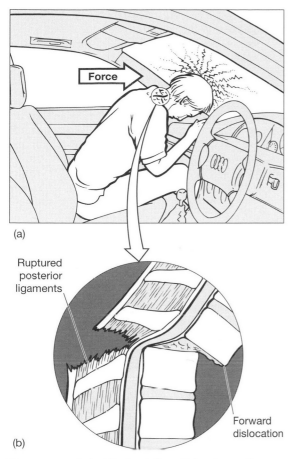

(a)

Ruptured posterior ligaments

Forward dislocation

(b)

Figure 6.2 – *Spinal flexion injury. (After Jaworski &* *Wirtz 1995.)*

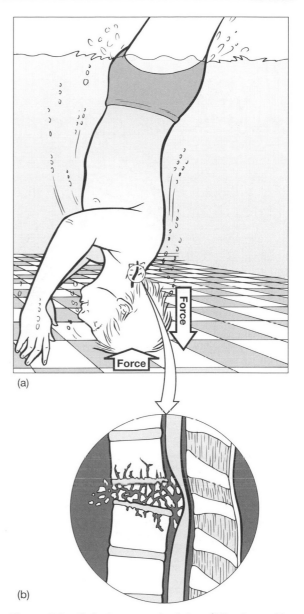

(a)

(b)

Figure 6.3 – *Spinal compression injury. (After Jaworski* *& Wirtz 1995.)*

be obtained from the ambulance personnel, police officers and others involved in the pre-hospital phase of patient care. If the patient has been injured as the result of a RTA, Polaroid pictures of the accident scene and the damage sustained to vehicles can provide valuable information about the mechanisms involved. If taken, these photographs should be included in the patient's hospital notes.

A high index of suspicion is needed if patients are to be managed correctly (Caroline 1983). Spinal cord injury should be suspected with any of the following:

■ a history of significant trauma and altered mental status from intoxication
■ a history of seizure activity since the accident
■ any complaint of neck pain or altered sensation in the upper extremities
■ a complaint of neck tenderness
■ a history of loss of consciousness
■ an injury above the clavicle

■ a fall greater than three times the patient's height
■ a fall that results in a fracture of the heels
■ an unrestrained (no seat belt) person with a facial injury
■ significant injuries in a RTA that result in chest and intra-abdominal injuries.

The patient may complain of a feeling of 'electric shock' or 'hot water' running down his back. A history of incontinence before arrival in A&E may be reported

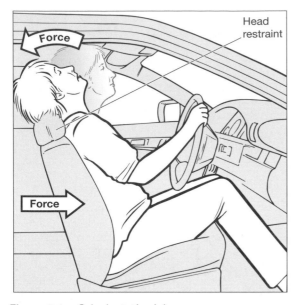

Force

Head
restraint

Force

Figure 6.4 – *Spinal rotation injury.*

Table 6.1 – *Categories of movement that may result in spinal cord injury (Semonin-Holleran 1998)*

Category	Mechanism of injury
Hyperextension	The head is forced back and the vertebrae of the cervical region are placed in an overextended position
Hyperflexion	The head is forced forward and the cervical vertebrae are placed in an overflexion position
Axial loading	A severe blow to the top of the head causes a blunt downward force on the vertebrae and the spinal column
Compression	Forces from above and below compress the vertebrae
Lateral bend	The head and neck are bent to one side, beyond the normal range of motion
Overrotation and distraction	The head turns to one side and the cervical vertebrae are forced beyond normal limits

(Semonin-Holleran 1998). Priapism may be noted in male patients due to parasympathetic nervous system stimulation and loss of sympathetic nervous system control. Failure to suspect a spinal injury will lead to failure in its detection, with potentially devastating consequences for the patient.

The patient's ability to walk should not be a factor in determining whether he needs to be treated for spine injury. Not all patients will have a dramatic entrance into the A&E department; in one American study 17% of patients who required surgical repair of unstable spine injuries were found 'walking around' at the accident scene or walked into the A&E department in the local hospital (McSwain 1992). A nod of the head or a sneeze in such patients could easily push an unstable fragment of vertebra against the spinal cord. Therefore an unstable spine can only be ruled out by X-ray examination or a lack of any potential mechanism.

Examination

Spine immobilisation

When the patient arrives in the A&E department, extreme care is required in the transfer from the ambulance stretcher to the trauma trolley: total spinal immobilisation is the goal. The use of a 'scoop' stretcher is ideal for the transfer of such patients.

Once the patient is on the trauma trolley, protection of the cervical spine should be given the same priority as the airway (American College of Surgeons 1997). All accident personnel involved in caring for the patient must be continually aware that imprudent movement of the spine has the potential to cause secondary injury. The patient must have the cervical spine immobilised in a semi-rigid well-fitting cervical collar (Aprahamian *et al.* 1984), have sandbags either side for lateral stabilisation and have the forehead taped to the trauma trolley. Semi-rigid cervical collars alone are inadequate.

It should also be noted that in children the head is large and the posterior musculature is not well developed. If placed on a rigid board or trolley, a child's head is typically moved to severe flexion. When immobilising children, significant padding under the torso is usually necessary to maintain the immobilis-ation (Pre-Hospital Trauma Life Support Committee 1994).

One member of the A&E team must remain at the patient's head and ensure total in-line immobilisation of the spine and airway patency. This team member should communicate with the patient, explaining what is happening and why. The patient is in an unnatural environment, probably surrounded by strangers, and is likely to feel out of control of his situation, because of carer interventions. Reassurance and support are therefore vital in gaining the patient's cooperation. If the patient is confused, agitated and restless, it is advisable to leave only the semi-rigid cervical collar on and not to use forcible restraint. Otherwise the patient will be liable to twist and thrash, causing unwanted movement of the neck and trunk and a possible total transection of a partially transected spinal cord. Once the patient has become settled, full immobilisation can be initiated (Tippett 1993).

Maintaining airway patency

Obstruction of the airway is an ever-present threat in managing patients with suspected cervical spine injuries. Normal efforts used for maintaining airway patency are liable to exacerbate the injuries (Aprahamian *et al.* 1984). If the patient can talk in a normal voice and give appropriate answers to questions, the airway is patent and the brain is being perfused (Skinner *et al.* 1996). In an unconscious patient, potential problems come from the tongue falling back against the posterior pharyngeal wall and causing an obstruction. Foreign bodies, such as loose teeth and broken denture plates, and the risk of regurgitation and aspiration all put the airway at risk.

Obstruction caused by the tongue is corrected by the chin lift. The airway can then be maintained by the insertion of an oropharyngeal airway (Safar & Bircher 1988). To perform the chin lift, place the fingers of one hand under the mandible and gently lift the chin upward; the thumb of the same hand lightly depresses the lower lip to open the mouth. The chin lift is the method of choice for the patient with a suspected spinal injury since it does not risk aggravating a possible fracture.

The jaw thrust is another technique. This is performed by grasping the angles of the lower jaw, one hand on each side; forward displacement of the mandible will open the airway. Again, great care must be taken not to flex or extend the neck. All debris, such as broken teeth or loose denture plates, must be removed in order to prevent potential problems. These can be removed using Magill forceps under direct vision.

Blood and vomit must be removed immediately. A rigid wide-bore suction device, with head-down tilt of the trauma trolley, will help to prevent aspiration. The semi-prone recovery position is contraindicated since it involves cervical rotation. Endotracheal intubation with a cuffed tube is the definitive method of securing a patent airway, preventing aspiration and aiding ventilation, oxygenation and suctioning. If intubation is required, it must be performed by a suitably skilled and experienced member of the team (Safar & Bircher 1988). During intubation, in-line cervical spinal immo-

bilisation must be maintained. Cricoid pressure can be applied through the aperture in the front of the semi-rigid collar. Stimulation of the oropharynx during intubation or suctioning may cause a vagal discharge, resulting in profound bradycardia. The heart rate should be closely monitored during intubation and supported if necessary with intravenous atropine.

Primary survey

Once the patient has a safe patent airway and full cervical spine precautions are in place, further examination can proceed. All clothing needs to be removed to facilitate examination; this should cause minimum discomfort and not aggravate potential injuries (Rutherford 1989). Under no circumstances must the neck or trunk be flexed, extended or rotated during this process. Extending the arms to the side or elevating them above the head causes angulation of the shoulder girdle and substantial movement of the cervical spine. Therefore, to ensure no disruption to the cervical immobilisation, it is often safest to cut away clothing. Clothing that remains under the patient can be removed during the later log roll.

Once the airway and cervical spine are protected, a full set of baseline vital signs must be recorded:

- the patient's neurological status
- respiratory rate
- pulse
- blood pressure
- temperature
- blood glucose levels
- 12-lead electrocardiograph.

In patients who are potentially haemodynamically unstable, cardiac monitoring and measurement of oxygen saturation should be considered.

Secondary survey and the log roll

As part of the secondary survey, the patient's back must be fully examined. Obviously this involves turning the injured patient. Without losing control of the in-line cervical spine immobilisation, this can be safely accomplished by using the log roll technique (Tippett 1993). Four members of the team are required to safely execute this procedure (see Fig. 6.5). The senior team member assumes manual control of the cervical spine; only then are tapes and sandbags removed. The remaining three members of the team take responsibility for the thorax, pelvis and legs. The senior person at the patient's head coordinates the roll. The person holding the leg keeps the lateral malleolus in line with the hip, preventing adduction.

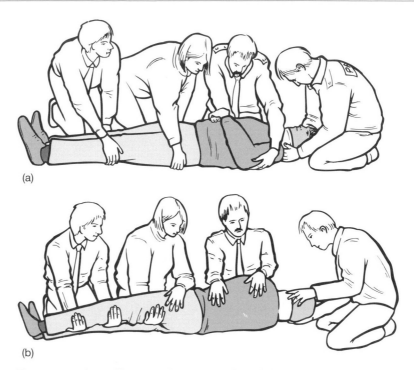

(a)

(b)

Figure 6.5 – *Log rolling the spinal patient. A: Initial position. B: Patient on side during roll. (From Greaves et al. 1997.)*

The patient is then smoothly rolled in a well coordinated move, avoiding any rotational movements of individual spinal segments.

The cervical, thoracic and lumbar spines are all examined for areas of deformity, grating crepitus, haematomas and areas of increased pain on palpation. An assessment for paraesthesia is made, noting the location and level. Finally a rectal examination is performed, the aim of which is to assess rectal sphincter tone, and thereby the sacral nerves. If voluntary sphincter contraction occurs, the spinal injury is classified as incomplete (Jaworski & Wirtz 1995). Before the patient is returned to the supine position, all remaining clothing that may have been left under the patient can be removed at this stage. Debris such as windscreen glass fragments can easily be cleared away with the aid of a portable car vacuum, thus minimising further risk to the patient's skin and pressure areas.

Once full posterior examination of the patient has been performed, the person holding the head gives the command for all members of the team to return the patient to the supine position. Once returned, sandbags and tape are reapplied and manual immobilisation can then be discontinued.

Cervical Spine Fractures

The cervical spine is the most mobile part of the entire vertebral column and as such is liable to considerable injury. Sudden violent forces can move the spine beyond its normal range of movement, either by impacting on the head and neck or by pushing the trunk out from under the head. Since extreme forces are required to damage the cervical spine, patients will often present with severe head and maxillo facial wounds. Despite what may look like horrific injuries, the ATLS principles of patient care should be applied: airway and cervical spine management is first and foremost, followed by breathing and circulatory support as appropriate.

Good quality X-rays are essential for accurate diagnosis of spinal injury (Swain *et al.* 1996). There are only three radiographs that are mandatory in the resuscitation room and these can be obtained as soon as life-threatening problems have been identified and controlled. The first is a lateral cervical spine view, and the other two are of the chest and pelvis. The lateral cervical spine views can be obtained without interrupting immobilisation (Aprahamian *et al.* 1984).

All seven cervical vertebrae, C1 to the C7/T1

junction, must be identified on the lateral film (Grundy 1993). If problems are encountered viewing C7, the application of downwards traction on the arms will pull the shoulders down and should make viewing easier. Sometimes this proves impossible. If this is the case a 'swimmer's view' of the lower cervical spine and upper thoracic areas can be obtained (Kirby 1991). The lateral radiographs will normally show any fractures, dislocations or subluxations. The type of vertebral injury most likely to produce neurological damage is a fracture-dislocation. Inadequate or misinterpreted radiographs of the cervical spine are potentially devastating for the patient. It is vital that the A&E nurse insists on continued c-spine immobilisation until all radiographs have been reviewed and C1 to C7 have been cleared of abnormality.

All cervical spine fractures should be treated as unstable in the A&E department and, depending upon neurological examination, be referred to the orthopaedic, neurosurgical or specialist spinal unit teams.

Thoracolumbar Spine Fractures

Fractures of the thoracic spine between T2 and T10 are usually the result of hyperflexion which produces a wedge compression of one or more vertebrae. Wedge compression fractures of the thorax are rarely unstable because the rib cage provides fairly rigid support; however, these fractures can be rendered unstable if there are associated fractures of the ribs and sternum. Fractures of the thoracic vertebrae tend to be slightly more common in elderly patients, where they are often associated with a degree of osteoporosis and can sometimes occur with minimal trauma. In younger patients, severe trauma is required to cause these fractures (Segelov 1986). Fractures of the thoracolumbar region are frequently due to the relative immobility of the thoracic spine compared with the lumbar spine. The mechanism of injury is usually acute hyperflexion and rotation, and hence these fractures are commonly unstable.

Falling from a height and landing on the feet can result in compression and axial loading. The impact of landing forces the weight of the head and thorax down against the lumbar vertebrae, while the sacral vertebrae remain stationary. Fractures of the lumbar vertebrae are reasonably common, especially at the T12/L1 and L4/S levels (Kirby 1991). Twenty per cent of falls greater than 15 feet involve associated fractures of the lumbar vertebrae (McSwain 1992).

Isolated sacral fractures are uncommon and are frequently associated with much more serious fractures of the pelvis. As with cervical spine injuries, the patient must be kept in the neutral position and complete spinal immobilisation maintained. The log roll must be employed to facilitate examination of the back.

Spinal Cord Injury

The main risk factor associated with spinal fractures is damage to the spinal cord. If the fracture is stable, the cord is safe, but if the fracture is unstable the possibility of cord injury is present. Stable fractures are not likely to displace further than at the time of injury; an unstable fracture or dislocation is, however, liable to further displacement, therefore posing considerable risk to the spinal cord (Crawford-Adams 1987).

The spinal cord is the communication pathway between the brain and the body. A transection of the cord will render all nerves distal to the injury useless. A conscious patient will be able to identify pain at the site of the injury but have no sensation below it; from the moment of injury the patient feels cut in two. Voluntary movement below the level of the cord injury is lost immediately and the muscles become flaccid. The bladder and rectum are paralysed, however the bladder sphincter subsequently recovers and causes acute urinary retention.

The position of the cord injury has a direct effect on the patient's prognosis. Complete transection of the cord at levels C1, 2 or 3 is incompatible with life. Damage to the cord at this level causes both intercostal and diaphragmatic movement to cease, and only intermittent positive pressure ventilation (IPPV) will keep the patient alive. Lower cervical cord damage may leave the phrenic nerve sufficiently intact to maintain diaphragmatic breathing. Diaphragmatic breathing only, provided from C4 to T6, is liable to reduce vital capacity and a subsequent compensatory tachypnoea will develop. If tidal volume and vital capacity are reduced, consideration must be given to intubating and providing IPPV (Robertson & Redmond 1994).

If the patient is unconscious, the following clinical findings will indicate a cervical cord injury:

- diaphragmatic breathing
- hypotension with bradycardia
- flaccid rectal sphincter
- evidence of painful stimuli above the clavicles
- ability to flex, but not extend, the elbows
- priapism.

Since the urinary bladder is paralysed when the cord is damaged, acute urinary retention will occur.

Insertion under strict aseptic technique of an indwelling urinary catheter will be required to decompress the bladder in order to monitor the patient's haemodynamic status. Short periods of local pressure result in pressure sores. It is essential that all clothing and debris are removed from under the patient at the earliest opportunity, ideally during the secondary survey log roll procedure. Loss of gastrointestinal tone will result in the cessation of peristaltic activity with subsequent gastric distension and a paralytic ileus, necessitating the use of a nasogastric tube. High dose methylprednisolone given during the first 8 hours after spinal cord injury has been shown to improve neurological function (Swain 1997). Advice concerning steroid treatment should be sought from the local spinal injury unit.

Neurogenic shock

Neurogenic shock is the term used to describe hypotension associated with cervical or high thoracic spinal cord injury. It results from impairment of the descending sympathetic pathways in the cord between T1 and L2, resulting in the loss of vasomotor and cardiac sympathetic tone. Loss of vasomotor tone causes vasodilation and a pooling of blood in the lower extremities, resulting in hypotension. Loss of cardiac tone produces a bradycardia (Skinner *et al.* 1996).

Patients presenting to the A&E department may have extensive injuries that would normally be associated with a hypovolaemic shock state; bradycardia with hypotension – not tachycardia and hypotension – should increase suspicion of spinal cord injury. The peripheral skin is generally warm and dry because of peripheral vasodilation and may be either flushed or pale (Selfridge-Thomas 1995). Fluid resuscitation is required if circulatory volume is to be restored (Grundy 1993). Overloading the patient who is in purely neurogenic shock can precipitate pulmonary oedema, and therefore all patients must have careful monitoring of their vital signs in order to detect the physiological response to fluid resuscitation (Mitchell 1994). Insertion of an indwelling catheter will drain the dysfunctional bladder and provide information about overall tissue perfusion. Central venous pressure monitoring also provides an accurate method of determining response. Improved cardiac output may be indicated by a heart rate above 50 beats/min and a systolic pressure of greater than 100 mmHg.

Spinal shock

Spinal shock (or cord shock) is a temporary neurological condition that occurs after injury to the cord above the T6 level. The signs are a loss of all motor, sensory, reflex and autonomic responses below the site of the injury. There will be flaccidity and a positive Babinski sign, i.e. dorsal flexion of the first toe instead of plantarflexion, although all areas below the level of injury will not necessarily be permanently destroyed (Royle & Walsh 1992). Hypotension, bradycardia and hypothermia, because of the loss of sympathetic control and tone, are classic signs of spinal cord shock that occur immediately after injury.

Spinal shock may subside in a few days or may persist for much longer. Its end is marked by a return of reflex activity in the spinal cord. In areas where no function has returned, flaccid paralysis becomes spastic with increased tone. The diagnosis of spinal shock can only be formally made retrospectively. The immediate management in the A&E department is the same as for any cord-injured patient.

Conclusion

Spinal injuries are a common cause for presentation to the A&E department. The injuries range from simple muscle spasm, possibly with no history of trauma (as in a torticollis), to gross fracture-dislocations with associated spinal cord damage. Whatever associated injuries coexist, the priorities – airway with cervical spine control, breathing and circulatory support – remain unchanged, as hypoxia from an upper airway obstruction or transection of the upper cervical cord will kill before hypoperfusion.

The nurse should always listen carefully to the pre-hospital history to find out the mechanism of injury, maintain a high index of suspicion and if in doubt initiate full spinal immobilisation. A semi-rigid cervical collar alone will not provide adequate immobilisation; sandbags and tape must be used. The initial damage from the injury has already occurred, and A&E staff must prevent secondary injury by careful handling of the patient – one false move could result in quadriplegia or paraplegia. Failure to suspect spinal injury can lead to failure in its detection. All vertebral fractures should be treated as unstable in the A&E department until fully examined by senior A&E, orthopaedic or neurosurgical staff.

References

American College of Surgeons (Committee on Trauma) (1997) *Advanced Trauma Life Support, Student Manual*. Chicago: American College of Surgeons.

Aprahamian C, Thompson BM, Finger WA, Darin JC (1984) Experimental cervical spine injury model: evaluation of airway management and splinting. *Annals of Emergency Medicine*, **13**(8), 584–587.

Caroline N (1983) *Emergency Care in the Streets*, 2nd edn. Boston: Little Brown.

Crawford-Adams J (1987) *Outline of Fractures*, 8th edn. Edinburgh: Churchill Livingstone.

Greaves I, Hodgetts T, Porter T (1997) *Emergency Care: a Textbook for Paramedics*: London: WB Saunders.

Grundy D (1993) *ABC of Spinal Cord Injury*, 2nd edn. Bristol: BMJ Publications.

Jaworski MA, Wirtz KM (1995) Spinal trauma. In: Kitt S, Selfridge-Thomas J, Proehl JA, Kaiser J, eds. *Emergency Nursing – a Physiological and Clinical Perspective*. Philadelphia: WB Saunders.

Kirby N (1991) *Accidents and Emergencies*. London: Castle House Publications.

McSwain N (1992) *Advanced Emergency Care*. Philadelphia: JB Lippincott.

Mitchell M (1994) Spinal cord injury. In: Hudak C, Gallo BM, eds. *Critical Care Nursing: a Holistic Approach*, 6th edn. Philadelphia: JB Lippincott.

Perez-Avila C (1986) Spinal injuries. *Paramedic UK*, **1**(9), 256–257.

Pre-Hospital Trauma Life Support Committee (1994) *PHTLS: Basic and Advanced Pre-Hospital Trauma Life Support*. St Louis: Mosby Lifeline.

Robertson C, Redmond AD (1994) *The Management of Major Trauma*, 2nd edn. Oxford: Oxford University Press

Royle J, Walsh M (eds) (1992) *Watson's Medical-surgical Nursing and Related Physiology*, 4th edn. London: Bailière Tindall.

Rutherford W (1989) *Accident and Emergency Medicine*, 2nd edn. Edinburgh: Churchill Livingstone.

Safar P, Bircher N (1988) *Cardiopulmonary Cerebral Resuscitation*, 3rd edn. London: WB Saunders.

Segelov P (1986) *Manual of Emergency Orthopaedics*. Edinburgh: Churchill Livingstone.

Selfridge-Thomas J (1995) Shock. In: Kitt S, Selfridge-Thomas J, Proehl JA, Kaiser J, eds. *Emergency Nursing – a Physiological and Clinical Perspective*. Philadelphia: WB Saunders.

Semonin-Holleran R (1998) Spinal trauma. In: Newberry L, ed. *Sheehy's Emergency Nursing: Principles and Practice*, 4th edn. St Louis: Mosby.

Skinner D, Driscoll P, Earlam R (1996) *ABC of Major Trauma*, 2nd edn. London: BMJ.

Swain A (1997) Trauma to the spine and spinal cord. In: Skinner D, Swain A, Peyton R, eds. *Cambridge Textbook of Accident and Emergency Medicine*. Cambridge: Cambridge University Press.

Swain A, Dove J, Baker H (1996) Trauma of the spine and spinal cord. In: Skinner D, Driscoll P, Earlam R, eds. *ABC of Major Trauma*. London: BMJ.

Tippett J (1993) Providing comfort in the resuscitation room. *Accident and Emergency Nursing*, **2**(3), 155–159.

Chapter 7

Thoracic Injuries

Karen Castille & Lynda Holt

- Introduction
- Mechanism of injury
- Anatomy of the chest
- The physiology of respiration
- Principles of care
- Immediately life-threatening injuries
- Serious chest injury
- Sternum, ribs and scapular injuries
- Conclusion

Introduction

Thoracic injury is one of the most serious types of trauma and may result in disruption of the airway, breathing or circulation. It is responsible for approximately 25% of trauma-related deaths (Driscoll *et al.* 1993). Many patients who sustain severe chest injuries die immediately (Westaby & Brayley 1991). Patients who reach hospital alive, however, have a good chance of survival if a systematic approach to their assessment and treatment is adopted. Westaby & Brayley (1991) found that, in practice, less than 15% of patients with chest injuries required surgical intervention. The majority of patients improve dramatically following simple procedures. The management of patients with chest injuries can therefore be challenging and rewarding.

Mechanism of Injury

The A&E nurse is likely to be the first contact with the patient on arrival at the hospital. It is therefore imperative that the nurse obtains all available information about the patient and the incident. It is important to remember that serious intrathoracic injury can occur without obvious external damage to the chest wall. The mechanism of injury is an essential part of the history and can give crucial diagnostic clues to aid patient assessment. The main consideration is whether the chest injury was caused by blunt or penetrating trauma. In addition, an estimate of the velocity (speed) causing the injury may be gleaned from evidence of intrusion or vehicle damage. Known high-velocity trauma, the presence of other seriously injured or dead people, ejection from a vehicle or fall from a great height are indicative of the potential for serious injuries to be present.

In the UK, as ballistic injuries are relatively uncommon, blunt chest trauma is currently more common than penetrating trauma. Blunt chest trauma commonly results from rapid deceleration of the chest wall against a solid object. Typically, this is seen following road traffic accidents (RTAs) in which the chest strikes the vehicle steering wheel, causing a high-velocity blunt chest injury. Blunt chest trauma can also result from a fall from a height. This type of chest trauma may be associated with injuries to the great vessels, major airways, lung parenchyma and myocardium, as well as diaphragmatic rupture and fractures to the ribs and/or sternum. Crush injuries may also be caused by RTAs or industrial accidents. Frequently, fractured ribs and cardiac and pulmonary contusion may ensue. Other causes of blunt chest trauma include blast injury and low-velocity impact from direct blows to the chest. Most penetrating chest injuries in the UK are caused by stabbing (Castille 1993); gunshot wounds, farming, industrial and road traffic incidents are less common causes.

Although this chapter deals predominantly with chest injuries, it is imperative that the chest is not viewed in isolation, as other life-threatening injuries outside of the chest may be present. While chest trauma may occur in isolation, it is more common in patients with multiple injuries. Ingestion of alcohol or drugs is particularly noteworthy in patients with chest trauma because the pattern, depth and rate of respiration may be affected.

Anatomy of the Chest

The chest wall. Chest injury occurs when there is damage to the thoracic cage or its contents. The thoracic cage comprises ribs and intercostal muscles. It is divided by the central mediastinum which acts as a partition between the lungs. The outer surface of each lung is covered by the visceral pleura and this is reflected onto the chest wall as the parietal pleura (see Fig. 7.1). The two pleural layers are effectively sealed together by a film of pleural fluid which exerts a strong surface tension force that prevents separation of the membranes. This seal is essential since it enables the lungs, which themselves contain no skeletal muscle, to be expanded and relaxed by movements of the chest wall (Hinchliff *et al.* 1996). If the pleura is breached, e.g. as a result of penetrating trauma, the integrity of this system is disrupted and the lung will collapse.

The mediastinum forms the central part of the thorax and extends from the sternum to the vertebral column. The mediastinum contains the trachea, oesophagus and major blood vessels, such as the aorta. It also encases the heart. It is important in the assessment of a trauma patient because disruption of its shape, such as widening, is indicative of damage to one of the structures within it, most commonly the aorta.

The heart lies above the diaphragm at the base of the thoracic cavity, with two-thirds of its bulk to the left of the body's midline. The outer surface of the heart is covered by the visceral pericardium. This is reflected onto the surrounding fibrous sac to form the parietal pericardium. A thin film of fluid separates these pericardial surfaces allowing the heart to move freely, only being anchored by the great vessels (see Fig. 7.2). This potential space can become filled with blood

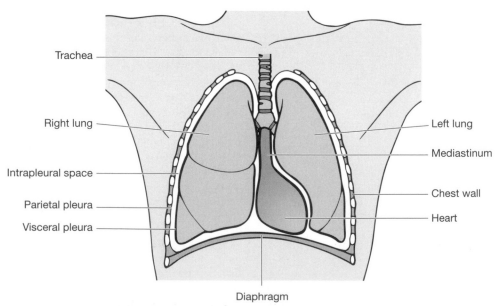

Labels (left): Trachea, Right lung, Intrapleural space, Parietal pleura, Visceral pleura

Labels (right): Left lung, Mediastinum, Chest wall, Heart

Label (bottom): Diaphragm

Figure 7.1 – *Relationship between lungs, thoracic cage and pleurae.*

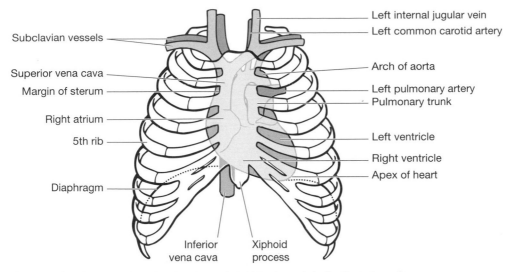

Figure 7.2 – *Location of the heart and associated blood vessels in the thoracic cavity.*

(haemopericardium) following trauma or myocardial infarction. As the fibrous pericardium is unable to distend, any fluid collecting within the potential space (pericardial cavity) will exert pressure on the heart and impair filling.

Below the level of the fourth inter-costal space, the thoracic cage surrounds the upper abdominal region, particularly when the diaphragm elevates during expiration. Any injury to the ribs at or below this level should alert the nurse that an intra-abdominal injury, specifically to the liver, spleen or diaphragm, may also be present.

The Physiology of Respiration

The key functions of respiration are oxygen uptake and carbon dioxide elimination. To enable this to happen, air is conveyed through the respiratory tract – this is called ventilation (see Fig. 7.3).

In addition, an adequate blood volume must circulate through the pulmonary capillaries. This is called perfusion. The exchange of oxygen and carbon dioxide between the alveoli and capillaries is called diffusion. Gases move from an area of high partial pressure to one of low partial pressure. When leaving the lungs via the pulmonary veins, blood has its highest partial pressure of oxygen (Po_2).

Oxygen diffusion requires: a high concentration of oxygen in the alveolus; a low blood concentration of oxygen; solubility of the gas; membrane thickness that the gas has to cross; perfusion pressure; and alveolar ventilation. Damage to either system leads to hypoxia or hypercapnia, which in turn threatens homeostasis. The

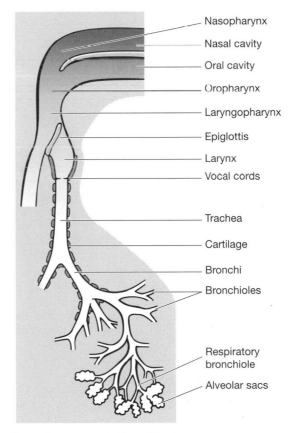

Figure 7.3 – *Organisation of the airways.*

ratio between ventilation and perfusion is fundamental to the success of respiratory function (see Fig. 7.4).

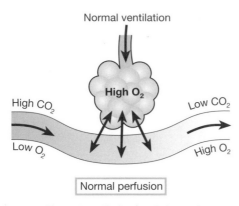

Figure 7.4 – *Normal ventilation/perfusion ratio.*

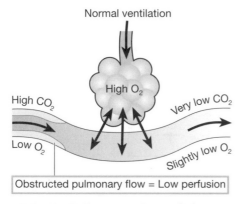

Figure 7.5 – *Ventilation greater than perfusion.*

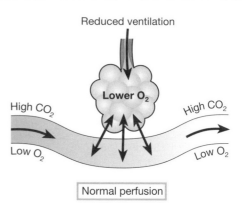

Figure 7.6 – *Ventilation lower than perfusion.*

If a problem occurs with pulmonary flow, most commonly a low circulatory volume in trauma, adequate oxygen cannot be taken up. This is because less blood passes the alveoli and there is subsequently less haemoglobin take-up of oxygen. This results in a decrease in tissue perfusion. Unbound oxygen is expired. This results in a high ventilation/perfusion ratio (see Fig. 7.5).

If ventilation decreases, most commonly with an obstructed airway, the amount of oxygen reaching the alveoli is reduced. When perfusion is normal this results in more blood and haemoglobin passing the alveoli than can be saturated with oxygen. As result, the blood leaving the lungs has a low oxygen content. This is a low ventilation/perfusion ratio (see Fig. 7.6).

Although the ventilation/perfusion ratio varies in different parts of the lung, a high ratio in one area will not offset a low ventilation/perfusion ratio in another. This is because of the reduction in haemoglobin saturation. In the trauma patient, particularly where chest injury has occurred, maintaining adequate ventilation is crucial in preventing hypoxia. A simple and vitally important nursing intervention is the early

administration of effective oxygen therapy. This is best achieved by using a reservoir bag attached to a face mask, which allows a high concentration of inspired oxygen. Oxygen therapy helps to prevent respiratory acidosis (Driscoll *et al.* 1993), which results from impaired ventilation associated with chest injury. Metabolic acidosis results from inadequate tissue perfusion secondary to airway, breathing and circulatory problems, further compounding the patient's condition.

Principles of Care

The trauma team

Many A&E departments have established a system of care for seriously injured patients based on a team approach which utilises Advanced Trauma Life Support (ATLS) principles and incorporates well established objectives of trauma management (see Ch. 2). The team leader is responsible for the coordination of care and the appropriate delegation of roles whilst maintaining an overview of the situation. The use of a standardised systematic approach not only expedites patient care, but also offers a format enabling less experienced staff to focus their activities in a predetermined order. Some hospitals have established trauma teams in which each member has a specific role.

Clearly, the A&E nurse's role is dynamic and directly related to the patient's needs. The key components of the nursing role when caring for patients with chest trauma are outlined in Box 7.1. The number and experience of other team members may influence the nurse's actual activities, but the needs of the patient and her family/friends must remain paramount. Ideally, a member of the care team will be allocated to care for and liaise with the patient's family and/or friends (see Ch. 13 for guidance on this issue).

Assessment of chest injury

The immediate management of the patient with chest injury should follow the principles laid down in the ATLS guidelines (American College of Surgeons 1997). A primary survey should be carried out to identify and treat any immediately life-threatening conditions (Box 7.2; the management of specific conditions will be discussed later in the chapter). A secondary survey, or head-to-toe examination should then be carried out to identify any other injury.

Nursing assessment of the patient's overall condition is part of the overall progress towards definitive care. Nursing observations should include:

- the rate and depth of respiration
- chest wall movement
- blood pressure
- pulse oximetry
- pulse rate and pressure
- pain assessment
- level of consciousness
- urine output.

Additional investigations include:

- cardiac monitoring
- chest X-ray
- ECG
- blood gas analysis
- blood chemistry
- full blood count and cross-match.

A specific chest injury assessment is listed in Box 7.3

Initial management of chest injury

Airway and breathing

Management of chest injury should include high-flow oxygen as described above. The method of delivery depends largely on the patient's condition; in a conscious patient without obvious compromise, use of a mask and non-rebreathing bag is the method of choice. If the patient is unable to maintain her airway, as is common after chest injury, supportive methods should be found (see Box 7.4).

Airway compromise occurs either because of damage to the airway, resulting in oedema, compression or

Box 7.4 – *Assessing and securing the airway in a trauma patient*

1. Seek verbal response from patient, by asking, for example, 'Are you all right?', while giving O_2 and stabilising the cervical spine.

2, 3 & 4 should be simultaneous
2. Look for chest movement – for 10 seconds minimum

3. Listen for breath sounds – for 10 seconds minimum (check simultaneously with chest movement)

4. Feel for expired air – for 10 seconds minimum

5. If the airway is compromised → chin lift or jaw thrust. If airway remains compromised repeat steps 3–5

6. Clear mouth of obvious debris, such as vomit, broken teeth, ill-fitting dentures

7. If airway remains compromised, repeat steps 3–5

8. Intubation with assisted ventilation. If airway remains compromised, repeat steps 3–5

Box 7.5 – *Indicators of airway obstruction*

- Apnoea
- Tachypnoea
- Increased respiratory effort
- Intercostal recession
- Use of accessory muscles
- Tracheal tug
- Stridor/noisy breathing
- Pallor/cyanosis (late sign)

Box 7.6 – *Indications for endotracheal intubation*

- Poor airway maintenance with other methods due to injury
- Loss of gag reflex with high risk of aspiration
- Compromised respiratory function due to chest injury
- Need for mechanical ventilation
- Anticipation of airway obstruction, such as increasing oedema
- Raised intracranial pressure

---

removed carefully with suction or angled forceps. It is important not to stimulate the gag reflex during suction because this can induce vomiting.

If the gag reflex is present, or the patient is conscious, a nasopharyngeal airway is best tolerated (Landon *et al.* 1994). This is inserted via the nostril to the pharynx. This type of adjunct should not be used where a base of skull fracture is suspected or where facial injuries prevent its use. The tube should never be forced. If oedema or potential haemorrhage is likely, alternative airway support should be used.

If the gag reflex is absent, the patient needs endotracheal intubation; however, an oropharyngeal or Guedel airway is the temporary support of choice (Landon *et al.* 1994). This will prevent the tongue from occluding the pharynx and provide an artificial airway. If simple airway management fails to secure a patent airway, because of either injury or vomiting, endotracheal intubation should be performed (see Box 7.6). It is important to stress the need for in-line immobilisation of the cervical spine. This is addressed in detail in Chapter 6.

bleeding, or through a deterioration in the patient's consciousness level, resulting in the loss of her gag reflex. If breathing is absent, the airway should be assumed to be blocked. Noisy breathing (stridor) may be indicative of partial upper airway obstruction. If the patient is able to give a verbal response, then the airway can be assumed to be patent (see Box 7.5).

A significant number of airway obstructions are caused by the tongue slipping back and occluding the oropharynx. These can be simply resolved by using a chin lift or jaw thrust manoeuvre. This will pull the tongue forward in the mouth and remove the obstruction. The mouth should be inspected with adequate light to identify any debris, which should be

The effectiveness of all airway management should be assessed by:

- *Looking* at chest movement
  — Is it symmetrical and bilateral?
  — Is there sufficient chest expansion?
- *Listening* to breath sounds
  — Are they present?
  — Is there stridor or gurgling from debris?
- *Feeling* for expired air.

Conditions which compromise breathing will be considered below.

Circulation

The patient's circulatory status should be assessed by:

- pulse rate and volume
- the speed of capillary return
- skin colour or pallor.

All patients should have i.v. access established with two wide-bore cannulae and a fluid regime appropriate to circulatory status. Blood should also be taken for cross-match, and baseline full blood count and urea and electrolytes during initial management. Conditions posing a specific threat to circulation will be discussed later.

Immediately Life-Threatening Chest Injuries

Pneumothorax

A pneumothorax can be caused by blunt or penetrating trauma. It occurs when the fluid seal between the parietal and visceral pleura is broken. Once the seal is broken, air rushes in, expands the space and the existing negative pressure is lost. The resulting positive pressure in the expanded intrapleural space is exerted onto the adjacent lung. This may result in partial or total collapse of the lung, and serious impairment of gaseous exchange. Because the pleural layers are separated by the mediastinum, the opposite lung continues to move with the chest wall and functions normally, unless it becomes compressed by the volume of air accumulating on the injured side (see Fig. 7.7).

> **Box 7.7** – *Classification of pneumothoraces*
>
> - **Simple** – Occurs spontaneously or as a result of blunt trauma. It is not initially life-threatening but has the potential to develop into a tension pneumothorax. A simple pneumothorax may compromise respiratory function, particularly on mild exertion
>
> - **Open** – Results from a penetrating injury, where the integrity of the chest wall is breached and air is sucked into the pleural cavity
>
> - **Tension** – Results from blunt or penetrating trauma, mechanical ventilation or from a simple pneumothorax. It occurs when air enters the pleural space and becomes trapped. The volume of air increases and causes compression of other organs

Pneumothoraces are classified in Box 7.7.

Tension pneumothorax

This is an immediately life-threatening chest injury and should be dealt with as soon as it is identified in the primary survey. Tension pneumothorax can result:

- from blunt or penetrating trauma
- from baro-trauma associated with positive pressure ventilation
- where chest injury such as rib fracture exists

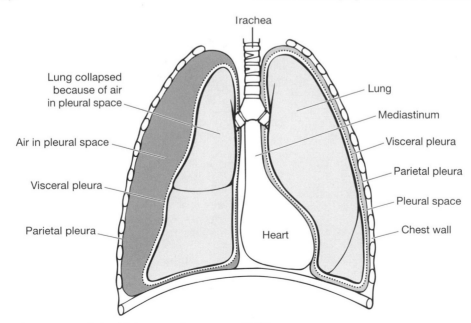

Trachea

Lung collapsed because of air in pleural space

Air in pleural space

Visceral pleura

Parietal pleura

Lung

Mediastinum

Visceral pleura

Parietal pleura

Pleural space

Chest wall

Heart

Figure 7.7 – *Right-sided pneumothorax, normal left lung.*

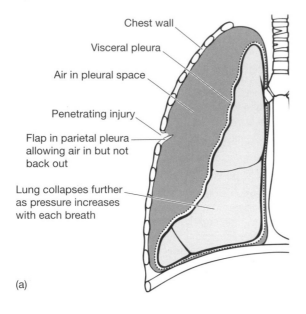

- Chest wall
- Visceral pleura
- Air in pleural space
- Penetrating injury
- Flap in parietal pleura allowing air in but not back out
- Lung collapses further as pressure increases with each breath

(a)

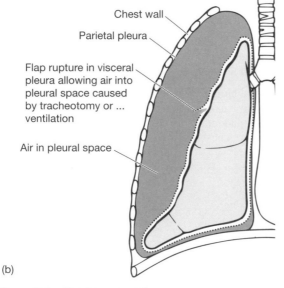

- Chest wall
- Parietal pleura
- Flap rupture in visceral pleura allowing air into pleural space caused by tracheotomy or ... ventilation
- Air in pleural space

(b)

Figure 7.8 – *Tension pneumothorax.*

- following invasive procedures, such as insertion of a central line
- as a complication of a simple pneumothorax.

It is imperative that the A&E nurse remains vigilant as a tension pneumothorax can occur at any stage of the patient's treatment.

A tension pneumothorax is a clinical diagnosis. It occurs when air is sucked into the pleural space, either from the lung or from outside the chest wall. The pleura acts as a one-way valve, trapping air in the pleural space, therefore allowing air in, but not out, of the cavity. The pressure of this causes a total collapse of the lung on the affected side. As the intrathoracic pressure increases, the mediastinum and trachea shift towards the unaffected side, causing impaired venous return and cardiac compression. This results in reduced cardiac output and severe hypotension. The increasing pressure also causes compression of the unaffected lung, compounding the patient's already compromised ventilation. A tension pneumothorax is a condition of rapid onset and demands immediate decompression of the pleural space to maintain life. Time should not be wasted by attempting to obtain a chest X-ray (see Fig. 7.8).

Assessment

Priorities for care of the patient with a tension pneumothorax lie with correct identification of the condition. A conscious patient will be very distressed because of the rapid worsening of the dyspnoea. Hypoxia may also make the patient confused, agitated and restless. Specific clinical features are highlighted in Box 7.8.

Box 7.8 – *Clinical signs of tension pneumothorax*

- Tachypnoea
- Tachycardia
- Shock
- Decreased air entry to affected side
- Hyperresonance on affected side
- Distended neck veins – if the patient is not hypovolaemic (late sign)
- Tracheal deviation away from affected side (late sign)
- Cyanosis (late sign)

A tension pneumothorax can expand rapidly. This increase in size correlates with a decrease in functional lung space. Therefore, as the condition worsens, the patient's dyspnoea, respiratory function and tissue oxygenation all deteriorate.

Immediate management

Immediate management entails maintaining oxygenation. This is a twofold activity. First, oxygen intake must be maintained either through a high-flow mask with oxygen reservoir or with assisted manual or mechanical ventilation. The second life-saving intervention is to remove the 'tension' from the pneumothorax to reduce further loss of lung capacity. This is achieved by providing an artificial escape route for the trapped air. To facilitate this, a needle thoracentesis is performed. While this is a rapid and simple procedure which buys time for the resuscitation team, it is not definitive treatment.

Chest decompression by needle thoracentesis is carried out by inserting a wide-bore (16g) cannula into the pleural space. The cannula is inserted in the second intercostal space midclavicular line over the superior aspect of the third rib. The cannula is attached to a syringe, and once *in situ*, the rapid release of air confirms initial diagnosis. This procedure should dramatically reduce the patient's discomfort and clinical symptoms.

At this stage, it is important to obtain intravenous access as bleeding may lead to hypovolaemia. A chest drain will facilitate the removal of remaining air from the pleural cavity. The chest drain is inserted in front of the midaxillary line through the fifth intercostal space. The drainage tube is connected to an underwater sealed system which allows air out of the pleural space, but not back in. Fluid levels in the drainage system should rise and fall with respiration (Landon *et al.* 1994). While a chest X-ray will verify the presence of collapsed lung and demonstrate a mediastinal shift towards the unaffected lung, if the patient has severe cardiopulmonary instability and a high suspicion of tension pneumonthorax exists, immediate treatment should be instituted without obtaining a chest X-ray film (Henneman *et al.* 1993).

Open pneumothorax

Open pneumothorax may occur following penetrating trauma in which the chest wall is pierced. When chest wall integrity is breached, e.g. by a stab wound, air can enter the pleural space creating a pneumothorax. This occurs because of a loss of negative pressure and an equalling of atmospheric and intrathoracic pressures. If the external damage to the chest wall is large enough, air will enter the pleural cavity via the wound rather than via the normal respiratory tract. This occurs if the disruption to the chest wall is greater than two-thirds of the tracheal diameter (Driscoll *et al.* 1993).

It is for this reason that an open pneumothorax is often referred to as a 'sucking chest wound', as air can be heard entering the pleural space on inspiration. As air enters the thoracic cavity by this route, respiratory efficiency is rapidly decreased. This is because of alveolar hypoventilation despite increased respiratory effort. This results in a low ventilation/perfusion ratio and tissue hypoxia.

Assessment

The mechanism of injury is the main factor in assessment. The patient will have a history of penetrating trauma and may or may not have an impaled object *in situ*. On examination, the patient will be tachypnoeic and tachycardic. The chest wound will have an audible sucking sound on inspiration. The actual size of the wound does not give significant indication of the extent of intrathoracic damage. This should be judged by the level of respiratory compromise (Rooney *et al.* 1996).

Immediate management

This is a potentially life-threatening condition and should be treated in the resuscitation phase of the primary survey. Initial management is relatively simple; it involves maintaining oxygen intake and temporary closure of the chest wound. Oxygen intake is supported by the use of high-flow oxygen via a mask and reservoir bag. If the patient is unable to maintain breathing, artificial ventilation is indicated. The chest wound is covered with a sterile occlusive dressing taped down on three sides to create a flutter valve. During inhalation, the dressing is sucked against the chest wall and acts as a seal, which prevents any further air from entering the pleural space. On expiration, the open side of the dressing pushes away from the patient's skin, allowing air to escape from the pleural space.

A dressing sealed on all sides would result in a tension pneumothorax, as air would enter the pleural space but would have no means of escape. If a tension pneumothorax is suspected, the occlusive dressing should be temporarily removed to allow air to escape (Driscoll *et al.* 1993).

Any impaled object should not be removed as this significantly increases the risk of respiratory compromise and circulatory collapse. After establishing i.v. access, a chest drain should be inserted through a surgically created hole, not via the wound, to facilitate decompression of the pleural space. The majority of patients with an open pneumothorax require surgical closure of the wound once their overall condition has been stabilised. It is at this stage that any impaled objects are usually removed.

Massive haemothorax

Haemothorax can result from penetrating trauma or

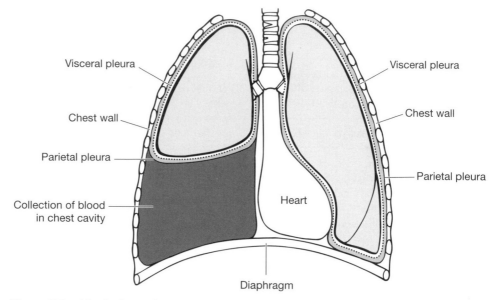

Visceral pleura

Chest wall

Parietal pleura

Collection of blood
in chest cavity

Visceral pleura

Chest wall

Parietal pleura

Heart

Diaphragm

Figure 7.9 – *Massive haemothorax.*

blunt injury where an intercostal vessel or internal mammary artery has been ruptured. It can be defined as a rapid accumulation of blood, greater than 1500 ml (Rooney *et al.* 1996), in the pleural cavity (see Fig. 7.9).

Assessment

The patient will present with tachypnoea, tachycardia and hypovolaemic shock. Specifically, chest examination will reveal decreased or absent breath sounds on the affected side. On percussion, dullness will be detected over the haemothorax due to the density of blood. Internal jugular veins should be observed; jugular venous pressure (JVP) may be elevated as a result of pressure in the thoracic cavity because of the accumulation of blood, or other associated injury, such as tension pneumothorax or cardiac tamponade. Conversely, neck veins may be collapsed as a result of hypovolaemia.

Immediate management

The patient should be given high-flow oxygen via a mask and reservoir bag. Intravenous access should be established and fluid resuscitation commenced. Once fluid replacement begins, a chest drain should be inserted to drain blood from the thoracic cavity and allow the lung to reinflate. Before a chest drain is inserted, a ruptured diaphragm should be excluded as the cause of reduced breath sounds and dull

resonance. This can be done by careful history-taking of the mechanism of injury. A chest drain should always be inserted by blunt dissection, so that any herniated abdominal organs can be felt with a finger prior to the insertion of a drainage tube, thus preventing further injury. Bleeding to the lung parenchyma usually stops once the lung is reinflated because of the drop in pulmonary perfusion (Driscoll *et al.* 1993). If bleeding persists at a drainage rate of greater than 200 ml/h, a thoracotomy is indicated to stop bleeding.

Flail chest

Flail chest usually results from blunt trauma, most commonly crush injuries (Rooney *et al.* 1996). It is defined as an injury from rib fractures, with or without sternal involvement, which results in a disruption in the continuity of chest wall movement. A segment of the thoracic cage loses its bony continuity because of the fractures and subsequently moves paradoxically to the rest of the chest wall. A flail segment results from the fracture of two or more adjacent ribs in two places, therefore disconnecting them from the rest of the thoracic cage (Fig. 7.10).

This paradoxical movement on inspiration reduces tidal volume, and therefore compromises ventilation. While this carries a risk of hypoxia, the primary danger to the patient stems from underlying lung injury. Lung contusion or penetrating injury can cause profound hypoxia, and rib fractures cause significant

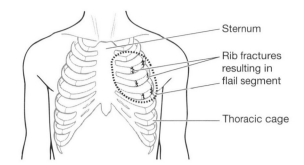

Sternum

Rib fractures resulting in flail segment

Thoracic cage

Figure 7.10 – *Flail chest.*

Box 7.9 – *Indications for mechanical ventilation*

- Respiratory rate of >30 breaths/min
- Exhaustion
- Falling Pao_2<10.5 kPa on O_2
- Rising $Paco_2$>6.0 kPa on O_2
- Associated head injuries
- Respiratory rate <10 breaths/min

hypovolaemia, particularly if there is sternal involvement.

Assessment

Rib fractures are extremely painful and the conscious patient will complain of severe chest pain and difficulty in breathing. The patient will be tachypnoeic with shallow breaths, tachycardic and will show early signs of hypoxia. Examination of the chest usually reveals a paradoxical segment not expanding with the rest of the chest wall on inspiration. Palpation of the area will reveal crepitus and instability of the rib cage.

Assessment should include careful monitoring for hypoxia. This should include rate and respiratory effort, tachycardia, skin colour, oxygen saturation and arterial blood gases.

Management

Management involves the restoration of respiratory function. Pain is a significant threat to respiratory function as it reduces respiratory effort, resulting in shallow breathing and reduced tidal volume. In addition, pain inhibits coughing, allowing bronchial secretions to build up, further jeopardising respiratory function. Adequate pain control is essential to recovery; often the method of choice is an intercostal nerve block which is performed as part of definitive care.

Both ventilation and perfusion are vital to respiratory function, so initial management should include adequate oxygenation and restoration of circulatory volume. Fluid replacement should be managed carefully, measured by heart rate, capillary refill and urine output. An injured lung is sensitive to underperfusion, which reduces the diffusion rate of oxygen. It is equally sensitive to circulatory overload, which can rapidly cause a raised central venous pressure (CVP) and left ventricular failure.

Unless profound hypoxia is present, many patients with a flail chest maintain their own ventilation, supported with high-flow oxygen via a mask and reservoir bag. The need for mechanical ventilation is determined by respiratory function and the level of hypoxia, not necessarily by the size of a flail segment (see Box 7.9).

Cardiac tamponade

Cardiac tamponade commonly results from penetrating injury, primarily stab wounds to the chest or upper abdomen (Robertson & Redmond 1994). It can also result from blunt trauma if the heart or great vessels have been damaged. Cardiac tamponade can be a rare complication of an expanding, untreated tension pneumothorax which causes mediastinal shift and eventually cardiac compression. Tamponade occasionally results from a myocardial infarction. The pericardium anchors the heart to the mediastinum, diaphragm and sternal wall. The risk of tamponade in trauma occurs because the pericardium is non-elastic and inflexible. This allows the heart to move without causing friction. The heart wall, consisting of myocardium and endocardium, lies beneath the pericardium and forms the muscle needed for cardiac function (see Fig. 7.11).

Cardiac tamponade occurs when injury to the heart or disruption of its blood vessels results in bleeding into the pericardial cavity. Because there is no elasticity in the pericardium, any additional fluid compresses the cardiac wall and chamber. This is primarily because filling capacity is reduced during diastole, and therefore venous pressure is elevated and there is a fall in stroke volume.

Assessment

The mechanism of injury should alert the trauma team to suspect a cardiac tamponade. If a penetrating injury has occurred to the thoracic area, anteriorly,

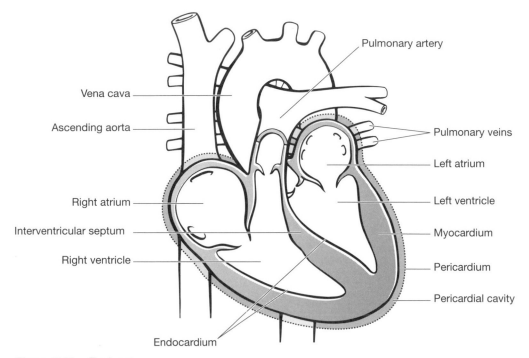

Figure 7.11 – *The heart.*

posteriorly or to the left lateral aspect, tamponade should be excluded as part of the primary survey. A patient with cardiac tamponade will be shocked, and therefore assessment of pulse and respiration are important. Specifically, patients will show signs of falling arterial pressure, because of reduced cardiac output, and increased venous pressure, because of cardiac compression. Venous pressure can be assessed by venous distension; time should not be spent inserting CVP lines in the initial stages of management (Driscoll *et al.* 1993).

Venous pressure is also influenced by hypovolaemia, and therefore absence of distended neck veins does not exclude cardiac tamponade. Kussmaul's sign, a paradoxical increase in JVP on inspiration (Rooney *et al.* 1996), may be found with tamponade but is a difficult sign to elicit. The classic diagnostic tool described as Beck's triad is only present in about a third of patients with tamponade, and so should not be too heavily relied upon (Driscoll *et al.* 1993) (see Box 7.10).

A 12-lead ECG trace is useful. It may indicate damage to myocardium, seen as ST elevation in the affected area. Continuous cardiac monitoring is recommended to detect any rhythm changes, commonly ventricular ectopics.

Management

Similar to all trauma patients, those with cardiac tamponade should be given high-flow oxygen, through a mask and reservoir bag. Initial attempts should be towards circulatory resuscitation to correct hypovolaemia. If there is no improvement in the patient's condition, pericardiocentesis should be performed to relieve the tamponade. This is a mechanism for draining fluid from the pericardial cavity and reducing cardiac compression. The patient's condition can be improved dramatically by the removal of as little as 20 ml of blood from the pericardial cavity (Rooney *et al.* 1996).

Pericardiocentesis is performed by inserting a wide-bore cannula, at least 15 cm in length, into the pericardial cavity. This is done 1–2 cm left of the

---

Box 7.10 – *Beck's triad*

1. *Raised CVP* – due to impaired venous return because of cardiac compression

2. *Hypotension* – low arterial pressure because of poor cardiac output

3. *Decreased, muffled heart sounds* – due to fluid in pericardial cavity

xiphochondral junction at a 45° angle, aiming the needle towards the tip of the scapula. The cannula should be attached to a three-way tap and syringe. Continous aspiration should take place during insertion. When blood flows freely into the syringe, the insertion should stop.

Continuous ECG monitoring is imperative during this procedure for a number of reasons. First, if the needle is inserted too far, myocardial irritation (seen as ventricular ectopics on the ECG monitor) or myocardial damage (seen as QRS complexes or ST segment changes) can occur. Should this happen, the needle should be withdrawn gradually until the ECG returns to normal. Secondly, as blood is removed on aspiration, cardiac decompression occurs and the myocardium expands back into its usual position.

The A&E nurse should watch the ECG monitor for signs that the myocardium is touching the cannula. Again, should this occur, the needle should then be gently withdrawn until the ECG returns to normal. Once blood has been withdrawn from the pericardial cavity, the cannula should be firmly taped in position in case further aspiration is required. If blood has clotted in the pericardial cavity, it is impossible to relieve symptoms of tamponade by pericardiocentesis. If the results of pericardiocentesis reveal blood in the pericardiac cavity, or if there is a strong clinical suspicion of tamponade, the patient should undergo urgent surgical exploration.

Survival rates from cardiac trauma resulting in tamponade are directly related to speed of definitive surgery (Robertson & Redmond 1994). This is, in part, because a fine balance exists between internal and external pressure during tamponade. Cardiac compression severely compromises circulatory activity and will lead to cardiac arrest if unchecked. However, by reducing cardiac compression, internal cardiac pressure is increased and profound haemorrhage can occur because the tamponade effect is lost. If cardiac arrest occurs, the mortality is linked to the speed at which cardiac bypass can be established; the faster this occurs, the lower is the rate of mortality (Robertson & Redmond 1994). Some A&E departments recommend emergency thoracotomy in A&E should cardiac arrest occur. Survival from this is rare unless cardiothoracic back-up is available and cardiac bypass can be quickly established.

Serious Chest Injury

The following injuries can be potentially life-threatening and should be diagnosed as part of the secondary survey and treated definitively (see Box 7.11).

> **Box 7.11** – *Serious chest injuries*
>
> ■ Pulmonary contusion
>
> ■ Blunt cardiac trauma
>
> ■ Aortic dissection
>
> ■ Ruptured diaphragm
>
> ■ Airway injury
>
> ■ Oesophageal rupture

Pulmonary contusion

Pulmonary contusion commonly occurs following a rapid deceleration injury. For example, a restrained passenger in an RTA may come to an abrupt stop on impact, but soft viscera such as the lung remain in motion, causing stretching, tearing and shearing. The resultant bruising and pain cause an insidious onset of respiratory distress, with decreased lung compliance and, rarely, increased airway resistance.

Assessment

The mechanism of injury and the time elapsed can give some clues to pulmonary contusion. Primarily, the A&E nurse should assess the respiration rate and depth. Patients will classically demonstrate an increasing tachypnoea and increasingly shallow breathing. Initially, the work of breathing is manifested by accessory muscles and intercostal recession. Because ventilation is poor, an imbalance in the ventilation/perfusion ratio occurs. This is demonstrated by a fall in PaO_2; serial arterial blood gas monitoring should take place. The nurse must look for any marks, e.g. abrasions or bruising on the chest wall, following the original injury. These may indicate pulmonary contusion.

Assessment is aided by chest X-ray, which will show hazy shadowing in the affected areas within a few hours post-injury (Driscoll *et al.* 1993). Pulse oximetry and ECG monitoring are also useful.

Management

Management principles entail maintaining respiratory function. High-flow oxygen should be given and the oxygen saturation carefully monitored. Adequate pain control aids respiratory function. Careful fluid balance is imperative to prevent secondary lung damage from pulmonary oedema, as a result of fluid overload, and to ensure fluid replacement is not underestimated; this would cause hypovolaemia and a subsequent reduction in pulmonary perfusion, compounding existing hypoxia.

Indications for mechanical ventilation are shown in Box 7.12.

Box 7.12 – *Indications for mechanical ventilation in patients with pulmonary contusion*

- Hypoxia and worsening respiratory function

- Impaired level of consciousness

- Progressive fall in Pao_2

- Progressive increase in $Paco_2$

- Pre-existing chronic lung disease

- Imminent surgery for associated injuries

- Other systems failure, e.g. renal failure

- Prior to transfer to another hospital

Blunt cardiac trauma

This usually results from RTAs and is exemplified by a driver who sustains an impact with the vehicle steering wheel causing a deceleration injury. It is a commonly undiagnosed condition (Rooney *et al.* 1996), sometimes with fatal consequences. Compression of the heart results in bleeding into the myocardium and ischaemia. The coronary arteries become occluded because of spasm or oedema. The physiological effect of this is similar to a myocardial infarction: the heart becomes ischaemic and, if not treated, necrosis and infarction occurs. Chest pain in patients following blunt cardiac trauma should be assessed like any other cardiac pain. A large percentage of these injuries are overlooked because pain is attributed to chest wall injury, e.g. with rib or sternal fractures.

Assessment

The mechanisms of injury should make the A&E nurse suspect a cardiac injury. Blunt trauma is associated with sternal fracture and wedge fracture of the thoracic vertebrae. Assessment should follow the same pattern as the assessment of a patient with a non-traumatic cardiac pain.

Baseline observations should be obtained and the patient should be observed on a cardiac monitor; a 12-lead ECG can be helpful in detecting myocardial damage. It may show a similar pattern to that of an evolving myocardial infarct (see also Ch. 27). However, myocardial damage can occur without ECG

changes. Sinus tachycardia and arrhythmias, such as ventricular ectopics and atrial fibrillation, are indicators of a 'stressed' myocardium.

Management

The priorities for management are to maintain adequate oxygenation and cardiac output. The patient should be given high-flow oxygen through a mask and reservoir bag, and oxygen saturation levels should be monitored. Pain control is important and intravenous morphine is the drug of choice, unless other injuries contraindicate its use. The patient should be managed by giving symptomatic support, i.e. treating dysrhythmias and maintaining blood pressure with drug therapy if necessary.

Aortic rupture

The descending thoracic aorta is particularly susceptible to rupture in rapid deceleration injury. Ninety per cent of patients die immediately (Driscoll *et al.* 1993). Those who survive do so because the adventitial layer of the aorta contains a haematoma which has a tamponade effect, preventing massive haemorrhage. Survival depends on rapid diagnosis and surgical repair.

Assessment

The history of deceleration injury should lead the A&E nurse to suspect a possible aortic rupture. Because of the tamponade effect, patients with this injury may have lost less than 500 ml of circulating volume, so they may not appear clinically shocked. If aortic injury is suspected, pulses should be checked in all limbs. Patients with an aortic injury will have higher pulse pressure in upper limbs than in lower limbs. Blood pressure may also vary between arms. Chest X-ray may show a widened mediastinum because of the tamponade effect. Conclusive assessment should include CT scan, angiography and/or transoesophageal echocardiography to show the extent and location of the tear.

Management

Initial management involves stabilising and resuscitating the patient in preparation for theatre. Definitive management demands rapid surgical repair of the aorta by grafting. Thoracic aortic surgery is carried out at a cardiothoracic centre, so many patients need to be transferred to alternative sites for surgery.

Patients should always be intubated prior to transfer and adequate fluid and analgesia should be available.

Ruptured diaphragm

A ruptured diaphragm can be caused by blunt or penetrating trauma. Generally, penetrating injuries are smaller and less serious; blunt injury however, can cause large tears. It is uncommon to injure both hemispheres of the diaphragm. The impact of large-scale tearing, particularly rupture to the left side, is that the abdominal viscera herniates into the thoracic cavity. Mortality following a ruptured diaphragm is high, up to 50% (Maddox *et al.* 1991). These patients often present with a clinical picture similar to a haemothorax, but if a ruptured diaphragm cannot be excluded, diagnosis should be confirmed on X-ray.

Assessment

The mechanism of injury will give a high index of suspicion that a ruptured diaphragm has occurred. This is important because some patients will be asymptomatic, which hampers diagnosis. More commonly, patients will present with respiratory difficulty and tachypnoea due to decreased lung capacity as a result of abdominal contents in the thoracic cavity. In addition to chest pain, patients may complain of dysphagia and dyspepsia because of shifting gastric contents, and shoulder tip pain because of phrenic nerve irritation. Chest auscultation will reveal reduced breath sounds on the affected side and bowel sounds may be present. A chest X-ray will complete assessment.

Management

The management priority is to maintain respiratory function. High-flow oxygen should be given via a mask with a reservoir bag. Unless contraindicated because of other injuries, a nasogastric tube should be inserted to decompress the stomach and give symptomatic relief. Chest drain insertion is by blunt dissection because of the risk of rupture to organs such as the liver or spleen. Early surgical repair is the treatment of choice; this minimises damage to lung tissue from gastric contents if gastric rupture or aspiration has occurred.

Tracheobronchial injuries

Injury to the major airways occurs following both severe blunt trauma and obvious penetrating trauma. Trauma to the major airways is rare, but in the case of blunt trauma it can be difficult to detect. It usually results in some degree of rupture to the airway at one of three anatomical levels (see Fig. 7.3).

The larynx

Injury results from RTAs where impact with the steering wheel or dashboard has occurred, or from direct blows from a fist or foot. Attempted hanging can sometimes result in a fractured larynx.

Assessment. In addition to pain and dyspnoea, the classic indications of laryngeal damage include hoarseness, crepitus and subcutaneous emphysema around the neck, because of air leaking into tissues.

Initial management entails the establishment and maintenance of a patent airway. Usually a formal tracheostomy is required.

The trachea

Mechanisms of injury are similar to those of laryngeal injury.

Assessment. Penetrating injury is usually obvious, but blunt trauma is more difficult to assess, particularly in a multiply injured patient. Respiratory distress is usually the only sign to guide the A&E nurse towards an airway injury. The patient may also have haemoptysis if conscious. Obstruction occurs in the airway because of oedema and bleeding.

Initial management is to maintain a patent airway. This normally requires endotracheal intubation. In penetrating injury this can sometimes be achieved through the wound site. Where available, bronchoscopy is useful both to confirm diagnosis and to remove tissue debris and blood. Early surgical repair is required.

The bronchi

The proximal bronchi are anatomically fairly immobile and therefore susceptible to rapid deceleration injury, which results in partial or complete tearing. Patients often have associated lung injuries and the mortality rate is around 30% (Rooney *et al.* 1996).

Assessment. The patient will show signs of severe respiratory distress, have haemoptysis and surgical emphysema. The patient may also have a pneumothorax on the injured side. Bronchoscopy will help to determine the extent of injury.

Initial management is similar to that in tracheal injury, except that oral intubation may be difficult because of oedema. If an adequate airway can be maintained, patients are often managed conservatively. If there is a complete bronchial tear, then surgical intervention is indicated.

Oesophageal injury

Penetrating trauma can cause a rupture to the oesophagus. Oesophageal injury may also be caused by gastric contents creating a tear from inside the oesophagus, often as a result of a blow to the stomach forcing gastric contents up the oesophagus under pressure. The gastric contents then leak into the mediastinum and can erode into pleural cavities.

Assessment

Specific signs include severe pain and shock which is not consistent with other injuries, pneumothorax without fractures, and gastric contents in chest drainage.

Initial management

This involves maintaining adequate ventilation, pain control and surgical repair of the oesophagus.

Sternum, Rib and Scapular Injuries

The ribs, sternum and scapula are most commonly damaged by blunt trauma. Such injuries may follow a direct blow to the chest, crushing or rapid deceleration as epitomised by RTAs. Typically, rib and sternal fractures occur on impact with a steering wheel. In comparison with injuries to the scapulae, rib injuries are much more common. Rib fractures are often associated with other injuries and therefore this suspicion should always be borne in mind. A fragment of a fractured rib may pierce the lung, pleura, pericardium or skin. Thus, subsequent complications include pneumothorax and haemothorax. Fracture of the first or second rib and/or scapula often occurs concurrently with serious head, neck, lung, great vessel and spinal cord injury and therefore is of great significance. Lower rib fractures are associated with spleen and liver injuries.

Although rib injuries vary in severity, they are all significant because of the associated pain with chest movement which may cause splinting of the chest and impair ventilation. Furthermore, this may lead to pneumonia and atelectasis. The mechanism of injury, together with chest wall contusions and bruising, should raise suspicion of rib or sternal fractures. The patient may be dyspnoeic and will have pain, localised tenderness, crepitus and deformity. Suitable analgesia to ensure adequate ventilation and deep breathing exercises are an essential part of the management of fractured ribs. An intercostal nerve block may be used and is often the most effective way of reducing pain and facilitating adequate inspiration.

Since seat belt legislation was introduced in 1983, an increasing number of patients with seat belt-related sternal fractures have been reported. As a great deal of force is required to fracture the sternum, underlying injury to the heart and great vessels should be suspected. Monitoring for cardiac dysrhythmias is required for patients with fractured sternum as there may be significant cardiac contusion.

Conclusion

In the A&E department the main focus for care of patients with chest injury must be to ensure a patent airway, adequate breathing and maintenance of a viable circulation. Essentials of nursing care include early administration of high-flow oxygen, careful monitoring of vital signs and judicious fluid resuscitation. Only when these fundamental elements have been secured can more specific management ensue.

References

American College of Surgeons (Committee on Trauma) (1997) *Advanced Trauma Life Support Programme.* Illinois: American College of Surgeons.

Castille K (1993) Penetrating Trauma in Manchester. *Accident and Emergency Nursing,* **1**(2), 65–72.

Driscoll PA, Grinnutt CL, LeDuc Jimmerson C, Goodall O, eds. (1993) Thoracic trauma. In: Driscoll PA, *Trauma Resuscitation: the Team Approach.* Basingstoke: Macmillan.

Fox HJ, Pooler J, Prothero D, Banmister GC (1994) Factors affecting the outcome after proximal femoral fractures. *Injury,* **25**, 297–300.

Henneman E, Henneman PL, Oman KS (1993) Ventilation and gas transport: pulmonary, thoracic and facial injuries. In: Neff JA, Stinson Kidd P, eds. *Trauma Nursing: the Art and Science.* St Louis: Mosby Year Book.

Hinchliff S, Montagne S, Watson R (1996) *Physiology for Nursing Practice,* 2nd edn. London: Baillière Tindall.

Holt E, Evans RA, Hindley CJ, Metcalfe JW (1994) 1000 femoral neck fractures: the effect of pre-injury mobility and surgical experience on outcome. *Injury,* **25**, 91–95.

Hyde J, Sykes T, Graham T (1997) Reducing morbidity from chest drains. *British Medical Journal,* **314**, 914–915.

Landon BA, Driscoll PA, Goodall JD (1994) *An Atlas of Trauma Management.* Carnforth: Parthenon.

LoCicerco J, Mattox KL (1989) Epidemiology of chest trauma. *Surgical Clinics of North America,* **69**(1), 15.

Maddox P, Mansel R, Butchat E, (1991) Traumatic rupture of the diaphragm: a difficult diagnosis. *Injury,* **22**, 299.

Robertson C, Redmond A (1994) *Major Trauma,* 2nd edn. Oxford: Oxford University Press.

Rooney S, Westaby S, Graham T (1996) Chest injuries. In: Skinner D, Driscoll P, Easlam R, eds. *ABC of Major Trauma*, 2nd edn. London: BMJ.

Westaby S, Brayley N (1991) Thoracic trauma. In: Skinner D, Driscoll P, Earlan R, eds. *ABC of Major Trauma*. London: BMJ.

Chapter 8

Abdominal Injuries

Paul Gee

- Introduction
- Anatomy and pathophysiology
- Types and patterns of injury
- Uncontrolled haemorrhage
- Assessment of abdominal trauma
- Abdominal injuries in children
- Conclusion

Introduction

Abdominal trauma has a relatively low incidence, but is associated with high morbidity and high mortality. Blunt abdominal trauma has been identified as a contributing factor in as many as 25% of all trauma deaths (Trunkey & Lewis 1986). Intra-abdominal injuries carry this high mortality rate because they are difficult to identify and, once identified, their severity is often underestimated.

This chapter will examine the priorities of nursing care for the victim of abdominal trauma. A systematic approach based on the Advanced Trauma Life Support Course (American College of Surgeons 1997) will be adopted. A rationale for the care proposed will be sought, examining the causes, patterns and likely outcomes of abdominal trauma and the relevant anatomy and physiology. It is hoped that this knowledge will assist the reader to function more effectively as a trauma team member in the assessment and resuscitation of the person with intra-abdominal injuries in the A&E setting.

Anatomy and Pathophysiology

The abdomen has three distinct anatomic compartments – the peritoneal compartment, the retroperitoneal compartment and the pelvic compartment. Bleeding from a damaged organ in one compartment is often contained within that compartment, and for this reason may not be revealed by diagnostic tests applied to other compartments. The abdominal organs are vulnerable to injury because minimal protective structures surround the area.

The peritoneal compartment extends superiorly into the bony thorax. The superior border of this compartment is the diaphragm, which may rise to the level of the fourth intercostal space on full expiration. Part of the peritoneal compartment may therefore be thought of as intrathoracic, and this part contains the liver, spleen, stomach and transverse colon. Portions of the colon and the small intestine (ileum and jejunum)

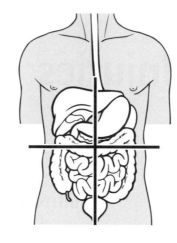

Right upper quadrant

Right lobe of liver
Gallbladder
Pylorus
Duodenum
Head of pancreas
Upper right kidney

Left upper quadrant

Left lobe of liver
Spleen
Stomach
Left kidney
Body of pancreas
Splenic flexure of colon

Right lower quadrant

Lower right kidney
Cecum
Appendix
Ascending colon
Right fallopian tube (female)
Right ovary (female)
Right ureter
Bladder (distended)

Left lower quadrant

Descending colon
Sigmoid colon
Left fallopian tube (female)
Left ovary (female)
Left ureter
Bladder (distended)

(a)

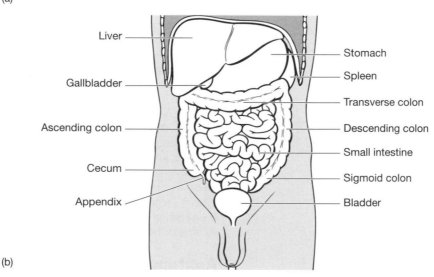

(b)

Figure 8.1 – *(a): Abdominal contents. (After Stillwell 1996.) (b): Gastrointestinal structures. (After Seidel et al. 1995.)*

lie within the abdominal part of the peritoneal compartment (see Fig. 8.1).

The retroperitoneal compartment contains the abdominal aorta and vena cava, the pancreas, kidneys, adrenal glands, ureters, duodenum and parts of the colon. The pelvic compartment contains the urinary bladder, the prostate gland, urethra, rectum, iliac vessels and the female internal genitalia.

Types and Patterns of Injury

Intra-abdominal injuries may be classified as penetrating or blunt.

Penetrating injuries

Penetrating injuries may be the result of stabbing or accidental impalement, or be caused by a high-velocity projectile, such as a bullet or a piece of disintegrating machinery. Stab wounds involve low energy but usually damage all the structures within their path (see Fig. 8.2). The site of surface penetration into the abdomen, together with a history giving the length of blade, should enable an accurate prediction of the organs likely to be injured. The liver, stomach, small and large bowel are commonly involved (Mills *et al.* 1995). Stab wounds should not be underestimated,

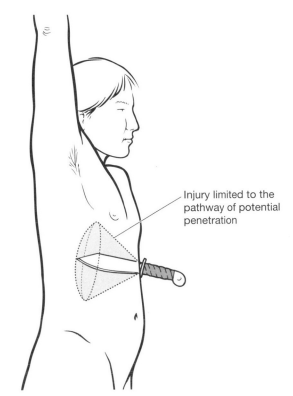

Injury limited to the
pathway of potential
penetration

Figure 8.2 – *Path of knife wound penetration in patient.
(After McSwain et al. 1996.)*

however, as up to 30% result in visceral injury. A negative physical examination is made in up to a third of patients found to have serious visceral injury at operation (Cope & Stebbings 1996).

Many surgeons perform exploratory laparotomy following a penetrating injury because of the unreliability of a negative physical examination. Alternatively, patients can be selected for laparotomy on the basis of local wound exploration and diagnostic peritoneal lavage (DPL; Box 8.1).

Gunshot injuries to the abdomen involve high energies and may damage organs remote from the site of penetration into the abdomen. Up to 95% of gunshot wounds to the abdomen result in visceral injury (Moore *et al.* 1980). The amount of energy released is proportional to the mass and velocity of the bullet and also depends on the density of tissue involved. A low-velocity bullet from a handgun will release less energy and cause less injury than a high-velocity bullet from a rifle (see Fig. 8.3). Similarly, a high-mass bullet will cause more damage than a low-mass bullet of similar velocity. An accurate history involving the type of weapon used and the range at which it was fired is

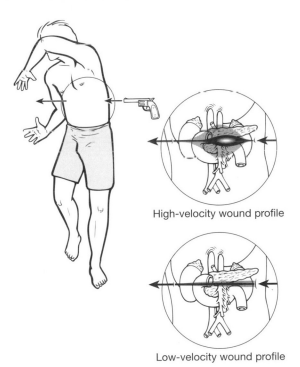

High-velocity wound profile

Low-velocity wound profile

Figure 8.3 – *Potential injury path of high- and low-velocity bullets. (After Neff & Kidd 1993.)*

essential in order to assess the likely magnitude of visceral injury.

A bullet will release its energy in the abdomen in two ways. First, it does so by direct contact with organs in its path. Bullets may take a non-linear path through the abdomen. A simple, straight line connecting entry and exit wounds may not indicate the actual path of the bullet. In cases where there is no exit wound, X-rays will locate the bullet. Secondly, bullets transfer energy in the form of pressure waves. These pressure waves may disrupt many organs not in the actual path of the bullet. Pressure waves result in cavitation, extending the diameter of injury to many times the actual diameter of the bullet. Dense, solid viscera are more susceptible to cavitation than hollow organs. The sudden formation of a cavity increases intra-abdominal volume, creating a negative pressure, which may suck debris such as clothing in through the entry wound, resulting in gross intra-abdominal contamination.

Penetrating injuries to the lower chest below the fourth intercostal space may result in additional penetration of the abdomen through the diaphragm. Significant intra-abdominal injury is found in up to 15% of stab wounds and up to 46% of gunshot wounds to the lower chest (Moore *et al.* 1981). It is important to establish the type of weapons used, whether handgun or rifle, and the distance between the patient and the gun. Gunpowder around the bullet entry site will suggest firing at close range and is usually associated with an increase in injury severity.

Blunt injuries

In the UK, blunt trauma to the abdomen is far more common than penetrating trauma (Sexton 1997). In addition, blunt trauma may present with incomplete data. Intra-abdominal injuries caused by blunt trauma may result from one or more of several traumatic forces, and these injuries are different in character from those caused by penetrating trauma (Dowds 1994). Direct blows to, or compression of, organs through the abdominal wall, sudden deceleration or acceleration, the crushing of organs between rigid structures and rapid changes of pressure within the abdomen may combine, or act in isolation, to damage organs. High-energy blunt trauma leads to more severe injuries. The commonest cause of high-energy blunt trauma to the abdomen is motor vehicle trauma.

The organs most commonly damaged through blunt abdominal trauma are the spleen, the liver, mesentery, urological structures and the pancreas (McAnena *et al.* 1990). These are 'solid' viscera, which cannot change shape or stretch and are therefore vulnerable to damage by direct blows, compression or crushing. These organs are given some protection by the thoracic skeleton, but when great force is applied, they may be crushed between the lower ribs and the anterior vertebral column or the paravertebral

muscles. Fractures of the lower ribs should therefore create a high level of suspicion of associated visceral damage. Although more commonly injured as a result of penetrating trauma, the pancreas may also be injured by crushing against the anterior spine.

The organs within the pelvic compartment are generally protected by the bony pelvis. A great deal of force is required to fracture the pelvis. This great force and the potential for haemorrhage from the adjacent vascular structures are reflected in the severe injuries and high mortality associated with pelvic fractures. Genitourinary injuries are seen in association with 15% of all pelvic fractures (Meyer 1989). The bladder, rectum and vagina may be punctured by fragments of a fractured pelvis, or the bladder may be ruptured by a direct blow if full of urine. The part of the male urethra that passes through the prostate is relatively immobile. The rest of the urethra passes through the urogenital diaphragm, which is attached to the pubic rami. If the pelvis is fractured, this portion may shear from the rest at the apex of the prostate. The prostate is then displaced upwards. Injuries to the female urethra are rare. Bleeding from fractured pelvic bones and vascular injuries associated with a pelvic fracture may constitute life-threatening haemorrhage, especially in the case of a compound injury. Stabilisation of the pelvis by external fixation is often used in the resuscitation room to limit blood loss (see also Ch. 5).

Changes of pressure in the abdomen may be produced by sudden external compression. Car seat belts can produce this compression during a collision involving sudden deceleration, especially if the lap belt is worn too high, above the superior/anterior iliac spines. The general increase in intra-abdominal pressure is reflected in an increase in pressure inside air-filled organs, notably the duodenum. As a result of peristalsis, a 'closed loop' of duodenum may exist which may rupture when compressed (DeMars *et al.* 1979). The diaphragm may also be ruptured by a sudden increase in intra-abdominal pressure. Abdominal viscera, especially the stomach and colon, may herniate through the rupture, compromising breathing and circulation by compression of the pleura and the mediastinum. Pericardial tears may be associated with diaphragmatic rupture.

The sudden, massive and catastrophic changes of pressure associated with blasts or explosions may damage the air-filled 'hollow' viscera of the gastro-intestinal tract. The air within the viscera will transmit the force of the blast equally in all directions, leading to a general disruption or 'bursting' effect (Halpern 1982). Victims of such severe trauma rarely survive the other injuries associated with blasts, and visceral contusion is much more commonly seen in the blast survivor.

Sudden deceleration injuries may be the result of motor vehicle trauma or falls from a height. The abdominal organs move at the same speed as the external framework of the body. The external framework may decelerate suddenly, as in the case of a car driver hitting the steering wheel, dashboard and windscreen during a high-velocity collision. The driver's abdominal organs will continue at the pre-collision velocity, putting strain on or disrupting their points of attachment, until they meet another structure such as the abdominal wall. Catastrophic injuries to the aorta can occur within the thorax by this mechanism. In the abdomen, disruption of the renal pedicle may lead to rupture of the renal vessels or tears to the ureter at the pelvic–ureteric junction. The duodenum may also be torn as it is only fixed at one end.

Uncontrolled Haemorrhage

Uncontrolled haemorrhage from damaged abdominal organs and vessels will cause hypovolaemia and death. Haemorrhage may remain uncontrolled because it is not detected. Early detection of haemorrhage is therefore essential for survival in any case of abdominal injury (Andrews 1989). Abdominal trauma carries a high mortality rate because detection of injury is not only essential, but also extremely challenging, for a number of reasons.

There may or may not be external signs of abdominal injury – bruising, grazes or penetrating wounds – but any intra-abdominal injury is invisible to the naked eye. This invisible space is full of highly vascular structures which bleed when damaged. Detection of this bleeding depends upon the results of a clinical examination, which may be unreliable due to the location of the injury, e.g. retroperitoneal haemorrhage, pain from adjacent injuries, intoxication, unconsciousness or high cervical injury in the victim. These factors often mandate time-consuming investigations such as DPL or CT scanning.

The need for urgent laparotomy should be determined by history, findings on examination and the results of investigations. This difficulty in determining a significant abdominal injury has led to the belief that some deaths due to abdominal trauma are preventable. The key to prevention of these deaths is intervention without delay (Anderson *et al.* 1988), and therefore profound hypotension unresponsive to fluid resuscitation, with no other obvious cause, is an indication for urgent laparotomy.

Assessment of Abdominal Trauma

The aim of assessment is to establish whether an intra-abdominal injury exists, not what the specific injury is.

Evidence of intra-abdominal injury mandates urgent surgical exploration of the abdomen, at which time an accurate diagnosis may be made. Assessment is made on the basis of a history, the results of a primary survey, the victim's response to treatment started as a result of that primary survey, a secondary survey including an abdominal examination, and the results of any diagnostic tests such as DPL or CT scan.

History

It is important to obtain an accurate history of the events leading to the injury. Awake patients may complain of abdominal pain or shoulder pain. Intra-abdominal blood irritates the inferior surface of the diaphragm and the phrenic nerve causing referred pain to the shoulder. Known as Kehr's sign, this finding should alert the nurse to the possibility of peritoneal bleeding (Feeman & Newberry 1998). The nurse should assess the patient carefully and continually reassess the haemodynamic status, level of consciousness and level of pain. Certain specific elements of the history are useful in assessing abdominal injuries (see Boxes 8.2 and 8.3).

Box 8.2 – *Useful information specific to penetrating injuries (Luckmann & Sorenson 1987)*

Stabbing or impalement injuries
- The size, shape and length of the weapon
- The number of stabbing attempts made
- Blood loss at scene and in transit
- Angle of penetration
- Height of assailant
- Sex of assailant (males tend to stab upwards)

Gunshot injuries
- The type of weapon involved
- High/low velocity and bullet size
- Weapon to victim distance
- Number of shots fired

Box 8.3 – *Useful information specific to blunt injuries*

- Motor vehicle speed, or height of fall
- Was the victim ejected from the vehicle on impact?
- Damage caused to vehicle and position of victim in vehicle
- Was the victim restrained by a seat belt?
- The impact configuration

The impact configuration in severe collisions of motor vehicles may help to suggest possible injuries. The likelihood of sustaining torso injuries, particularly of the spleen and pelvis, is higher in side impact collisions than in frontal impact collisions (Pattimore *et al.* 1992). Recording, collating and communicating all the elements of a history are key responsibilities of the A&E nurse in trauma care.

Primary survey

The primary survey and resuscitation are not examined in detail here (see Ch. 2). Only the following points with relevance to abdominal trauma are emphasised:

- *Airway maintenance with cervical spine control.*
- *Breathing and ventilation* – Injuries to the diaphragm or penetrating injuries involving the intra-thoracic abdomen and chest may compromise breathing.
- *Circulation with haemorrhage control* – Gross external haemorrhage from the abdomen is rare. The abdomen may, however, be a reservoir for a large volume of occult haemorrhage. Any hypovolaemia is treated with an intravenous fluid challenge.
- *Disability* – Neurological status.
- *Exposure* – Completely undress the patient, but do not cut clothes across stab or bullet holes as this may destroy crucial forensic evidence.

On completion of the primary survey, X-rays of the chest, cervical spine and pelvis should be taken. A rise in respiratory and pulse rates with a reduction in pulse pressure are clear and early indicators of haemorrhage. Similarly, the reverse indicates a response to fluid resuscitation. Traditionally, girth measurement has been taken. An increase in girth was used as an indicator of abdominal bleeding. It is, however, a late and unreliable method of assessing intraperitoneal bleeding and should not be used in initial trauma care (Robertson & Redmond 1994). The A&E nurse should rely on vital sign monitoring to assess intra-abdominal bleeding. The patient should be log rolled maintaining cervical spine immobilisation. This is necessary for complete assessment of the abdomen. Evidence of penetrating injury, surface bruising or grazing, or tenderness over the thoracolumbar spine may all indicate possible retroperitoneal organ injury.

While the patient is in a lateral position, a rectal examination should be performed. Bony fragments felt on rectal examination may indicate a fractured pelvis. Fresh blood in the rectum suggests a disrupted colon or rectum. A high-riding or absent prostate in the male may indicate an urethral transection, and contraindicates urinary catheterisation. A vaginal examination is necessary in the female patient. Fractures of the pelvis may be discovered by direct palpation, and the integrity of the vaginal wall can be assessed.

Other contraindications for urinary catheterisation are blood at the urethral meatus and the presence of a scrotal haematoma, both of which may indicate urethral injury. The urinary catheter allows monitoring of urinary output as an index of tissue perfusion. It also decompresses the bladder in preparation for an abdominal examination and possible surgical entry into the abdomen. If no contraindications exist, a urinary catheter should be inserted and a sample of urine should be tested for the presence of blood. Up to 65% of trauma patients with gross haematuria and hypovolaemia have intra-abdominal injuries, and the presence of microscopic haematuria should be viewed with a high index of suspicion (Knudson *et al.* 1992).

Insertion of a nasogastric catheter allows for decompression of the stomach and aspiration of stomach contents via the tube, avoiding possible regurgitation into the airway. If blood is aspirated from the tube, it may indicate upper oesophageal or stomach injury. Maxillofacial injuries may, however, be the source of any aspirated blood. Visualisation of the nasogastric tube within the thorax on chest X-ray may indicate gastric herniation through a diaphragmatic tear. The presence of free air or fluid in the upper abdomen also suggests visceral damage. Fractures of the lower ribs indicate great force applied to the spleen or liver, and should be viewed with a high index of suspicion.

Secondary survey

A physical examination of the abdomen is performed as part of a complete secondary survey of the whole victim. The physical examination consists of looking at, listening to and feeling the abdomen in a systematic manner. Fully exposing and log rolling the patient allow inspection of the whole external surface of the abdomen. Any bruising, grazes or penetrating wounds may indicate intra-abdominal injury. The lower chest overlying the intrathoracic abdomen, buttocks and perineum should all be examined.

The abdomen should be listened to (auscultated) for the presence of bowel sounds (McGrath 1998). Visceral injury may release blood or enteric contents into the peritoneal cavity. The resulting irritation of the bowel may produce a paralytic ileus and thus an absence of bowel sounds. Rib, spine and pelvic fractures may also cause pain, irritation and ileus. This possibility and the difficulty of hearing bowel sounds during a trauma resuscitation make the absence of bowel sounds an unreliable sign of intra-abdominal injury. The presence of bowel sounds does not exclude intra-abdominal injury.

Percussion, or gentle tapping of the abdomen, produces a slight movement of the peritoneum. If the peritoneum is injured or irritated by free fluid released as a result of injury to other viscera, this movement will cause pain – rebound tenderness. This is an unequivocal sign of intra-abdominal injury. The abdomen is felt, or palpated. This is done partly to discover if palpation causes pain. Pain from intra-abdominal injuries is usually poorly localised and is unreliable as an indicator of visceral injury. If the muscles of the abdominal wall are involuntarily tense to palpation (guarding) as a result of peritoneal irritation, this is an unequivocal sign of intra-abdominal injury. The abdominal examination may be equivocal, due to pain from other injuries such as fractured ribs, pelvis or lumbar spine. It may be unreliable because the victim is unconscious or insensitive due to alcohol, drugs (anaesthetic or recreational), head injury or spinal cord trauma.

Subsequent action

The action that follows the completion of the secondary survey is determined by the results of the physical examination and the circulatory status of the patient, i.e. whether there is any hypovolaemia and the nature of the response to any fluid challenge measured by frequent recordings of vital signs. All blunt trauma should carry an associated high index of suspicion of intra-abdominal injury. Constant reassessment of the patient is necessary as it may take several hours for symptoms to develop, particularly splenic injuries (Wilson & Flowers 1985).

A three-stage response to abdominal examination exists:

■ *No immediate action – observation only*. A negative abdominal examination with no hypovolaemia. The abdominal examination should be repeated at frequent intervals.
■ *Special diagnostic studies urgently required*. An equivocal or unreliable abdominal examination in a multiply injured patient.
■ *Immediate surgical exploration of the abdomen required*. Unequivocal evidence of intra-abdominal injury – rebound tenderness, involuntary guarding, chest X-ray shows free air in peritoneal cavity, or migration of abdominal organs into thoracic cavity (diaphragmatic injury); stab wounds or gunshot

wounds to the abdomen with associated hypotension; nil or transient response to resuscitation of hypovolaemia, with no obvious cause. Surgical exploration of the abdomen determines the exact location and extent of any visceral injuries. More importantly, it provides intervention to treat those injuries.

Special diagnostic studies

Diagnostic peritoneal lavage is an invasive surgical procedure. It involves making a small incision into the anterior abdomen, through a bloodless field. This is performed under local anaesthetic, with adrenaline to constrict the blood supply to the incised area. A catheter is inserted into the peritoneal cavity through the incision, and warm, sterile, isotonic fluid is infused rapidly. The fluid is then drained. Any blood present in the lavage fluid, visible or microscopically visible, indicates intraperitoneal bleeding.

DPL correctly identifies intraperitoneal bleeding, or the lack of it, in 90% of its applications (American College of Surgeons 1997). It will not, however, identify which organs are injured. Neither will it detect bleeding from retroperitoneal viscera, such as the kidneys or pancreas. It is quick and can safely be done in the resuscitation room by an experienced surgeon, with a minimum of preparation and surgical instruments. There are potential complications to the procedure, including mechanical injury to viscera during incision or during insertion of the catheter. These are serious, but rare.

Computed tomography (CT) scanning is a non-invasive radiological examination. It involves preparing composite images (by computer) which allow the abdomen to be viewed in a series of 'slices'. CT scanning requires expensive equipment and is not universally available. It is not as sensitive in detecting bleeding as DPL (Bell & Coleridge 1992), but will usually identify specific injuries when bleeding is detected. It is also more time-consuming than DPL. The equipment for CT scanning is not portable, and therefore the patient must leave the resuscitation room. During the scan, and during the journey to and from the scan room, any sudden deterioration in the condition of the victim may be difficult to manage. CT scanning is therefore only suitable for patients whose condition is entirely stable (Thomason *et al.* 1993). Careful monitoring during scanning is an important responsibility for the A&E nurse. Anticipation of resuscitation in CT scan rooms must be considered by A&E nurses.

Ultrasound. This may also help to diagnose a wide range of intra-abdominal injuries. It is valuable in detecting abdominal aortic aneuyrsms and intra and retroperitoneal fluid collections (Marx 1992). At least 70 ml of intraperitoneal fluid must be present for a diagnostic benefit (Finis 1995). Ultrasound is not very effective in detecting liver or spleen injuries, as the missed rate is 20–25% (Chambers & Pilbrow 1988). Ultrasound is an effective way to assess fetal viability in the pregnant trauma patient.

Ultrasound examinations are fast and injury-specific. Like CT scanning, they require expensive equipment and a trained operator. Unlike CT, however, they may be performed with portable equipment in the resuscitation room. Repeated studies may be carried out, unlike DPL which is a 'one-off' examination. Several studies indicate that ultrasound may be a useful examination in the evaluation of abdominal trauma (Bode *et al.* 1993, Visvanathan & Low 1993).

Other studies. Injuries to the urinary tract, i.e. the kidneys, ureters, bladder and urethra, which is entirely outside the peritoneal compartment, may not be detected by DPL. Contrast radiographic studies, such as cystography, intravenous urogram or ascending urethrography may be safely performed on a stable patient.

Abdominal Injuries in Children

Children are different, physically, emotionally, intellectually and socially, from adults. Only the differences significant to abdominal injuries are considered here.

Specific anatomy in children

Children are vulnerable to abdominal injury for a number of reasons. They are small and therefore any blunt trauma is likely to affect more body systems than in a similar incident involving an adult. The abdominal wall is thin and offers little protection to its contents. The ribs are more elastic, decreasing protection to the spleen, liver and kidneys. The diaphragm lies more horizontally, lowering and further exposing these organs. The kidneys are also more mobile and not shielded by perinephritic fat, as in adults. The bladder is superior to the protection of the pelvis, and therefore more vulnerable. Finally, abdominal injuries may cause diaphragmatic irritation and splinting, compromising ventilation (Advanced Life Support Group 1997).

Types and patterns of injury

The majority of abdominal injuries in children are caused by blunt trauma. Penetrating injuries are rare. Motor vehicle trauma and falls are the most common causes of abdominal injuries. As in adults, the spleen, liver and kidneys are the most commonly injured organs in the child victim of blunt trauma.

Assessment of abdominal trauma

The primary survey is carried out as in adults, with the same priorities and aims. An examination of the abdomen is carried out as part of the secondary survey. The examination is the same as that for adults, with the following special considerations. Care should be taken to be gentle on palpation, as any pain will produce voluntary guarding, making assessment difficult. Children swallow air when crying and upset. This produces distension of the stomach, which makes assessment difficult, and may mimic the rigidity and distension found in intra-abdominal injury. For this reason, a nasogastric catheter should be passed at an early stage, to aspirate any swallowed air (Lloyd-Thomas & Anderson 1996).

In children with multisystem trauma, a urinary catheter of appropriate size should always be passed, unless contraindicated, in order to decompress the bladder and allow measurement of urine output. The indications for DPL are the same as in adults. However, CT scanning is more frequently used in children. Many minor liver and spleen injuries are managed without operation in children (Luna & Dellinger 1987), making the more specific CT scan the study of choice.

Conclusion

The challenge of nursing the patient with abdominal trauma in the A&E department is in eliminating the preventable deaths which currently occur as a result of that trauma. Training in the systematic assessment and resuscitation of victims of trauma, such as the Advanced Trauma Nursing course or Trauma Nursing Core course, should be a basic requirement for A&E nurses. This training enables effective multidisciplinary teamwork, ensuring that where there is a need for urgent abdominal surgery, it is recognised and acted upon promptly – the key to eliminating preventable deaths.

References

Advanced Life Support Group (1997) *Advanced Paediatric Life Support*. London: BMJ.

American College of Surgeons (1997) *Advanced Trauma Life Support*. Chicago: American College of Surgeons.

Anderson ID, Woodford M, de Dombal FT, Irving M (1988) Retrospective study of 1000 deaths from injury in England and Wales. *British Medical Journal*, **296**, 1305–1308.

Andrews J (1989) Difficult diagnoses in blunt thoraco-abdominal trauma. *Journal of Emergency Nursing*, **15**(5), 399–404.

Bell C, Coleridge ST (1992) A comparison of diagnostic peritoneal lavage and computed tomography (CT scan) in evaluation of the haemodynamically stable patient with blunt abdominal trauma. *Journal of Emergency Medicine*, **10**(3), 275–280.

Bode PJ, Niezen RA, Van-Vugt AB, Schipper J (1993) Abdominal ultrasound as a reliable indicator for conclusive laparotomy in blunt abdominal trauma. *Journal of Trauma*, **34**(1), 27–31.

Chambers JA, Pilbrow WJ (1988) Ultrasound in abdominal trauma: an alternative to peritoneal lavage. *Archives of Emergency Medicine*, **5**(26), 26–33.

Cope A, Stebbings W (1996) Abdominal trauma. In: Skinner D, Driscoll P, Earlam R, eds. *ABC of Major Trauma*, 2nd edn. London: BMJ.

DeMars J, Bubrick M, Hitchcock C (1979) Duodenal perforation in blunt abdominal trauma. *Surgery*, **86**, 632–638.

Dowds P (1994) Blunt abdominal trauma. *Accident and Emergency Nursing*, **2**(2), 63–69.

Feeman LM, Newberry L (1998) Gastrointestinal trauma. In: Newberry L, ed. *Sheehy's Emergency Nursing: Principles and Practice*, 4th edn. St Louis: Mosby.

Finis NM (1995) Abdominal trauma. In: Kitt S, Selfridge-Thomas J, Proehl JA, Kaiser J, eds. *Emergency Nursing: a Physiological and Clinical Perspective*, 2nd edn. Philadelphia: WB Saunders.

Halpern JS (1982) Patterns of trauma. *Journal of Emergency Nursing*, **8**(4), 170–175.

Knudson MM, McAninch JW, Gomez R, Lee P, Stubbs HA (1992) Hematuria as a predictor of abdominal injury after blunt trauma. *American Journal of Surgery*, **164**(5), 482–485.

Lloyd-Thomas AR, Anderson I (1996) Paediatric trauma. In: Skinner D, Driscoll P, Earlam R, eds. *ABC of Major Trauma*, 2nd edn. London: BMJ.

Luckman J, Sorenson KC (1987) *Medical Surgical Nursing*. Philadelphia: Saunders.

Luna GK, Dellinger EP (1987) Non-operative observation therapy for splenic injuries: a safe therapeutic option. *American Journal of Surgery*, **153**, 462–468.

McAnena OJ, Moore EE, Marx JA (1990) Initial evaluation of the patient with blunt abdominal trauma. *Surgical Clinics of North America*, **70**(3), 495–510.

McGrath A (1998) Abdominal examination and assessment in A&E. *Emergency Nurse*, **6**(4), 15–18.

McSwain N *et al.* (1996) *The Basic EMT: Comprehensive Prehospital Patient Care*. St Louis: Mosby.

Marx JA (1992) Abdominal trauma. In: Rosen P, Barkin RM, Braen G *et al.* eds. *Emergency Medicine: Concepts and Clinical Practice*. St Louis: Mosby Year Book.

Meyer PS (1989) Urologic complications associated with pelvic fractures. *Orthopaedic Nursing*, **8**(4), 41–44, 68.

Mills K, Morton R, Page G (1995) *Colour Atlas and Text of Medical Emergencies*, 2nd edn. London: Mosby-Wolfe.

Moore EE, Moore JB, Van Duzer-Moore S (1980) Mandatory laparotomy for gunshot wounds penetrating the abdomen. *American Journal of Surgery*, **140**, 847–851.

Moore JB, Moore EE, Thompson JS (1981) Abdominal injuries associated with penetrating trauma in the lower chest. *American Journal of Surgery*, **140**, 724–730.

Neff JA, Kidd PS (1993) *Trauma Nursing: the Art and Science*. St Louis: Mosby.

Pattimore D, Thomas P, Dave SH (1992) Torso injury patterns and mechanisms in car crashes: an additional diagnostic tool. *Injury*, **23**(2), 123–126.

Robertson C, Redmond AD (1994) *The Management of Major Trauma*, 2nd edn. Oxford: Oxford University Press.

Seidel HM *et al.* (1995) *Mosby's Guide to Physical Examination*, 3rd edn. St Louis: Mosby.

Sexton J (1997) Trauma epidemiology and management. *Emergency Nurse*, **5**(1), 14–16.

Stillwell S (1996) *Mosby's Critical Care Nursing Reference Guide*, 2nd edn. St Louis: Mosby.

Thomason M, Messick J, Rutledge R, Meredith W (1993) Head CT scanning versus urgent exploration in the hypotensive blunt trauma patient. *Journal of Trauma*, **34**(1), 40–45.

Trunkey D, Lewis F (1986) *Current Therapy of Trauma*. Philadelphia, BC: Decker

Visvanathan R, Low HC (1993) Blunt abdominal trauma – injury assessment in relation to early surgery. *Journal of the Royal College of Surgeons Edinburgh*, **38**(1), 19–22.

Wilson DH, Flowers MW (1985) *Accident and Emergency Handbook*. Oxford: Butterworths.

Chapter 9

Facial Injuries

Elspeth Richie

- Introduction
- Anatomy and physiology
- Mechanism of injury
- Assessment
- Le Fort fractures
- Mandibular fractures
- Orbit floor fractures (blow-out fracture)
- Temporomandibular joint (jaw) dislocation
- Frontal sinus fractures
- Nasal fractures
- Facial wounds
- Conclusion

Introduction

This chapter deals with facial trauma, highlighting those injuries most commonly identified in A&E departments. It will explain how these injuries are sustained, the treatment and nursing care required and any problems which are likely to arise thereafter.

Anatomy and Physiology

The face contains all the special structures and centres for breathing, speech, vision, hearing, mastication and deglutition and ingestion, and is highly vulnerable to a wide variety of injuries (see Box 9.1 and Fig. 9.1). These injuries can often be dramatic and are frequently

---

Box 9.1 – *The facial bones*

The skeleton of the face is formed by 14 bones including the frontal bones:

- **Zygomatic** – the two bones commonly referred to as the cheek bones

- **Maxilla** – forms the upper jaw, the anterior part of the roof of the mouth, the lateral walls of the nasal cavities and part of the floor of the orbital cavities

- **Nasal** – the paired bones form part of the bridge of the nose. The lower and major part of the nose consists of cartilage

- **Lacrimal** – the two bones are thin and roughly resemble a fingernail in size and shape. They are the smallest bones of the face

- **Palatine** – two L-shaped bones form the posterior portion of the hard palate

- **Turbinate** – two scroll-like bones which project into the nasal cavity. Their function is the filtration of air before it passes into the lungs

- **Vomer** – roughly resembles a triangle in shape and forms the lower and back part of the nasal septum

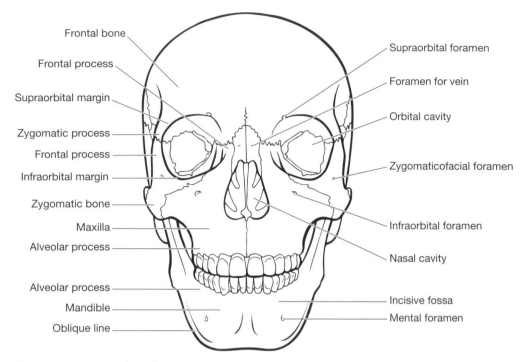

Frontal bone
Frontal process
Supraorbital margin
Zygomatic process
Frontal process
Infraorbital margin
Zygomatic bone
Maxilla
Alveolar process
Alveolar process
Mandible
Oblique line

Supraorbital foramen
Foramen for vein
Orbital cavity
Zygomaticofacial foramen
Infraorbital foramen
Nasal cavity
Incisive fossa
Mental foramen

Figure 9.1 – *Normal facial/skull anatomy.*

disfiguring, leading to considerable psychological damage. Facial injuries often disrupt the appearance and the ability to express emotions. Resultant medicolegal problems may arise if these patients are not handled with the utmost skill and competence.

The diagnosis and treatment of facial fractures depends on the type of injury involved. Therefore it is crucial to establish an early clear understanding of the mechanism of injury. Combined with a detailed knowledge of the anatomy and physiology of the injured area and immediate proper care, the result for the patient should be one of optimum management.

Mechanism of Injury

Most facial injuries are caused by motor vehicle accidents, sports injuries and altercations. Falls and industrial and domestic accidents account for the remainder. Generally it is accepted that the greater the speed of the vehicle, the greater the injury. A history of broken windscreen and damaged dashboards is associated with head and most facial injuries. A bent or collapsed steering wheel should almost certainly make the nurse consider facial or larnyngotracheal injuries. In motorcyclists, the necessity for full face helmets with correctly mounted chin straps which do not allow the helmet to pivot forwards and fly off is highlighted (Richards 1984).

Interpersonal violence continues to be a source of many A&E attendances. The diagnosis and treatment can often be made more complex as alcohol intoxication plays a major part in many altercations; however, injuries tend to be less severe than those following road traffic accidents.

The facial bony structures and sinus cavities have been constructed to offer protection to the brain and will collapse under force, absorbing energy which would otherwise be transmitted into the brain. The attachments of facial muscles also assist in absorbing energy by exerting downward and backward forces on the maxilla. The mandible is often described as one of the strongest bones of the body; however, the condylar necks are frequently fracture sites as they absorb energy forces directed towards the brain. Bony facial injuries are less common in children because of the resilience and elasticity of their facial tissues. When injury does occur, the pattern differs from adults because the relatively large cranium of the child protects the facial bones.

Assessment (Box 9.2)

Maxillofacial trauma is defined as any structure or functional alteration of the bones, nerves, blood vessels or soft tissues of the face that results from accidental or intentional injury (Brown-Stewart 1989). It covers a wide spectrum of disease, ranging from the simple isolated laceration to massive facial trauma with haemorrhage and airway obstruction accompanied by multisystem involvement.

Initial assessment should involve a rapid but thorough examination of the mouth and throat to identify and eliminate any foreign material. Obstruction may occur instantaneously or slowly, as oedema and bleeding progressively occlude the airway. Upper airway obstruction is most commonly due to the tongue and foreign bodies, including vomitus, blood, broken dentures, oedema of the area surrounding the epiglottis, and more uncommonly injury to the larynx. During unconsciousness tone is lost in the muscles which normally hold the tongue away from the pharyngeal wall. Abnormal or prolonged relaxation of these muscles will allow the tongue to prolapse back, obstructing the upper airway. The nurse must be alert for signs and symptoms of airway obstruction, including agitation, intercostal retractions, dyspnoea, cyanosis, gurgling, stridor and a S_aO_2 less than 90% (Henneman *et al.* 1993).

Intubation of the patient may be inevitable where there is a decreased level of consciousness, and it is often very difficult as the head must be maintained in a neutral position. Performance of non-traumatic intubation is vital, as traumatic insertion causes increased intracranial pressure which underlines the need to obtain experienced specialist help. The nasopharyngeal route should normally be avoided

unless basilar skull fracture has been excluded, thus leaving cricothyrotomy as the method of choice for many patients.

Airway obstruction can be alleviated by manoeuvring the mandible anteriorly, thereby moving the tongue anteriorly. This manoeuvre can be accomplished by the chin lift or jaw thrust technique. As neither one will compromise a possible cervical spine fracture, both methods should be used in the treatment of trauma victims. Whilst suctioning remains the primary method of clearing secretions, extreme care should be taken not to stimulate the gag reflex or aggravate existing injuries with overactive suctioning techniques. Where appropriate, the fully conscious patient may be allowed to hold her own suction catheter, thereby controlling the build-up of secretions and eliminating the risk of overstimulation.

If no airway obstruction is present and the patient is haemodynamically stable, a systematic examination of the head and face can be performed. Alterations in skin integrity are often readily observable, and their size and location, as well as the amount of associated bleeding and surrounding tissue swelling, should be determined. Careful inspection and palpation of the scalp should be undertaken for injuries disguised by the hair. The head and face should be palpated for crepitus, bony irregularity, tenderness and swelling. Visual acuity and extraocular movements are assessed to detect cranial nerve damage, globe rupture and extraocular muscle injury or entrapment. Diplopia may indicate the presence of an orbital floor fracture (see Box 9.3).

The ears and mastoid areas should be inspected for ecchymosis (Battle's sign), lacerations or discharge. Perforation of the eardrum, bloody or serous rhinnorhoea or otorrhoea, haemotympanum and bilateral periorbital haematomas ('panda eyes') are important findings suggestive of a basilar skull fracture (Criddle 1995). The nose should be examined for alignment, deformity, pain, swelling, septal haematoma, epistaxis and difficulty in breathing. If bleeding and leakage of cerebrospinal fluid are present, an anterior cranial fossa fracture at the cribriform plate should be suspected. Nasal endotracheal or nasogastric tubes should not be passed in case the fracture is further aggravated. Prophylactic sulphonamides or chloramphenicol to prevent meningitis should be prescribed.

Teeth should be examined for fractures, subluxations and avulsions. A tongue blade and good light source can be used to inspect the oral cavity for lacerations. Jaw occlusion should be assessed, checking for pain, malalignment and range of motion.

Because of the location of the seventh cranial (facial) nerve, one or more of its branches are frequently

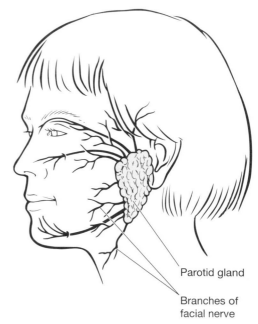

Parotid gland

Branches of facial nerve

Figure 9.2 – *Anatomy of facial nerves.*

superficial lacerations do not usually require a transfusion, there is a danger in overlooking the continuous trickle of fresh blood from a puncture wound.

damaged in maxillofacial trauma. Therefore, facial motor and sensory motor function should be assessed before analgesia or anaesthetics are administered. Assessment of the facial nerve includes testing for muscle strength, symmetry and taste sensation on the anterior two-thirds of the tongue (Criddle 1995). Motor function of the facial nerve is checked by having the patient wrinkle her forehead, frown, smile, bare the teeth and close the eyes tightly. All three major branches of the trigeminal nerve should also be tested for sensation on each side of the face. Loss of sensation in any one of these areas may imply a fracture in the vicinity of that branch (see Fig. 9.2).

Correct positioning of the patient with facial injuries is crucial. After cervical spine injury has been eliminated by clinical examination or lateral cervical X-ray, the fully conscious patient may be allowed to adopt a suitable position for both adequate airway management and comfort. Elevation of the trolley head between 15° and 30° will assist the drainage of blood and secretions from the nasopharynx and decrease the amount of oedema (LeDuc Jimmerson & Lomas 1994).

Soft tissue injuries must be fully inspected. Unexpected foreign bodies are not infrequently found in facial and scalp wounds. Additionally, while extensive

Le Fort Fractures

In 1901, Rene Le Fort published the results of his experiments in which he inflicted blows to the heads of 35 cadavers by striking them with a wooden club and throwing them at the edge of a table. Le Fort fractures make up the classification of maxillary fractures commonly used today (Tiner & Luce 1994) (Fig. 9.3).

Le Fort I. This can be described as a horizontal fracture through the maxilla and nasal septum, below the level of the malar. This compartment is mobile but produces minimal deformity and will be evidenced by epistaxis, damage to the dental surface and teeth, and crepitus on palpation.

Le Fort II. In this case, the pyramid fracture line passes through the lateral orbital rim, zygomatic arches, roof of the nose and high in the pterygoid plates. This is clinically obvious if displaced, as in the 'stove in' face. The middle third of the facial skeleton becomes detached and is usually driven backwards and downwards, thus compressing the airway and producing an open bite.

Le Fort III. This fracture line passes through the lateral orbital rim, zygomatic arches, roof of the nose and high in the pterygoid plates. It results in complete separation of the facial skeleton from the cranial

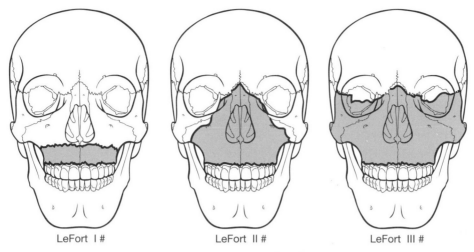

LeFort I #   LeFort II #   LeFort III #

Figure 9.3 – *Le Fort fractures. A: Le Fort I. B: Le Fort II. C: Le Fort III.*

skeleton. It is not unusual for patients to sustain different combinations of these fractures, such as a Le Fort II on one side with a Le Fort III on the other. Maxillofacial expertise may be required to make an accurate assessment.

Clinical evidence

Because the force required to create a Le Fort fracture is quite significant, patients with these injuries usually have a history of severe facial trauma. Clinical findings associated with Le Fort fractures include pain, swelling, nasopharyngeal bleeding, flattening and/or elongation of the facial features, tenderness, mobile maxilla and malocclusion – the patient may describe the teeth as feeling different. Anaesthesia of the cheek, caused by damage to the infraorbital nerve, is also a common finding. A cerebrospinal fluid leak may occur in 25–50% of Le Fort II and III fractures (Manson 1984) and indicates the presence of an open fracture.

Patients with Le Fort III fractures, in particular, tend to have massive facial oedema and ecchymosis and occasionally suffer complete airway obstruction secondary to dissection of a haematoma into the palate, pharyngeal wall or tonsillar pillars. Le Fort fractures are frequently associated with mandibular fractures, causing prolapse of the tongue and intraoral haematoma formation (Crumley 1990).

Management

This is initially directed at maintaining the airway which may be compromised secondary to oedema or haemorrhage. Other causes of obstruction include the accumulation of vomit or other foreign material within the mouth; oedema of the lips, tongue or pharynx resulting from direct trauma; chemical or thermal injuries; and instability of the mandible. It may be necessary to pass an endotracheal tube to secure the patient's airway. In extreme cases, where the airway is severely compromised, placing the fingers in the mouth and lifting the soft palate forward may be life-saving. While assessing the airway, the A&E nurse should note the respiratory rate, evaluate breathing patterns and provide supplemental high-flow oxygen (Ritchie 1994).

Conscious patients should be nursed in an upright position with the head well forward (high Fowler's) allowing any fluid to run freely from the mouth, provided no medical contraindications exist, such as cervical spine injuries or hypovolaemic shock. Unconscious patients should be nursed on their side, allowing fluids to drain unrestricted from the oral cavity.

If a CSF leak is present, anterior cranial fossa and basilar skull fracture should be suspected. Thin, watery, nasal discharge should be considered to be CSF leakage until proven otherwise and the halo or Dextrostix test should be undertaken. Whether there is a CSF leak or not, position, suction and, if required, endotracheal intubation may be satisfactory in securing the airway. Tracheostomy should be considered if the middle third of the face is impacted and cannot be brought forward manually or in the case of uncontrollable postnasal haemorrhage or severe oedema of the glottis.

Definitive treatment of Le Fort fractures is usually delayed for several days until the oedema subsides. Nasal and pharyngeal packing may be necessary where severe haemorrhage is present. Wound care should be carried out as soon as possible and facial lacerations should be repaired within 24 hours. Application of ice packs to minimise oedema formation should be considered as soon as practicable. Prophylactic antibiotic therapy should be initiated if CSF leak is suspected or present and adequate analgesia should be administered.

Mandibular Fractures

The mandible is a horseshoe-shaped structure suspended from the cranium at the temporomandibular joint (Hinchcliffe *et al.* 1996). The prominent position of the mandible predisposes it to trauma and it may be fractured or displaced as a result of a direct blow to the lower third of the face (see Fig. 9.4 for fracture sites). This may cause a fracture at the site or indirect fracture near the temporomandibular joint. The severity of the fracture may depend upon the mechanism of injury and the dentition of the jaw (the more teeth, the less severe the fracture). Displacement of the fragments depends on the shape of the fracture and the action of muscles. Contre-coup injuries are common in mandibular fractures. A blow sustained on the right mandible frequently results in left mandibular fracture. The majority of mandibular fractures occur in the adolescent or young adult population and are due to interpersonal violence, sports injuries, road traffic accidents and falls (Jones 1997).

Clinical evidence

The importance of correct diagnosis of mandible fractures cannot be stressed enough, particularly in the case of children. If mismanaged or even undetected, they may lead to gross asymmetry of growth or ankylosis of the joint. Although clinical manifestations

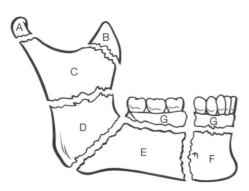

Figure 9.4 – *Mandibular fracture sites. A: Condyle. B: Coronoid process. C: Ascending ramus. D: Angle. E: Body. F: Symphysis. G: Alveolar process.*

of mandibular fractures will vary depending on the location, assessment usually reveals malocclusion, pain, difficulty in speaking and swallowing, facial asymmetry and decreased range of motion. Bruising of the floor of the mouth is highly suggestive of mandibular fracture. Mandibular injuries are classified as open or closed. Fractures are considered open whenever a communication with either the oral cavity or the skin surface is present.

Evaluation of occlusion is the most important aspect of the mandibular examination. Patients with only mild pain and full range of motion, including lateral motion, a normal bite and no loss of strength, are unlikely to have a mandibular fracture (Criddle 1995). Radiographic diagnosis of a fracture is most easily made with a dental panoramic X-ray film, but regular films will detect most fractures. Fractures in the area of the condyles may be visible only on CT scan (Cantrill 1988).

Management

Management of mandibular fractures begins with maintenance of a clear airway, as described for Le Fort fractures above, and administration of antibiotics if the fracture is compound, which includes a tooth-bearing area. Application of ice packs to reduce swelling, wound care and repair of oral lacerations to prevent contamination by saliva are also important considerations. Adequate analgesia should be given and the patient prepared for admission to hospital for surgical fixation. This is usually intermaxillary wiring for simple fractures and open reduction with interosseus wiring for more complex fractures. Generally, mandibular fractures will require some sort of jaw immobilisation for approximately 6 weeks to promote both healing and comfort. Fixation is usually delayed until the patient is stable.

Orbit Floor Fractures (Blow–Out Fracture)

These are caused by a sudden rise in intraorbital pressure and are usually sustained as a result of a direct blow to the globe when an object more than 5 cm in diameter, such as a ball, dashboard or fist, hits the rim of the orbit (see Fig. 9.5). Smaller objects tend to cause penetrating injuries. The orbital rim is not usually damaged but the bone of the orbital floor gives way under pressure of the eyeball, which can sustain considerable force without rupturing, resulting in the inferior oblique and inferior rectus muscles herniating with some periorbital fat through into the maxillary antrum.

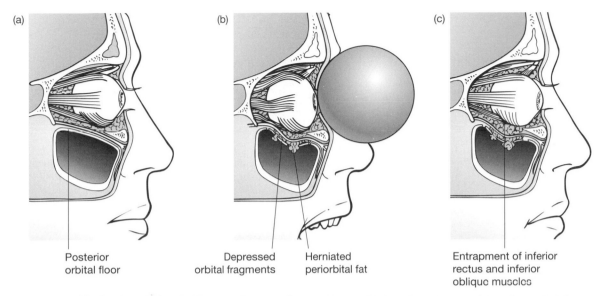

Posterior orbital floor

Depressed orbital fragments

Herniated periorbital fat

Entrapment of inferior rectus and inferior oblique muscles

Figure 9.5 – *Mechanism of injury in blow-out fractures (lateral view, sagittal section through orbit and associated structures). 1, Force causing increased intraorbital pressure; 2, posterior orbital floor; 3, depressed orbital floor fragments; 4, herniated periorbital fat; 5, entrapment of inferior rectus and inferior oblique muscles. (After Gerlock et al. 1981.)*

Clinical evidence

Entrapment of nerves and muscles produces the signs and symptoms associated with this injury. The only evidence of a blow-out fracture may be a 'tear drop' of soft tissue seen on X-ray hanging down into the antrum. On examination, enophthalmus, a limited upward gaze, may be detectable, and on asking the patient to adopt an upward gaze, diplopia may be observed. Globe injury occurs in 10–25% of blow-out fractures, with vision loss in 8% of patients (Tintannalli *et al.* 1996). Pain, periorbital bruising and sub-conjunctival haemorrhage are regarded as reliable signs of a blow-out fracture.

Management

Treatment includes the application of cold compresses to reduce oedema formation, antibiotic cover to prevent orbital cellulitis and the administration of analgesia. Regular monitoring of vital signs and recording of neurological observations should also be carried out. To avoid further haemorrhage, the patient should be made aware of the need to avoid blowing the nose. Surgical elevation of the orbital floor may be required after the release of any trapped nerves, usually after 24 hours. As the patient may be acutely anxious about the loss of vision, the nurse should provide reassurance and information about the treatment and care plans.

Temporomandibular Joint (Jaw) Dislocation

Temporomandibular joint (TMJ) dislocations are commonly caused by yawning, chewing and, laughing, typically occurring with an audible 'pop' during maximal jaw opening (see Fig. 9.6). Occasionally they occur as a result of trauma. Although dislocation can be unilateral, it is more commonly bilateral and is always anterior. Many patients with TMJ dislocation have anatomical conditions which predispose them to recurrent episodes.

Clinical evidence

Dislocations of the jaw are relatively easy to diagnose, as the patient will present with a drooling mouth which is propped open and unable to be closed or moved. It is usually very painful and the patient will also find it difficult to speak. If the patient presents with a history of trauma, X-rays should be taken; otherwise they are unnecessary.

Management

The treatment of TMJ dislocation is directed towards relocation of the jaw. Reduction usually requires analgesia and some form of sedation. Short-acting

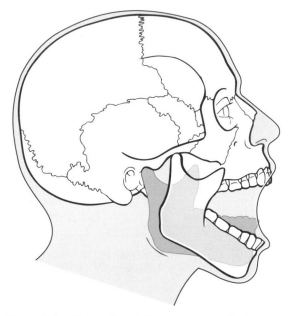

Figure 9.6 – *Dislocation of the temporomandibular joint.*

parenteral muscle relaxants, such as diazepam or midazolam, are useful for relaxing jaw spasms and only rarely is there a need to resort to general anaesthesia or open reduction.

Reduction is accomplished by sitting the patient in a chair or on the floor with her back to the wall. A physician or nurse practitioner with well-padded thumbs stands directly in front of the patient and places his thumbs on the third molars of the mandible with the fingers curled under the symphysis of the mandible. Downward pressure is then applied on the molars with slight upward pressure on the symphysis to lever the condyles downward. As soon as the condyles are past the articular eminence, the strong jaw muscles will cause the mandible to shut suddenly into the normal closed position – hence the need for well-padded thumbs (Amsterdam 1988).

Post-reduction X-rays should be taken if this is the first dislocation for the patient. The patient should be advised to avoid yawning or otherwise stressing the temporomandibular ligaments for several weeks after TMJ dislocation. This will include advice to take a soft diet for several weeks to reduce the risk of further dislocations.

Frontal Sinus Fractures

Frontal sinus fractures frequently occur as a result of blows to the face, sports injuries and falls on the side of the face. The frontal, zygomatic and nasal bones are affected. They are frequently found to be depressed and can be compound or closed.

Clinical evidence

The patient with a frontal sinus fracture will present with a history of trauma, tenderness and swelling at the site of the injury. Periorbital ecchymosis and severe lateral, subconjunctival haemorrhage are often present. Physical examination is usually hampered by oedema, and these injuries are notorious for appearing insignificant until the oedema resolves (Smith 1991). Related complications, e.g. eye injuries, supraorbital anaesthesia and CSF rhinorrhoea, may also be present.

Management

This involves wound care and ice packs to reduce swelling. Antibiotic cover will be required if a compound is present. Elevation of the depressed fracture will be required when the patient's condition is stable. Most zygomatic fractures are significant enough to require open reduction and stabilisation with internal wire fixation for 4–6 weeks.

Nasal Fractures

The nose is the most common site for facial fractures and is frequently associated with other fractures of the middle third of the face. Usually they are the result of blunt trauma because of the prominence and lack of supportive structures. The nasal bones may be displaced laterally or posteriorly depending on the direction of the traumatic force (Fig. 9.7).

Clinical evidence

Patients with nasal fractures usually present with a history of trauma, oedema, tenderness, ecchymosis and obvious deformity. Periorbital haematoma and subconjunctival haemorrhage may also be present. Epistaxis may or may not be present and is usually minor. It is usually due to bleeding from Little's area and is easily halted by pressure with the thumb for several minutes. It is important to examine the inside of the patient's nose for the present or absence of a septal haematoma and to observe for CSF rhinnorhoea, an indicator of fractures of the cribriform plate (Cantrill 1988).

Management

There is no treatment required for undisplaced fractures, however the ENT department may wish to see the patient 5–10 days later, when any swelling has

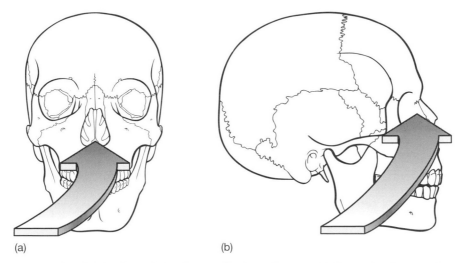

(a)   (b)

Figure 9.7 – *Mechanism of injury in nasal fractures. A: Tangential forces displace nasal bones laterally. B: Posteriorly directed blows displace fracture fragments into other facial structures. (After Criddle 1995)*

resolved but before the fracture has united. Conventional packing of the nose may be sufficient, although a postnasal pack may be required and advice should be sought from an ENT specialist if available.

An X-ray is not essential in diagnosis but is often requested for medicolegal reasons. If haemorrhage has been severe or persistent then vital signs and haemoglobin level should be checked. For comfort, the patient should be given analgesics and advised to apply a cold compress to the nose.

Facial Wounds

The face is highly vascular and, as a consequence, most wounds, even when contaminated, heal well if careful wound management is carried out. Infection is usually rare but haemorrhage can be severe and may result in the patient requiring transfusion. Small puncture wounds that scarcely seem to require suturing may cause life-threatening haemorrhage if they should involve an artery such as the facial or superficial temporal arteries.

Wounds should be assessed regularly for blood loss. If there is continued haemorrhage all wounds, however small, should be explored, and if necessary blood vessels should be ligated or clipped. Significant haemorrhage can occasionally occur in patients with closed middle-third injuries of the face. This normally presents as a steady flow of blood from the nose and mouth; bleeding into the soft tissues of the face gradually produces marked facial swelling and the skin is shiny and tense. As road traffic accidents are

frequently the cause of facial wounds, glass may be present from a shattered windscreen, and therefore it is wise to have soft tissue X rays taken before any attempt is made at wound closure.

Irregular skin edges should be trimmed, although large areas of skin should not be incised. Dirty abrasions should be scrubbed thoroughly and occasionally general anaesthesia may be required in order to achieve the best result. As facial wounds heal faster than wounds elsewhere, fine monofilament nylon or polypropylene, which causes less tissue reaction, should be used and removed after approximately 4 days. If required, adhesive strips may be applied when the sutures have been removed. This provides a little extra support and eliminates the risk of scarring caused by suture marks. Repair of complicated wounds may require the skills of an experienced plastic surgeon and attempts by the inexperienced casualty officer should be avoided whenever possible. Wound care is examined in detail in Chapter 34.

Eyelids

Wounds of the lids frequently occur but are rarely dangerous. The lids, when closed tightly in reaction to a threat, have nearly half an inch (13 mm) of tissue in front of the eyeball providing adequate cushioning and protection (London 1991). Nevertheless, eyelid wounds caused after a fall or of a penetrating nature may create complications and require meticulous attention. They should therefore be referred to an ophthalmic or plastic surgeon.

Lips

A blow on the lip can sometimes split it cleanly against the teeth, but if the blow is angled it can cause a shearing of the lip from its attachment to the gum. It is particularly important that perfect alignment of the mucocutaneous junction of the lip is achieved in order to avoid a step resulting in the lip margin. It is possible for injected local anaesthetic to cause distortion of the tissues and the picture may be confused as a result. However, careful attention by an experienced senior doctor or plastic surgeon can produce excellent results.

Infection is common where a penetrating wound is caused by the teeth when both sides of the lip have been involved. It is important that the laceration should be repaired inside and out. Careful examination is required where broken teeth are present, to eliminate any fragments which may be retained within the lip.

Eyebrows

Eyebrows should *never* be shaved as they may never regrow properly and can cause unnecessary distress. As in the treatment of the lip, the aim is to achieve perfect alignment. Modern methods include the use of tissue adhesive for many types of wound closure (Davis & Cordeaux 1994). Careful assessment of the type, size and location of the wound must take place before any attempt is made and only those well practised should undertake this task.

Ears

Lacerations involving cartilage will need careful reconstruction, but it should be the skin alone which is sutured and not the cartilage. Avulsion of the pinna is not uncommon as a result of interpersonal altercations. The skin slips and the cartilage is pulled out. If adequate blood supply is retained in the flap which is formed then the cartilage can be tucked back in and the skin sutured.

Haematomas (cauliflower or rugby player's ear) require urgent aspiration, followed by pressure pads bandaged or strapped to press the ear against the head. This procedure may have to be carried out every few days until no reaccumulation of blood occurs, thereby allowing the perichondrium to grow back onto the cartilage. If this is not achieved then it will die and shrivel, resulting in a cauliflower ear.

Rupture of the ear drum can occur from sustaining a blow to the side of the head. After the diagnosis is confirmed, the patient should be warned not to allow water into the meatus. The ear should not be packed and no ear drops are required; only referral to an ear, nose and throat clinic is necessary (see Ch. 43).

Teeth

Care must be taken not to miss an inhaled tooth, and if in any doubt an X-ray must be arranged. Lacerations of the lip should be carefully examined for small pieces of broken tooth which may have become embedded there. Tooth sockets which continue to bleed may require packing; this should be done using adrenaline-soaked gauze. Failure to arrest the haemorrhage may result in suturing and/or packing of the socket, with surgical referral to a dentist.

Injuries to the inside of the mouth and tongue

These are most commonly seen in children after a fall, when the teeth penetrate the tongue. Small lacerations can be left untouched and they will heal quickly. Larger lacerations often result in prolonged haemorrhage and can be distressing to both patient and parent. Suturing of the wound is often necessary, especially if the edge of the tongue is involved, causing a flap. Absorbable suture material is often used, thereby obviating the need for a return visit for removal. However, this procedure in children is frequently difficult and occasionally general anaesthesia has to be administered if optimum results are to be achieved.

It is important to examine the patients intraorally for haematoma, especially under the tongue as this is indicative of a mandibular fracture. The patient or parent should be advised of the need to adopt meticulous oral hygiene care when injury to the tongue or the inside of the mouth occurs.

Fauces

Injury to the tonsillar fossa is often the result of a child falling while holding an object in her mouth. As the internal carotid artery is close by and traumatic thrombosis can ensue, this situation should be taken seriously from the outset. The mechanism of injury must be clear before a final conclusion is reached regarding the treatment of cases presenting with this type of injury. The patient should be closely observed for signs of developing retropharyngeal abscess post-injury.

Conclusion

All facial injuries should be treated as a head injury. Therefore neurological and vital signs should be checked and recorded at regular intervals (see Ch.

26). Continuous reassurance from both nursing and medical staff will be required due to the distressing nature of the injury. The patient is likely to be very anxious and the nurse will play a major part in the early provision of both physical and psychological care.

Detailed initial assessment of the patient with facial injuries is crucial and will consequently influence the final outcome. Correct airway management is essential and extreme care and continuous monitoring of the patient are imperative if a satisfactory result is to be achieved. Severe facial injuries ideally should be managed by an experienced maxillofacial surgeon, if the patient is to receive the best possible care with the best possible outcome.

References

Amsterdam JT (1988) Dental emergencies. In Rosen P, Barkin RM, Braen G, *et al.*, eds. 2nd edn. *Emergency Medicine: Concepts and Clinical Practice*. St Louis: Mosby.

Brown-Stewart P (1989) Maxillo-facial trauma: Implications for critical care. *Critical Care Nurse*, **9**(6), 44–57.

Cantrill SV (1988) Facial trauma. In Rosen P *et al.*, eds. 2nd edn. *Emergency Medicine: Concepts and Clinical Practice*. St Louis: Mosby.

Criddle LM (1995) Maxillofacial trauma and ear, nose and throat emergencies. In: Kitts, Selfridge-Thomas J, Proehl JA, Kaiser J, eds. *Emergency Nursing: a Physiologic and Clinical Perspective*, 2nd edn. Philadelphia: WB Saunders.

Crumley RL (1990) Maxillofacial and neck trauma. In: Ho MT, Saunders CE, eds. *Current Emergency Diagnosis and Treatment*. Norwalk: Appleton & Lange, pp. 228–244.

Davis JE, Cordeaux S (1994) Tissue adhesive: use and application. *Emergency Nurse* **2**(2), 16–18.

Gerlock AJ, McBride KL, Sinn DP (1981) *Clinical and Radiographic Interpretation of Facial Fractures*. Boston: Little Brown.

Henneman EA, Henneman PL, Oman KS (1993) Ventilation and gas transport: pulmonary, thoracic and facial injuries. In: Neff JA, Stinson Kidd P, eds. *Trauma Nursing: the Art and Science*. St Louis: Mosby Year Book, p. 167.

Hinchliff S, Montague S, Watson R (1996) *Anatomy and Physiology*, 2nd edn. London: Baillière Tindall.

Hutchinson I, Lawlor M, Skinner D (1996) Maxillofacial injuries. In: Skinner D, Driscoll P, Earlam R, eds. *ABC of Major Trauma*, 2nd edn. London: BMJ.

Jones N (1997) Facial fractures. In: Jones N, ed. *Craniofacial Trauma*. Oxford: Oxford University Press.

LeDuc Jimmerson C, Lomas G (1994) Facial, ophthalmic and otolaryngeal trauma. In: Driscoll PA, Gwinnutt CL, LeDuc Jimmerson C, Goodall O, eds. *Trauma Resuscitation: the Team Approach*. Basingstoke: Macmillan.

London PS (1991) *The Anatomy of Injuries and its Surgical Implications*. Oxford: Butterworth Heinemann.

Manson PN (1984) Maxillo-facial injuries. *Emergency Medicine Clinics of North America*, **2**, 761–768.

Richards PG (1984) Detachment of crash helmets during motor cycle accidents. *British Medical Journal*, **288**, 758

Ritchie E (1994) Management of facial fractures. *Emergency Nurse*, **2**(3), 10–15.

Smith RG (1991) Maxillorfacial injuries. In: Harwood-Nuss A, Linden C, Luten RC, Sternbach G, Wolfson AB, eds. *The Clinical Practice of Emergency Medicine*. Philadelphia: JB Lippincott.

Tiner BD, Luce EB (1994) Facial fractures. In: Montgomery MT, Redding SW, eds. *Oral-Facial Emergencies: Diagnosis and Management*. Portland: JBK.

Tintannalli B *et al.* (1996) *Emergency Medicine: a Comprehensive Study Guide*. New York: McGraw Hill.

Chapter 10

Burns

Steve Harulow & Lynda Holt

- Introduction
- Assessment
- Specific burns injuries
- Burn wound care
- Pain control
- Escharotomies
- Psychological considerations
- Transfer to specialist units
- Minor burn wound care
- Conclusion

Introduction

Despite legislative attempts to improve safety and increase public awareness, patients with burn injuries remain a significant proportion of trauma patients attending A&E departments. Each year in the UK, it is estimated that more than 10 000 people need admission to hospital because of burn-related problems; 600 of these subsequently die from their injuries (Arturson 1993). Add to this the number of individuals treated as outpatients and the scale of the problem becomes apparent. Although the mortality rate from major burns has been reduced enormously in the latter part of the 20th century, because of a better understanding of the mechanisms of injury, the control and prevention of infection, and earlier and more effective surgery, the potential for death still exists (Settle 1995). Without pertinent and urgent treatment, the chances of surviving a major burn are greatly reduced. Burn injuries are more than 'skin deep'; they represent a complicated assault on the body's vital organs and systems (Arturson 1993). Management of major burn injury must reflect this, and through effective organisation and prioritisation of care, potentially life-threatening problems can be dealt with successfully, or in some cases avoided in the first instance.

This chapter aims to unravel some of the complexities of burn injury management. Mechanisms of injury with specific first aid measures, implications of a burn injury in the assessment of airway, breathing and circulation, and immediate psychological care needs will all be covered in detail. The chapter will also consider burn wound management, treatment of more minor injuries and indications for transfer to specialist burns units.

Assessment

First aid overlaps the initial A&E management of burn injuries, especially when first aid has not been commenced at the scene of the incident. Prompt, appropriate first aid, besides being life-saving, can lessen the severity of burn injury (Lowry & Gill 1992). In a stressful situation, confusion often exists over what constitutes safe first aid, particularly for the lay person (Lawrence 1987). Appropriate action can be summarised as:

- safe removal from the source of the burn
- maintenance of airway
- arresting the burning process by application of cold water to reduce residual heat in body tissues or to remove corrosive substances
- reduction of pain
- protection of damaged skin from desiccation and infection.

During this period it is important to obtain a brief, accurate history of the event (Settle 1995). Establishing what, where, when, why and how injuries happened will enable appropriate, prioritised care to be commenced promptly (Kemble & Lamb 1987). This can be taken from the patient, relatives or ambulance crew (Box 10.1)

Box 10.1 – *Information about patient/incident*

- Circumstances of the incident (e.g. explosion, RTA or fire)
- Time of injury, to allow accurate estimation of circulatory fluid loss
- First aid measures undertaken
- Distribution of burns
- Presence of other injuries: fractures, head injury
- Relevant medical history, including tetanus status and current drug therapy

---

The principles of ATLS should be applied to the assessment and immediate care of patients with major burn injuries.

Airway and breathing

The first priority in the management of a burn-injured patient is to secure the patency of the airway and provide adequate ventilation (Judkins 1992). Inhalation injury and respiratory complications are two of the leading causes of fatality in the early period following burn injury. The presence of one or both of these greatly increases the risk of mortality (Mosley 1988). The early detection and treatment of airway or breathing problems must be paramount in the patient's overall management. Direct heat and chemical pro-

ducts pose the greatest threat to airway and breathing. A direct heat injury will be evident soon after injury. Unless steam inhalation has occurred, the damage is usually limited to the upper airway. Direct heat injury causes face, neck and intraoral burns and leads to a rapid development of oedema, resulting in complete airway obstruction within hours (Wilding 1990).

Chemical inhalation usually involves the by-products of combustion, carbon monoxide and hydrogen cyanide, which affect the lower airways. The chemicals cause alveolar damage, pulmonary oedema and surfactant insufficiency. They reduce the circulatory availability of oxygen because carbon monoxide has a much greater affinity for haemoglobin than oxygen, and subsequently induce acidosis. Chemical inhalation should be suspected following a loss of or altered consciousness, history of fire within an enclosed space, the presence of intraoral burns and soot in the mouth, nose and sputum, and where a confirmed history of smoke inhalation exists (Judkins 1992).

Acute airway obstruction is diagnosed by the presence of dyspnoea, wheezing, hoarseness, stridor, loss of voice and even minimal evidence of laryngeal swelling. Once this has been detected, early intubation is essential to allow effective airway management. In less severe cases, where there is no direct evidence of airway involvement, close and careful observations should be continued. The A&E nurse should not be misled by the apparent mildness of symptoms. This is often an inaccurate indicator of the degree of damage occurring and the patient's condition should be reviewed on an ongoing basis for increasing shortness of breath, feelings of tightness, wheezing or hoarseness, (Judkins 1992). All patients with suspected inhalation injuries should be given high-flow, humidified oxygen therapy (at least 60%) as soon as possible (Kinsella 1993).

The administration of high levels of oxygen, either via mask or endotracheal tube, greatly reduces the half-life of carboxyhaemoglobin (HbCO) and increases its rate of elimination from the body. This reduces systemic hypoxia. Measuring this can prove difficult in A&E because usual methods such as oxygen saturation monitoring are rendered ineffective as they do not discriminate between oxy- and carboxyhaemoglobin and are therefore misleading (Langford & Armstrong 1989). The actual diagnosis of an inhalation injury is often difficult to confirm in the initial stages of care (Clark *et al.* 1989). Investigations include arterial blood gas analysis, although values initially remain within normal limits, with a gradual decline in P_aO_2 developing on repeated analysis (Judkins 1992).

Chest X-rays are usually obtained, but they do not often show early signs of respiratory problems, although they may highlight other injuries (Clark *et al.* 1989). Measurement of HbCO and cyanide levels is important, but results are not always immediately available to A&E staff. Fibre-optic bronchoscopy is valuable as a secondary investigation to confirm the presence of soot in the lower respiratory tract (Kinsella 1993). Because of the difficulty in diagnosis, objective observation and reporting of respiratory changes by the A&E nurse provide the subtle indicators needed to decide the treatment needed. Burn injuries result in a significant increase in respiratory tract secretion as part of the histamine response. If the patient has a compromised airway or is intubated, regular suctioning may be necessary to clear the airway of excessive secretions (Swearingham & Keen 1991). Circumferential full-thickness burns to the neck and chest may compromise the mechanism of breathing and necessitate emergency escharotomy (Settle 1995).

Circulation

The patient with major burns will develop severe hypovolaemic shock within 3–4 hours from the time of injury, unless adequate fluid resuscitation measures are initiated (Settle 1995). Damage to the capillary network in the skin leads to loss of water, proteins and electrolytes from the circulation. There are three reasons for this: wound secretion, evaporation and localised oedema; in severe cases, generalised oedema in surrounding, apparently uninjured, areas also occurs (Arturson 1993). The oedema occurs because of changes in permeability of capillaries and tissues affected by heat. Fluid consists mostly of dilute plasma, which increases the viscosity of the remaining intravascular fluid and slows or stops blood flow to capillaries. Poor tissue perfusion increases the extent of the burn because of low oxygen (Cook 1997). If this process is left unchecked, severe shock is likely, but given the predictability of fluid loss, the principal aim of care is to anticipate it and compensate with fluid resuscitation (Settle 1995).

Loss of circulating volume always occurs following a major burn injury. Cardiac output is reduced by about a third within the first hour of injury (Cook 1997). Normal compensatory mechanisms allow homeostasis to be maintained initially, but fluid resuscitation is vital if this is to be maintained. Rapid initial transfusion may result in little improvement. It does, however, reduce the impact of a further reduction of cardiac output around 6 hours post-injury. Although haemoglobin becomes more fragile and has a shorter life span following a significant burn injury, blood transfusion is not recommended in initial management as it may increase the viscosity of intracellular fluid. Haemolysis will occur in transfused blood, therefore reducing its effectiveness.

Fluid replacement

To accurately determine the amount of fluid required, it is necessary to assess the area of body surface damaged by burn injury. The 'rule of nines' (Fig. 10.1) is a convenient tool for a quick initial assessment, but has been largely superseded by the Lund and Browder assessment guide (Fig. 10.2). This toll is more accurate, as it allows for surface area variations with age. If the surface area burned exceeds 15% in adults (10% in children) intravenous fluid resuscitation is indicated; over 30% and this resuscitation becomes urgent (Settle 1995). It is also possible to estimate the patient's likelihood of survival based on the percentage area of body burned (Table 10.1).

Fluid replacement is calculated from the time the burn is sustained, rather than the time resuscitation

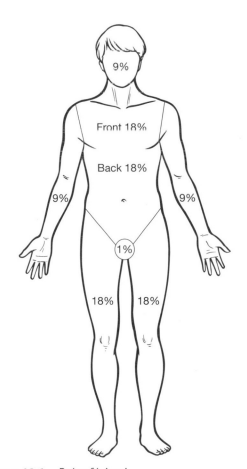

Figure 10.1 – *Rule of 'nines'.*

NAME _____ WARD _____ NUMBER _____ DATE _____

AGE _____ ADMISSION WEIGHT _____

LUND AND BROWDER CHARTS

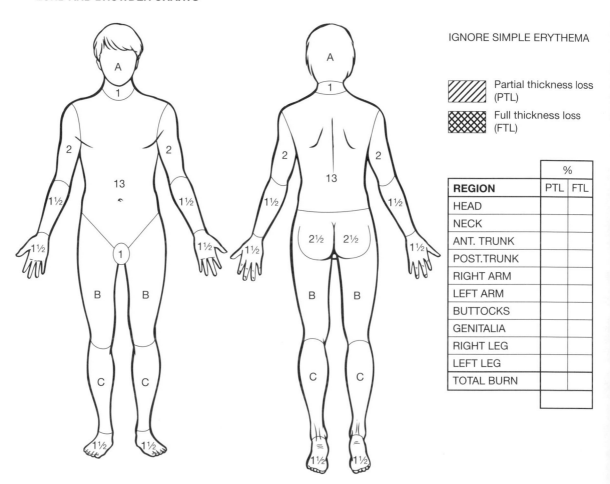

IGNORE SIMPLE ERYTHEMA

| | Partial thickness loss (PTL) |
| | Full thickness loss (FTL) |

	%	
REGION	PTL	FTL
HEAD		
NECK		
ANT. TRUNK		
POST.TRUNK		
RIGHT ARM		
LEFT ARM		
BUTTOCKS		
GENITALIA		
RIGHT LEG		
LEFT LEG		
TOTAL BURN		

RELATIVE PERCENTAGE OF BODY SURFACE AREA AFFECTED BY GROWTH

AREA	AGE 0	1	5	10	15	ADULT
A = ½ OF HEAD	9½	8½	6½	5½	4½	3½
B = ½ OF ONE THIGH	2¾	3¼	4	4½	4½	4¾
C = ½ OF ONE LEG	2½	2½	2¾	3	3¼	3½

Figure 10.2 – *Lund and Browder charts.*

begins. In the UK, the most commonly used fluid replacement tool is the Muir & Barclay formula:

$$\frac{\text{Percentage Area of burn} \times \text{Weight in kg}}{2}$$

This gives the amount of fluid needed for each time period of resuscitation (see Box 10.2). The first 36

hours after injury are divided into the following time periods:

- 3×4 hours
- 2×6 hours
- 1×12 hours

Any delay in hospitalisation is significant because the fluid replacement in the first time period should be

Table 10.1 – *Statistical values of mortality with age and percentage area of body burned. (From Bull 1971)*

Area of body burned (%)	Age (years)								
	0–4	5–14	15–24	25–34	35–44	45–54	55–64	65–74	75+
93+	1.0	1.0	1.0	1.0	1.0	1.0	1.0	1.0	1.0
83–92	0.9	0.9	0.9	0.9	1.0	1.0	1.0	1.0	1.0
73–82	0.7	0.8	0.8	0.9	0.9	1.0	1.0	1.0	1.0
63–72	0.5	0.6	0.6	0.7	0.8	0.9	1.0	1.0	1.0
53–62	0.3	0.3	0.4	0.5	0.7	0.8	0.9	1.0	1.0
43–52	0.2	0.2	0.2	0.3	0.5	0.6	0.8	1.0	1.0
33–42	0.1	0.1	0.1	0.2	0.3	0.4	0.6	0.9	1.0
23–32	0	0	0	0.1	0.1	0.2	0.4	0.7	1.0
13–22	0	0	0	0	0	0.1	0.2	0.4	0.7
3–12	0	0	0	0	0	0	0.1	0.2	0.4
0–2	0	0	0	0	0	0	0	0.1	0.3

0.1 = 10% mortality; 0.9 = 90% mortality.

Box 10.2 – *Example of Muir & Barclay fluid replacement formula*

A 60 kg woman with 20% burns would need the following fluid replacement in the first 36 hours:-

$$\frac{20 \times 60}{2} = 600$$

She would therefore need 600 ml per 4 hours for the first 12 hours, 600 ml per 6 hours for the second 12 hours, and 600 ml for the last 12 hours – totalling 3600 mls over the first 36 hours post-injury.

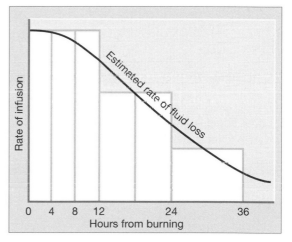

Figure 10.3 – *Estimated rate of fluid loss. (After Bosworth 1997.)*

Table 10.2 – *Maintenance fluid requirements for children*

Body weight	Fluid requirement
< 10 kg	100 ml/kg per hour
10–15 kg	90 ml/kg per hour
15–20 kg	80 ml/kg per hour
20–25 kg	70 ml/kg per hour
25–30 kg	60 ml/kg per hour

adjusted to equate to volume for the first 4 hours post-injury, not the first 4 hours following admission (Fig. 10.3). A fluid resuscitation formula can help to reduce inaccuracies in fluid replacement, particularly when assessment has to be made by inexperienced staff, but these formulae only act as a guideline for infusion (Arturson 1993). Actual amounts of fluid administered should reflect the condition of the patient and vary from the predicted forecasts, dependent on the nursing and technical observations of the clinical situation as it develops.

There is no agreement on the type of fluid which should be used for resuscitating the burn-injured patient. In the UK, most resuscitation attempts use colloid plasma proteins, such as human albumin solution (Settle 1995). This replaces the proteins and water lost through the burn. In addition, fluid must be given to supplement that used by metabolic requirements, which tend to increase following injury. In adults, 50 ml/h of sodium base crystalloid should be given to maintain metabolic function. In children, fluid replacement should be titrated by the child's weight (Wilson 1997) (Table 10.2).

In the resuscitation phase, even seemingly well patients with a major burn should be kept nil by mouth because of the risk of developing paralytic ileus. If this occurs, gastric aspiration via nasogastric tube may be necessary to prevent persistent vomiting (Swearingham & Keen 1991). During resuscitation, frequent monitoring is necessary to detect changes and to attempt to maintain the patient's stability. By using several indicators to give a picture of the patient's overall condition, appropriate clinical decisions can be made.

Pulse, respiration and blood pressure. These give an indication of changes to the patient's homeostasis, level of pain and anxiety. Any increase in pulse or respiration rate should be closely monitored and its cause established. Changes to blood pressure are a late sign in most cases of haemodynamic compromise, but monitoring is still valuable.

Altered level of consciousness. This can have a variety of causes, from primary injury to substance abuse, but hypoxia and hypovolaemia should not be disregarded. A sudden onset of restlessness, particularly in children, should be treated with suspicion and other indicators of stability should be checked.

Skin colour. This is used to detect shock, as well as the level of injury to specific areas. A pink skin tone is indicative of a well perfused patient, whereas pallor indicates arteriole constriction and a blue skin tone indicates venous stagnation consistent with severe shock (Wilson *et al.* 1987).

Skin and core temperature. This is useful for determining the level of vasoconstriction – the greater the difference, the poorer the level of perfusion. In a well person, this different is between 1° and 4°C.

Urinary output. Patients with major burn injuries should be catheterised at an early stage, unless specific contraindications exist. Urine output will vary in early resuscitation because of hormones secreted as part of the stress response to injury. Adequate fluid resuscitation should yield 0.5–1 ml/kg of body weight per hour. Less than this indicates inadequate resuscitation and large volumes of low concentration urine indicate overtransfusion.

Central venous pressure. Although this is useful in the monitoring of most cases of major trauma, its value for the burns patient is limited. Changes to CVP are gradual and the risk of infection is high (Copley & Glencorse 1992).

Frequent laboratory analysis of haematocrit level. This gives an indication of the ratio of red cells to plasma volume. An increased haematocrit level indicates a low plasma volume and therefore inadequate fluid replacement.

Specific Burn Injuries

Thermal burns

These account for a large percentage of minor burn injuries, and a significant proportion of major burn injuries. They can be subdivided into three groups (Box 10.3):

Prehospital management

The source of the burn should firstly be removed, i.e. flames should be extinguished and contact with hot substances reduced. Cold water should be applied to the affected area for approximately 10 minutes to dissipate heat and relieve pain (Kinsella & Booth 1991). This should not exceed 20 minutes because of a significant risk of hypothermia, and the patient should be protected from environmental heat loss (Harulow 1995). Care should be taken if removing molten clothing, as the risk of devitalising healthy tissue is high.

Box 10.3 – *Thermal burns*

■ **Scalds**
Injuries from hot fluids, such as tea, bath water, kettles etc., are the most common causes of all burns. Most of these cause skin damage or loss and are extremely painful. Exposure to water at 60°C (140°F) for 3 seconds can cause a deep partial-thickness or full-thickness burn. If the water is 69°C (156°F), the same burn occurs in 1 second. As a comparison, freshly brewed coffee is about 82°C (180°F) (Wraa 1998). Steam can cause deeper injuries because of its heat. Hot fat also causes more severe injury because of its temperature and, usually, a more prolonged contact with skin.

■ **Contact**
The most commonly treated are injuries from contact with hot objects, such as irons, ovens, hot metal or bitumen. Friction contact, e.g. with road surfaces, causes more superficial burn injuries.

■ **Flame**
Ignition of clothing by petrol, barbecues, bonfires, house fires etc. causes severe injury because of the prolonged contact of the source with the patient's skin. Flash burns from lightning or other electrical sources cause brief exposure to very high temperatures and therefore can result in significant injury (Thayre 1995).

Chemical burns

Common injuries occur from contact with acids and alkalines, as well as domestic substances, such as bleach and cleaning agents. The severity of the burn injury will be determined by the type of chemical, its concentration and the length of time it is in contact with the patient's skin (Cook 1997).

Prehospital management

The treatment priority lies with removal of caustic chemicals from the patient's skin. After rapid removal of soaked clothing, the patient should be showered by large amounts of running water to dilute and remove the chemical. Dry powders should be brushed off before decontamination with water commences (Kemble & Lamb 1987). Water has advantages over specific neutralising solutions. The principal aim of decontamination is to minimise the period of contact between the contaminant and the skin. Time taken searching for particular antidotes leads to deeper levels of injury (Herbert & Lawrence 1989). More importantly, neutralising reactions are exothermic; they generate sufficient heat to exacerbate the injury process. In most cases, adequate dilution reduces the risk of further damage.

Litmus testing of wet skin will indicate acidity or alkalinity, and a neutral buffer solution can be applied, if necessary, once the chemical is diluted sufficiently. In extensive chemical burns, absorption can have systemic effects, including alteration of the blood's acid–base and electrolyte balance, together with renal and hepatic damage (Herbert & Lawrence 1989). Where possible, the identity of the chemical should be established and local poison unit facilities contacted to provide information on specific reactions and antidotes (Settle 1995).

Chemical eye injuries require *immediate* attention (Glenn 1995). Signs and symptoms include:

- pain
- oedema and irritation of the eyelids
- reddened sclera
- loss of or blurred vision.

Periorbital skin irritation or damage should always increase suspicion of eye problems (Brooks 1989). Alkaline injuries are more serious than those involving acids because they rapidly penetrate the conjunctiva through to the cornea, causing significant long-term damage. In all chemical injuries, the eyes should be irrigated, with water initially and with the eyelids held open, until the contaminant is removed. This can be checked by gently placing litmus paper on the eye surface. Insertion of a buffer neutralising solution may be necessary to halt the injury process.

Ensure contact lenses are removed prior to irrigation to prevent a film of contaminant remaining between lens and cornea. The use of a local anaesthetic will relieve pain, reduce anxiety and allow easier examination and treatment (Brooks 1989). Once decontamination has been completed, antibiotic ointments should be prescribed and applied to reduce corneal scarring. All chemical eye injuries must be referred for specialist ophthalmological opinion (Okhravi 1997) (see also Ch. 30).

Electrical burns

These are sometimes more serious than they first appear, as there may be little superficial tissue loss; however, massive muscle injury may be present beneath normal looking skin. Contact with high voltage cables can lead to propulsion injuries. Domestic injury, although of lower voltage, can cause significant damage. The electrical current takes the path of least resistance through the body. Small entry and exit points on the skin's surface may belie the amount of damage to the blood vessels, muscles and bone tissue beneath. In addition to direct heat damage caused by the progression of the current, injury can be sustained by blood vessel necrosis, severe tetany of muscles, conductivity problems in the myocardium, and the force of propulsive impact, often severe enough to cause bone fractures. These patients often suffer secondary 'flash' burns.

Following electrical injury, cardiac monitoring should be used to detect possible arrhythmias. Depending on the path of the current, a 12-lead ECG should be performed to detect myocardial damage, which may occur at the time of injury or several hours afterwards as myocardial tissue breaks down. In serious cases, close attention should be paid to renal function, which will be severely impaired by the release of proteins (myoglobin) from massive tissue breakdown. Hourly urine output should be observed after insertion of a urinary catheter. Darkened urine indicates that myoglobin is, present and warrants immediate action to maintain renal function including intravenous fluid therapy and possibly mannitol to create a high urine output and quickly flush out proteins from the kidneys (Settle 1995).

Cold burns (frostbite)

Although relatively uncommon in the UK, frostbite can be seen in individuals who have had prolonged exposure to extreme cold conditions. Immediate management of the patient concentrates on the monitoring and gradual increase of core body temperature. The extreme cold causes the formation of ice crystals and disrupts cell membranes; vasoconstriction of blood vessels leads to tissue necrosis and an increase in blood viscosity impairs capillary blood flow (Kemble & Lamb 1987). This occurs most commonly on exposed extremities such as fingertips, ear lobes and toes. With superficial frostbite, the frozen part is waxy white and does not blanch or show capillary refilling after mild pressure. The tissue below is soft and resilient on pressure and the affected part is anaesthetic. Rewarming is usually painful, and afterwards the appearance is initially erythematous and oedematous, progressing to a mottled purple colour. Blisters appear, lasting approximately 5–10 days, and eventually dry out leaving a black eschar associated with pain. Demarcation and separation occur over the next month leaving a delicately epithelialised area which is the site of long-term hypersensitivity.

Deep frostbite occurs when the temperature of a limb is lowered (Morris 1998). The frozen part is waxy white and does not blanch or show capillary refilling after mild pressure. The tissue below is hard and cannot be compressed. The affected part is numb. Rewarming is often painful and afterwards the appearance is usually mottled blue (Mills *et al.* 1995). Frostbitten areas should be protected from further trauma, quickly reheated in warm water (around 38°C), dried and maintained at room temperature. Thawing frozen tissue is extremely painful, so intravenous analgesia may be given. Heparin therapy may be commenced together with intravenous Dextran 40 to improve peripheral blood flow. Swelling of the whole limb occurs or appears at the demarcation line several weeks later. If necrosis has occurred, the areas are usually allowed to demarcate before amputation surgery is carried out.

Radiation

These are most commonly caused through overexposure to sunlight or sunbeds. The burns are usually superficial but slow to heal due to injury thromboangitis. More serious injury occurs from exposure to nuclear substances or accidents in radiotherapy. Acute radiation syndrome is a symptom complex that occurs following whole-body irradiation. It varies in nature and severity depending on dose, dose rate, distribution and individual susceptibility.

Pre–hospital management

Decontamination is necessary in cases of nuclear exposure. If the patient's condition permits, this should be initiated at the scene. Ambulance personnel should wear protective clothing, including rubber gloves and shoe covers. The patient's clothing should be removed and placed in plastic bags, and if possible, soap and water cleansing of exposed skin should be performed. Performing these tasks will minimise contamination of the ambulance and A&E department, most of which are not currently well designed for decontamination patients.

Assessment and management

The receiving hospital should be given as much information as possible about the numbers and types of patients involved in a radiation exposure incident, as a decision will need to be made regarding implementation of a full disaster plan versus a limited response. Ideally, contaminated patients should enter the department through a separate, protected entrance. All health care personnel should wear protective, disposable clothing, including surgical gloves and shoe covers. If not already done, the patient should be immediately undressed and washed and all clothing placed in sealed containers labelled 'radioactive waste'. If the patient has open wounds, the surrounding skin should be decontaminated by scrubbing with soap and water. Wounds should be irrigated with copious amounts of saline. The normal principles of wound closure should be followed. No danger to health care personnel should exist if proper precautions are carried out (Markovchick 1992).

Burn Wound Care

Initial management of burn wounds

The aims are:

- to limit further damage with appropriate first aid measures
- to assess the depth of injury, in order to determine treatment plan
- to maintain perfusion and protect damaged tissue from desiccation and infection.

Measurement of burn depth

Burns can be divided into two categories: partial- and full-thickness skin damage. Partial-thickness burns are subcategorised into superficial and deep.

Superficial injuries involve skin loss from epidermis only (Fig. 10.4). The dermal capillaries dilate and fluid leaks into the surrounding tissues. This causes increased pressure on intact nerve endings

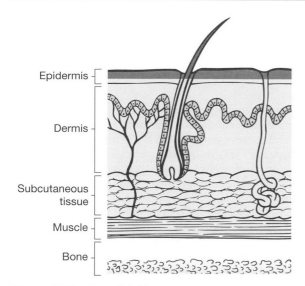

Epidermis

Dermis

Subcutaneous
tissue

Muscle

Bone

Figure 10.4 – *Superficial burn.*

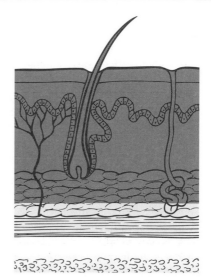

Figure 10.6 – *Full-thickness burn.*

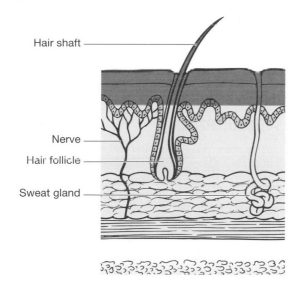

Hair shaft

Nerve

Hair follicle

Sweat gland

Figure 10.5 – *Partial-thickness burn.*

which results in a reddened painful wound, with good capillary refill. It will heal by epithelialisation over a period of about 7 days. These burns usually leave no scarring.

Deeper partial-thickness burns involves both epidermal and dermal damage of varying depths (Fig. 10.5) Capillary destruction occurs which results in fluid escaping to form blisters or a shiny wet wound surface. The wound appears less red than a superficial injury and may have some white avascular areas. Nerve supply is sometimes damaged and generally these wounds are less painful than superficial wounds. Sensation is not lost and the patient should be able to

distinguish between blunt and sharp. These burns heal by regeneration, usually within 14 days.

Full-thickness burns involve all of the dermal layer and may involve underlying structures like muscle, tendon and bone. (Fig. 10.6) The upper skin layers are destroyed, the wound is avascular and appears white or charred, capillary return is absent, and wound exudate is minimal. Sensation is reduced or absent in full-thickness burns. These injuries heal by granulation. Because of the vascular damage, blood supply is reduced and so necrosis and infection are common. Full-thickness burns often require surgical debridement.

Protection of wound

Asepsis is of paramount importance with burn injuries because of the inherent infection risk. Wounds should be cleaned by irrigation with saline. Irrigation reduces the risk of tissue damage when compared with other cleaning methods, and is less painful for the patient. As saline is isotonic, it is unlikely to cause irritation to tissue. Burned clothing, dirt and devitalised tissue should be carefully removed as part of the cleaning process (Copley & Glencorse 1992). Controversy exists over the treatment of wound blisters. Although the fluid contained in blisters promotes healing, and the roof of the blister provides an effective cover to protect new structures forming underneath (Arturson 1993), the size and weight of the blister create a risk of traumatic shearing which can increase the extent of the wound. To remove this risk, blisters can be treated as devitalised tissue and be deroofed (Settle 1995). The optimum approach is to aspirate blister fluid, removing the shearing risk and leaving the blister roof in place to act as a natural dressing (Copley & Glencorse 1992).

Exposed wounds have a faster rate of fluid loss than covered wounds (Dziewulski 1992). Wound care should focus on reinstating the functions lost by the destruction of skin, control of body temperature, maintenance of fluid balance and providing a barrier to infection (Clarke 1992a). For major burn wounds, the replacement of skin functions is the only reason for dressings; they should be simple and not include creams or lotions. The treatment of choice is PVC clingfilm (Wilson & French 1987). It reduces evaporate fluid loss and provides a protective barrier to infection. Clingfilm can be used next to skin or over wet compresses. It is easy to apply and painless to remove. The patient needs additional protection against heat loss. It is important to check the patient's tetanus status and administer tetanus toxoid if the patient is not covered. Systemic antibiotics have not proven effective in preventing wound infections (Dziewulski 1992). They should not be used as a prophylactic measure because they increase the risk of resistant bacteria developing (Lawrence 1992).

Pain Control

Most patients with burn injuries will experience pain, and after immediate life-saving interventions, pain control should be treated as a priority (Kinsella & Booth 1991). The psychological response to burn injury should not be underestimated when assessing a patient's pain. The euphoria of survival and ignorance or denial of the full impact of injury can result in a transient period of little or no pain. Fear and insight into potential outcomes can also have an effect on the extent and type of pain the patient feels. It is imperative that the A&E nurse recognises psychological influences and uses both pharmacological and psychological methods to achieve pain control.

Assessment of pain should include:

- psychological state
- verbal responses
- facial expression
- mobility
- protecting injured areas
- posture.

It is uncommon for an injury to be solely full-thickness (Settle 1995). It is more likely that the wound will be of mixed depth, and therefore some nerve endings will be intact, causing pain. Pain relief starts with the application of cold water. Initial treatment in A&E can include the use of inhaled nitrous oxide (Entonox) in the conscious patient unless associated injuries prevent this. Nitrous oxide has a rapid effect and gives the patient control over his own pain relief (Toulson 1990). Because it is self-administered, there is an inherent safeguard against overdose.

For major burn injuries, patients should be given small, frequent doses of intravenous opioids until pain relief is achieved (Copely & Glencorse 1992). Intramuscular or subcutaneous routes are inappropriate because of hypovolaemia, which causes reduced peripheral circulation and results in poor absorption of the drug and inadequate pain control. Intramuscular and subcutaneous routes also carry the risk of respiratory or CNS depression. This is because a delayed absorption of the drug takes place as circulation improves. Because this happens rapidly, an overdose effect can occur (Kinsella & Booth 1991).

Assessment of pain should include the observation of non-verbal behaviour, such as facial expressions, distorted posture, splinting and impaired mobility, in addition to verbal responses (Kinsella & Booth 1991). This may also give an indication of other traumatic injuries, especially if the patient has been involved in an RTA, explosion or high voltage injury (Bueno & Demling 1989) (see also Ch. 24).

Escharotomies

Escharotomies are carried out where circumferential full-thickness burns occur around limbs, chest, neck, digits or penis. As oedema develops in the tissue beneath, the relatively inflexible full-thickness injury cannot compensate for the increase in tissue volume and exerts a tourniquet effect. If the increasing pressure is not released at an early stage, usually within 3 hours, ischaemic damage will occur in tissues distal to the burn (Settle 1995). In the case of the chest and neck, the rigidity compromises the expansion of the lungs (Judkins 1992). The procedure is carried out by making longitudinal incisions with a sterile blade through the burned skin to bleeding tissue. The release of tension forces the wound to gape open. An absorbent haemostatic dressing, such as calcium alginate, can be placed into the wounds to arrest bleeding. Because the burns are full-thickness in nature, relatively little analgesia is required (Kinsella & Booth 1990).

All burned limbs should be closely observed for signs of impaired circulation, looking at perfusion, capillary refill, temperature and sensation (Molter & Greenfield 1997). Rings, watches, restrictive clothing and tight dressings should be removed and the limbs elevated above heart level to reduce swelling.

Psychological Considerations

Burn injuries produce highly emotive responses because of their association with loss of life, pain and scarring. The psychological impact can be devastating for the patient, relatives and those required to deal with the aftermath (Alexander 1993).

The patient

Initial reactions vary, and some patients will exhibit 'shock', bewilderment and disorientation, with an apparent denial of injury linked to internal defence mechanisms to reduce the anxiety associated with severe injury (Blumenfield & Schoeps 1993). Many patients also experience an initial euphoria associated with survival (Copley & Glencorse 1992). Often the significance of injury is not appreciated, particularly where full-thickness damage is involved or where respiratory complications have not had time to develop. Others may be distressed because of pain and anxiety caused by an awareness of the seriousness of their condition (Kinsella & Booth 1991).

Relatives

The fact that the patient is alert, able to talk and not in any great distress can often lead friends and family into a false sense of security, reinforcing a denial that serious injury has taken place (Konigova 1992). For some, the sight of the patient in pain or with facial or hand burns can be very distressing and cause relatives to fear much worse consequences than will actually be the case. Honest, informative support from experienced A&E staff is necessary.

Staff

Burn injuries, particularly those as a result of fires, have characteristics that are not shared with other forms of trauma. The smell of burned skin and degree of suffering witnessed, especially where death occurs, can be very upsetting even to experienced staff. Staff support is crucial, however the nature of support needs to be tangible and flexible in order to respond to individual needs (Regel 1997) (see also Ch. 12).

Transfer to Specialist Units

Although policies for admission vary, Box 10.4 lists the types of burn injury considered serious enough to warrant specialist attention.

Burns units offer a concentration of resources, in terms of experienced staff and specialised facilities.

> **Box 10.4** – *Burn injuries requiring transfer to specialist units. (From Kemble & Lamb 1987)*
>
> ■ **Major burns** – partial- or full-thickness burns involving more than 5% of of the total body surface area in babies, 10% in children or 15% in adults.
>
> ■ **Burns involving inhalation injury**
>
> ■ **Full-thickness burns** – greater than 2.5 cm in diameter, where skin grafting or flap reconstruction will be necessary to facilitate healing and improve scarring
>
> ■ **Electrical and chemical burns** – both are often more serious than they at first appear and require specific care
>
> ■ **Burns involving specific problematic areas** – these include the hands and feet, face, perineum and major joints
>
> ■ **Burns in those with other problems** – e.g. diabetes, epilepsy, the elderly or where child abuse is suspected

---

Each unit tends to be highly individualised, with its own protocol for admission. For this reason it is difficult to draw up a definitive etiquette for transferring burn-injured patients. It might, however, be useful to consider the following points when planning a transfer. And remember: *Safety is more important than speed.*

Any attempt at transfer must not be considered until the patient is in a stable condition and prepared in such a way that any risk of deterioration in transit is greatly reduced. The airway must be fully assessed and measures must be taken to maintain a patent airway during transfer to reduce the risk of obstruction. An experienced escort, including an anaesthetist where there is airway and respiratory involvement, is essential and the transfer vehicle must be suitably furnished with oxygen, suction and resuscitation equipment (Settle 1995). Intravenous access must be established using two wide-bore cannulae (Ellis & Rylah 1990). Adequate fluid replacement should be commenced and sustained throughout transfer. Similar attention must be paid to analgesia (Arturson 1993). The patient should be transferred in a warm vehicle, well insulated with blankets. Wet dressings are not necessary at this stage (Ellis & Rylah 1990).

Although the initial referral is carried out by medical staff, verbal communication between nursing personnel in the A&E department and receiving burns unit, prior to transfer, is essential. It is worth drawing up a list of local units and their telephone numbers for ease of reference. Confirm with the nurse in charge that a bed is available. Give preliminary verbal information including:

- the name and age of the patient
- relevant medical record
- brief history and time of the incident
- extent, i.e. percentage area involved
- nature of other injuries sustained, particularly any inhalation involvement
- first aid and other subsequent measures undertaken
- ascertain whether the patient should be transferred directly to the burns unit or the A&E department.

It is difficult to convey large amounts of complex information by verbal means alone. Therefore, when handing over to burns unit staff, the escorting nurse must have clearly written details, documenting the points outlined above and specifically:

- the patient's clinical observations
- fluid input and urine output, including that during the transfer
- laboratory results
- any medications given.

Accurate and effective communication improves the continuity of care and allows burns unit specialists to make early decisions about the future course of treatment. It may prove useful to obtain constructive feedback from the burns unit about the transfer procedure and the patient's recovery. This information can be used either to improve the department's future performance or to confirm to those involved that they fulfilled their roles to a satisfactory standard.

Minor Burn Wound Care

Minor burns tend to be classified as those which can be treated on an outpatient basis. The injury usually represents less than 5% of the body surface area and excludes some of the problematic body areas (Duncan & Driscoll 1991) (see Box 10.5).

Box 10.5 – *Areas of special concern*

- Circumferential injury of a limb
- Face
- Eyes
- Ears
- Hands
- Feet
- Perineal injury

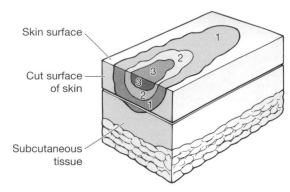

Figure 10.7 – *Pathophysiology of a burn wound. 1, zone of hyperaemia; 2, zone of stasis; 3, zone of necrosis.*

The patient's social circumstances should be considered and his level of support/aid assessed before a decision to discharge is taken. The initial burn injury causes significant disruption to normal skin function. Heat causes cellular injury, resulting in a breakdown of the skin's protective barrier and a susceptibility to infection. The wound itself is initially controlled by the body's natural inflammatory response. Oedema and exudate are rapidly produced, which can to some extent be minimised by cooling the wound and reducing further cellular damage (Clarke 1992b).

The area of the injury has three specific parts (Rylah 1992) (Fig. 10.7):

- *The zone of necrosis* – this is non-viable, or dead, tissue usually found at the centre of the wound.
- *The zone of stasis* – this is the area of the wound which is most vulnerable. It consists of viable tissue, but is at risk of ischaemic damage because of reduced tissue perfusion.
- *The zone of hyperaemia* – this is the area immediately surrounding the damage, which is undergoing the inflammatory phase to injury. The tissue itself is undamaged and develops an increased blood flow in an attempt to control the extent of injury.

The healing of a burn wound depends very much on the depth of injury. Superficial and partial-thickness burns involving the epidermis and upper dermal layers will only heal spontaneously by epithelialisation and regeneration over a period of 7–14 days (Clarke 1992b). It is this group of injuries which are best treated on an outpatient basis. Deeper partial-thickness burns, with damage to all but the deep dermal layers, will heal much more slowly over a period of 3–4 weeks. Full-thickness burns heal by granulation, a process which can take several weeks or months depending on the size of the injury, its site and the patient's general health and age. This group of patients

Table 10.3 – *Stages of wound healing*

Stage	Features of healing
Inflammatory (0–3 days)	Initial response to injury causes redness, heat, pain and swelling with copious exudate
Destruction (2–5 days)	Clearing of devitalised tissue and bacteria and development of fibroblasts
Proliferation (3–24 days)	Production of collagen and granulation tissue which fills the wound space. Although it may looked 'healed' the wound remains very fragile
Maturation (24 days–1 year)	This focuses on restructuring scar tissue; vascularity decreases and redness fades. The wound area strengthens and by 6 weeks scar tissue has about 50% of the tensile strength of uninjured skin
Contraction (4 days onwards)	Process whereby the wound naturally reduces in size. Usually only occurs in large wounds with considerable tissue loss

benefit from referral to specialist units for excision and grafting of wounds.

For those patients who can be discharged, wound care and appropriate advice are paramount. The primary aim is to foster an environment which is appropriate to the healing needs of the wound at a particular stage (see Table 10.3).

Wound cleaning, as discussed above, should be as rigorous for small or minor wounds as for major burns. Differences in management occur in the assessment of wound dressings needed. Most major injuries will not have their full extent and depth assessed for 48 hours until oedema begins to subside (Pankhurst 1997). For smaller wounds, the aims of burns dressings are to prevent colonisation of bacteria, to provide a warm, moist environment for cellular reconstruction, to absorb exudate and to protect the area from further injury.

A&E care usually focuses around the inflammatory stage, where copious exudate is present, and the destructive phase where autolysis demands a moist environment. Initially, a multiple layer of paraffin tulle type dressing, applied under copious padding and bandages, will provide a warm non-adherent, protective dressing for the inflammatory phase. The disadvantage with this method is that, if the dressing soaks through, a tract for infection is created and the patient will need to return to A&E for renewal. These types of dressing should be changed at least daily. Antibacterial agents such as silver sulphadiazine cream are useful in preventing Gram-negative or *Pseudomonas* infections in the initial stages. To remain effective, cream should be reapplied every 24–48 hours (Holt 1998).

After 48 hours, as the wound enters the destructive phase, exudate begins to reduce and the wound benefits from less frequent dressing changes (Clarke 1992b). Hydrocolloid dressings are most effective for this stage of healing. They provide a warm and moist environment which facilitates autolysis and natural debridement of the wound. For maximum effectiveness, these dressings should be left in situ for 4–7 days depending on the site and extent of the wound. Hydrocolloid dressings are also valuable in the treatment of granulating wounds.

Facial burns. Burns to facial areas should be kept moist with soft paraffin ointment and left exposed. Antibacterial creams should not be used as they can cause skin staining when in contact with oxygen. Ears are the exception to this. Silver sulphadiazine should be applied and the area covered with paraffin tulle and padding. This is because the risk of complications from infection includes ear deformity and internal structural damage.

Hands and feet. One of the treatment priorities is to maintain movement. For this reason, wounds are treated with antibacterial cream and covered with polythene bags or gloves. This allows for observation of the wound as well as movement of digits. Wounds treated in this way require daily dressing changes. For further information on wound care see Chapter 23.

Discharge information should include advice about wound care and when to return to A&E, but should also include advice on:

- nutrition to promote wound healing
- exercise regimes to restore normal function
- wound progress and scarring.

Psychological support should also be provided at this time, by allowing the patient to express fears or uncertainty about management of the injury as well as to ask any general questions he may have about care.

Conclusion

Caring for a patient with burn injuries represents a multifocal challenge to A&E staff. Priorities of care must be with the systematic assessment and implementation of life-saving activities, such as airway management and fluid resuscitation. Protection of burn wounds is imperative if secondary injury and infection are to be prevented. The initiation of wound care and patient education are important for those with minor injuries. All patients need time and psychological support to come to terms with their injury. Even minor wounds create high levels of anxiety about scarring.

References

Alexander DA (1993) Burn victims after a major disaster: reactions of patients and their care-givers. *Burns* **19**(2), 105–109.

Arturson G (1993) Management of burns. *Journal of Wound Care* **2**(2), 107–112.

Blumenfield M, Schoeps MM (1993) Psychological reactions to burn and trauma. In: Blumenfield M, Schoeps MM, eds. *Psychological care of the burn and trauma patient* Boston: Williams & Wilkins.

Bosworth C (1997) *Burns Trauma: Management and Nursing Care.* London: Baillière Tindall.

Brooks J (1989) Managing eye injuries. *Practice Nurse* **4**, 451–452.

Bueno R, Demling RH (1989) Management of burns in the multiple trauma patient In: Manll KI, ed. *Advances in Trauma* Vol. 4. Philadelphia: Year Book Medical Publishers.

Bull JP (1971) Revised analysis of mortality due to burns. *Lancet* **ii**, 1133.

Clarke JA (1992a) Burns and the burn wound. *Care Of The Critically Ill* **8**(6), 233.

Clarke JA (1992b) *A Colour Atlas of Burn Injury.* London: Chapman & Hall.

Clark WR, Bonaventura M, Myers W (1989) Smoke inhalation and airway management at a Regional Burn Unit 1974–83. *Journal of Burn Care and Rehabilitation* **10**(1), 52–60.

Cook D (1997) Pathophysiology of burns. In: Bosworth C, ed. *Burns Trauma: Management and Nursing Care.* London: Baillière Tindall.

Copley J, Glencorse C (1992) The nursing management of burns. *Care of The Critically Ill* **8**(6), 246–251.

Duncan DJ, Driscoll DM (1991) Burn wound management. *Critical Care Clinics of North America* **3**(2), 255–267.

Dziewulski P (1992) Burn wound healing: James Ellsworth Laing Memorial essay for 1991. *Burns* **18**(6), 466–478.

Ellis A, Rylah LTA (1990) Transfer of the thermally injured patient. *British Journal of Hospital Medicine* **44**(3), 200–206.

Glenn S (1995) Care of patients with chemical eye injury. *Emergency Nurse* **3**(3), 7–9.

Harulow S (1995) Assessment of burn injuries. *Emergency Nurse* **2**(4), 19–22.

Herbert K, Lawrence JC (1989) Chemical burns. *Burns* **15**(60), 381–384.

Holt L (1998) Assessing and managing minor burns. *Emergency Nurse* **6**(2), 14–16.

Judkins KC (1992) Burns and respiratory system injury. *Care of the Critically Ill* **8**(6), 238–241.

Kemble JV, Lamb BE (1987) *Practical burns management.* London: Hodder & Stoughton.

Kinsella J (1993) Smoke inhalation injury. *British Journal of Intensive Care* **3**(1), 8–14.

Kinsella J, Booth MG (1991) Pain relief in burns: James Laing Memorial essay 1990. *Burns* **17**(5), 391–395.

Konigova R (1992) The psychological problems of burned patients: the Rudy Hermans Lecture 1991. *Burns* **18**(3), 189–199.

Langford RM, Armstrong RF (1989) Algorithm for managing injury from smoke inhalation. *British Medical Journal* **299**, 902–905.

Lawrence JC (1987) British Burns Association recommended First Aid for burns and scalds. *Burns* **13**(2), 153.

Lawrence JC (1992) Infective complications of burns. *Care of the Critically Ill* **8**(6), 234–236.

Lowry M, Gill A (1992) Taking the heat out of burns. *Professional Nurse* **10**, 26–30.

Markovchick M (1992) Radiation injuries. In: Rosen P, Barkin RM, Braen G *et al.* eds. *Emergency Medicine: Concepts and Clinical Practice* 3rd edn. St Louis: Mosby.

Mills K, Morton R, Page G (1995) *Colour Atlas and Text of Emergencies* 2nd edn. London: Mosby-Wolfe.

Molter NC, Greenfield E (1997) Burns. In: Hartshorn JC, Sole ML, Lamborn ML, eds. *Introduction to Critical Care Nursing* 2nd edn. Philadelphia: WB Saunders.

Morris J (1998) Environmental emergencies. In: Newberry L, ed. *Sheehy's Emergency Nursing: Principles and Practice* 4th edn. St Louis: Mosby.

Mosely S (1988) Inhalation injury: a review of literature. *Heart and Lung* **17**(1), 3–9.

Okhravi N (1997) *Manual of Primary Eye Care.* Oxford: Butterworth Heinemann.

Pankhurst S (1997) Wound care. In: Bosworth C, ed. *Burns Trauma: Management and Nursing Care* London: Baillière Tindall.

Regel S (1997) Staff support on the burns unit. In: Bosworth C, ed. *Burns Trauma: Management and Nursing Care* London: Baillière Tindall.

Rylah LTA (1992) *Critical Care of the Burned Patient* Cambridge: Cambridge University Press.

Settle JAD (1995) *Burns: the First Five Days* Romford: Smith and Nephew.

Swearingham P, Keen J (1991) *Manual of Critical Care* 2nd edn. St. Louis: Mosby Year Book.

Thayre K (1995) Lightning strike injuries. *Emergency Nurse* **3**(3), 16–18.

Toulson S (1990) More than a lot of hot air. *Nursing* **4**(2), 23–26.

Wilding PA (1990) Care of respiratory burns: hard work can bring spectacular results. *Professional Nurse* **5**, 412–420.

Wilson D (1997) Management in the first 48 hours following burn trauma. In: Bosworth C, ed. *Burns Trauma: Management and Nursing Care.* London: Baillière Tindall.

Wilson GR, Fowler CA, Housden PL (1987) A new burn area assessment chart. *Burns* **13**(5), 401–405.

Wilson GR, French G (1987) Plasticised polyvinyl chloride as a temporary dressing for burns. *British Medical Journal* **294**, 556–557.

Wraa C (1998) Burns. In: Newberry L, ed. *Sheehy's Emergency Nursing: Principles and Practice*, 4th edn. St Louis: Mosby.

Part 3

Psychological Dimensions

11. Aggression `175`

12. Stress and Distress `183`

13. Care of the Bereaved `189`

14. Psychiatric Emergencies `199`

Chapter 11

Aggression

Barbara Neades

- Introduction
- Why aggression occurs in A&E
- Prevention of aggression in A&E
- Recognising potential aggression
- Defusing aggression in A&E
- Managing the violent individual
- Follow-up care after an aggressive violent incident
- Conclusion

Introduction

Violence and aggression are now recognised as major hazards for staff within the health care sector. The fields of mental health, learning disability and A&E, unsurprisingly, report the highest incidence of verbal and physical threats to staff (Health & Safety Commission 1997). Although most would agree that prevention is better than cure, it may not always be possible to prevent violence and aggression occurring in the A&E environment. This may be a result of the wide variety of factors which can influence the development of aggression in the A&E department, some of which are beyond the control of the department.

The A&E nurse will care for all sorts of human conditions and problems every day of his working life, most of which will be a result of sudden illness or injury. The nature of these events will produce intense emotions and reactions, some of which will be displayed as aggression (Wright 1986). Over 20 years ago, the Royal College of Nursing (RCN) and the Casualty Surgeons Association (CSA) (1977) demonstrated that most aggressive incidents within A&E departments are not recorded. It is a situation which, while improving, is likely to remain the same, and therefore it will continue to be difficult to measure the problem accurately. Whittington & Wykes (1989) demonstrated that verbal abuse and minor injuries can have a significant effect on the individuals involved, including staff and other individuals who are witnesses or who are involved in an incident.

If staff are to attempt to resolve aggression in A&E, it is necessary to assess and manage the problem from a holistic and caring viewpoint, maintaining the safety and dignity of everyone involved. This requires the nurse to identify the factors which influence aggression in the A&E situation, develop strategies designed to prevent it occurring and manage the aggressive situation effectively when it does occur, protecting the patient, staff and any other individuals involved. This chapter will discuss the problem from these perspectives and offer some suggestions to assist the A&E nurse to resolve this increasing difficulty.

Why Aggression Occurs in A&E

Assessing the source of an aggressive situation in the A&E department offers particular difficulties to the staff, as there can be a number of factors influencing its development. These include attitudes of staff, the internal state of the individual and the environment of the A&E department. Standing & Nicolini (1997) argued that the highest risks of violence at work are associated with:

- dealing with the public
- providing care or advice
- working with confused older people
- working with those who have mental health problems
- alcohol or drug misuse
- working alone
- handling valuables or medication
- working with people under stress.

The Royal College of Nursing (1998) noted that many or all of these features are present in the work undertaken by most nurses. Inadequate resources, low staffing levels and inappropriate skill mix also form significant contributory factors. The A&E department can appear a very hostile and threatening place to a patient or relative in an emotionally charged state. Brennan (1998), in examining the range of theories of aggression and violence, suggested that providing satisfactory definitions or an explanation as to where or how these behaviours originate is a complex task. From a psychological perspective the occurrence of a sudden crisis resulting from a serious illness or accident, with the hurried removal of an individual to an A&E department, can often trigger strong emotions (Hildegard *et al.* 1987). These emotions of fear, anxiety, confusion and loss of control often result in stress reactions within the patient or relative and can be displayed in a variety of ways (Farrell & Gray 1992). Many individuals view the A&E department as an anxiety-provoking and hostile environment.

Wright (1986) suggested that individuals develop their own coping mechanisms to deal with stress and that it is when these coping mechanisms fail that aggression may be displayed. Freud (1932) argued that aggression was an innate, independent, instinctual tendency in humans. Bandura (1973) identified the way in which children learn aggressive responses, by role modelling what they had observed in adults. Bateson (1980) argued that an individual is only aggressive when assessed in relation to the other people/surroundings affecting that individual.

Contributing physiological factors in the development of aggression in A&E include the consumption or withdrawal from alcohol or drugs (Kaplan & Sadock 1993). Intoxication with these drugs not only reduces the individual's capacity to understand and interpret events but also reduces inhibitory responses in times of stress. Other organic reactions seen in acute confusional states, e.g. metabolic disorders or hypoxia, may result in altered perceptions for the patient. These alterations in perception may also result in a confused aggressive patient arriving in the A&E department. When admitting these patients, the A&E nurse may be required to repeat information and instructions several times before the patient understands what is happening and how she should conduct herself. The frustration of not understanding can result in aggression as a self-defence mechanism (Taylor & Ryrie 1996).

From a sociological viewpoint, the location of the A&E department, near to the public street, and with 24-hour access may also attract a number of hostile individuals. Distressed or psychologically disturbed patients often attend A&E departments aware of the immediate access to medical and nursing care for crisis intervention (Ambrose 1996). Their confused or distressed state may also result in aggressive responses to the A&E department staff (Brown *et al.* 1990). Hostility can also be a response to pain, the severity of which often increases with long waits to see medical staff in A&E (Wright 1986). In the UK's culturally diverse society, not every member of the public is as conversant with the organisation of the A&E department as the health care worker. The frustration which results from unrealistic expectations of the A&E service may produce conflict and confrontation between the nurse and the patient or relative.

From an organisational perspective the A&E department itself can also influence the level of aggression displayed by patients and relatives who attend. Lack of information about the well-being of a loved one or long waiting times for treatment as a result of poor staffing levels can lead to frustration and anger. Poor waiting environments with lack of stimulation have also been suggested as being influential in developing aggression (Walsh 1996). Judgmental attitudes adopted by staff and poor understanding of the individual's emotional state can result in confrontation between the nurse and the patient or relative (Rix 1985, Warburton 1982). In particular, a sense of lack of control in the individual can precipitate aggression (Moran 1984). The nurse's verbal and non-verbal communications with the patient or relative are very important in conveying a caring understanding attitude to an individual in times of stress or crisis, and in averting confrontation.

Negative non-verbal cues displayed by the nurse stemming from judgmental attitudes can precipitate aggressive outbursts in patients or relatives (Warburton 1982). Berkowitz (1964) suggested that people are more likely to behave aggressively if cues for aggression are provided by others. Poor staffing of A&E departments, where there is a considerable workload, may also contribute to an atmosphere of tension. In these conditions, the nurse may be under pressure to care for a large number patients at any given time. This lack of time to care for the patient adequately may convey an impression of lack of interest in the patient and relatives, resulting in negative non-verbal cues from the nurse and provoking aggressive confrontations.

It is clear that not all aspects of aggression in the A&E are preventable, although a number of influential factors do prevent aggression occurring (Ward 1995). If nurses are to resolve the problem of aggression, a comprehensive review of the preventable factors must be undertaken.

Prevention of Aggression in A&E

The environment into which the patient or relative is received can have a major effect on the response to the stressful events experienced. Poor communication between staff and patients on admission, and in-adequate waiting areas with little or no facilities for stimulation or refreshments can cause frustration in both the patient and relatives (Walsh 1986). Lack of information and increasing waiting times to see a doctor can often trigger aggressive confrontations between the A&E nurse and the patient/relative.

Simple measures that provide the patient or relative with information, such as clear displays of waiting times and comfortable surroundings in which to wait, can relieve the anxiety and tension that may result in aggression. Careful consideration of seating arrangements and decor of the A&E department can help to reduce stress in those waiting to be treated. Other measures such as providing up-to-date reading material and a TV or radio within the waiting area can reduce the boredom and frustration so often experienced while waiting in A&E departments. The use of videos explaining the A&E department's organisation can reduce tension and anxiety in the waiting area. These measures can also be employed to provide health promotion advice to the public. The provision of information is easily the most important issue to stressed relatives and friends (see Box 11.1).

The increase in the number of departments providing a nurse triage system has been invaluable in improving the communication between the nurse and the public in the A&E department. During triage the patient can be assessed and gain information with regard to the illness or injury and the expected waiting times (Williams 1992). This initial assessment allows a

---

Box 11.1 – *Reducing the risk of violence*

ENVIRONMENTAL FACTORS
Environmental calming features

- All areas should look clean and welcoming, paying special attention to reception areas
- There should be adequate warmth/ventilation
- Noise should be minimised, e.g. by keeping the TV volume at a comfortable level
- Designate separate smoking areas as appropriate
- Overcrowding, as far as possible, should be avoided
- Natural daylight and fresh air should be maximised
- Privacy for staff and patients must be provided
- There should be clear direction signs

Providing a secure environment

- There should be a safe room for severely disturbed people as appropriate
- Consider the weight, size and construction of movable objects
- Allow unimpeded sightlines with access points in sight of staff
- Install alarm, communication and monitoring systems where appropriate
- Clinical areas should be lockable to prevent intruders

POLICIES, PROTOCOLS AND STAFFING

- Violent incidents should be audited
- Make provision for incidents, injuries, sickness and time out to be recorded
- Ensure adequate numbers of trained and experienced staff, including arrangements for meal breaks
- There must be appropriate staff mix, including adequate supervision for newly registered and non-registered staff
- Specify who is responsible in the event of an incident
- Ensure adequate support systems in the event of incidents
- Policy should be in place for the assessment and management of substance misuse given its association with violent assaults
- Draw up policies for the avoidance and management of violence
- Ensure that policies are implemented and periodically reviewed

relationship to be formed between the nurse and the patient and can provide an opportunity for the nurse to reduce the stress experienced by the patient. Access to the triage nurse keeps patients or relatives in constant communication with their progress through the department, further reducing stress and anxiety (Dolan 1998).

The provision of adequate numbers of medical and nursing staff in the A&E department prevents long waiting times and allows good communication and the development of good patient–staff relationships. Less aggression is usually demonstrated if the patient or relative is satisfied with the level of care provided by the A&E department and good patient – staff relationships are formulated. This cannot occur in areas where patients and staff are underresourced and pressured. Dolan *et al.* (1997) found that the use of nurse practitioners in A&E, which led to reductions in waiting times, also led to a reduction in aggressive incidents at the times when nurse practitioners were on duty.

In some inner city A&E departments it has been necessary, however, to provide increased security measures to limit the risk of aggression to staff. These measures have included the provision of security screens for reception staff, closed circuit TV cameras, security guards, direct links to police stations via panic buttons and personal attack alarms. Although these measures are not often conducive to conveying a caring, trusting attitude to the public, in some instances they have been required to protect the staff from injury.

Recognising Potential Aggression

Recognising the potential for aggression requires the A&E nurse to have an awareness of the contributing factors in the development of aggression. In addition, the nurse must also have an ability to spot physical signs of impending aggression in order to manage it successfully. Aggressive outbursts in A&E departments rarely occur without warning and are almost always preceded by clear indications that the individual is becoming agitated or aggressive. Jones & Littler (1992) suggested that there are often signs of impending aggression, both verbal and non-verbal, which if left to go unheeded may result in violent outbursts. In the patient or relative, these signs include:

- appearing tense and agitated
- rapid breathing/sweating
- increasing voice pitch and volume
- replying to questions abruptly, very often using abusive gestures

- dilating pupils
- altered body posture, demonstrating muscular tension in the face and limbs
- invasion of other patients'/staffs' personal space
- balled fists
- banging of fists against the palm of the opposite hand or onto nearby objects
- use of obscenities and sarcasm when discussing the staff.

In the A&E environment, the nurse may not be the intended object of the aggressive individual's outburst, but merely an obstacle in the path of the patient or a vehicle for releasing pent-up emotions. This, however, may be of little comfort to the nurse who experiences an aggressive outburst or who is injured by an agitated patient or relative. The nurse therefore has a responsibility to develop an awareness of the patients'/relatives' emotional status through good communication, in order to prevent potentially aggressive incidents occurring.

Defusing Aggression in A&E

Inexperience and lack of skill in some nurses in dealing with aggression may result in their avoidance of the agitated person until a violent situation occurs. Indeed, not all nurses are equipped or able to deal with aggressive or violent individuals. Student nurses are particularly vulnerable to verbal or physical injury (Wondrak 1989). Moran (1984) suggested that even in a situation involving an experienced nurse, there are sometimes only seconds for the nurse to assess the cause of the frustration or aggression within the individual.

Good verbal communication with the aggressive individual is vital in defusing the situation. This attempt to engage the aggressive patient or relative should only be undertaken after summoning assistance, either verbally or via an agreed call system. No nurse should approach an agitated individual unsupported (Farrell & Gray 1992). A calm, confident non-threatening attempt to engage the individual in conversation is viewed as the first step to restoring order to the situation. Wright (1988) suggested that an empathetic approach is useful, listening carefully to the individual's complaint in a private but safe area away from an audience. It is critically important that other staff can find their colleagues quickly in this situation. Encouraging the patient to discuss the problem may assist in defusing the tension of the moment. During this attempt to deal with an aggressive individual, the nurse's voice pitch, volume and tone need to remain within normal conversational range.

If the aggressive individual is confused or under the influence of alcohol or drugs, the nurse may have to repeat the message several times before being understood. Intoxicated thinking often proceeds by association rather than logic. Key phrases such as, 'let us work together' are recommended. Conversely, negative phrases such as, 'you're not going to fight or give us trouble' are generally inflammatory as the patient may associate with the words 'fight' and 'trouble' (Taylor & Ryrie 1996). Nothing will be gained by the nurse responding to the patient or relative negatively despite the provocation from the aggressor. The nurse should listen carefully to the complaint and attempt to offer an explanation or agree a plan of action with the individual to resolve the situation. The use of solutions which are unachievable and the use of inaccurate information to pacify the individual are to be avoided. When these promises are not forthcoming, aggression is more likely.

Walsh (1996) also warned against engaging in communication with large groups of people in an attempt to defuse aggression. He suggested that aggression is amplified by large groups of people, especially in large groups of young males anxious to demonstrate their position by acts of bravado. The aggressive individual should be interviewed in a quiet area, offering privacy and dignity to the patient or relative and, allowing them to express the source of their grievance. Glasson (1993) suggested that the approach of the nurse to caring for the aggressive individual is vital in resolving the problem and protecting the nurse from danger of physical injury. She also suggested that non-verbal communication with the patient via body language is an important factor in reducing tension.

The nurse should also be aware of personal space and stand at least an arm and a half's length away from the individual, allowing a means of escape should it be required. Moran (1984) suggested positioning the feet slightly apart with the body weight on the slightly flexed back leg allowing quick escape. This position poses minimal threat to the aggressive individual. Direct eye contact with the individual can also be interpreted as being provocative by the aggressive individual. The nurse's attention is best concentrated away from the face to just below the larynx area; however, attentive facial expressions suggest interest to the individual and allow good peripheral vision for the nurse. It is also important for the nurse to be aware of the danger in being trapped in an enclosed area while this conversation is in progress. The nurse should always ensure there is a clear method of exit should it be required.

The room where the interview is conducted should be free of objects which could be used as weapons against the nurse. Sharp objects carried by the nurse, such as scissors, can be easily grabbed and used against him. Neck chains, ties and an inappropriately draped stethoscope can all quickly become weapons against the nurse. These should all be removed before approaching the individual. In today's society, weapons such as knives and guns are frequently used by aggressive individuals. The nurse should be aware of suspicious bulges in clothing which may be concealed weapons.

Managing the Violent Individual

Many A&E departments now employ security guards to assist in dealing with violent incidents and issue staff with personal attack alarms to reduce the risk's to their person. This support is certainly useful to staff, but if a caring approach is to be adopted for all individuals within the A&E department, the nurse cannot discharge the responsibility of managing the violent patient/relative to other colleagues. Learning to deal with this challenging and stressful situation is not easy for the A&E nurse. The appropriate knowledge and skills must result from a combination of role modelling of good management strategies and education and training (Paterson *et al.* 1999).

If violence does erupt while the nurse is alone, it is unwise to attempt to restrain the individual. Assistance from other departmental staff, security or local police should be summoned via agreed methods. Until assistance is available, the nurse should make every attempt to avoid physical contact, even if this means there is some damage to property. The nurse would be well advised to place a substantial object between himself and the aggressive person while attempting to discreetly remove any object that could be used as a weapon.

If assistance is not forthcoming, it is better for the nurse to withdraw and observe the individual than to engage that person alone. This can only be done if other patients and staff are not put at risk. If a member of staff is attacked, there should be an attempt made to break away, endeavouring not to put anyone else at risk in doing so. If the situation escalates and restraint is required to contain the aggressive individual, this should be carried out in a coordinated manner with a minimum of four staff. A show of strength in this way is enough to subdue some agitated individuals.

One experienced staff member should be nominated as team leader and maintain verbal communication with the aggressive patient/relative throughout the response. The individual should be invited to place any weapon in a neutral location. No attempt should be made to grapple with a weapon. The aggressor should be approached in force and moved to the ground as quickly as possible. The method of restraint will vary, depending on the incident. Clothing rather than limbs should be held to restrain. If limbs require to be grasped, it is useful to remember the following points:

- Always ensure there is a sufficient number of staff members available to restrain the patient, who are all experienced in restraint.
- Pinion the aggressive individual's arms to her sides.
- Legs and arms should be grasped near major joints. This may require a staff member at each limb.
- Make sure that the airway and circulation to the extremities are not impaired.
- Weight should be placed on hips and abdomen by lying across the body.
- If there are attempts at biting, the head should be grasped firmly and held still.
- If possible, the aggressive individual should be moved to a quiet environment.
- The individual should only be released on the assessment of the team leader that it is safe to do so.

Throughout this procedure, it is the team leader's responsibility to maintain communication with the individual, clearly providing instructions and support which may result in a resolution of the situation by the aggressive individual. In so doing, the patient's airway and physical status can also be observed (Merson & Baldwin 1995). Restraining the patient in this manner will reduce the possibility of dislocation or fracture and the long-term discomfort caused. The individual's dignity will also be respected, while reducing the risk of harm to the staff involved.

Physical restraint should be used for the minimum amount of time required to control the individual until further action is decided upon. This may include sedation or observation and counselling of the individual by staff. The decision to release the individual must be made by the team leader and carried out in a controlled, co-ordinated fashion to minimise the risk of injury to the violent individual and staff. At the earliest opportunity, the aggressive individual should be examined by senior medical and nursing staff so that a fuller assessment of the individual's condition may be undertaken. The psychiatric/psychological response of the aggressive individual may help to determine whether she is calm enough to be released, whether she requires further intervention, e.g. a psychiatric assessment, or whether she is to be released into the custody of the police.

It is acknowledged that in extreme instances the degree of reasonable force necessary to control a violent individual may be of concern to the staff involved. In line with the duty of care to the individual highlighted in the *Code of Professional Conduct* (UKCC 1992), the degree of force should be the minimum required to control the violence in a manner appropriate to calm rather than provoke further violence. Staff injured in the attempt to restrain the violent individual must also be reviewed by a doctor at the earliest opportunity and be made aware of their entitlement to criminal injuries compensation, if appropriate.

Follow-up Care after an Aggressive Violent Incident

In accordance with good professional practice procedures and nursing accountability, any aggressive or violent incidents should be reported to the senior nurse and medical officer and recorded appropriately within the documentation. In recognition of the growing levels of violence in A&E (Sheehan 1991), most departments now require completion of an incident form specifically designed to record verbal or physical abuse of the staff.

In addition, Jones & Littler (1992) suggested that a full written report will be required if any of the following occurs:

- any incident involving physical violence and injury by a patient to herself, other patients, members of staff or any other person, or any allegation of such an incident
- any incident which necessitates the use of physical restraint of a patient by members of the department staff
- any incident causing significant damage to hospital property or to the property of other patients or relatives
- any incident of verbal aggression to members of staff.

In making the report it is important to provide as much detail as possible about the circumstances of the incident. Analysis of this information may be useful in the prevention of further incidents safeguarding future A&E patients and staff. (see Box 11.2).

In addition to the care of the aggressive individual, the A&E nurse also has a responsibility for the psychological care of the staff and patients who may have been involved in or witnessed the incident. Distressed staff or patients/relatives should be afforded an opportunity to discuss their fears and anxieties arising from the incident. In some cases following extreme events, post-traumatic counselling may be required by individuals involved in incidents of aggression or violence. It is not a sign of weakness or failure in the A&E nurse to admit the need for this support to

Box 11.2 – *Information to be recorded on incident form*

- When and where the incident occurred

- The names, addresses and status of the people involved

- A brief factual account of the incident, including the main direction of the aggression

- The action taken to resolve the incident

- The names of all additional people bearing professional responsibility

- Observations on the mental state of the aggressive individual involved

- Any injury or damage that occurred

- Any additional comments

overcome the trauma of such incidents. Ward (1995) noted that nurses who experience assault or who witness distressing events, either regularly or in a one-off situation, are just as at risk of suffering the effects of post-traumatic stress as any other member of the public. Critical incident stress debriefing should also be available for involved members of staff (Whitfield 1994) (see also Ch. 12).

Conclusion

Glasson (1993) suggested that there should be a coordinated approach to dealing with aggression and violence in A&E departments, similar to the coordinated approach adopted in dealing with a critically ill patient or a cardiac arrest situation. Planning and resourcing

in the prevention of aggression and violence in A&E should, therefore, be as detailed as the planning and resources provided for the prevention of death from cardiac arrest.

For this to be achieved there must be a planned policy of response to a violent or aggressive outburst which is known to all the staff within the department and practised on a regular basis. The purpose of this response must be to control the violent or aggressive outburst as efficiently as possible, thereby minimising the danger to the aggressive individual, other patients/relatives and to the staff involved. The achievement of this objective has staffing and educational implications for the A&E management team.

To respond to aggressive or violent incidents in the A&E department requires the provision of adequate levels of staff (Neades 1994). Failure to provide the staffing levels renders any policy to deal with aggression redundant. The knowledge and skills required by the nurse to deal with such incidents are not common-place among A&E nurses. These skills must be developed through experience and by undertaking specialist training designed to inform the A&E nurse and build confidence in coping professionally with these challenging incidents for the betterment of the staff and patients.

Opportunities must be provided for all staff in A&E to undertake suitable education programmes and to practise the acquired knowledge and skills regularly. These specialist courses provide education and training in staff attitudes, communication skills and techniques in restraining violent individuals. By undertaking these measures, the problem of aggression in A&E will not be totally eradicated but the nurse will have the means to deal with the situation in a professional and appropriate manner.

References

Ambrose K (1996) Mental health care in A&E: expanding nursing roles. *Emergency Nurse*, **4**(3), 16–18.

Bandura K (1973) *Aggression: a social Learning Analysis.* Englewood Cliffs, NJ: Prentice-Hill.

Bateson G (1980) *Mind and Nature.* London: Fontana.

Berkowitz L (1964) Aggressive cues in aggressive behaviour and hostility catharsis. *Psychological Review*, **71**, 104–122.

Brennan W (1998) Aggression and violence: examining the theories. *Emergency Nurse*, **6**(2), 18–21.

Brown TM, Scott IF, Pullen IM (1990) *Handbook of Emergency Psychiatry.* Edinburgh: Churchill Livingstone.

Dolan B (1998) Waiting times (editorial). *Emergency Nurse*, **6**(4), 1.

Dolan B, Dale J, Morley V (1997) Nurse practitioners: role in A&E and primary care. *Nursing Standard*, **11**(17), 33–38.

Farrell GA, Gray C (1992) *Aggression: a Nurses' Guide to Therapeutic Management.* London: Scutari Press.

Freud S (1932) *The Complete Psychological Works of Sigmund Freud.* London: Hogarth Press.

Glasson L (1993) The care of the psychiatric patient in the emergency department. *Journal of Emergency Nursing*, **19**(5), 385–391.

Health & Safety Commission Advisory Committee (1997) *Violence and Aggression to Staff in the Health Services* London: HSE Books.

Hildegard ER, Hildegard R, Atkinson RC (1987) *Introduction to Psychology.* New York: Harcourt Brace Jovanovich.

Jones D, Littler A (1992) *Management of Violent or Potentially Violent Persons* 2nd edn. Cardiff: South Glamorgan Health Authority.

Kaplan HI, Sadock BJ (1993) *Pocket Handbook of Emergency Psychiatric Medicine.* Baltimore: Williams and Williams.

Merson S, Baldwin D (1995) *Psychiatric Emergencies.* Oxford: Oxford University Press.

Moran J (1984) Aggression management: responses and responsibility. *Nursing Times*, **80**(14), 28–31.

Neades B (1994) How to handle aggression. *Emergency Nurse*, **2**(2), 21–24.

Paterson B, McCormish AG, Bradley P (1999) Violence at work. *Nursing Standard*, **13**(21), 43–46.

Rix G (1985) Compassion is better than conflict. *Nursing Times*, **81**(38), 53–55.

Royal College of Nursing (1998) *Dealing with Violence against Nursing staff: a RCN Guide for Nurses and Managers*. London: RCN.

Royal College of Nursing Accident and Emergency Forum and The Casualty Surgeons Association (1977) Violence in the A&E department. *Discussion paper*. London: RCN/CSA.

Sheehan A (1991) RMNs have a part to play: mental health nurses within A&E facilities. *Nursing*, **4**(37), 35–42.

Standing H, Nicolini D (1997) *Review of Workplace Related Violence*. London: HSE Books.

Taylor R, Ryrie I (1996) Chronic alcohol users in A&E. *Emergency Nurse*, **4**(3), 6–8.

United Kingdom Central Council for Nursing Midwifery and Health Visiting (UKCC) (1992) *Code of Professional Conduct* 3rd edn. London: UKCC.

Walsh M (1986) On the frontline. *Nursing Times*, **82**(37), 55–56.

Walsh M (1996) *Accident and Emergency Nursing: a New Approach* 3rd edn. London: Heinemann.

Warburton JM (1982) Violence and the nurse. *Nursing*, **36**, 1533–1534.

Ward M (1995) *Nursing the Psychiatric Emergency*. Oxford: Butterworth-Heinemann.

Whitfield A (1994) Critical incident debriefing in A&E. *Emergency Nurse*, **2**(3), 6–9.

Whittington R, Wykes T (1989) Invisible injury. *Nursing Times*, **85**(42), 32.

Williams DG (1992) Sorting out triage. *Nursing Times*, **88**(30), 34–36.

Wondrak R (1989) Dealing with verbal abuse. *Nurse Education Today*, **9**, 276–280.

Wright B (1986) *Caring in Crisis: a Handbook of Intervention Skills for Nurses*. Edinburgh: Churchill Livingstone.

Wright B (1988) Encountering hostility and aggression. In: Wright B, ed. *Management and Practice in Emergency Nursing*. London: Chapman and Hall.

Chapter 12

Stress and Distress

Bob Wright

- Introduction
- Coping
- Distress in A&E nursing
- Approaches to support and care
- Defusion
- Demobilisation
- Critical incident stress debriefing (CISD)
- Responses to burn-out
- Conclusion

Introduction

The development of the stress concept has contributed to an understanding of the nature and causes of disease, as well as to its psychological implications. It would not be useful to focus only on the psychological 'distress'. Basic issues connected with stress have been applied to biological, psychological and social behaviours. Cannon (1935), Wolfe (1950), Selye (1976) and Lazarus (1966) are among the theorists who have made a significant contribution to the development of the concept of stress.

In his work on homeostasis, Cannon (1935) discussed stress as a causative factor of disease. He described how stresses place pressures on specific mechanisms of the body and how they are necessary to maintain a steady state. Cannon called this state homeostasis – maintaining a correct balance of temperature control, fluid and electrolyte balance, nervous system control and immune system response. The homeostatic response is therefore described as a mechanism to maintain equilibrium and sustain life. Cannon viewed disease as a fight to maintain the homeostatic mechanisms that help to maintain equilibrium.

Wolfe (1950) described stress as a dynamic state within the organism rather than an external stressor. He defined stress as 'an internal force produced by external forces', and viewed it as an interaction between the external environment and the individual. According to Wolfe, past experiences would be a contributing factor in determining the response to the stress.

He described a 'protective reaction pattern' as a concept for the development of his ideas on stress. This pattern causes a complex reaction to rid the body of threat, symbolic and physical threats initiating similar responses. The pattern involves alteration in feeling, body processes and behaviour.

Selye (1976) focused his attention on the bio-chemical and physiological functioning. He described the body's response as non-specific, in that all or most parts of the body must try to adjust to any agent of stress. Selye related stress to homeostasis when he described shivering as the body's adaptive response to cold, the goal being to return the body to its previous steady state.

Selye described the 'general adaptive syndrome' (GAS) by which all people adapt to stress throughout life, but he also stated that hereditary factors play some part. He described three stages of adaptation:

- the alarm reaction
- the stage of resistance
- the state of exhaustion.

The alarm reaction is the early response of the body's defence mechanism. This reaction cannot be maintained for too long or death will follow. The resistance stage leads to homeostasis and survival. The exhaustion stage results from this activity when it is prolonged, and in turn leads to ageing.

Selye believed that with most short-lived, more manageable stressors, only the first and second stages are apparent. Repeated encounters with the first and second stages lead to people learning to adapt to the environment. Severe exhaustion is only initiated by more serious threat, and it is not experienced as often as the other stages. Selye argued that an individual's adaptability is the most unique characteristic of life, allowing him in all the complexities of life, to resist stress and return to homeostasis.

Lazarus (1966) described how the degree of reaction to a stressor is related to the subjective appraisal each individual makes of the event as being threatening or non-threatening. The 'Lazarus cognitive model of stress' involves three phases:

- appraisal
- coping
- outcome.

Appraisal occurs when the stressor and the degree of danger are evaluated. Secondary appraisal involves assessing the availability of adequate coping devices. Direct action, by meeting or avoiding the approaching threat, may be a coping mechanism. The other coping mechanism is to alter the distress the person feels, by working with his response to the event. The effectiveness of these two appraisals leads to the outcome, i.e. the effect the stressor has upon the person.

From these concepts, it can be seen that stress is an essential component of life and does not always have the negative connotation regularly placed upon it. This negative connotation should, perhaps, be more accurately described as distress. The very nature of work in A&E must mean that nurses experience both stress and distress.

Coping

The definitions for coping are many, and are as varied as those for adaptation to stress. Some authorities identify coping more readily in the context of crisis or in adjustment to adverse conditions. This is defined as involving problem solving efforts in situations which are perceived as very important to the individual and which make demands on his adaptive resources (Lazarus & Folkman 1984). This approach considers coping to be primarily a cognitive process, whilst Levin et al. (1978) recognised the relationship between psychosocial and cognitive processes and defined the ultimate goal of coping as the reduction of physiological activity.

In general terms, coping refers to processes or skills used to deal with situations or events which are out of the ordinary. In the integrated process, 'gut feelings' influence cognition of the need to cope. Stimuli to coping also arise in the external environment, in the form of physical stimuli, interpersonal relationships and community, national and international events. Stimuli in the internal environment arise in terms of thoughts, feelings and physical illness.

Distress in A&E Nursing

For even the most competent A&E nurse, continued exposure to particularly difficult and emotionally draining situations can result in serious emotional crisis. The diversity of A&E work, although valued by the nurses, can be difficult to tolerate, especially as it covers such a wide range of conditions.

The bleeding, multiply injured patient, followed by a patient with a minor cut of the hand, demands rapid changes in energy and focus. Concern about a patient's physical or psychological condition can lead to feelings of frustration at being unable to do more. The nurse begins to lose emotional objectivity and control. Some patients are demanding, unappreciative, hostile and difficult. The A&E nurse may feel there is little she can do to intervene, and can be left feeling ineffective and helpless.

While personal responses have been identified as a predictor of burn-out in nurses, so also are organisational factors (Hare et al. 1988). Concern about the negative effects of stress and the need to minimise acute distress have influenced research to identify and analyse the various working environments of A&E nurses (Blunt 1984, Caldwell 1976, Keller 1990, Phipps 1988).

Much of the literature is anecdotal. There is, however, a lot of discussion concerning deaths, violence, pain and hostility. A survey by Burns et al. (1983)

identified organisational issues as a great stressor, with unit management being cited as the greatest source of stress. Care issues ranked second to inadequate staffing and inexperienced medical staff. Hawley (1992) showed that, although stress relates to a variety of sources, inadequate staffing and resources, and non-nursing tasks have a negative impact on nurses' ability to provide quality care. This is a major source of distress.

This book confronts us with a range of life crises encountered in A&E departments. As a result of these crises, A&E nurses run a higher risk of victimisation than either the general public or other human service workers (Mahoney 1991). Cudmore (1998) recommended that staff educators should include the recognition of burn-out, coping skills and recognition of post-traumatic distress in the curriculum for emergency nurses.

When assessing personality types of emergency nurses, Atkins & Piazza (1987) found that on the introvert/extrovert scale, the majority of these personalities were independent, diligent, task-orientated and enjoyed working alone. This does not appear to fit in with the needs of A&E nursing. On the judgement/perception scale these individuals were able to make rapid decisions, plan, order, control and remain with the task. The other extreme of this scale indicates a tendency to be stubborn, inflexible, unadaptable and judgmental. A&E nurses who are at this end of the scale are at risk of burn-out. The knowledge that certain personality characteristics can affect work performance may aid staff selection. It should also influence education about responses to A&E work.

Responses to distress

There may be a high turnover of staff in response to the distress encountered in the A&E department. In addition, an increase in illness may be recorded in these workers (Mitchell & Resnik 1986). One of the final stages of this distressing and distressed state is called burn-out, signs of which include (Wright 1992):

- unrealistic expectations
- inability to respond to change
- resentment and suspicion
- intolerance
- being judgmental
- a feeling of being undervalued
- lack of direction or goals
- physical manifestations
- illness and absenteeism.

These symptoms may have crept up on the nurse insidiously and may be felt as a long 'burning up'

process. The symptoms of burn-out can leave nurses feeling drained, exhausted and unable to tolerate even minor stresses. These problems loom large not only at work, but also invade personal lives. If the problems are not dealt with, demoralisation and damage begin to affect other staff and personal relationships. In a study using the Maslach burnout inventory (MBI), Walsh *et al.* (1998) showed that lack of staff, pressure of work and patient aggression were the main stressors for A&E nurses, coupled with a perceived lack of managerial support and inadequate resources. They found that participants in the study were on the borderline between moderate and high levels of depersonalisation, one of the three components of burn-out identified by the MBI subscales. They also showed that nurses experienced moderate levels of emotional exhaustion. This was reflected in the fact that about half of the 134 nurses in the sample reported feeling used up at the end of the day, frustrated by their job and emotionally drained at least once a week.

In order to identify the signs and symptoms of a stress reaction, the five dimensions of a person can be explored. When dealing with acute or chronic stress reactions, these help to break down symptoms into definite areas and clarify the confusion and perplexity.

Approaches to Support and Care

Listening

Listening is a basic and perhaps simple response, and its value should not be underestimated. Talking and sharing difficulties with a colleague are well used and caring responses. Trust is imperative, as self-disclosure is involved, and insight into the person behind the nursing role will increase the value of sharing (Wright 1992).

How the story is told and heard, and how the storyteller hears his own story are emphasised in other work on coping with stressful incidents (McKechnie 1993). This process helps to clarify and identify difficulties, and often alters the teller's perception of the event. It has long been recognised that certain critical incidents may be difficult for student nurses to tolerate. After the incident, they have been sought out to check whether they were managing their feelings. This response is equally important for trained and experienced staff.

Nurse counsellors

The need for nurse counsellors is now well established in health care organisations. The availability of an independent, confidential counselling service is essential in the high-stress work that is nursing. The provision of nurse counsellors could be seen as a recognition by management of the serious problems that might emerge from this work. Nurses' own responsibility towards self-care can motivate them to bring pressure on the organisation to provide this clinical service.

Self-support groups

These will be explored later, in the less formally structured defusing sessions. Here the more formal groups will be discussed. Groups which meet regularly to discuss cumulative stress have been found to be useful (Wright 1991). Groups meeting to consider the aftermath of a traumatic event must be handled very carefully. Those involved in an acute traumatic incident may be afraid of expressing the intensity of their feelings and the intimacy of the experience. How these more critical incidents should be handled will be discussed under the headings of defusion, demobilisation and debriefing.

At times, a group crisis intervention may be helpful if the whole group has suffered the same impact of the same event. In these instances, the shared experience of the group can be an important resource for recovery (Herman 1992). A multidisciplinary group means that everyone's contribution is recognised and that common fears, problems and anxieties are shared.

Time set aside for airing views and feelings about some difficulties, particularly about how the whole team works, will allow common difficulties to be examined. Rapid decisions and change in pace and demands mean it is not at all unusual for hostility, aggression and scapegoating to occur. The group work setting can be very useful for allowing a healthy confrontation of the issues, instead of carrying around internalised resentment. The groups should therefore be set up regularly to deal with general issues, rather than be used solely for critical incident stress debriefing.

Defusion

Defusion may best be described as a short type of crisis intervention. Its aim is to make a critical incident less harmful, a critical incident being any situation faced by the A&E team members that causes them to feel strong emotional reactions. These feelings could potentially interfere with their ability to function, at the time or later. Defusion helps to restore control and provides immediate support and assistance. It should reduce tension, focus on strengths and skills and help staff to regain emotional control. This focus on skills

helps to ensure a return to normal functioning and to start the recovery process. A return to cognitive functioning enables the person to think rather than to react.

The facilitator maintains a low profile and mostly provides the right conditions for the defusing to occur. This will usually be to send all or as many people as possible who were involved in the incident for a tea or coffee break. They will then, naturally and spontaneously, go over the details of the event. They take charge of the level of emotional ventilation and take it as far as they want to, and then return to normal functioning.

Most nurses will recognise how the report or handover of a shift is used to defuse. Although the whole shift is to be reported on, or a group of patients in a certain order, any critical incident will receive immediate attention. Details of other events or other information will not be shared until the whole story has been told. Any attempts made to curtail disclosure of a critical incident will cause it to emerge later. Time and attention given to those involved will, on the other hand, allow the incident to be laid to rest or ended more appropriately (Wright 1993).

Demobilisation

Demobilisation provides staff with a structure to end a span of duty. While most people will end a shift together, some, because of workload, will leave at a different time. Their needs should not be ignored. Large-scale incidents benefit most from this approach. A room will be needed to hold large numbers of staff. Ideally the group should be multidisciplinary. These people should be expected to remain no more than 15 minutes, and this time should be part of their working span of duty.

The team leader should have up-to-date, accurate information about the whole event from its beginning to the present time. There is no room for rumours or guesswork. Everyone should be ordered to attend the demobilisation; it is not just for the vulnerable or sensitive or those who think they need it. It is for the whole team and it should be made clear that it is an issue for the whole team. It is designated to facilitate an end to a stressful working period.

The aims of the demobilisation are:

■ to regain emotional control and cognitive functioning and to reduce tension
■ to focus on strengths and skills, to re-evaluate the incident and to receive some factual information
■ to begin the recovery process and leave behind some of the stress
■ to begin to be educated by the incident.

The process of demobilisation is begun by saying, for example: 'At 13.40 hours today an explosion occurred at Blake's Foundry, resulting in six seriously injured patients.' All available information is then given as to services concerned, types of casualties and personnel involved. Different members of staff will have worked in different aspects of the incident but will generally not have been involved in the whole. For this reason, information about the whole event will be useful.

For staff, this complete picture reduces the possibility of unanswered questions before they leave the hospital. The difference between a demobilisation and defusion is that, although they have similar aims, the demobilisation is clearly time-limited and focused. On this occasion, staff are told that anyone may seek and will be given further help if they have further difficulties about the event.

At the end of the demobilisation, the opportunity should be used to thank everyone for their contribution to a difficult and demanding event. They are then given permission to leave, hopefully with reliable information about the event and a better overall perception of the incident. The focus of demobilisation is primarily on cognitive functioning rather than on emotional ventilation. If demobilisation is a positive event, staff are more likely to return for debriefing if they think this is necessary. Assuring them that this was an abnormal event will be more likely to help them to seek further support if needed. Some A&E departments have set up critical incident stress debriefing teams, which include all the emergency services involved. They feel that this explores the incident more thoroughly (Rubin 1990). This approach can be more difficult to expedite.

Critical Incident Stress Debriefing (CISD)

This is a more formal type of debriefing and should ideally be done by someone with knowledge of counselling skills. A formal debriefing occurs 24–48 hours after the event and should be a short, well-focused type of intervention. A format for CISD could consist of three 1-hour sessions to be completed within 10 days.

Session 1. After introductions, rules about confidentiality should be explained. This confirms that no information about the debriefing will be disclosed to anyone. The client is then asked to give a factual account of the whole incident and her part in it. This first session involves mostly factual information, but asks the client for a detailed account.

Session 2. Return to the incident and begin the story again, but ask about some of the sounds, smells, visual images and things she felt. Ask questions about feelings: 'How did you feel when it was happening?', 'How has it left you feeling?'; 'Have you ever felt like this before?'. These questions are intended to help the client to get nearer some of the distress of the incident. This often includes feelings of frustration, helplessness, fear, guilt, anger and ambivalence at being involved. There may be a major focus on what appears to be a trivial aspect of the incident. The client will often apologise for this. This whole session should allow some of the more disturbing aspects of the incident to be explored.

Session 3. This final session is used to teach something about stress, the emphasis being on the normal and the natural. Common physical symptoms will be identified and then connected to an abnormal experience. The last session is often called the re-entry phase because it is working towards normal function and 'closing off' the incident. Any outstanding issues are dealt with and loose ends tied up. A plan of action may be discussed, i.e. what the client would do differently next time in a similar incident. Questions highlighting the education aspects of the event are useful in this final session: 'What have you learnt about yourself?'; 'How will this influence your work in future incidents?'.

This type of approach to debriefing a critical incident will be short-term if the only problem presented concerns the incident. If the event returns the client to a previous life crisis, a much longer period of counselling will be required, as CISD is aimed solely at reducing stress reactions and returning quickly to normal functioning (Whitfield 1994). Some would question its effectiveness in group settings (Kleber & Brom 1992), as people are often reluctant to participate in intervention programmes. CISD is more likely to be accepted if offered on an individual basis and to those for whom defusing and demobilisation did not offer enough to enable them to disengage from the incident.

Responses to Burn-out

Burn-out does not mean irreparable damage. The following options exist to alleviate some of the distress.

Re-education or further education. This can help to clarify the A&E nurse's role as well as providing an update on current trends and practice. It can be very stressful to feel left behind in the area of knowledge. It is important that A&E nurses know the eventual outcome of what they do. Since only a short time is spent with the patient and his condition, nurses do not often have the chance to see the final outcome. This greater overall awareness of patient care may make us more aware of the end result of our intervention.

Life outside work. There are many diversions outside work. Lack of stimulation and interest in other activities can itself contribute to burn-out. It may be that a personal relationship or life problem continually affects our ability to work to full potential. It is also possible to blame all difficulties on work when the answer lies elsewhere.

Ask for a move. It may be that something less demanding or different is needed. It is worth considering working in a different area or with a different kind of client, perhaps with longer transactions. An alternative to a move is a change to the existing working environment.

Encourage support systems. It is essential to recognise and use formal and informal support networks in caring for and supporting each other.

Expectations of the clients. Patients, clients and relatives will not always match up to nurses' expectations of them. They have a right to reject what nurses have on offer and may not always do this graciously. Nurses' plans will be changed and disrupted despite a major investment in them. We may feel let down and disillusioned. It could be useful to check whether we remain realistic about the work.

Conclusion

Nurses' thoughts, feelings and vision about A&E practice may change, but this is evolution not failure. Personal philosophies about nursing work and roles are not static. The fact that A&E nurses are continually exposed to pain, suffering, stress and trauma makes them vulnerable. Work on post-traumatic stress disorder (PTSD) suggests that A&E nurses are capable of suffering from it (Chandler 1993) and that nurses need to create healing communities for themselves as well as for patients.

Departmental policies which address the issues of defusing, demobilisation and debriefing make a clear statement that it is the department's philosophy to care for its staff and acknowledge the difficulty of the work. These strategies dispel some of the myths, such as that only the weak go to the wall, and will help to confirm that stress and distress are issues affecting all emergency personnel.

References

Atkins J, Piazza D (1987) Personality types of emergency nurses. *Journal of Emergency Nursing*, **13**(1), 33–37.

Blunt C (1984) A very stressful place. *Nursing Times*, **80**(7), 28–32.

Burns AK, Kirilloff LH, Close JM (1983) Sources of stress and satisfaction in emergency nursing. *Journal of Emergency Nursing*, **4**(9), 329–336.

Caldwell MM (1976) Staff stress: what you can do about it. *Journal of Emergency Nursing*, **2**(2), 21–23.

Cannon W (1935) Stresses and strains of homeostasis. *American Journal of Medical Sciences*, **189**(1), 1.

Chandler E (1993) Can post traumatic stress disorder be prevented? *Journal of Accident and Emergency Nursing*, **1**(2), 87–91.

Cudmore J (1998) Critical incident stress management strategies. *Emergency Nurse*, **6**(3), 22–27.

Hare J, Pratt CC, Andrews D (1988) Predictors of burnout in professional nurses working in hospitals. *International Journal of Nursing Studies*, **25**(2), 105–115.

Hawley MP (1992) Sources of stress for emergency nurses in four urban Canadian emergency departments. *Journal of Emergency Nursing*, **18**(3), 211–216.

Herman J (1992) *Trauma and Recovery*. New York: Basic Books.

Keller KL (1990) The management of stress and prevention of burnout in emergency nurses. *Journal of Emergency Nursing*, **2**(16), 90–95.

Kleber RJ, Brom D (1992) *Coping with Trauma*. Amsterdam: Swetz & Zetlinger.

Lazarus RS (1966) *Psychological Stress and the Coping Process*. New York: McGraw Hill.

Lazarus RS, Folkman S (1984) *Stress, Appraisal and Coping*. New York: Springer.

Levin S, Weinberg J, Ursin H (1978) *Psychology of Stress: a Study of Coping Mechanisms*. New York, Academic Press

McKechnie R (1993) Earwitness to disaster. *Journal of Accident & Emergency Nursing*, **1**(3), 149–153.

Mahoney BS (1991) The extent, nature and response to victimisation of emergency nurses. *Journal of Emergency Nursing*, **1**(5), 282–294.

Mitchell JT, Resnik HLP (1986) *Emergency Response to Crisis*. London: Prentice Hall.

Phipps L (1988) Stress among doctors and nurses in the emergency department of a general hospital. *Canadian Medical Association Journal*, **4**(139), 375–376.

Rubin JG (1990) Critical incident stress debriefing: helping the helpless. *Journal of Emergency Nursing*, **16**(4), 255–258.

Selye H (1976) *The Stress of Life* 2nd edn. New York: McGraw Hill.

Walsh M, Dolan B, Lewis A (1998) Burnout and stress among A&E nurses. *Emergency Nurse*, **6**(2), 23–30.

Whitfield A (1994) Critical incident stress debriefing. *Emergency Nurse*, **2**(3), 7–9.

Wolfe H (1950) *Life Stress and Bodily Diseases*. Baltimore: Williams & Wilkins.

Wright B (1991) *Sudden Death*. Edinburgh: Churchill Livingstone.

Wright B (1992) *Communication Skills: Skills for Caring*. Edinburgh: Churchill Livingstone.

Wright B (1993) *Caring in Crisis* 2nd edn. Edinburgh: Churchill Livingstone.

Chapter 13

Care of the Bereaved

Brian Dolan

- Introduction
- Background
- Preparing for receiving the patient and relatives
- Witnessed resuscitation
- Breaking bad news
- Viewing the body
- Organ donation
- Legal and ethical issues
- Sudden infant death syndrome
- Staff support
- Conclusion

Introduction

It is estimated there are some 25 000–30 000 resuscitation attempts in the UK every year (Resuscitation Council 1996). Dealing with the suddenly bereaved in A&E is difficult for all staff, no matter how much experience they have. This chapter will consider approaches to the management of sudden death in A&E. It will examine the literature surrounding this subject, before exploring the process of care for those who have been suddenly bereaved. It will also outline the care of staff who have cared for the suddenly bereaved.

Background

The literature surrounding the subject of sudden death is vast (McGuinness 1988, Royal College of Nursing and British Association for Accident and Emergency Medicine 1995, Wright 1996). Death is the permanent cessation of all vital functions, the end of human life, an event and a state. Dying is a process of coming to an end: the final act of living (Thompson 1994). Wright (1993) defined sudden deaths as those occurring without warning – the unexpected death. It is these sudden deaths that are most frequently encountered in A&E.

The Royal College of Nursing (RCN) and British Association for Accident and Emergency Medicine (BAEM) (1995), in the largest study of its kind, considered the facilities in A&E departments for the bereaved. A questionnaire was sent to all 267 A&E departments in England and Wales to identify the systems, facilities and training provided. Of the 248 (93%) departments that responded, it was possible to estimate that two to three attendances per 1000 new attendances involved relatives who were bereaved following a patient dying in A&E. Forty per cent of the departments that responded stated they had two to three deaths per week, with a further 25% having four to five deaths per week. In terms of workload and impact on the average A&E department, sudden death can be significant for staff as well as relatives. As Caldwell & Weiner (1981) noted, caring for critically ill and dying people is a major stressor for nurses.

The concept of a trajectory of death was developed by Glaser & Strauss (1965, 1968) to refer to the pattern of death. They distinguish between 'quick' and 'slow' dying trajectories. Generally, in A&E, the patients have a 'quick' death trajectory, which is unexpected by the family, even when it is the result of a long-standing medical condition, such as heart disease. Lindemann (1944), in a classic study of bereavement, suggested that people who fear the death of a loved one often begin the process of grieving before any loss actually occurs. The acute reactions to loss include an initial period of shock followed by intense emotional pangs of grief. Lindemann identified the following symptoms of normal grief:

- somatic distress, such as feelings of tightness in the throat or chest
- preoccupation with the image of the deceased
- guilt
- hostile reactions
- loss of patterns of conduct.

These symptoms will not be unfamiliar to A&E staff who have looked after recently bereaved relatives. Lindemann's work stemmed from a fire at the Coconut Grove night club in 1942 which claimed the lives of 474 people. He found that the fire resulted in a crisis for all individuals closely involved, including staff. Scott (1994) suggested that caring for distressed relatives following a sudden death is perhaps one of the most emotionally draining of nursing interventions. Wright (1996), in a study of relatives' responses to sudden death, found nine common emotional responses identified by nurses as difficult to manage, including:

- denial
- withdrawal
- anger
- acceptance
- isolation
- bargaining
- crying, sobbing, weeping.

It is noteworthy that five of the emotional responses that cause difficulties for A&E nurses also correspond with what Kubler-Ross (1973) described as the stages of grief, i.e. denial, anger, isolation, bargaining and acceptance. Kubler-Ross was careful to point out that these stages do not happen in a particular order, and can occur side by side. These stages do not just affect dying patients but, as can be seen above, affect relatives and staff as well.

Preparing for Receiving the Patient and Relatives

With growing improvements in communications technology, staff are increasingly informed of the impending arrival of critically ill or injured patients by ambulance control or the ambulance crew en route from the scene. This enables staff to prepare the resuscitation room and contact the on-call medical, paediatric and anaesthetic teams as appropriate. In accordance with advanced life support principles, staff should be designated specific roles for the management of the patient (see also Ch. 2).

The 5–10 minutes' forewarning also serve to mentally prepare staff for the arrival of patient's and their relatives. This time can also be used to provide support and guidance for more junior staff about what they might expect. A member of staff should be allocated to receive relatives. This nurse should not have any clinical responsibilities in the management of the resuscitation (see Box 13.1).

> **Box 13.1** – *Guidance for nursing staff dealing with grieving relatives*
>
> The nurse allocated with this task should, where possible, be experienced in dealing with grieving relatives or feel confident to do so. His sole purpose in resuscitation is to support the relatives and he must not become involved in the procedure, except to have the opportunity to give an opinion on stopping the resuscitation. The rest of the team must recognise this as a role and must not pressure him to carry out any procedure or run for any equipment. The relative must not be left unaccompanied.
>
> This nurse must be given adequate time to deal with the relatives following the death of their loved one. Debriefing should take place after the relatives have left the vicinity.

When anxious relatives arrive, they should be met by a named link nurse and not be kept waiting around at reception for the department's communications to be established. While the term 'relatives' is used throughout this chapter, it is important to note that in some instances close friends or partners of either sex may be severely distressed and should be handled in the same way as the relatives.

Witnessed Resuscitation

Witnessed resuscitation, the practice of enabling relatives to stay in the resuscitation room while their loved one is being resuscitated, remains controversial

(Back & Rooke 1994, Bloomfield 1994, Chalk 1995, Higgs 1994, Williams 1996). A report by the Resuscitation Council (1996) suggested that although many nurses and doctors working in A&E departments do not allow relatives to be present in the resuscitation room, the majority of relatives and close friends want to be there. While Dolan (1997) argued that 'enabling witnessed resuscitation is about having enough faith in ourselves as carers to show we are not afraid of others seeing us losing the battle for someone's life', Connors (1996) suggested that the advantages of allowing relatives to be present in the resuscitation room appear to outweigh any potential disadvantages. Boxes 13.2 and 13.3 outline health care professionals' concerns about allowing relatives into resuscitations rooms as well as reasons why relatives should be allowed in the resuscitation room.

Witnessed resuscitation was first documented by the Foote Hospital Michigan, after they introduced the system in 1982, following two incidents when family members insisted on being present (Hanson & Strawser 1992). They questioned recently bereaved

---

Box 13.2 – *Health care professionals' concerns about allowing relatives in resuscitation rooms*

- Family members' uncontrollable grief would disrupt smooth functioning of the resuscitation team

- Family members would become physically involved in the resuscitation attempt

- The team's emotions would be too strongly evoked by family presence

- Fear that some observed action or remark by the medical or nursing staff may offend grieving family members, such as use of humour as a stress reliever (Jezierski 1993)

- Witnessing a resuscitation is an experience that is non-therapeutic and traumatic enough to haunt the surviving family members as long as they live (Osuagwn 1993)

- There would not be enough adequately trained staff to implement a supportive role for all families (Back & Rooke 1994)

- The relatives may become cardiac arrest victims themselves (Osuagwn 1993)

- Fear that allowing observation of the activity and procedures would increase the legal risk (Hanson & Strawser 1992)

- Relatives may feel pressured into attending a resuscitation

---

Box 13.3 – *Reasons why relatives should be allowed in the resuscitation room*

- The relative is able to see rather than being told that everything possible is being done. This comes from the belief that the reality of the resuscitation room is far less horrifying than the fantasy

- The relative is able to touch the patient while she is still warm – to the general public, warm means alive (Connors 1996)

- Relatives can say whatever they need to while there is still a chance that the patient can hear them

- The grieving process is long and hard enough without eliminating any elements that might help adjustment (Martin 1991)

- The family is viewed more as part of a loving family and less as a clinical challenge

- Closer relationships are formed between nursing staff and the patient's relatives (Hanson & Strawser 1992)

- Reduces the legal risk as families can see for themselves that no-one is trying to hide anything (Renzi-Brown 1989)

- The relatives feel that they are doing something in a hopeless situation

---

relatives and found that 72% would have liked to have witnessed the resuscitation attempt. As a result, a programme of witnessed resuscitation began; however, there was resistance from many staff members (Hanson & Strawser 1992). In an audit 3 years later, staff were questioned about their views and 71% endorsed the practice even though they felt it had incurred an increased stress level.

Witnessed resuscitation is likely to become more common and relatives will, in future, insist on being present. It is already seen as good practice by the working group of the Royal College of Nursing and British Association for Accident & Emergency Medicine (1995). Nurses should anticipate the changing needs of the community and plan this change carefully. Hampe (1975) found that family members expressed three main needs:

- to be with the dying patient
- to be kept informed
- to know that the dying person was not in pain.

It was also found that the least supportive measure was to remove the family members from the bedside. For staff who have, or wish to develop, a witnessed

Box 13.4 – *Suggested guidelines for staff on what to say to relatives prior to witnessing a resuscitation*

■ Relatives should be informed that their loved one is very ill and that at present the heart has stopped, so the doctors and nurses are having to breathe for the patient and artificially make her heart pump by pressing on her chest wall. If there is any signs that the heart is starting to function again, then the team may have to give an electrical shock to try to kickstart the heart again

■ Relatives should be informed that the prognosis is very grim and it is very unlikely that their loved one will live. Should the patient come out of this event then the next 24 hours will be critical and there is the likelihood that this event will recur

■ Relatives should be given the choice of going into the resuscitation room; they should never be made to feel that they must go in

■ Relatives should be informed that it is acceptable for them to come in for a couple of minutes at a time and leave whenever they wish

■ Relatives should be informed that even though their loved one cannot respond to them it is possible that she might be able to hear them. This information should only be given to relatives who have decided to enter the area

■ Relatives should be informed that no more than two to three relatives are allowed into the resuscitation room at any one time, as more might distract and hamper the resuscitation attempt. This number is suggested as it would be very difficult and distressing to the relatives to allow two out of three attending the department into the resuscitation area. The third person would then be lacking in support

■ Relatives should be informed that the doctors may ask them to wait outside while some investigations, such as X-rays or invasive procedures, are carried out

■ Relatives should be informed that at some point the team will feel that they have done everything possible to regain life, and that unfortunately their loved one is going to die. When this decision has been reached, the carer should say something like. 'We're going to have to stop soon, we've tried everything and nothing is helping'

■ Before all attempts have ceased, the team should try to accommodate the relatives and give them an opportunity to be able to get close to their loved one to say 'goodbye' etc.

Box 13.5 – *Guidance for team leader, doctors and nurses on how to stop an arrest with relatives present*

■ The relatives must be supported by an experienced trained nurse, and this must be this nurse's only role. The relatives should have been informed before entering the scene that the prognosis is very poor and that the chances of successful resuscitation are very slim

■ The decision to stop resuscitation should be made quietly. All staff involved should be consulted and, if feasible, the relatives should be included in this

■ The team leader, with the help of the support nurse, will inform relatives that the resuscitation attempt has failed and that they are about to stop

■ Gradually, one by one, staff should leave the scene, those with no active involvement leaving first. The team leader should stay to support the relatives and the nurse looking after them. When most of the staff have left, the staff member carrying out cardiac massage should stop and leave quietly. The anaesthetist should then turn off the ventilator and cardiac monitor and, when possible, remove the ET tube, stop all i.v. lines and then leave the area

■ When ready, the nurse should then escort the relative out of the area and follow the local bereavement guidelines

■ The team leader will talk to the relatives in the relatives room, answering any questions that may arise. The support nurse should still be with the relatives

■ All staff should be involved in the debriefing

resuscitation policy, Box 13.4 offers guidance on what to say to relatives prior to witnessing a resuscitation. Box 13.5 provides guidance for the team leader, doctors and nurses on how to stop an arrest with relatives present.

Breaking Bad News

For relatives who are waiting in the 'sitting room' or 'relatives room', it should be sensitively decorated, bright and well lit (see Box 13.6). Frequent updates on the patient's condition are important. The link nurse should liaise with staff in the resuscitation room to maintain communication between the relatives and the resuscitation team. Concise terms like 'critical', 'serious', 'good' and 'fair' appear to be reasonably understood by lay and professionals alike.

Box 13.6– *Facilities for the bereaved in the A&E department*

In the room there should be:

- Comfortable, domestic chairs and sofas. In recognition of people with speical needs, for example, the elderly, appropriate furniture should be provided

- Tissues

- Ashtrays

- A telephone with direct dial access for incoming and outgoing calls

- Telephone directories

- A washbasin, with soap, towel, mirror and freshen-up pack

- TV/radio available, but not prominent

- Hot and cold drinks should be available. A fridge and kettle point enable independence, and are convenient for staff. A non-institutional tea/coffee set should also be available

- Toys and books should be available

Table 13.1 – *Phrases to be avoided when breaking bad news*

What is said	What the relative may understand
We have lost him	He has gone missing in the hospital
She has passed on	She has been transferred to another ward
He has slipped away	He has sneaked out of the department
She suffered irreversible asystole	Nothing!

In the event of cessation of resuscitation, if relatives are not present when the patient dies, or if they arrive after the death, staff will have to break the news to them. McLauchlan (1996) suggested that breaking bad news has to be tailored to the situation and particular relatives; however, the following principles apply:

- On leaving the resuscitation room, the breaker of bad news, who is usually a doctor but may also be nurse, should take a moment to gather his composure. Removal of plastic aprons, stethoscopes around the neck and other obviously clinical paraphernalia is recommended.
- It is important to confirm that the correct relatives are being addressed. It can be a simple but traumatic mistake to inform the wrong people of the death of a relative.
- On entering the relatives room, it is important for the nurse and doctor to introduce themselves. Sitting down to talk with relatives gives the impression that the bearers of bad news are not in a rush to leave.
- During the interview, it may be helpful and natural to touch or hold the hand of the bereaved relative(s). While various social and cultural factors

may influence the appropriateness of this, if it feels appropriate then it probably is right.
- Getting to the point quickly is important.
  When providing information and answering questions, keep it honest, direct and simple. Phrases like 'dead' and 'died' should be used as they are unambiguous. Giving the news thoughtfully, showing concern will enable the relatives to understand the event as reality.
- Euphemisms should be avoided at all costs. Table 13.1 outlines phrases that should *not* be used when breaking bad news.
- After breaking the bad news, allow time and silence while the facts sink in, re-emphasising them if appropriate.
- Be prepared for a variety of emotional responses or reactions. Some may appear unmoved, while others will sob and wail. These reactions are not the fault of the bearer of bad news, but are a reaction to the news itself.
- Offer the relatives the opportunity to view the deceased.

Communication is a dynamic, complex and, continuous exchange (Wright 1993, Winchester 1999). Frequently, however, the person communicating the bad news feels that it has been done badly. In a health profession which still sees death as a failure, this is not surprising, especially when it is compounded with the powerful feelings evoked by sudden death. Thayre & Hadfield-Law (1995) noted that, when preparing to give bad news, it is essential that the nurse is aware that increasing urbanisation, advances in medical technology and skills, and the declining size and importance of the extended family have all decreased people's experience of close death. In addition, changing cultural and religious practices mean that nurses may not always be aware of family needs in this respect.

Telephone notification

Where possible, telephone notification of bereavement should be avoided as it can cause acute distress to the receiver as well as the person delivering the news. Wright (1993) noted that the feelings of a person receiving information over the telephone frequently include the following:

- 'They knew more than they said'
- 'I am not sure what they said'
- 'It cannot be as bad as they say'
- 'I am not sure what they want me to do'
- 'It does not make sense'.

Fears of the individual giving information over the telephone may include:

- 'I hope I have identified and am speaking to the right person'
- 'What if they collapse when I tell them, and they are alone?'
- 'Panic may prevent them hearing me'
- What will I say if they ask me outright if their relative is dead?'
- 'People just should not hear this over the phone'.

Thayre & Hadfield-Law (1995) suggested that information given over the telephone should be in small units. Following the shock of bad news, people tend to respond only to simple questions or instructions and may be slow to take in involved explanations. Jones & Buttery (1981) found that relatives only rarely asked over the telephone whether their loved one was dead. Box 13.7 outlines the information that should be given to those who ring or are contacted about death or critical illness of a relative.

Viewing the Body

The opportunity to see the dead person should be always be offered and gently encouraged. While some well-meaning friends or relatives may discourage this act, it is an important part of accepting the reality of the situation. Jones & Buttery (1981) found that relatives of sudden death victims who spent time with the body in A&E department concluded that the viewing process was helpful.

The environment in which the relatives view the body should be made as non-clinical as reasonably possible. Monitors should always be switched off. Drips and invasive treatment aids, such as ET tubes, catheters and cannulae, should be removed. A blanket should cover the patient up to the upper shoulder. Leaving the deceased person's arm(s) over the covers and respectful washing of the face and combing of the

---

Box 13.7 – *Information to give to relatives over the telephone*

- Clear, concise communication is vital

- The caller should state his name, designation and the hospital from which he is calling

- The caller should be clear about who he is speaking to, by asking for the person's name and relationship with the patient

- If this is not the most significant relative, it is important to ascertain where this person can be found

- Give the name of the ill or injured person and her condition

- If there is doubt about the identity of the patient, tell the relative it is believed to be this person

- After giving this information, the caller should check that the relative is clear about:
  - which hospital
  - how to get there
  - what has been said

- The relative should be advised:
  - to get someone to come to the hospital with them
  - to drive carefully, and preferably get someone else to drive
  - to inform other close relatives or friends where they are heading

- Records of the time of the call, who made the call, who responded, and how, are important. After a death, some relatives may want to clarify details

---

hair should be done before relatives attend. Religious insignia can be added as appropriate. Sufficient chairs should be available for relatives to sit down.

When the dead person is disfigured or mutilated, the relatives' wishes are paramount. Gentle, honest explanations beforehand can inform the relatives' decision about whether they wish to see the dead person (McLanchlan 1990). The relatives should be encouraged to touch, hold, kiss, hug or say goodbye to their loved one. Unless there are suspicious circumstances and the police wish to remain with the body, the relatives may also like to be left alone with the body and must be given permission to stay as long as they wish or as is practically possible (Morgan 1997).

Organ Donation

Body organs and tissues, such as the kidneys, heart, liver, pancreas and corneas, may be donated by the patient for availability for transplant. There is, however, a great shortage of organs for transplant, which continues to limit transplant efforts, and the demand is growing at a much greater rate than the supply. The usage of potential organs from A&E departments is very low (Riker & White 1991). Sweet (1996) noted that there are two types of donors of organs and tissues for transplantation. First, there are the 'beating heart' donors, who constitute either those who have been declared brain dead – i.e. where respiratory and circulatory functions are maintained solely by mechanical ventilation – or those who are living, who can only donate kidneys and bone marrow. If they fit the criteria, brain dead donors can be multi-organ donors, i.e. their organs and tissues can be used in transplantation. Secondly, there are the 'non-beating heart' donors, where death with cessation of circulatory and respiratory function has occurred. This is the type of donor usually found in A&E. Wellesley *et al.* (1997) noted that the organs that can be donated from A&E include corneas, heart vales and, in certain departments, kidneys. For heart valves there must be no congenital valve defect, no systemic infection, no hepatitis B or C, and the donor must not be HIV-positive. For corneas, there are even fewer contraindications: no scarring of the cornea, no infection in the eye and no invasive brain tumours. Both organs are very successfully transplanted, with at least 85% success for corneas and even higher for heart valves, due to the absence of rejection problems.

Consent from the coroner may be a limiting factor to tissue retrieval in A&E. Unless a doctor is prepared to sign a death certificate to state that a patient died of natural causes then the coroner must give consent prior to removal or any organ or tissue, as stated in the Human Tissue Act 1961 (DHSS 1961).

Many nurses believe relatives should not be approached about organ donation in A&E, feeling that they have been through enough (Coupe 1990). However, a recent small-scale study by Wellesley *et al.* (1997) highlighted that 27 (72.9%) of the 37 recently bereaved respondents to a questionnaire would not have minded being asked about organ donation following a sudden death. They suggested that the subject could be broached by having leaflets in the room where relatives are given the bad news, as a way of introducing this delicate subject and providing more information. They believe the interview with bereaved relatives needs to be carried out sensitively by senior nurses, registrars or, in some cases, the consultant, who have been appropriately trained and who have access to staff support within the A&E department (see also Ch. 39).

Legal and Ethical Issues

Contact with the coroner's officer may occur in the A&E department or in the home when the notification of the death and identification of the body are established. It is important to distinguish between a coroner's officer who gathers and records details related to the death, e.g. by attending postmortems, and the coroner, usually a doctor or lawyer, who responds to the results of the details by concluding on the circumstances of the death and reaching, if necessary, a verdict at inquest.

Scott (1995) suggested that relatives are often devastated by the news of the death and that these feelings are intensified at the thought of the purposeful mutilation of the body at autopsy. In fact, the autopsy is a legal requirement for most deaths that occur in A&E (see Box 13.8). This information needs to be conveyed to patients in a dignified, sensitive way.

Box 13.8 – Criteria for investigation of a death by a coroner

---

The coroner is a doctor or lawyer responsible for investigating death in the following situations:

- The deceased was not attended by a doctor during the last illness or the doctor treating the deceased had not seen her after the death or within 14 days of the death

- The death was violent or unnatural or occurred under suspicious circumstances

- The cause of death is not known or is uncertain

- The death occurred in prison or in police custody

- The death occurred while the patient was undergoing an operation or the patient did not recover from the anaesthetic

- The death was caused by an industrial disease

Controversy exists over whether personal possessions, and in particular jewellery and precious metals, should be given to relatives. Should relatives wish to remove any rings or special belongings, they should be enabled to do so. Legally, a witnessed signature is sufficient to corroborate the act of handing over or retaining property and this may be obtained from another nurse, doctor or coroner's officer (Cooke *et al.* 1992). Clothing should be carefully folded and itemised along with any other possessions such as jewellery and money. The nurse should seek permission from the family to dispose of badly damaged clothing. This should be recorded in the patient's notes.

Sudden Infant Death Syndrome

This issue is addressed in detail in Chapter 15.

Staff Support

Cudmore (1998) believes that A&E nurses are 'at risk' of developing post-traumatic stress reactions because of their exposure to traumatic events as a routine part of their job, which for most people would be outside the range of human experience. Walsh *et al.* (1998) argued that if stress is the main cause of burn-out, then understanding coping mechanisms is the key to minimising the problem. Coping strategies employed by those working with trauma include the following:

- suppressing emotions and feelings
- mutual staff support
- promoting a sense of unreality
- mental preparation for tasks
- feeling competent and capable
- regulating exposure to the event
- having a sense of purpose
- humour.

Box 13.9 outlines the effects of traumatic events on carers. The following are methods that staff working with dying people can use to improve their coping skills:

- the encouragement of personal insight to understand and acknowledge one's own limits
- a healthy balance between work and outside life
- the promotion of a team approach to care
- an ongoing support system within work and outside work
- for those working in isolation, continuing guidance and support, from peers and superiors.

(Defusion, demobilisation and critical incident debriefing skills for staff are discussed in detail in Ch. 12.)

Conclusion

Sudden death, by whatever cause, is a stressful and distressing event for staff as well as patient's relatives. While A&E departments may be geared towards saving lives, death should not be seen by staff as a

---

> **Box 13.9** – *The effects of traumatic events such as failed resuscitation attempts on carers*
>
> - **Emotional effects** – anxiety, depression, anger, guilt, irritability and feelings of helplessness
> - **Cognitive effects** – memory/concentration changes, nightmares, intrusive thoughts and imagery
> - **Behavioural effects** – altered use of drugs, alcohol, nicotine, caffeine etc., social withdrawal and loss of interest in usual activities
> - **Relationship effects** – changes in work, social, intimate and sexual relationships through irritability, inability to share feelings, isiolation and conflict of loyalty between work and home
> - **Somatic effects** – changes in sleeping and eating habits, altered energy levels, an increase in accidents and physical health problems
> - **Motivational effects** – viewing life from a different perspective, often as more tenuous. Values may be reorientated to less materialistic ones

failure. No matter how confident or experienced the practitioner, it is never easy to tell relatives or friends that a loved one has died (Kendrick 1997). In relation to the needs of relatives, Dolan (1995) argued that:

> *...in so many respects, it seems worth the effort and distress of the trip to know that everything that could be done was done. The tacit transfer of responsibility from patient and family to health carers highlights that while caring costs, our compassion must never get sacrificed as the cost of our caring.*

This chapter has highlighted the process of care for those who have been suddenly bereaved. Within an ageing society, it is likely that more people will require the resuscitative efforts of A&E staff; however, many will not survive. Their relatives are particularly vulnerable in this traumatic situation and require the nurse to advocate for them at this time, enabling them to witness the resuscitation if they wish and receive the news of death with compassion and understanding. For A&E personnel, training and ongoing support will enable them to deal with the challenges of caring for such vulnerable people. The unexpected end of one person's life is the beginning of someone else's grief. A&E nurses are in a key position to enable a relative's last memory of a loved one to become a lasting memory of compassionate support and care.

Further reading

Benefits Agency (1995) *What to Do after a Death in England and Wales* (D49). London: Department of Social Security.

Brewis E (1995) Issues in bereavement: there are no rules. *Paediatric Nursing*, **7**(9), 19–22.

Cook A (1995) 'Blue light' patients: resuscitate or not? *Emergency Nurse*, **3**(2), 24–25.

Dear S (1995) Breaking bad news: caring for the family. *Nursing Standard*, **10**(11), 31–33.

Jacobson FW, Kindleman M, Shoemark A (1997) *Living Through Loss: a Manual for Those Working with Issues of Terminal Illness and Bereavement* London: Jessica Kingsley Publishers.

Keizer B (1996) *Dancing with Mister D: Notes on Life and Death* London: Black Swan.

Kung H, Jens W (1995) *A Dignified Dying* London: SCM Press.

Lugton J (1987) *Communicating with Dying People and their Relatives* London: Austen Cornish.

Marshall F (1993) *Losing a Parent* London: Sheldon Press.

Murray Parkes C, Relf M, Coudrick A (1996) *Counselling in Terminal Care and Bereavement* Leicester: BPS Books.

Pritchard C (1995) *Suicide – the Ultimate Rejection?: a Psychosocial Study* Buckingham: Open University Press.

Scott T (1995) Sudden death in A&E. *Emergency Nurse*, **2**(4), 10–15.

Stewart A, Dent A (1994) *At a Loss: Bereavement Care When a Baby Dies* London: Baillière Tindall.

Tschudin V (1997) *Counselling for Loss and Bereavement* London: Baillière Tindall.

References

Back D, Rooke V (1994) The presence of relatives in the resuscitation room. *Nursing Times*, **90**(30), 34–35.

Bloomfield P (1994) Good information and time with the body are more important. *British Medical Journal*, **308**, 1688–1689.

Caldwell T, Weiner MF (1981) Stresses and coping in ICU nursing. *General Hospital Psychiatry*, **3**, 119–127.

Chalk A (1995) Should relatives be present in the resuscitation room? *Accident and Emergency Nursing*, **3**(2), 58–61.

Connors P (1996) Should relatives be allowed in the resuscitation room? *Nursing Standard*, **10**(44), 44–46.

Cooke MW, Cooke HW, Glucksmann EE (1992) Management of sudden bereavement in the accident & emergency department. *British Medical Journal*, **304**, 1207–1209.

Coupe C (1990) Donation dilemmas. *Nursing Times*, **86**(27), 34–36.

Cudmore J (1998) Critical incident stress management strategies. *Emergency Nurse*, **6**(3), 22–27.

DHSS (1961) *Human Tissue Act*. London: HMSO.

Dolan B (1995) Drama in crisis. *Journal of Clinical Nursing*, **4**(5), 275.

Dolan B (1997) Editorial. Underlining compassion in casualty. *Emergency Nurse*, **5**(2), 1.

Glaser BG, Strauss AL (1965) *Awareness of Dying*. Chicago: Aldine Press.

Glaser BG, Strauss AL (1968) *Time for Dying*. Chicago: Aldine Press.

Hampe SO (1975) Needs of the grieving spouse in a hospital setting. *Nursing Research*, **24**, 113–120.

Hanson C, Strawser D (1992) Family presence during CPR: Foote Hospital Emergency Department's nine year perspective. *Journal of Emergency Nursing*, **18**(2), 104–106.

Higgs R (1994) Relative's wishes should be accommodated. *British Medical Journal*, **308**, 1688.

Jezierski M (1993) Foote Hospital emergency department: shattering a paradigm. *Journal of Emergency Nursing*, **19**(3), 266–267.

Jones WH, Buttery H (1981) Sudden death: survivors' perceptions of their emergency department experience. *Journal of Emergency Nursing*, **7**(1), 14–17.

Kendrick K (1997) Sudden death: walking in a moral minefield. *Emergency Nurse*, **5**(1), 17–19.

Kubler-Ross H (1973) *On Death and Dying*. New York: Macmillan.

Lindemann E (1944) Symptomatology and management of acute grief. *American Journal of Psychiatry*, **101**, 141–148.

McGuinness S (1988) Sudden death in the emergency department. In: Wright B, ed. *Management and Practice in Emergency Nursing*. London: Chapman & Hall

McLauchlan CAJ (1990) Handling distressed relatives and breaking bad news. *British Medical Journal*, **301**, 1145–1147.

McLauchlan CAJ (1996) Handling distressed relatives and breaking bad news. In: Skinner, D, Driscoll P, Earlam R, eds. *ABC of Major Trauma*, 2nd edn. London: BMJ.

Martin J (1991) Rethinking traditional thoughts. *Journal of Emergency Nursing*, **17**(2), 67–68.

Morgan J (1997) Introducing a witnessed resuscitation policy to A&E. *Emergency Nurse*, **5**(2).

Osuagwn CC (1993) More on family presence during resuscitation. *Journal of Emergency Nursing*, **19**(4), 276–277.

Renzi-Brown J (1989) Risk management specialist. *Nursing*, **19**(3), 46.

Resuscitation Council (1996) *Should relatives witness resuscitation?* London: Resuscitation Council.

Riker RR, White BW (1991) Organ and tissue donation from the emergency department. *Journal of Emergency Medicine*, **9**, 405–410.

Royal College of Nursing and British Association for Accident and Emergency Medicine (1995) *Bereavement Care in A&E Departments*. London: RCN.

Scott T (1995) Sudden death in A&E. *Emergency Nurse*, **2**(4), 10–15.

Sweet A (1996) Organ donation and transplantation. *Emergency Nurse*, **3**(4), 6–9.

Thayre K, Hadfield-Law L (1995) Never going to be easy: giving bad news. *Nursing Standard (RCN Nursing Update supplement)*, **9**(50), 3–8.

Thompson D (1994) Death and dying in critical care. In: Burnard P, Millar B, eds. *Critical Care Nursing*. London: Baillière Tindall.

Walsh M, Dolan B, Lewis A (1998) Burnout and stress among A&E nurses. *Emergency Nurse*, **6**(2): 23–30.

Wellesley A, Glucksmann EE, Crouch R (1997) Organ donation in the accident and emergency department: a study of relatives' views. *Journal of Accident and Emergency Medicine*, **14**, 24–25.

Williams K (1996) Witnessing resuscitation can help relatives. *Nursing Standard*, **11**(3), 12.

Wright B (1993) *Caring in Crisis* 2nd edn. Edinburgh: Churchill Livingstone.

Wright B (1996) *Sudden Death: Intervention Skills for the Caring Professions*, 2nd edn. Edinburgh: Churchill Livingstone.

Winchester A (1999) Sharing bad news. *Nursing Standard*, **13**(26), 48–52.

Chapter 14

Psychiatric Emergencies

Barbara Warncken & Brian Dolan

- Introduction
- Aetiology of mental illness
- Assessment of psychiatric patients in A&E
- Acute organic reactions
- Acute psychotic episode
- Anxiety states
- Alcohol-related emergencies
- Munchausen's syndrome and Munchausen's syndrome by proxy
- Suicide and deliberate self-harm (parasuicide)
- Individual at odds with society
- Learning disability clients and mental health problems
- Elderly clients presenting to A&E with mental health problems
- Child and adolescent psychiatry
- Patients attending A&E with eating disorders
- Social problems
- Iatrogenic drug-induced psychosis
- Monoamine oxidase inhibitors (MAOIs)
- Conclusion

Introduction

Patients with psychiatric emergencies constitute a significant percentage of those who visit an A&E unit annually. A psychiatric emergency is any disturbance in the patient's thoughts, feelings or actions for which immediate therapeutic intervention is necessary (Kaplan & Sadock 1993). The reasons most frequently given by patients for emergency psychiatric visits include (Gillig *et al.* 1990):

- a need to talk things over so decisions can be made
- to help get control over themselves
- treatment for 'nerves'
- to obtain or adjust medications.

People who come to A&E range from those with specific requests for help to those who are brought in against their will for reasons they do not understand. In either case, the patient or carers may believe that the patient is no longer able to maintain coping abilities at his usual level of functioning.

The reasons why many of these patients attend A&E are multifactorial. A primary reason, however, is the deinstitutionalisation of the mentally ill, due to the introduction of psychotropic medication in the 1950s and the changing focus on treatment and rehabilitation within the community. As a consequence, for many in society, their only access to health care is through A&E (Ambrose 1996).

For the A&E nurse who deals with various life-threatening emergencies on a routine basis, these needs may not appear to be true emergencies; however, it is a crisis that brings the psychiatric patient to the A&E department and the nature and degree of a crisis are defined by the person experiencing it. It is also to be seen as an opportunity, because prompt and skilful interventions may prevent the development of serious long-term disability and allow new coping patterns to develop (Aguilera & Messick 1986).

Aetiology of Mental Illness

It is recognised that genetic, biological and biochemical dyscrasiais play a significant role in the causes of major psychiatric illness. It is therefore difficult to discuss psychiatric disorders as having a purely organic or functional basis. However, for the purpose of this chapter, organic disorders will be considered as those disorders that have a grossly identifiable and potentially reversible physiological cause, such as endocrine and metabolic disorders, neurological causes and drug-induced states. Functional disorders will be considered as those disorders without a grossly identifiable physiological cause.

Assessment of Psychiatric Patients in A&E

The goals of A&E psychiatric evaluation are to conduct a rapid assessment, including diagnosis of any underlying medical problems, to provide emergency treatment and to arrange appropriate disposition (Greenstein & Ness 1990). These goals will be hampered by various obstructions and restrictions, such as time and space, departmental milieu, inability to obtain a history from a disturbed or distressed patient and experience of staff. Information collected must be concise and methods of assessment flexible enough to take into consideration the patient's and the unit's needs. Relevant details must be documented as they may be the only recorded evidence of symptoms displayed by the patient in the acute phase. This forms the baseline for the management and treatment plan. Records are also important for medicolegal reasons. The nurse should make full use of any information source available, such as family, escorts, ambulance personnel, community staff, police, hospital notes and other staff who may know the patient from previous attendances or admissions. Once an assessment is made, the patient should be given the appropriate triage category using the triage system employed by the unit, e.g. the Manchester triage guidelines (Mackway-Jones 1996).

History

History is usually initiated by the triage/assessment nurse, who must speedily determine the urgency of the crisis for which the person is seeking care and his capacity to wait. The nurse at this time has to determine how much of a risk the patient poses to himself and to others, such as violent tendencies, suicide, self-mutilation, impaired judgement, etc. The history should include:

- reason for attendance
- history of presenting illness
- past general medical/psychiatric history
- social history
- family history.

The triage/assessment nurse may be the patient's first contact with the health care system, and an attitude of acceptance, respect and empathy, with a desire to help, should be conveyed to the patient. This first contact may significantly influence the patient's acceptance of emergency care and his receptivity to future treatment. Ward (1995) suggested the following as a reasonable focus to begin with:

- What does the patient want?
- Who is in danger?
- What has caused this behaviour?

And, if the patient is already known:

- What has happened in previous situations like this?
- What did this mean to the patient the last time it happened?

Mental state examination

Examination of the mental state in psychiatry is analogous to the physical examination in a general medical or surgical practice (Merson & Baldwin 1995). At a minimum the nurse should note:

- *Appearance and general behaviour* – especially if the patient is disturbed and no history is available. Describe motor behaviour, impulse control, orientation, eye control, attention/concentration, memory.
- *Mood* – blunting/flattening of effect, agitation, hypomania, diurnal mood variation (depressed in the mornings, but feeling brighter in the evenings or vice versa), sleep pattern, appetite, weight loss/gain.
- *Speech and thought* – this assessment should include form and content of speech, anxieties, suicidal/future references, evidence of formal thought disorder, thought broadcasting, thought insertion, pressure of speech, ideas of reference, delusions (for glossary of terms see Box 14.3)
- *Abnormal perceptions and related experiences* – hallucinations, derealisation, depersonalisation.
- *Cognitive state* – if an organic diagnosis is suspected, a more formal and detailed examination is required.
- *Insight and judgement* – Does the patient recognise that he is ill and in need of assistance? Is he able to make rational judgements?

■ *Impulse control* – Is the patient capable of controlling sexual, aggressive or other impulses? Is he a potential danger to himself or others? Is this as a result of an organic mental disease or of psychosis or chronic character defects?

■ *Physical assessment* – a complete physical assessment is required to rule out a physical cause. This will include neurological observations, BM stix, glucose, U&Es, FBC, LFT(DAX), ECG etc.

Formulating and agreeing a nursing and medical management framework of aims and objectives are important, i.e.:

■ main features of presenting complaint
■ physical examination and consultation
■ investigations undertaken
■ provisional and differential diagnosis, e.g. organic cause, acute functional psychosis (schizophrenia, affective states), neurosis, personality disorders
■ any immediate intervention taken.

If admission is not recommended or required, the A&E nurse should be aware of local services and agencies that the patient may be referred to, such as:

■ chemical dependency/detox services
■ outpatients
■ crisis telephone numbers
■ day hospital facilities
■ social services
■ facilities available for the homeless
■ hostels
■ ethnic minority advisory groups
■ interpreters
■ rape counselling centres
■ needle exchanges
■ sexual health and associated conditions services
■ police/probation officers.

Acute Organic Reactions

Frequently, acute organic reactions present to A&E as psychiatric emergencies when the aetiology is unknown and there is loss of behavioural control (All Box 14.1). The most consistent symptom of an acute organic reaction is impairment in the consciousness, worsening symptoms at night, and good pre-morbid personality.

Nursing and medical management

A treatment plan, both nursing and medical/psychological, will be based on the cause and presenting behavioural disturbance. If possible, medication should be withheld, as this may mask or

---

Box 14.1 – *Causes of acute organic reactions*

■ Trauma

■ Infection

Local
  – cerebral abscess
  – meningitis
  – encephalitis
  – syphilis
  – cerebral malaria

General
  – systemic infection
  – septicaemia
  – typhus
  – typhoid

■ Cerebrovascular
  – cerebrovascular accident
  – transient ischaemic attack
  – subarachnoid haemorrhage
  – subdural haemorrhage
  – hypertensive encephalopathy
  – systemic lupus erythematosus
  – cervical arteritis

■ Epilepsy

■ Tumour
  – primary secondary metastastic effects

■ Organ failure
  – renal, cardiac, hepatic, respiratory

■ Anaemia

■ Metabolic
  – U&E imbalance
  – acid–base imbalance
  – uraemia

■ Endocrine
  – hypo/hyperthyroidism,
  – hypo/hyperparathyroidism, hypopituitarism
  – hypo/hyperglycaemia

■ Deficiency disorders
  – thiamine, nicotinic acid, folic acid, vitamin B_{12}

■ Toxic causes
  – drug overdose
  – alcohol withdrawal
  – lead, arsenic, carbon monoxide/disulphide, mercury

---

distort neurological signs, unless the patient's presenting behaviour warrants it.

A physical examination should be performed on all patients presenting with a psychiatric crisis in order

Box 14.2 – *Organic illnesses or conditions that mimic psychiatric symptoms*

■ Thyrotoxicosis

■ Hypoparathyroidism

■ Hypoglycaemia

■ Phaeochromocytoma

■ Carcinoid syndrome

■ Brain tumours or bleeding

■ Head trauma

■ Seizure disorders, such as, epilepsy

■ Drug ingestions or poisoning
  – amphetamines
  – hallucinogens
  – lead poisoning
  – steroid toxicity
  – atropine

■ Myxoedema

■ Cushing's syndrome

■ Porphyria

■ Hyperparathyroidism

■ Addison's disease

■ Systemic lupus erythematosus

■ Carcinoma

to rule out common physical illnesses that mimic psychiatric disorder (see Box 14.2). People with mental health problems have a higher morbidity rate for physical illness than the general population, so their physical symptoms and complaints need to be taken seriously and investigated (Gournay & Beadsmore 1995). Diagnostic tests to confirm or rule out physical conditions masking psychiatric disorders or vice versa should be performed as necessary.

Acute Psychotic Episode

Psychotic patients experience impaired reality testing as they are unable to distinguish between what is real and what is not. Their thought processes are often disordered and often characterised by hallucinations, delusions, ideas of reference, thought broadcasting and thought insertion (Kaiser & Pyngolil 1995) (see Box 14.3). It is essential that the A&E nurse is able to differentiate between a psychosis with an organic cause, e.g. delerium, and a functional psychosis, e.g.

Box 14.3 – *Acute psychotic episode symptoms*

■ **Ideas of reference**
Referring to him in their gestures, speech, mannerisms

■ **Delusions, delusional mood**
A fixed false idea or belief held by the patient which cannot be corrected by reasoning

■ **Hallucinations**
Apparent perception of external object not actually there involving any of the special senses, e.g. visual, auditory, third person auditory, voices arguing, commenting, commanding, gustatory, tactile, olfactory

■ **Disorder of experience of thought**
Thought insertion: patient believes others are inserting, placing thoughts into his mind
Broadcasting: person believes his thoughts are being broadcasted and that all are aware of what he is thinking
Blocking: interruption of a train of speech as a result of the person losing his train of thought

■ **Experience of passivity**
A delusional feeling that the person is under some outside control and therefore must be inactive

■ **Disturbance of speech**
Tangential speech: a style of speech containing oblique or irrelevant responses to questions asked, e.g. the person will talk about world hunger when asked about his breakfast
Poverty of content: restriction of speech, so that spontaneous speech and replies to questions are brief and without elaboration
Word salad: a characteristic of schizophrenia – a mixture of words that lack meaningful connections

■ **Emotional disturbance**
Emotional flattening: without normal 'highs' or 'lows' of feelings
Inappropriate affect: incongruous responses to situations, e.g. laughing at hearing sad news

■ **Motor disturbance**
Excitement; bizarreness, in response to hallucinations; stupor

schizophrenia. Psychotic patients may present to A&E on an emergency basis when it is:

■ an acute psychotic episode, first presentation
■ the exacerbation of a chronic state
■ a long-term problem where the patient is requesting admission, support or medication
■ a catatonic excitement/stupor.

Schizophrenia

There are circumstances, as mentioned above, where patients with schizophrenia may present as an emergency to A&E.

Clinical features

Clinical features will depend to a certain extent on the type of schizophrenia – paranoid, hebephrenic, simple or catatonic. The distinction between subtypes will be based on a full assessment and is less relevant in A&E. These acute symptoms may be superimposed on those of a chronic illness, e.g. apathy, impaired social network etc. Personal hygiene in the psychotic patient is frequently neglected. He may be incontinent and have a poor diet intake.

Long-term patients frequently attend A&E as a 24-hour walk-in service for requests of admission, social support or medication. Often these patients are in need of reassurance and support. If the delusions or hallucinations are a re-emergence in a long-term patient, the patient may be referred to outpatients for adjustment of medication. It is important to ensure that the patient's consultant and community team are aware of his attendance and changes, and that appropriate referrals are made (see Box 14.3).

Kaiser & Pyngolil (1995) suggested that the following therapeutic principles be used in guiding the A&E nurse caring for patients who are experiencing distortions in thought content and perception (which are often associated with great fear):

■ Attempt to establish a trusting relationship. The nurse should reassure the patient that she wants to help and that the patient is in a safe place and will not be harmed.
■ Attempt to determine whether there was a precipitating event that triggered the psychotic episode. If so, evaluate it accordingly.
■ If an organic, reversible cause is identified, reassure the patient that his feelings and thoughts are temporary.
■ Minimise external stimulation. Psychotic people may be having trouble processing thoughts and often hear voices. By decreasing external stimulation, the nurse may decrease sensory stimulation to which the patient may be responding.
■ Do not attempt to reason, challenge or argue the patient out of his delusions or hallucinations. Often these patients need to believe their delusions in order to decrease their anxiety and maintain control.
■ The nurse should not imply that she believes the patient's hallucinations or delusional system in an attempt to win his trust. Statements to the effect that the nurse does not hear these things the patient is hearing but is interested in knowing about them are recommended.
■ Do not underestimate the significance of a patient's psychotic thoughts. They are very real to the patient, and he cannot just 'put them aside'.
■ Unless restraint is required, physical contact with psychotic patients or sudden movements should be avoided as they may induce or validate the patient's fears.

Puskar & Obus (1989) suggested the following questions be asked when assessing a possibly schizophrenic patient:

■ Do your thoughts make sense to you?
■ Do you have ideas that come into your head that do not seem to be your own?
■ Do you worry about what other people think about you?
■ Do you think other people know what you are thinking?
■ Do you hear your own thoughts spoken out loud?
■ Do you sometimes feel that someone or some outside influence is controlling you, or making you think these things?

Once an organic cause has been ruled out, admission from A&E will generally be required if the patient is disturbed, suicidal/homicidal or experiencing command hallucinations telling him to harm himself.

Depression

Depression is a period of impaired functioning associated with depressed mood and related symptoms, including sleep and appetite changes, psychomotor changes, impaired concentration, fatigue, feelings of hopelessness, helplessness and suicide (Kaplan & Sadock 1993). Although estimates vary, approximately 20% of women and 10% of men will suffer from depression at some point in their lives. Community surveys indicate that 3–6% of adults are suffering from depression at any one time (Merson & Baldwin 1995).

Clinical features

Clinical features may include many of the following: depressed mood and affect feelings of hopelessness, helplessness and worthlessness; guilt and inappropriate self-blame; suicidal ideation; decreased energy and activity agitation/stupor; psychomotor retardation; anorexia; weight loss; and early morning wakening/

difficulty getting to sleep. In more severe cases the patient may have somatic delusions and/or auditory hallucinations.

Nursing and medical management

Kaplan & Sadock (1993) proposed the following guidelines for evaluation and management of depression in A&E:

- Treat any medical problems that may have resulted from suicide attempts or gestures.
- Maintain a safe environment for the patient.
- Rule out organic and pharmacological causes of depression.
- Make an assessment of the severity of depression to determine the patient's disposition.

It is important to convey an attitude of compassion, empathy and understanding to the depressed patient. It is also worth reassuring the patient that depression is reversible. However, it is pointless attempting to talk the patient out of depression as he cannot snap out of it any more than he could snap out of a diabetic coma. The patient's social networks should be identified and mobilised where appropriate. The patient should be placed in a safe room, especially if he is at high risk of suicide. The room should be free of any objects which can be used to selfharm, e.g. glass, telephone cords etc. The patient will need admission if he is suicidal, stuporous, hyper-agitated or lacks social support. Referral to the psychiatric outpatient department or other services should be arranged if the patient does not require admission, and his GP and/or community psychiatric nurse (CPN) should be informed of the attendance at A&E.

Postpartum psychiatric problems

In the postnatal period, the patient may present with:

- acute organic reaction
- affective psychosis
- schizophreniform psychosis.

Affective puerperal disorder episode. Problems may range from 'the blues' to a clinical depression severe enough to require admission.

Puerperal psychosis. Symptoms may occur within 2 weeks to approximately 9 months following the birth of a child. There may be clouding of consciousness, perplexity, delusions and hallucinations.

Management

If after assessment in A&E the patient can be managed on an out-patient basis, adequate home support should be initiated and the presenting complaint treated as appropriate. Generally, patients presenting with puerperal psychosis or severe clinical depression will require admission from A&E and arrangements should be made for both mother and baby. Medication in A&E will need to be selective to prevent drugs being prescribed which are secreted in breast milk if the mother is breast-feeding.

Hypomania/mania/acute or chronic mania

Hypomania is the term used to describe a syndrome involving sustained and pathological elevation of mood, accompanied by other changes in function, such as disturbances of physical energy, sleep and appetite. Mania is a similar syndrome in which the patient additionally holds delusional ideas, i.e. he is psychotic (Merson & Baldwin 1995). The patient who frequently attends A&E does so when he has become too disruptive for family life. He may have a history of mania or depression with his behaviour becomingly increasingly disruptive over a few days. As a result, if mania is not controlled, the patient is at risk of harming himself or others. Drugs such as steroids and amphetamines may also trigger mania.

Clinical features

The key component of manic disorders is a persistent elevation of mood. However, these feelings of euphoria and elation may vacillate with feelings of irritability and hostility. The patient may experience racing of thoughts and pressure of speech and it may be very difficult to sustain conversations with patients in a manic state due to the constant pressure of bubbling and exciting ideas. Grandiose delusions are common and can lead to dangerous activities by the patient; for instance, he may believe he (and others) can fly and want to jump off a building. Such patients are therefore at high risk of suicide or homicide and should be assessed accordingly.

Nursing and medical management

Nursing care of these patients must centre on protecting them and others from injury while measures to control mania are instituted. If the patient has a history of mania, he is likely to be prescribed lithium carbonate. This is a metallic salt, identified as controlling mood swings in the 1970s. It has the ability to stabilise mood, thus reducing the possibility of elation and severe depression. If the patient is on lithium therapy, the levels and dosage may require adjustment as necessary. Lithium toxicity usually occurs at greater plasma concentration levels of 1.5 mmol/L Li$^+$, although it can occur at therapeutic levels (0.4–1.0 mmol/L Li$^+$). Toxic levels may result from deliberate overdose, inappropriate usage or non-compliance. It can lead to electrolyte disturbance through water loss, diarrhoea, vomiting and polyurea. Early symptomatology also includes nausea, sweating, tremor and twitching. With plasma concentrations above 2.0 mmol/L (severe over-dosage), symptoms displayed include convulsions, oliguria/renal failure and hypokalaemia. ECG changes (inverted/flat T wave) may also be present. Lithium should be stopped and urea and electrolytes checked. The patient should be admitted and haemodialysis or peritoneal dialysis may be required. In acute overdose much higher serum concentrations may be present without features of toxicity, and measures to increase urine production are necessary.

The manic patient requires patience in handling and tolerant, tactful, kindly authority to make it as restful and unstimulating as reasonably possible. It is essential to make appropriate arrangements to provide close observation and to protect the patient from danger and over-exhausting himself. As this kind of close observation can be quite exhausting for staff, one-to-one nurse contact is advised, with each nurse taking turns for a maximum of 30 minutes each. The A&E nurse must provide fluids and snacks of high calorific value for this patient, in order to reduce the risk of dehydration and hypoglycaemia.

Management of a manic patient outside hospital is only possible when the patient is sufficiently insightful to comply with treatment and where there is con-siderable and dependable informal support (Merson & Baldwin 1995). Admission to hospital is usually indicated.

Bipolar disease

This is a major mental illness characterised by mood swings, alternating between periods of excitement and an overwhelming feeling of sadness, misery, gloom and despondency. Management in A&E is directed towards presenting symptoms.

Anxiety States

Anxiety is an emotional sense of impending doom, a mental sense of unknown terror or fear of losing one's mind (Kaiser & Pyngolil 1995). The patient may present to A&E when symptoms are no longer tolerable or when there is a marked deterioration in ability to carry out day-to-day activities. Patients may also present with panic attacks.

Clinical features

Anxiety is characterised by both psychological and physiological features (Merson & Baldwin 1995):

- *Psychological symptoms and signs*
  - apprehensiveness
  - unfounded worrying
  - fearfulness
  - inner restlessness
  - irritability
  - exaggerated startle response
- *Physiological features*
  - autonomic in origin; e.g. palpitation, breathless-ness, epigastric discomfort, diarrhoea and urinary frequency
  - musculoskeletal, e.g. tension, stiffness and tremor.

Patients may be brought to A&E with an acute anxiety attack, exhibiting signs associated with sympathetic nervous system stimulation, such as tachycardia, palpitations, sweaty palms and hyperventilation. This change in respiration can produce serious biochemical changes due to the lowering in blood CO_2 levels that occurs with overbreathing. This in turn upsets the pH balance, making the blood more alkaline, which in turn upsets the calcium balance causing muscle spasm (tetany) and tingling in the fingers. There is a characteristic carpopedal spasm of the fingers and abdominal cramps that are associated with hysterical hyperventilation. Their effect is to make the patient even more anxious and therefore more likely to hyperventilate. The solution is to reassure the patient and encourage him to use a rebreathing bag to increase the CO_2 levels to normal as he rebreathes exhaled CO_2. After about 15 minutes, the respiratory rate will be back to normal and the muscle cramps will resolve (Walsh 1996).

Tachycardia is a common feature of anxiety attacks; however, in attempting to rule out organic causes of anxiety, it should be noted that tachycardia in patients experiencing anxiety attacks usually does not exceed 140 beats/minute, whereas in paroxysmal supra-ventricular tachycardia the heartbeat is usually above 140 beats/minute (Urbaitis 1983). In addition, supra-ventricular tachycardia is more likely to respond to vagal stimulation than tachycardia due to anxiety.

Nursing and medical management

The patient may respond to explanation, reassurance and a feeling of security. Admission may be required to break the cycle; if medication is required, 10 mg diazepam i.v. is usually given. If admission is not required, the aim should be for symptomatic relief and psychological support. Reassure the patient and allow him to discuss problems at his own pace. Arrange follow-up appointments for further treatment as appropriate.

Alcohol–related Emergencies

Alcoholic patients may present with a variety of problems:

- intoxication
- withdrawal states – delirium tremens
- morbid jealousy
- alcoholic hallucinations
- physical consequences of alcohol abuse, e.g. tuberculosis, GI bleed.

It is dangerous and unrealistic to attempt to conduct a satisfactory psychiatric interview when someone is intoxicated. While this may occasionally leave A&E staff feeling frustrated, on-call psychiatrists will rarely attend A&E while the patient is intoxicated on the grounds that no meaningful psychiatric interview can take place. Clinical management of patients with alcohol intoxication is often confounded by the potentially disruptive and violent behaviour associated with intoxication (Royal College of Psychiatrists 1986).

Alcohol is a central nervous system (CNS) depressant. Measures of alcohol are described in units, with one unit being equal to half a pint of ordinary beer, one standard glass of wine or one-sixth of a gill of spirit (a pub measure) at 40% alcohol concentration. Blood alcohol concentration (BAC) is a measure of the amount of alcohol (mg) present in the bloodstream (per 100 ml), with a standard unit containing approximately 15 mg of alcohol. As with any drug, the effect of a certain dose will vary with the physical and psychological condition of the user (Kennedy & Faugier 1989). Degrees of intoxication may be classified as mild, moderate or severe.

Mild intoxication occurs in individuals with a BAC of up to 80 and is usually achieved with between one and five units. The typical reaction in an emotionally stable person is a feeling of warmth and cheerfulness accompanied by impairment of both judgement and inhibition. Apart from an increased susceptibility to accidents and the risk of post-intoxication headache and mild gastritis there is negligible health risk from a single episode of intoxication at these levels.

Moderate intoxication occurs in individuals with a BAC of between 80 and 150, who will exhibit a loss of self-control, slurred speech, double vision and memory loss. This is usually achieved with doses of up to 10 units. These symptoms are similar to those of raised intracranial pressure, diabetic hypoglycaemia and drug overdose (Skinner *et al.* 1996). These and other possible aetiologies must therefore be excluded prior to such behaviour being ascribed purely to alcohol intoxication.

Accurate assessment and diagnosis of a patient's condition at this level of intoxication may be confounded due to alcohol's desensitising effect on pain response and its disruption to levels of consciousness. Other health problems from this level of intoxication include vomiting, severe gastritis, pancreatitis, hepatitis and interactions with medication and/or existing medical problems (Taylor & Ryrie 1996).

A BAC of between 200 and 400 leads to sleepiness, oblivion and coma, with possible cough reflex depression and airway obstruction from vomit or tongue. Such patients require constant neurological observation and may well require airway and cardiovascular support.

With a BAC of more than 400, death from severe CNS depression, particularly respiratory depression, is possible. Full emergency resuscitation with endotracheal intubation and cardiovascular support may be necessary. Stomach lavage should be considered with extreme caution since chronic alcohol abuse may result in peptic ulceration and/or oesophageal varices. In very severe alcohol poisoning, some patients may require transfer to intensive care units for haemodialysis or haemoperfusion. A BAC of over 600 is usually fatal and is generally only achieved by ingestion of large amounts of spirits.

Nursing management

Due to the behavioural component of moderate intoxication, these patients have the potential to become uncooperative, disruptive and violent, making assessment and treatment very difficult. Gilmore (1986) suggested a variety of behavioural management techniques which A&E staff may employ in such situations. As with any patient, a friendly interest and recognition as a person are essential. Staff are also advised to pace their interactions to suit the impaired cognitive processing of the patient, allowing him to comprehend what is required or suggested. Intoxicated thinking often proceeds by association rather than logic. Key words such as 'let us work together' or involving the patient in actions such as helping with dressings is recommended. Conversely, negative phrases such as 'you're not going to fight or give us trouble' are generally inflammatory, as the patient may associate with the words 'fight' and 'trouble'. In addition, adopting a non-authoritarian but confident manner, acting calmly and quietly, separating opposing groups and removing the injured person from his accompanying friends are valuable approaches.

Levels of intoxication are not static but exist on a time continuum line in relation to blood concentration of the drug. Alcohol is metabolised at approximately one unit or 15 mg of blood alcohol per hour, which is slower than most people drink alcohol. Nurses should therefore be aware that patients can move rapidly from mild to life-threatening intoxication while in the A&E department as they absorb previously ingested alcohol and/or drugs. Conversely, the aforementioned behavioural problems associated with moderate intoxication may follow treatment for the physical effects of severe intoxication.

The easiest way to determine risk levels is to ask patients how much they drink. While there is a general belief that people are reluctant to accurately disclose their drinking patterns, there is good evidence to suggest this is not so and that information on the whole is sufficiently truthful (Watson 1996). Information should be sought in a sensitive but matter-of-fact way when asking about other lifestyle factors such as diet and smoking. Patterns of consumption are also important since a man who drinks 21 units on 1 or 2 days a week is likely to experience different problems from someone who drinks as much, but in smaller amounts, on a more regular basis.

A more subjective approach to assessment, which provides information on an individual's experience of his alcohol use, is the CAGE questionnaire which includes the following four questions:

- Have you ever had to **C**ut down your alcohol intake?
- Have you ever become **A**nnoyed with the amount of alcohol you drink?
- Have you ever felt **G**uilty about how much alcohol you drink?
- Have you ever used alcohol as an **E**ye opener in the morning?

A positive response to two or more of these questions is considered to indicate an unhealthy attitude towards drinking which warrants some form of intervention (Kennedy & Faugier 1989).

Management of acute alcohol intoxication, the identification of potential problem drinkers and the provision of brief interventions do not require the skills of the specialist practitioner. Some basic knowledge and specific nursing actions are necessary, which may be employed as part of standard A&E service provision; however, there is evidence to suggest that the profession, while acknowledging its role in the detection and management of alcohol-related problems, often fails to address such issues adequately (Watson 1996).

Munchausen's Syndrome and Munchausen's Syndrome by Proxy

This is characterised by a patient frequently and repeatedly seeking admission, usually travelling to out of area A&E units. Munchauser's syndrome and Munchausen's syndrome by proxy are characterised by a person simulating physical or mental illness, either in himself or, in the case of Munchausen's by proxy, in a third person, e.g. a child. The carer, usually the mother or both parents, fabricates symptoms or signs and then presents the child to hospital. These is an overlaps with other forms of child abuse (see also Ch. 16).

The symptoms are supported by a plausible history and convincing physical signs. Motivation derives from a desire for attention. Physical examination may reveal multiple scars. Walsh (1996) identified five broad types of presentation by patients with Munchausen's syndrome:

The acute abdominal type. These patients will manifest acute abdominal symptoms and swallow objects, including safety blades and safety pins, in order to obtain the surgery and hospitalisation they crave. Nuts, bolts, coins and other paraphernalia are also swallowed. In well-documented cases, individuals have obtained well over 100 admissions and laparotomies in double figures.

The haemorrhagic type. This presentation is characterised by complaints of bleeding from various orifices. One eye-watering approach is for the patient to insert a coat hanger or needle into the penis, causing trauma and bleeding to the urethra. The positive test for haematuria, along with proclaimed symptoms of renal colic, usually lead to an injection of the desired pethidine. Presentations of haemoptysis and haematemesis are also lent further credibility by self-inflicted wounds to the back of the tongue with needles or razor blades.

The neurological type. This type of the syndrome is characterised by patients presenting with convincing (and not so convincing) epileptic fits or complaints of migraine. Men more frequently present with pseudo-fits than women. The practice of sternal rubs and squeezing the nail bed with a biro smacks of punishment and cannot be condoned under any circumstances. A more humane and equally effective means of assessing a pseudo-fit is to gently stroke the eyelashes in an unsuspecting 'unconscious' patient. It is difficult for them not to reflexively flicker their eyes, an action which would not occur in the genuinely unconscious patient (Dolan 1998).

The cardiac type. Here, the patient will present with a classic, textbook display of central chest pain. Many such patients will be aware that i.v. diamorphine is administered for cardiac-related chest pain, and hence their behaviour.

The psychiatric type. In some instances, patients will imitate various forms of mental illness in order to gain admission to psychiatric units and hospitals.

Clinical features and management

The diagnosis is generally not apparent at first presentation, although characteristic features may be noticeable in retrospect:

- The patient may be unwilling to provide significant personal details, such as an address or that of the next of kin.
- Patients may claim to be in transit and offer elaborate and seemingly implausible explanations for their movements (pseudologia fantastica).
- The presentation of symptoms may be classical, reflecting careful rehearsal – leading to retrospective opinions among professionals that symptoms were 'too good to be true'
- There may be signs of recent i.v. sites or cut-downs. Multiple abdominal scars should rate a very high probability of Munchausen's, especially if the first two points are present.
- The patient's manner and behaviour, especially when he thinks he is not being observed, give cause for suspicion (Walsh 1996).
- The patient may have significant links with the health care profession, either through family connections, a paramedical occupation or as a result of prolonged hospital stays earlier in life (Merson & Baldwin 1995).

Management within A&E is usually difficult due to time restrictions on obtaining a full history. The patient/carer, when confronted with the factitious nature of the symptoms (his own or a third person's), usually discharges himself. Communication with other A&E units and mobilisation of services are required, e.g. the health visitor or GP.

Suicide and Deliberate Self–harm (Parasuicide)

Suicide occurs when a person knowingly brings about his own death (Kreitman 1977). Parasuicide is a non-fatal act of self-injury or the taking of substances in excess of the general recognised or prescribed therapeutic dose. The incidence of self-harm, of which 90% of cases involve self-poisoning, now accounts for around 20% of admissions to general medical wards and is the most frequent reason for admission to hospital in young female patients (Merson & Baldwin 1995). Although potentially lethal drugs are regularly consumed, the overall hospital mortality rate is less than 1% (Valladares 1996). Ryan *et al.* (1996) noted that there is a significant association between suicide and previous attendance at A&E with deliberate self-harm. It is now commonly held that those who commit suicide and those who undertake acts of deliberate self-harm are two distinct groups (Vaughan 1985). Box 14.4 outlines the high-risk factors associated with suicidal behaviour; Box 14.5 highlights Beck's suicide scale which has been used to identify the seriousness of suicidal intent; and Boxes 14.6 and 14.7 provide assessment tools of suicidal ideas and risk (Hughes & Owens 1996).

The risk of suicide is increased by a factor of 100 compared with that in the general population where there is both a recent history of deliberate self-harm and persistent, distressing suicidal ideation. Many of the suicide intent scales depend on the balance between lethality and rescuability (Pritchard 1995). Lethality is the medical danger to life; methods such

---

Box 14.4 – *High-risk factors associated with suicidal behaviour*

Demographic factors
- Adolescence or older than 45 years
- Male
- White
- Protestant
- Separated, divorced or widowed
- Living alone
- Unemployed

Antecedent life circumstances
- Previous suicide attempts
  - recent attempt(s) with serious intent
  - previous attempt(s) with resultant physical or mental sequelae
  - previous attempt(s) that did not effect desired response(s)
- Family history of suicide or suicide attempts
- Inadequate or unavailable support systems
- Major life changes
  - major losses, e.g. spouse, job, money
  - major illness (of self or others)

Psychiatric conditions
- Depressive illnesses
- Alcoholism
- Schizophrenia

Box 14.5 – *Beck suicide risk scale (Beck et al. 1974)*

Preparation
- Act planned in advance
- Suicide note written
- Action in anticipation of death, for example, writing a will

Circumstances of the act
- Patient was alone
- Timed such that intervention was unlikely
- Precautions taken against discovery

Sequelae of the act
- Did not seek help
- Stated wish to die
- Stated belief that the act would be proven fatal
- Sorry the act failed

Box 14.6 – *The assessment of suicidal ideas: progressively specific questions*

- How do you see the future?
- Do you ever feel hopeless, like giving up?
- Do things ever seem so bad that you feel you cannot go on?
- Have you ever wished you could go to sleep and not wake up?
- Have you ever thought of doing anything to harm yourself?
- Have you made any plans for that?
- Have you done anything about it?

Box 14.7 – *Assessing suicidal risk following deliberate self-harm*

- What happened before and during the self-harm event?
- Did the patient intend to die?
- Does the patient still intend to die?
- Does the patient have a psychiatric disorder?
- What are the patient's problems?
- What are the patient's resources for dealing with this crisis?

---

as shooting and jumping from a high building have high lethality values, whereas a tranquilliser overdose will have a lower lethality value. Conversely, someone who takes an overdose of tranquillisers and alcohol,

and then disappears into the sea has a low likelihood of rescuability. The person who is drunk and attempts to take a large number of tablets in front of their partner has a high likelihood of rescue. The overall level of intent depends on the balance between lethality and rescuability (Jones 1995).

Obtaining a history from a patient following a suicide attempt is frequently very difficult. The patient may also give false information to avoid embarrassment (Zull 1995). A patient has the right to refuse treatment, and any treatment which is enforced on a patient is considered assault or battery (Dimond 1990). Under common law, treatment can be given without the consent of the patient in cases of necessity: circumstances in which immediate action is required and necessary to preserve life or prevent a serious or immediate danger to the patient or others. The treatment or physical restraint used must be reasonable and sufficient only to the purpose of bringing the emergency to an end. Medical treatment should be administered under the specific direction of a medical practitioner (Hughes & Owens 1996). This duty is imposed by statute and the UKCC *Code of Conduct* (1992) and is underpinned by the principles of civil law relating to negligence.

Stockbridge (1993) noted that the feelings of A&E staff towards patients with self-inflicted injuries appear to be predominantly negative. Ward (1995) suggested that the nurse has to make sense of the patient's behaviour from the patient's point of view, rather than the nurse's. The key to a successful nurse/patient relationship lies in establishing a positive rapport from the initial assessment. A strategy for achieving this was suggested by Burnard (1990) in relation to interviewing technique. He proposed the acronym 'SOLER' to remind the interviewer of the following:

- **S**it squarely opposite the patient, not behind a desk, and avoid distraction.
- **O**pen positioning, feet apart and palms resting on thighs.
- **L**ean forward towards the client.
- **E**ye contact – show attention and give feedback. This helps to establish a relationship. No staring or glaring.
- **R**elax – tension or fidgeting may convey impatience or lack of interest.

This position helps to make the nurse appear warm and empathetic. By adopting this strategy the nurse should be able to dissociate herself from prejudicial feelings, and the patient is more likely to feel accepted and worthwhile.

If the patient is determined to be at continued risk, the nurse should not leave him alone. If the patient is considered to be at high risk and is not willing to accept hospitalisation, involuntary admission will be necessary. If doubt exists, caution should be exercised and admission arranged.

Self-mutilation

Destructive acts against the self, such as putting a fist through the window and wrist cutting, may occur as behaviour secondary to personality problems. Patients are usually in their 20s or 30s and may be single or married. Most patients who cut themselves have a history of self-injury. The wrists, arms and thighs are common sites, and instruments such as razor blades, knives, broken glass or mirrors may be used. The wounds are usually relatively superficial and the patient may describe that the act brings relief of tension and depersonalisation. Patients who self-mutilate tend to have low self-esteem but the lethality of the intent is usually low.

Nursing management

Treatment in A&E should revolve around immediate care of the injury, evaluating the risk of suicide, protecting the patient from further self-harm and assisting in crisis resolution (Repper 1999). Patients who attend regularly following acts of deliberate self-harm may leave staff feeling frustrated and hostile towards them. However, such beliefs and attitudes must not be allowed to interfere with the care of the patient (van den Bent-Kelly 1992). The environment of care should be supportive and non-confrontational for patients who deliberately self-harm, and care should be delivered non-judgmentally. Given the degree of aggression which is channelled internally into acts of deliberate self-harm, the A&E nurse should also exercise caution when caring for these patients as the aggressive tendencies exhibited may be directed towards staff. Referral to appropriate agencies, such as community psychiatric nurses (CPNs), is encouraged so that the patient can ventilate and discuss feelings and explore other ways of coping more appropriately (McElroy & Sheppard 1999, Perego 1999).

Individual at Odds with Society

Sociopathy refers to a group of well defined anomalies or deviations of personality which are not the result of either psychotic or any other illness. Numerous theories have been put forward as to why this disorder should develop (Bowlby 1965, Cleckly 1967, Sim 1974).

The patient may present to A&E with depression, suicidal gestures, abuse of drugs, alcohol and sex, or

as a result of aggressive and violent behaviour and lack of impulse control etc. Management requires a complete history to be taken to exclude epilepsy, hypoglycaemia or any other acute organic reaction. Treatment is directed at managing the presenting condition with a firm and consistent approach. Reference to mental health teams is as appropriate.

Violent patients

Violence or threats of violence may be associated with a variety of disorders, e.g. psychosis, chemical intoxication, sociopathy etc., or with a specific situation, such as lack of communication. The nurse should be alert for violence, particularly if the patient has a previous history of violent behaviour or poor impulse control, if he has been brought in by the police or if he is verbally or physically threatening.

There are several management points in A&E:

- Always manage the patient with the required number of staff to do so appropriately and beware of uniform limitations.
- Be familiar with the alarm/security system.
- If entering a room, do so letting a colleague know where you are. See the patient in a non-isolated room and leave yourself and the patient an exit.
- Maintain a quiet, calm but firm approach. Avoid any contact which may be misinterpreted.
- Monitor both your own and the patient's reactions.

Management

If circumstances allow, try to establish whether a psychiatric disorder is present: is the patient demanding; is conscious level fluctuating? If a psychiatric disorder is present, assess the need for admission and suitability of facilities available. Give medication as appropriate

If no clinical reason for admission is elicited and the patient remains disruptive, security and/or the police should be contacted (see also Ch. 11).

Learning Disability Clients and Mental Health Problems

Patients with learning disabilities may present with:

- self-mutilation
- schizophrenia
- depression
- anxiety.

The patient should be assessed as appropriate and a history taken from the escort. If admission is not required, referral to local learning disability services and social services may be required to provide an emergency service. If behaviour is disturbed and the patient requires medications, low doses of neuroleptics should be given because of susceptibility to side-effects.

Elderly Clients Presenting to A&E with Mental Health Problems

Psychiatric emergencies arising '*de novo*' or super-imposed upon dementia include:

- acute confusional states
- mania – usually a history of bipolar disease is present
- depression and deliberate self-harm
- paranoid disorder.

In health care for the elderly, the decision as to whether to admit a patient is usually made after careful assessment. Ideally, problems presented by the elderly client will be assessed by the health care for the elderly team (mental health) on a domiciliary visit. In reality, elderly patients may be referred or present directly to the A&E department. Therefore the nurse must be alert to social admission. Dementia *per se* is not a sole reason for admission.

Assessment should be directed towards:

- evidence of an acute organic reaction, such as recent confusion, disorientation etc.
- in the absence of an acute organic reaction, whether mental illness is present, e.g. clinical depression, paranoid psychosis
- strength of family support, if any; respite need
- whether behaviour is disturbed.

If admission is necessary, the appropriate team should be contacted. If immediate treatment is required, medication should be limited to low doses, particularly if there is evidence of renal or hepatic improvement (see also Ch. 21).

Child and Adolescent Psychiatry

Children and adolescents will present to A&E as emergency referrals. The A&E nurse should be familiar with the procedure to contact the duty child and adolescent mental health team and management should be discussed with them. Any child or adolescent present with psychiatric pathology should be taken as seriously as any other age group and managed according to the presenting condition.

Common psychiatric presentations include:

- chemical abuse
- suicidal behaviour/deliberate self-harm
- depression – reactive and endogenous

- early schizophrenia
- adolescent behavioural disorders
- eating and nutrition disorders.

Management

- Assess, treat and admit as appropriate
- Referral to child psychiatric team
- Support and reassurance for the patient and family
- Institute appropriate follow-up.

Patients Attending A&E with Eating Disorders

The most common of these are:

- anorexia nervosa
- bulimia nervosa
- compulsive eating/food addiction – severe over-weight.

Patients with eating disorders may present to A&E with problems such as osteoporetic fractures, collapse, infection, dehydration, oedema, cardiac failure, fatigue, cyanosis, bradycardia, hypotension, weight loss, obesity, hypoglycaemia, hypocalcaemia/kalaemia, infertility, amenorrhoea, constipation and vomiting, or may be referred by dental practitioners for dental problems. In addition, they may present with agitation, depression or acopia.

Management

Treatment is aimed at the presenting symptoms and includes a complete physical work-up. Admission in the acute phase is usually required. In A&E, basic nursing care as well as care of malnutrition/dehydration needs to be addressed.

Social Problems

Some people tend to use A&E as a crisis walk-in clinic, e.g. someone who has become acutely disturbed or who is blamed as the cause of a crisis and is brought to A&E as the patient. Although these incidents may not be true psychiatric emergencies, A&E is seen as a 24-hour emergency unit, when no other help or assistance is perceived to be available. The presence of an impartial observer and environment may enable the patient and his family/carers to discuss the problems for the first time. Referral to agencies for follow-up is required, e.g. to counselling services in general and/or for specific needs, such as HIV, rape, social worker or probation officer.

Other social problems that may present to A&E are those people searching for a trolley, bed, shelter or food, often with no apparent psychiatric or medical illness. These patients can be very difficult or manipulative and require limit-setting and firm handling. The opportunity to discuss problems may help but the nurse should attempt to clarify what type of assistance the person requires and be familiar with telephone numbers of agencies able to help, such as crisis centres, social security, local hostels, emergency social workers, etc.

Iatrogenic Drug-induced Psychosis

Non-specific psychosis may occur, including mania, delirium, schizophreniform psychosis or depression in patients on maintenance therapy for a physical condition, e.g. Cushing's syndrome. If a patient's condition precludes reducing the dose of medication, antipsychotics can be administered concurrently to control symptoms.

Psychotropic drugs have served to revolutionise the treatment and care of the mentally ill. However, these drugs can also have side-effects which may require management in the A&E department. All antipsychotic agents may produce acute dystonias, akathisia, Parkinsonism, and akinesia.

Acute dystonia

Symptoms usually occur 1 hour to 5 days after commencement of antipsychotic medication, especially with high-potency neuroleptics such as haloperidol or trifluperazine. Dystonic reactions are prolonged tonic contractions of muscle groups. When the muscles of the neck, tongue and jaw are involved, this is called torticollis. Torticollis combined with contractions of the extraocular muscles, whereby the eyes are rolled upwards with the head turned to one side, is called occulogyric crisis.

Although these muscle contractions can be very frightening for the patient, they can usually be easily reversed with the intramuscular administration of 2 mg of benztropine mesylate or 10 mg of procyclidine. The nurse should stay with the patient and provide reassurance that the reaction can be reversed usually within 5–20 minutes of injection.

Akathisia

Symptoms of akathisia usually occur within 2–3 months of commencement of medication. The patient complains of an inability to sit still, pacing and fidgeting. While this is not an emergency, it can be distressing for the patient and be mistaken for agitation associated with the patient's primary disorder. Anti-Parkinsonian agents such as benztropine mesylate provide relief.

Akinesia

Akinesia is an extrapyrimidal reaction characterised by signs and symptoms of decreased motor activity. The patient experiences fatigue and muscle weakness. It can easily be controlled with an anti-Parkinsonian agent (Kaiser & Pyngolil 1995).

Monoamine Oxidase Inhibitors (MAOIs)

MAOIs inhibit monamine oxidase, therefore causing an accumulation of amine neurotransmitters. The metabolism of some amine drugs and tyramine found in some foods may cause a dangerous rise in the blood pressure. MAOIs also interact with opiates, lithium and tricyclic antidepressants. The danger of interaction persists for up to 14 days after treatment with MAOIs is discontinued.

Hypertensive crisis may occur if MAOIs are taken in combination with:

- amphetamines
- appetite suppressants
- dietary amines, cheese, marmite, broad beans, chocolate, bananas, Chianti wine, whiskey, beer, caffeinated tea or coffee
- proprietary cold and allergy remedies containing sympathomimetics, e.g. adrenaline, phenylephrine.

Hypertensive crisis is characterised by the sudden onset of severe throbbing headache, nausea, vomiting and dizziness. The patient's blood pressure can be as high as 350/250 mmHg, and chest and neck pain, palpitations and malignant hyperthermia, the usual cause of death in patients experiencing hypertensive crisis, may occur.

Nursing and medical management

Hypertensive crisis is an emergency, and therefore the patient's vital signs should be monitored closely and 12–15 L of oxygen administered via a tight-fitting reservoir mask. Intravenous phentolamine 5–10 mg should be given to reduce the patient's blood pressure and repeated as necessary. Supportive measures include forced diuresis, and therefore urine output should be monitored. Hypertensive crisis should resolve 1–3 hours after initiation of treatment.

Conclusion

Psychiatric emergencies present a particular challenge to A&E nurses as they may be a result of physical or functional disorders and increasingly present for the first time to A&E departments for initial management. This chapter has considered the more common psychiatric emergencies and identified a range of interventions for nurses to employ when caring for these distressed and frequently distressing patients. Recognising and understanding these emergencies will help the nurse meet the challenges of psychiatric emergency care in A&E.

References

Aguilera D, Messick J (1986) *Crisis Intervention: Theory and Methodology*, 5th edn. St Louis: Mosby.

Ambrose K (1996) Mental health care in A&E: expanding nursing roles. *Emergency Nurse* **4**(3), 16–18.

Beck AT, Morris JB, Beck A (1974) Cross-validation of the suicidel intent scale. *Psychological Reports* **34**(2), 445–446.

Bowlby J (1965) *Child Care and the Growth of Love*. Harmondsworth: Penguin.

Burnard P (1990) *Learning Human Skills: an Experiential Guide for Nurses*. Oxford: Heinemann.

Cleckly B (1967) *The Mask of Sanity*. New York: Basic Books.

Dimond B (1990) *Legal Aspects of Nursing*. London: Prentice Hall.

Dolan B (1998) The hospital hoppers. *Nursing Times* **94**(30), 26–27.

Gilig P, Dumaine M, Hilard JR (1990) Who do mobile crisis services serve? *Hospital and Community Psychiatry* **41**, 804–805.

Gilmore G (1986) Behavioural management of acutely intoxicated patients in the emergency department. *Journal of Emergency Nursing* **12**(1), 13–17.

Gournay K, Beadsmore A (1995) The report of the clinical standards advisory group: standards of care for people with schizophrenia in the UK and implications for mental health nursing. *Journal of Mental and Psychiatric Nursing* **2**, 359–364.

Greenstein RA, Ness DE (1990) Psychiatric emergencies in the elderly. *Emergency Medicine Clinics of North America* **8**, 429–441.

Hughes T, Owens D (1996) Management of suicidal risk. *British Journal of Hospital Medicine* **56**(4), 151–154.

Jones L (1995) Assessing suicide risk in A&E. *Emergency Nurse* **2**(4), 7–9.

Kaiser J, Pyngolil MJ (1995) Psychiatric emergencies. In: Kitt S, Selfridge-Thomas J, Proehl JA, Kaiser J, eds. *Emergency Nursing: a Physiologic and Clinical Perspective*, 2nd edn. Philadelphia: WB Saunders.

Kaplan HI, Sadock BJ (1993) *Pocket Handbook of Emergency Psychiatric Medicine*. Baltimore: Wilkins & Wilkins.

Kennedy J, Faugier J (1989) *Drug and Alcohol Dependency Nursing*. Oxford: Heinemann Nursing.

Kreitman N (1977) *Parasuicide*. London: John Wiley.

McElroy A, Shepperd G (1999) The assessment and management of self-harming patients in the accident and emergency department: an action research project. *Journal of Clinical Nursing* **8**(1), 66–72.

Mackway-Jones K. (ed.) (1996) *Emergency Triage: Manchester Triage Group*. London: BMJ.

Merson S, Baldwin D (1995) *Psychiatric Emergencies*. Oxford: Oxford University Press.

Perego M (1999) Why A&E nurses feel inadequate in managing patients who deliberately self-harm. *Emergency Nurse* **6**(9), 21–27.

Pritchard C. (1995) *Suicide – the Ultimate Rejection?: a Psychosocial Study*. Buckingham: Open University Press.

Puskar KR, Obus NL (1989) Management of the psychiatric emergency. *Nurse Practitioner* 14, 7, 9–10, 12, 14, 16, 18, 23, 26.

Repper J (1999) A review of the literature on the prevention of suicide interventions in accident and emergency departments. *Journal of Clinical Nursing* **8**(1), 3–12.

Royal College of Psychiatrists (1986) *Alcohol: Our Favourite Drug*. London: Tavistock.

Ryan J, Rushdy A, Perez-Avilla CA, Allison R (1996) Suicide rate following attendance at an accident and emergency department with deliberate self harm *Journal of Accident and Emergency Medicine* **13**, 101–104.

Sim M (1974) *Guide to Psychiatry* Edinburgh: Churchill Livingstone.

Skinner D, Driscoll P, Earlam R, eds. (1996) *ABC of Major Trauma*, 2nd edn. London: BMJ.

Stockbridge J (1993) Parasuicide: does discussing it help? *Emergency Nurse*, **1**(2), 19–21.

Taylor R, Ryrie I (1996) Clinical management of acute and chronic alcohol use in A&E. *Emergency Nurse* **4**(3), 6–8.

UKCC (1992) *Code of Conduct*. London: UKCC.

Urbaitis JC (1983) *Psychiatric emergencies*. Norwalk, CT: Appleton-Century Crofts.

Valladeres P (1996) Comparing clinical management of over-doses. *Emergency Nurse*, **4**(1), 6–8.

van den Bent-Kelly D (1992) Too busy for trivia: patients who self harm. *Nursing: Journal of Clinical Practice, Education and Management*, **5**(5), 32–33.

Vaughan P (1985) *Suicide Prevention*. Birmingham: PEPAR.

Walsh M (1996) *Accident and Emergency Nursing: a New Approach*, 3rd edn. Oxford: Butterworth-Heinemann.

Ward MF (1995) *Nursing the Psychiatric Emergency*. Oxford: Butterworth Heinemann.

Watson H (1996) Minimal interventions for problem drinkers. *Journal of Substance Misuse for Nursing, Health and Social Care* **1**(2), 107–110.

Zull DN (1995) Poisoning and drug overdose. In: Kitt S, Selfridge-Thomas J, Proehl JA, Kaiser J, eds. *Emergency Nursing: a Physiologic and Clinical Perspective*, 2nd edn. Philadelphia: WB Saunders.

Part 4

Life
Continuum

15. Infants   217

16. Pre-school Children   233

17. Ages 5 to Puberty   251

18. Adolescence   257

19. Young Adults   269

20. Middle Years   275

21. The Elderly   283

Chapter 15

Infants

Cathryn Bird & Lindsey Lorkin

- Introduction
- Assessment
- The critically ill infant and child
- Causes of respiratory difficulty
- The febrile infant
- Meningitis
- Dehydration in infants
- Failure to thrive
- The vomiting infant
- The injured infant
- Sudden infant death syndrome
- Conclusion

Introduction

Parents often bring their baby to A&E because it offers 24-hour access to advice and health care. To the A&E nurse, this may not always seem appropriate, however, if a therapeutic relationship is to be established with the family, nurses must learn to see the problem through the parents'/carers' eyes as well as from a professional perspective. Some families experience problems in accessing health care, particularly within inner cities and areas of ethnic diversity (Bedford *et al.* 1992). A number of factors could account for this. Knowledge regarding health care provision of out-of-hours GP services affects parents' decision-making, as does the workload and availability of the GP or health visitor. The proximity of an A&E department to patients' homes also influences uptake of facilities.

Parental anxiety plays a large part in determining appropriate action in accessing health care. Social isolation makes decision-making more difficult, as does inexperience, e.g. a first baby. These groups of carers are more likely to use A&E for support and advice once offered in the extended family structure. It is important for A&E nurses to remember that many parents bring their baby to A&E because they have assessed their baby's condition and have actively decided that A&E or hospital care is needed.

Assessment

Whatever the parents' reasons for choosing the A&E department for their baby, the A&E nurse should attempt meet the family's needs by aiming to establish a rapport during the initial assessment. This helps to reduce parental anxiety and fretfulness in the infant, and prevents some of the tensions which hinder assessment and subsequent treatment. The A&E nurse should approach the family in a calm and confident way. A crying baby at 3.00 a.m. may seem trivial or 'inappropriate' to A&E staff who are knowledgeable professionals, but to young parents who are tired, anxious and inexperienced, it is a frightening and emotional time.

Initial assessment or triage allows the nurse to collect information about the infant's condition and factors leading to admission. Parents' fears and anxieties can be explored. Honest, informative communication can provide a realistic view of waiting times and help parents to understand the likely treatment of their baby. This enables them to begin to trust the nurse and to believe that the care they have sought will be effective. Parent/carer cooperation relies on the formation of therapeutic relationships. Sometimes the A&E nurse is, in fact, caring for a well infant whose parents/carers are anxious or concerned. Effective care from the A&E nurse can go a long way towards meeting the needs of these families.

Development of the normal infant

For an A&E nurse to accurately assess and care for an infant, he must be aware of infants' expected development milestones. Developmental tables are a useful guide to infant development (Table 15.1).

The accurate assessment and recognition of a seriously ill or injured infant occurs during triage. The A&E nurse relies on parents or carers to give an accurate history of the presenting complaint. At this stage, it is useful to clarify who is accompanying the infant. The confidence and cooperation of parents or carers should be sought by allowing them to express concerns and disclose information about the infant's health problems. It is important for the assessing nurse to check information; for example, if the parent/carer says the infant has a rash, the nurse should look at it to determine its relevance, or if a parent/carer says the infant is sleepy, the nurse should handle the infant during the initial assessment (see Box 15.1).

Encourage the parent or carer to stay with the baby and, where possible, get the adult to hold the baby on her lap. This has a dual benefit of making the baby feel more secure because of familiarity (Bernado & Schenkel 1995) and helping the parent/carer to retain some control over the proceedings. The nurse should speak in soft tones and avoid sudden movements, so that the infant is less likely to become distressed. Accurate assessment of infants is dependent on gaining trust and cooperation, and this approach can optimise the process. For example, an infant can only focus on one thing at a time. Successful assessment can therefore be aided by distraction, e.g. diverting the infant's attention with a toy can make taking an axillary temperature easier (Morcombe 1998). It is also worth remembering that, while loud crying clearly signals an infant's distress, such an obvious

Table 15.1 – *A brief outline of developmental milestones*

Age	Stage of development
4–6 weeks	Smiles to social stimuli
2 months	Smiles and vocalises when talked to Eyes follow moving person/object
3 months	Holds a rattle when placed in hand Turns head to sounds on level with ear
5 months	Laughs aloud Pulled to sit – no head lag Able to reach and grasp objects
6 months	Sits on floor with support Rolls prone to supine Begins to imitate, e.g. cough When held in standing position, puts weight on legs
9 months	Crawls on abdomen Stands holding onto furniture
10 months	Waves goodbye Helps parent/carer when being dressed, e.g. by holding arms for coat Pincer grip used to pick up fine objects
12 months	Walks holding onto furniture or with one or two hands held Speaks two or three words with meaning

Box 15.1 – *Assessment of the infant*

- Rapid cardiopulmonary assessment – ABC
- Length of current illness
- Symptoms and additional circumstances surrounding the illness/injury
- Immunisation status
- Medical problems
- Prescribed medication/over-the-counter medication
- Known allergies
- Feeding and sleeping patterns
- General demeanour and condition should be assessed
- Interaction/response to accompany adult

sign may not always be present; the disinterested, lethargic and quiet infant, for example, is always a cause for clinical concern.

Table 15.2 – *Vital signs in infants*

Age (months)	Average weight (kg)	Normal BP	Heart rate	Respiratory rate
1	4	60–90/45–60	120–160	30–60
3	5	74–100/50–70	120–160	30–60
6	7	74–100/50–70	120–160	30–60
9	9	74–100/50–70	120–160	30–60
12	10	80–112/50–80	90–140	24–40

Vital signs

Normal parameters for an infant's vital signs change with age, and therefore a knowledge of normal ranges at specific ages is necessary in order to detect abnormalities (see Table 15.2).

Respiration

The anatomy of an infant's airway differs significantly from that of an adult or older child (Gilbert *et al.* 1993). The tongue is proportionately bigger in the mouth, thus increasing the risk of oral obstruction. Infants are obligatory nose breathers and become distressed when their nose is blocked with mucous secretions or a foreign body. The upper airway is smaller and narrower than that of an older person, and therefore they are more quickly distressed. Respiratory obstruction can occur as a result of oedema, mucus, blood or constriction (Chameides 1990). Stridor can be created by minimal oedema or obstruction but acts as an indicator of imminent respiratory distress. Infants have less respiratory reserve, despite a greater oxygen uptake, due to their faster metabolic rate. The increased activity of breathing during illness is not aided by poorly developed intercostal muscles and cartilaginous ribs. As a result, infants will develop respiratory distress more quickly.

It is important that infants presenting with a history of respiratory difficulty are assessed carefully. Parents or carers may hold important clues to the cause of perceived or actual respiratory problems. The A&E nurse must be able to listen, reduce the parents'/carers' fears and rapidly assess the physiological state of the infant's respiratory function (Box 15.2).

The Critically Ill Infant and Child

Caridiopulmonary arrest in infants and children is seldom sudden and rarely due to a primary cardiac event. It is often the end result of progressive

Box 15.2 – *Respiratory assessment*

- Rapid cardiopulmonary assessment – ABC

- Observe the baby's respiratory rate

- Look at skin colour – is the baby pink, pale or cyanosed; is the colour different centrally and peripherally?

- Listen to breathing – is there stridor, wheezing or grunting?

- Look at chest movements – are they equal on both sides; is there intercostal recession; is the baby using shoulders and head bobbing to aid respiratory effort; is there nasal flaring?

- Check pulse – is it within normal ranges; is the baby tachycardic or bradycardic; what is the pulse pressure?

- Is the baby pyrexial?

- Avoid distressing the baby – usually the parent or carer can hold the infant as she will have often found the position most comfortable for the baby. This is usually semi-upright

- Determine the infant's responsiveness – does she react to stimulus from the nurse; is she interacting with the parent/carer; is the baby aware of her surroundings?

- Is the baby easily distracted, upset, irritable, fretful, restless, floppy or unconscious?

- Is a blood glucose test indicated?

deterioration in respiratory and circulatory function. It usually results from a period of hypoxia and acidosis which has been caused by respiratory and/or circulatory failure (Bruce-Jones 1994). If pulseless cardiac arrest occurs, the outcome is bleak. Early recognition and treatment to prevent cardiopulmonary

Table 15.3 – *Paediatric differences in airway, breathing and circulation. (After Cosby 1998)*

Factor	Nursing considerations
Airway	
Large tongue	Airway is easily obstructed by tongue; proper positioning is often all that is necessary to open the airway
Smaller diameter of all airways (in a 1-year-old child, tracheal diameter is less than child's little finger)	Small amounts of mucus or swelling easily obstruct the airways; child normally has increased airway resistance
Cartilage of larynx is softer than in adults; cricoid cartilage is narrowest portion of neck	Airway of infant can be compressed if neck is flexed or hyperextended; provides a natural seal for endotracheal tube
Breathing	
Sternum and ribs are cartilaginous; chest wall is soft; intercostal muscles are poorly developed; infants are obilgatory nose breathers for first 4 weeks of life; increased metabolic rate (about twice that of an adult); increased respiratory demand for oxygen consumption and carbon dioxide elimination	Infant's chest wall may move inwards instead of outwards during inspiration (retractions) when lung compliance is decreased; greater intrathoracic pressure generated during inspiration; anything causing nasal obstruction can produce respiratory distress; respiratory distress increases oxygen demand, as does any condition that increases metabolic rate, i.e. fever
Circulation	
Child's circulating blood volume is larger per unit of body weight, but absolute volume is relatively small; 70–80% of a newborn's body weight is water, compared with 50–60% of an adult body weight; about half of this volume is extracellular	Blood loss considered minor in an adult may lead to shock in a child; decreased fluid intake or increased fluid loss quickly leads to dehydration
Increased heart rate, decreased stroke volume; cardiac output is higher per unit of body weight	Tachycardia is the child's most efficient method of increasing cardiac output if the heart rate is greater than 180–200 beats/min

arrest are fundamental to successful resuscitation. Thus cardiopulmonary arrest can often be prevented if the clinical signs of respiratory failure and shock are recognised promptly.

Every infant and child attending A&E should be thoroughly and continually assessed, using a structured rapid cardiopulmonary assessment. Blood volume in a child is 80 ml/kg, with total blood volume much less than in an adult. Loss of one cup of blood in a 10 kg child is equivalent to blood loss of almost 1 L in an adult. A child responds to increased cardiac output with tachycardia. Tachycardia may initially increase cardiac output during periods of distress; however, prolonged tachycardia of more than 200 beats/min for infants and 170 beats/min for children causes decompensation and decreased cardiac output. Close attention to heart rate, skin signs and mental status is the key to early recognition of compensated shock. Cardiopulmonary failure may be present in any child with respiratory distress, cyanosis, impaired conscious level or those who suffer severe trauma. The A&E nurse should develop expertise and skills to identify subtle changes in a child's condition in order to conflate them into a meaningful picture (see Table 15.3).

Paediatric primary and secondary assessment

Primary assessment consists of evaluation of ABCs and neurological status. The primary survey should include assessment of respiratory effort, skin colour and temperature, heart rate and quality and level of consciousness. Secondary assessment consists of vital signs and a head-to-toe survey.

Respiratory rate

The infant and young child's respiratory muscles are not well developed, so the diaphragm plays an essential role in breathing. Observation of the rise and fall of the abdomen are the best methods for assessing respiratory rate in patients less than 2 years old. As respiratory rates are often irregular in small children, the rate should be carefully assessed for a full minute. A neonate has a normal respiratory rate of 30–40 breaths/min, which slows as the child grows older. A resting rate faster than 60 breaths/min is a sign of respiratory distress in a child, irrespective of age (Cosby 1998). Other clinical signs of distress include nasal flaring, use of accessory muscles, recession, grunting, stridor and wheezing.

Skin perfusion and temperature

The skin colour and temperature should be consistent over the trunk and limbs. However, when assessing the patient, consider the ambient temperature. Decreased skin perfusion can be an early sign of shock. Clinical signs of poor perfusion include peripherally cool skin, pallor, mottling, peripheral cyanosis and capillary refill > 2 seconds.

Heart rate and blood pressure

Sinus tachycardia is a common presentation in most unwell, anxious children. Further assessment will be needed to determine and treat the cause. Bradycardia in a sick child is a pre-terminal sign and indicates imminent cardiopulmonary arrest. Vital signs should be documented as part of the baseline assessment. Children in early shock may have a normal blood pressure reading initially because of their ability to compensate. A dropping blood pressure is a serious sign warranting immediate intervention, as a child can lose a significant amount of blood before the blood pressure decreases (Hazinski 1992).

Conscious level

Normally, parents are often the first to recognise decreased levels of consciousness, often stating that their infant is 'not right'. An accurate history from parents is important and it is important to ask about trauma, previous medical problems, ingestions, and signs and symptoms of infection. Evaluation of the history and level of consciousness can be enough to classify the child's condition as an emergency. An altered level of consciousness in any child is an emergency condition. Signs of an impaired conscious level include drowsiness, difficulty to arouse, agitation, failure to recognise or interact with parents, and failure to respond to stimuli.

Management priorities

Using a structured approach, such as paediatric advanced life support (PALS), the A&E nurse must determine the relevance of the clinical signs found and prioritise further management. The child should be categorised as:

- in cardiopulmonary failure
- in definite respiratory failure/shock
- in potential respiratory failure/shock
- stable.

Paediatric basic and advanced life support interventions may be required (see Figs 15.1 and 15.2).

Paediatric advanced life support

Establish basic life support (European Resuscitation Council 1998a). Oxygenate and ensure the provision of positive pressure ventilation with a high inspired oxygen concentration. Attach a defibrillator or monitor and monitor the cardiac rhythm. Check the pulse: in the case of an infant, feel for the brachial pulse on the inner aspect of the upper arm; in the case of a child feel for the carotid pulse in the neck, taking no more than 10 seconds. Assess the rhythm on the monitor as being:

- non-ventricular fibrillation (non-VF) or non-pulseless ventricular tachycardia (non-VT) (asystole or electromechanical dissociation)
- ventricular fibrillation (VF) or pulseless ventricular tachycardia (VT).

Non-VF/VT (asystole, electromechanical dissociation) is more common in children. Administer adrenaline/epinephrine and carry out 3 minutes of basic life support and repeat the cycle at least twice more. Consider the use of other medications and treat reversible causes.

VF/VT is less common in paediatric life support but the nurse must always be aware of the possibility of treating this arrhythmia rapidly and effectively. Defibrillate the heart with three defibrillation shocks of 2, 2/and 4 J/kg. Place the defibrillator paddles on the chest wall, one just below the right clavicle and the other at the left anterior axillary line; for infants, when using this method of monitoring, it may be more appropriate to apply the paddles to the front and back of the infant's chest. If VF/VT persists, carry out 1 minute of basic life support and then defibrillate with

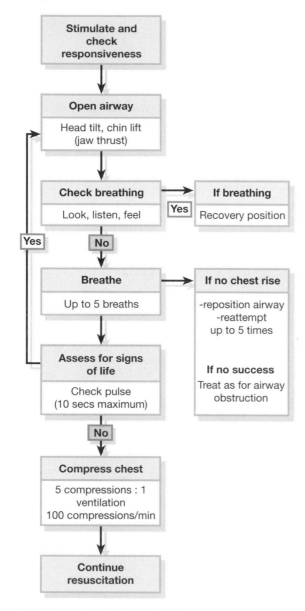

Figure 15.1 – *Paediatric basic life support.*

three defibrillation shocks of 4 J/kg. Repeat the cycle of defibrillation and 1 minute of basic life support until defibrillation is achieved. Consider the use of other medication and treat reversible causes, which include (European Resuscitation Council 1998b):

- hypoxia
- hypovolaemia
- hyper/hypokalaemia
- hypthermia
- hypothermia

- tension pneumothorax
- tamponade
- toxic/therapeutic disturbances
- thromboemboli.

Causes of Respiratory Difficulty

Inhalation of foreign body

Inhalation of a foreign body (FB) should always be considered if an infant presents with a sudden onset of cyanosis, stridor or choking. This is more common in toddlers than in infants. Timely treatment will prevent severe complications. It is not recommended that the Heimlich manoeuvre is used on children of less than 1 year as it could cause liver damage. (Gatch *et al.* 1987). Infants with total airway obstruction should be placed prone with their head being well supported by the operator, and five back blows should be given in rapid succession to relieve the obstruction. If this is not successful, place the infant supine on a firm surface and give five chest thrusts (European Resuscitation Council 1998b).

Bronchiolitis

Bronchiolitis is an acute lower respiratory tract infection and around 90% of cases are attributed to the respiratory syncytial virus (RSV) (Barkin & Rosen 1994). It is most prevalent in winter and is the most frequent cause of pneumonia in infancy (Dinwiddie 1990). Bronchiolitis is often precipitated by an upper respiratory tract infection. The virus causes an inflammatory response in the bronchioles, thus causing constriction of the airway. The resultant secretions begin to accumulate as exudate cannot be easily expectorated because of damage to ciliated cells. This results in impaired gaseous exchange (McFarlane 1992).

Infants present with a history of 'runny nose', cough and low-grade pyrexia worsening over a period of a few days. This leads to irritability, poor feeding and eventually to dehydration and respiratory distress (Barkin & Rosen 1994). Initial assessment will reveal an infant with dyspnoea and tachypnoea, and an expiratory wheeze. There may be signs of respiratory distress with intercostal recession, use of accessory muscles and nasal flaring. Infants under 6 months, or those born prematurely, are at greatest risk of respiratory failure or apnoeic episodes (Wolfram 1992).

Nursing interventions include reassurance of parents/carers and maintenance of a calm environment. The infant should be given oxygen by the least distressing route – via nasal cannulae or a face mask,

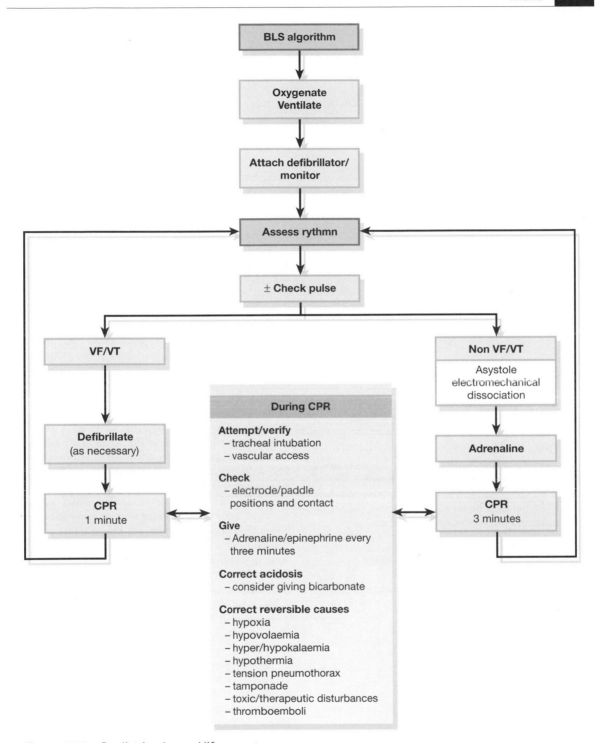

Figure 15.2 – *Paediatric advanced life support.*

blowing close to the infant. Pulse oximetry will indicate the effectiveness of the treatment. Nebulised beta-antagonists can be effective bronchodilators (Sanchez *et al.* 1993). The infant's respiratory function should be carefully monitored by the A&E nurse. If the infant responds well to nebulisers, tachypnoea reduces and the infant is feeding, it is appropriate for parents/carers to continue care at home in most cases. They should, however, be advised to return if the infant's condition worsens or is reluctant to feed. The infant should be admitted to hospital if she is lethargic, dehydrated, not feeding or there has been suspicion of apnoea.

Feeding is an important landmark in the severity of bronchiolitis. As dyspnoea increases, the infant becomes fatigued and the effort required to feed and maintain respiration is too great. At this stage the infant begins to demonstrate signs of respiratory distress. Young babies do not have a great fluid reserve and can become rapidly dehydrated. This results both from the reduced fluid intake and from increased insensible loss due to tachypnoea. These infants may require i.v. or nasogastric fluid replacement and in severe cases mechanical ventilation (Barkin & Rosen 1994). Infants with suspected bronchiolitis should be nursed away from other babies and stringent cross-infection measures should be employed as RSV is particularly contagious (Hay 1996).

The Febrile Infant

All infants presenting to the A&E department with fever/temperature should be thoroughly assessed at triage. Fever is indicated by a rectal temperature of 38°C (100.4°F) or higher. Hyperpyrexia, i.e. a temperature above 41°C (105.8°F), is an uncommon but serious problem, with approximately 20% of children experiencing convulsions (Surpure 1987). A concise but detailed history of the illness should be taken, gathering the following information:

- sequence of events
- accompanying symptoms such as vomiting
- fluid intake and output
- present medications and regularity, including dosage of antipyretics
- immunisation status.

Nursing activities should include:

- airway, breathing and circulation
- observe skin circulation, colour and rashes
- weight
- assess general handling and alertness as the infant is undressed
- distraction therapy helps in ascertaining whether the infant is either hot and miserable but responsive, or acutely ill
- a newborn with an axillary temperature of less than 36°C should have a BM stick recorded
- place a urine bag in situ for specimen collection.

Do not dismiss an infant as being well if she is not pyrexial. Check when antipyretics were last administered and ensure that the infant's temperature is within the normal acceptable range. Check heart rate, skin colour and capillary refill to ensure that the baby is truly apyrexial, and not peripherally shut down, septic or in shock. One of the most common reasons for pyrexial infants attending A&E is a simple viral illness and these often do not need medical intervention. The most important intervention from the A&E nurse is discharge advice to the parents about temperature control and the use of antipyretic drugs, such as paracetamol or ibuprofen, in those older than 6 months. It is useful to support this advice with written instructions for parents.

Febrile Convulsions

Febrile convulsions are seizures which occur in a child with a febrile illness. They are common but usually benign events occurring in infants, toddlers and young children. Witnessing a convulsion is, however, extremely distressing for parents. Approximately 2–5% of all children are affected. The seizures are of a generalised tonic-clonic nature, usually lasting less than 10 minutes, and complete recovery usually occurs within 1 hour (Valman 1993). The onset of a febrile convulsion is often the first sign that an infant is unwell, as seizures usually occur near the onset of a fever rather than after prolonged fever (Brunner & Suddarth 1991). The peak incidence occurs between 8 and 20 months; febrile seizures are uncommon after 5–6 years (Zukin & Grisham 1992). Upper respiratory tract infections are commonly present, representing more than 70% of underlying infections (Barkin & Rosen 1994).

Infants who arrive in the A&E department still convulsing obviously need urgent assessment and intervention. Maintaining a clear airway and providing adequate oxygenation are the first priorities for the A&E nurse. Clothes should be removed and temperature recorded. Rectal administration of anticonvulsants and antipyretics should be considered. Rectal diazepam (0.5 mg/kg) produces an effective blood concentration of anticonvulsant within 10 minutes (Valman 1993). Most febrile convulsions are self-limiting, but if an anticonvulsant has been used, careful monitoring of the infant's respiratory function and blood pressure should be carried out until an adequate conscious level is regained.

As most infants will arrive 'post-ictal', respiratory function and temperature should be assessed and antipyretics administered if necessary. Parents/carers need a lot of reassurance and support during this period. Infants with simple febrile seizures may be discharged after appropriate fever control has been achieved, although many paediatricians will admit a child for 24 hours' observation following a first convulsion. Before discharge parents need to be advised about temperature control at home and shown how to manage any further convulsions. Evidence suggests approximately 40% of children who have a febrile seizure will have a recurrence, half of which occur within 6 months of the first episode (Barkin & Rosen 1994).

Meningitis

Meningococcal meningitis/septicaemia is a serious disease which accounted for 110 childhood deaths in England and Wales in 1991, making it the commonest cause of death from infectious disease. (National Meningitis Trust 1992). Peak incidence is between 3 and 12 months, although the mortality remains above that of other age groups until around the age of 2 years, when numbers fall (Wilson & Lilley 1994). Meningitis is a consequence of inflammation of the meninges and is most commonly caused by infective agents such as viruses and bacteria. Bacterial meningitis is spread between people by droplet infection, whereas some viral infections can be found in other agents such as polluted water (Kumar & Clark 1990). Common causes of bacterial meningitis are *Streptococcus pnuemoniae*, *Nisseria meningitides* and *Haemophilus influenzae*, the latter being reduced by the introduction of the Hib vaccine in childhood immunisations.

Acute bacterial meningitis in infants is a paediatric emergency. In the newborn, it has a mortality of 25% (Kelnar *et al.* 1995). Early recognition and treatment are vital, since any delay in recognition can prove catastrophic for the infant. The disease has a rapid onset and, left undiagnosed, death may occur in less than 48 hours. One aid to recognition is the use of cascade protocols for detecting meningitis; however, it should always be considered in any infant with unexplained pyrexia or illness. Protocols for the management of bacterial meningitis will aid rapid treatment once suspected; these should be agreed with the paediatric department and made readily available to A&E staff. The triage nurse will be the first person to assess an infant, and therefore accurate and thorough recordings are vital. Pyrexial lethargic infants should always be fully assessed.

Signs and symptoms of bacterial meningitis are given in Box 15.3.

Infants with suspected meningitis require immediate urgent care. If a petechial or purpuric rash is present, deterioration will be rapid. The rash is distinctive and easily identifiable as it will not diminish or

---

Box 15.3 – *Signs and symptoms of bacterial meningitis*

Non specific signs and symptoms
- Drowsiness
- Irritability
- Off feeds
- Distressed when handled
- Vomiting
- Pyrexia

Specific signs and symptoms
- Neck stiffness
- Tense bulging fontanelle
- Purpuric or petechial rash
- Mottled appearance
- Hypothermic

Late signs and symptoms
- High-pitched moaning cry
- Reduced level of consciousness/coma
- Neck retraction/arched back
- Shock
- Widespread haemorrhagic rash.

---

blanch on pressure. Skin with a mottled pale appearance can be a sign of shock and sepsis.

If symptoms are vague or suggestive of possible early meningitis, a rapid septic screening should be performed. This should includes strict monitoring of vital signs including respirations and blood pressure, physical examination for obvious sources of infection e.g. ears or upper airway, blood analysis and culture, urine microbiology and lumbar puncture. Intravenous access should be established and fluid administration commenced at an appropriate rate for the infant's weight and physical condition. Rapid administration of antibiotics can be life-saving; it is recommended these are administered prior to the sometimes lengthy process of lumbar puncture.

A lumbar puncture is performed to detect the presence of bacteria in the cerebrospinal fluid. The administration of antibiotics immediately prior to lumbar puncture rarely alters the cerebrospinal fluid enough to interfere with interpretation or detection of bacteria (Bernardo & Schenkel 1995). Lumbar puncture is contraindicated if raised intracranial pressure is suspected as it enhances the risk of producing cerebral herniation. The infant should be attached to a cardiac monitor and respiratory effort should be closely watched by the A&E nurse during the procedure, as critically ill infants are at risk of cardiopulmonary arrest. Holding the infant in the necessary position for lumbar puncture increases this risk, and therefore the

Table 15.4 – *Degree of dehydration in infants*

Sign	Mild	Moderate	Severe
Increased pulse	–	+	+
Rapid respiration	–	+/–	+
Hypotension	–	+/–	+
Dry mucous membrane	+/–	+	+
Reduced skin turgor	+/–	+/–	+
Sunken eyeballs	–	+	+
Depressed anterior fontanelle	–	+	+
Urine output	Reduced	Oliguria	Oliguria/anuria
Blood pH (usually tested in moderate to severe dehydration)	7.40–7.30	7.30–7.00	< 7.10

procedure should be carried out with care and vigilance (Bernardo & Schenkel 1995).

This assessment period is obviously distressing for parents. During the septic screening and particularly when performing invasive investigations, it is important to explain the nature of these procedures and give the parents the option to stay with the infant or leave. This will prevent unnecessary anxiety and allow the parents to remain actively involved should they wish.

Depending on the causative organisms, i.e. the type of meningitis, prophylactic treatment may be required for the immediate family. The A&E nurse should ensure this is not overlooked and, where possible, should facilitate its prescription by medical staff.

Dehydration in Infants

Dehydration occurs when fluid loss exceeds fluid intake over a period of time, leaving the body in negative fluid balance. It is a consequence of many illnesses in infancy, particularly those involving the gastrointestinal tract. Initial assessment should include a history from the parent/carer leading up to A&E attendance, including changes in feeding pattern, the infant's intake during the last 24 hours, whether she is off feed, or whether she appears more thirsty than usual. Is there a history of vomiting, diarrhoea, or constipation? What is the urine output like? Has there been obvious weight loss?

Physical assessment of the infant should include:

- Airway, breathing and circulation
- Is the infant obviously dehydrated, with dry mucous membranes, absent tears and saliva, poor skin turgor, sunken eyes or depressed anterior fontanelle?

The percentage of body water in an infant is greater than that in an older child or adult, and thus dehydration in infants is more rapid in onset and potentially more serious. It is paramount to accurately assess the degree of dehydration in order to determine the treatment regime. Dehydration can be classified as mild (<5%), moderate (10%) or severe (15%). Rapid assessment of the degree of dehydration can be made by using the information in Table 15.4.

The fluid deficit per kg can be determined by multiplying the percentage dehydration by the weight of the infant. For example, a 10 kg infant who is 10% dehydrated has a fluid deficit of 100 ml/kg or a total deficit of 1000 ml, to be replaced over 24 hours (Barkin & Rosen 1994). If moderate or severe dehydration is present, intravenous fluid therapy should be commenced. In the case of mild dehydration, oral fluid replacement should be attempted unless specific contraindications exist. Oral rehydration solutions (ORS) are easily metabolised fluid and electrolyte replacements. If the infant does not tolerate oral fluid, either because of poor feeding or vomiting, she may be admitted for fluid replacement. If the infant is discharged, parents should be advised about fluid maintenance and monitoring. The use of clear fluids often needs to be stressed to parents who are worried about their baby being hungry because she is not taking milk feeds.

Failure to Thrive

This is a term used to identify an infant who has growth and developmental failure. The weight of the infant falls below that expected for the gestational and postnatal age (Brunner & Suddarth 1991). These infants have a history of failure to gain weight and loss of subcutaneous fat or muscle mass. Failure to thrive is not often the primary reason for A&E attendance. Parents may bring their baby because of related symptoms such as lethargy, weight loss or poor feeding; similarly they may be unaware of a developmental problem. Initial recognition of failure to thrive often relies on the familiarity of the A&E nurse with normal infant development. The actual intervention will depend on the severity and the social circumstances surrounding A&E attendance. Hospital admission is not always indicated; empowering parents to care for their baby at home is often more appropriate. Adequate community support is imperative, and the health visitor and the family's GP should be informed. In addition to the physical reasons for failure to thrive, it is often a feature in infants who suffer from emotional abuse and neglect (Skuse 1997)

The Vomiting Infant

Vomiting is a common symptom of many presentations of infants in A&E. The most common cause of vomiting is acute gastroenteritis. Other infections include urinary and respiratory tract infections, ear infections and tonsillitis. Poor feeding techniques or excessive feeding may also lead to vomiting.

Assessing the infant with vomiting

- Airway, breathing and circulation.
- Record birth weight and present weight. As a general rule, infants double their birth weight by 5–6 months and triple their weight by 1 year.
- Urine output.
- Bowel actions.

Management

Management of infantile vomiting should focus on correcting fluid deficits as well as definitive treatment of the underlying cause. Most well-hydrated infants with a self-limiting problem can usually be discharged home with appropriate advice regarding feeding.

Gastroenteritis

Acute gastroenteritis is a clinical syndrome characterised by the onset of diarrhoea and/or vomiting which is often accompanied by fever (Khatib 1986). Gastroenteritis is not uncommon in infants. Parents bring their children to A&E in varying stages of ill health, the majority of whom can be managed at home. An accurate history should be taken to rule out chronic illness. The following information should be gathered:

- commencement of illness
- diet and fluids taken
- episodes of vomiting since onset
- episodes of diarrhoea since onset
- urine output
- relevant medical history
- any recent visits abroad
- prescribed or over-the-counter medication.

The priority is to assess for dehydration (see Table 15.4). Vital signs should be recorded and oral rehydration should be initiated to replace the fluid loss and assess tolerance. Small amounts of clear fluid, preferably oral rehydration solution, should be given at frequent intervals. Most infants with a gastrointestinal infection can be treated at home with oral rehydration, but infants under 6 months and those living in poor social conditions are particularly vulnerable and may require hospital admission (Wharton et al. 1988).

Gastro-oesophageal reflux

This is a persistent regurgitation of feeds in a well baby which presents within the first few weeks of life. These infants may present with failure to gain weight or weight loss. Gastro-oesophageal reflux can result in recurrent pulmonary disease due to the acid erosion.

Intussusception

Intussusception is a telescoping of a portion of the intestine. The onset is sudden. It causes severe intermittent attacks of screaming and abdominal pain, often with associated drawing up of the legs, vomiting and pallor. The infant is irritable or lethargic. Diarrhoea is mucous-laden, and bloodstained 'red currant jelly' stools are passed. An infant presenting with this history should be seen as a matter of urgency; however, classic symptoms are absent in up to 50% of babies with intussusception (Barkin & Rosen, 1994). If an infant presents with an unaccountable change in behaviour, listlessness or altered level of consciousness, intussusception should be suspected.

The infant with intussusception is extremely unstable, and therefore intravenous access should be established and referral to a paediatric surgeon should be swift. Intussusception can be diagnosed on X-ray in some patients, but barium enema is both diagnostic and therapeutic in up to 75% of cases, particularly when early intervention occurs (Stephenson et al. 1989). During this procedure, close monitoring of the infant's vital signs are necessary, as shock and perforation of the bowel are potential side-effects. If a barium enema does not result in a reduction of the intussusception, surgery is indicated as a matter of urgency.

Pyloric stenosis

Pyloric stenosis is a disorder which usually becomes apparent during the first few weeks of life, although it can go undiagnosed for as long as 6 months. There is progressive hypertrophy of the pylorus, causing partial or total obstruction of the pyloric sphincter. Typically, the infant has poor weight gain or weight loss due to the projectile vomiting that occurs after feeds. The infant is excessively hungry and shows a willingness to feed immediately after vomiting. This can be very distressing for parents, particularly those caring for their first baby. Many parents blame their feeding technique, and careful intervention from A&E staff is needed to establish diagnosis and reduce feelings of anxiety or guilt the parents may have.

Pyloric stenosis does have a familial incidence, so parents of a second or subsequent baby may already suspect what is wrong and come to A&E seeking confirmation and action from staff. The infant may or may not be dehydrated on admission to A&E; this largely depends on the duration and severity of the stenosis. A test feed is indicated to help establish diagnosis. These babies will be admitted to hospital and undergo surgery once rehydrated and stable.

The Injured Infant

Infants are totally dependent on their parents/carers, and accidents that occur to infants are a reflection of this fact (Mead & Sibert 1991). As infants develop, their mobility increases together with a growing susceptibility to injury. Constant supervision is not always possible, but parental behaviour and education can help to reduce the serious consequences of injury.

Assessment of the injured infant

Parents are often distressed and anxious and may feel guilty or responsible for the infant's injury. Assessment therefore needs to be done carefully if a therapeutic relationship is to be established. The following information should be collected:

■ airway, breathing and circulation
■ time elapsed since injury
■ whether the accident was witnessed
■ cause and mechanism of injury
■ accident environment and whether indoors or outdoors
■ examine wound/injury
■ analgesia
■ relevant medial history, immunisation status, medications.

This assessment gives the A&E nurse an insight into the history leading to injury and the family dynamics, and should highlight any areas of concern relating to the family's psychosocial setup, as well as determining the actual severity of the injury. A&E nurses must remain vigilant for possible or evident non-accidental injuries (see also Ch. 16). The majority of injuries to infants are minor, requiring a one-off visit to A&E. On discharge, written advice to support nursing and medical intervention should be given.

Head injuries

These injuries normally occur when a baby is dropped or has fallen. The risk of head injury following a fall is likely, as infants have relatively large heads in proportion to their bodies. Most head injuries are minor and the majority of infants recover uneventfully; however, head injuries remain a significant cause of death among infants. A thorough history of events prior to admission should be obtained, which will give an indication of the degree of trauma. A list of the information to be collected is outlined in Box 15.4.

Treatment for most infants attending with head injury revolves around observation and advice to parents, but nurses must be able to detect and act upon findings indicative of a more serious injury (see also Ch. 4).

Sudden Infant Death Syndrome

This is undoubtedly one of the most traumatic and emotionally devastating events ever to happen to a family. One baby in every 500 live births dies suddenly and unexpectedly between the ages of 1 week and 2 years. There are about 2000 sudden infant deaths each year, accounting for half of all deaths in this age group (Royal College of Nursing 1990). Sudden infant death syndrome (SIDS) remains a mystery, but it is more common in the winter months among boys and babies of low birth weight. The peak incidence is in the age range 2–6 months and it usually occurrs during sleep, as a result of which it is sometimes called 'cot death'. It encompasses all social classes and there is no singular cause, although often a collection of predisposing factors is evident (Foundation for the Study of Infant Deaths (FSID) 1991). A common scenario is one where the infant is found dead a few minutes or hours after being put to rest in her cot.

Suffocation, electrolyte imbalances, mineral deficiencies, cardiac dysrythmias, infection, anaemia, seizures, hyperthermia, hyperthyroidism, upper airway obstruction, congenital abnormalities and occult trauma are but a few of the possible explanations for

Box 15.4 – *Assessment of head-injured infant*

- Was the accident witnessed and how long ago did it occur?

- Were there external forces involved, such as RTA, trauma to head by moving object, or a fall from one surface to another?

- What surface did the infant fall onto, e.g. linoleum floor, pavement, carpeted floor?

- How was the infant immediately following the accident? Did she cry immediately, lose consciousness or fit?

- Has the infant vomited? Infants often vomit as a normal reaction to a stressful event; persistent vomiting is considered significant

- Is she drowsy or unable to be roused? Sleeping is an automatic response to injury for an infant, particularly if the time coincides with a normal sleep time or if the infant is in an environment with rhythmic noise or movement, such as a car. For drowsiness to be significant the child must have reduced movements during sleep, or be slow to respond to stimuli which would normal wake her. Parents can often be the best judge of this as they are used to their baby's sleep pattern; emotion can, however, render the parent/carer less objective

- Establish any relevant medical history, immunisation status and medications

Physical assessment of the infant's condition should include:
- Airway, breathing, circulation

- Examination of the scalp for evidence of injury, lacerations or haematomas

- Palpate for tenderness, bony deformity and check the anterior fontanelle

- Observe the nose and ears for evidence of bleeding or fluid leak

- Examine the infant for any other injuries

---

sudden infant death. Although these factors may play a role in a small number of what appear to be SIDS deaths, the majority of these deaths remain unexplained (Gausche 1992). The infant who has suffered a cot death experiences irreversible cardiac and respiratory arrest. Recent evidence suggests that well infants who are born at term and have no complications should be placed down to sleep on either the side or the back to reduce the incidence of SIDS (Barkin & Rosen 1994).

Initial response

On admission, active resuscitation may have been initiated by paramedics or parents. The infant is assessed quickly while resuscitation continues. Parents should be given the choice of either staying with the baby during resuscitation or waiting in a relatives' room close by. Whatever the parents decide, an experienced nurse should accompany them. This nurse must ensure that the parents are fully informed about what is happening with their baby. It is essential that they are not given false hope, which can easily be done inadvertently by using phrases like 'it will be all right'. If other siblings or children have been brought to hospital with the parents, it is often appropriate for them to be looked after by a suitable person away from the immediate resuscitation area or in a relatives' room: A&E staff must be guided by the parents' wishes about this.

The A&E nurse accompanying the parents should try to obtain a brief history of the infant's age, general health, development and events leading up to the incident, including the circumstances of how the infant was found and when or if resuscitation was initiated. A calm, unhurried manner will usually help in getting this information, given that the atmosphere will be fraught and tense. The nurse should establish whether the parents would like spiritual support and, if required, contact the appropriate religious leader.

When breaking the news of an infant's death to parents, avoid the use of euphemisms. It is important that the words 'death' or 'died' are used. This avoids any potential misconceptions and finalises what has happened. For many younger parents, this may be their first experience of a close bereavement, and it is important to explain the coroner's duty to investigate all sudden deaths. Parents should be told that they will be asked to make a statement and that the coroner's officer or police may visit their home and may take the baby's bedding for examination to help establish the cause of death. This is routine procedure and it is important to stress that this does not mean anybody will be blamed or that an inquest will necessarily be held. The nurse caring for the parents should stay with, or be available to, the family up until they leave the department.

Continuing care

Ensure that a quiet area is made available for parents to spend time with their baby to say goodbye. Never hurry them to see the baby or go home. Acknowledge that families may remain in the department for a considerable amount of time. The nurse must be patient and offer reassurance that fault cannot be attributed to anything or anyone, especially those whose care the infant was in at the time of the incident. If possible, take a photograph of the baby and obtain a lock of hair; also take foot- and handprints. Although parents may not want them at this time, they may be grateful for them later on (RCN and BAEM 1995). If the mother is breast-feeding, she will need immediate advice on suppression of lactation.

Discharge advice and information

Provide written information on what will happen next, as little of what is said may actually be heard by the grief-stricken parents or family. The family should be offered either the FSID and the hospital's own guidelines on unexpected infant deaths as well as information about the patient's liaison officer who can offer guidance on funeral arrangements etc. The GP and health visitor should be informed as soon as possible.

Staff grief

The impact of a baby's death on A&E staff is enormous. Time must be made for critical incident debriefing (Cudmore 1998). Staff dealing with the family need to acknowledge their own grief. Crying or brief withdrawal is an acceptable reaction.

Conclusion

This chapter has outlined some of the more common and distinctive infant complaints that may present in the A&E department. Some important and useful considerations in respect of infants presenting in A&E have been noted. The infant's presenting complaint should be addressed together with the family as a whole unit. Always consider the infant's home and social circumstances when assessing and treating injuries or ailments. Parental anxiety may be a major manifestation of presenting infants.

Parents often feel guilty and/or inadequate in relation to their baby's injury or illness, especially when the baby is acutely unwell or seriously injured. Parents may not be familiar with the hospital environment and they may feel helpless, lost and anxious. Discharge advice must be given clearly and in a language suitable for the parents' understanding, and wherever possible this should be supported by written information. Community services, such as the Paediatric Home Care Team and particularly the family's health visitor, should be informed of any concerns and can assist the family after discharge. Thorough assessment is essential at all times to ensure the infant's safety, comfort and quality of care. A&E nurses are the key carers and the formation of a therapeutic relationship with the family is invaluable.

References

Barkin RM, Rosen P (1994) Pulmonary disorders. In: Barkin RM, Rosen P, eds. *Emergency Pediatrics: a Guide to Ambulatory Care*. 4th edn. St Louis: Mosby.

Bedford HE, Jenkins SM, Shore C, Kenny PA (1992) Use of an east end children's accident and emergency department for infants: a failure in primary health care. *Quality in Health Care*, 1, 29–33.

Bernardo LM, Schenkel KA (1995) Pediatric medical emergencies. In: Kitt S, Selfridge-Thomas J, Proeh JA, Kaiser J, eds. *Emergency Nursing: a Physiologic and Clinical Perspective*, 2nd edn. Philadelphia: WB Saunders.

Bruce-Jones J (1994) PALS: paediatric resuscitation. *Emergency Nurse*, 2(1), 7–9.

Brunner LS, Suddarth DS (1991) *The Lippincott Manual of Paediatric Nursing*, 3rd edn. London: Chapman and Hall.

Chameides L (1990) *Textbook of Paediatric Advanced Life Support*. Dallas: American Heart Association and American Academy of Paediatricians.

Cosby C (1998) Pediatric Emergencies. In: Newberry L, ed. *Sheehy's Emergency Nursing: Principles and Practice*, 4th edn. St Louis: Mosby.

Cudmore J (1998) Critical incident stress: Management strategies. *Emergency Nurse* 6(3), 22–27.

Dinwiddie R (1990) *The Diagnosis and Management of Respiratory Disease*. Edinburgh: Churchill Livingstone.

European Resuscitation Council (1998a) Paediatric basic life support. *Resuscitation* 37, 97–100.

European Resuscitation Council (1998b) Paediatric advanced life support. *Resuscitation*, 37, 101–102.

Foundation for the Study of Infant Deaths (1991) *Unexpected Infant Deaths. Guidelines for Accident and Emergency Departments*. London: FSID.

Gatch G, Myre L, Black RE (1987) Foreign body aspiration in children. *AORN Journal*, 46(5), 850–861.

Gausche M (1992) Sudden infant death syndrome. In: Rosen P, Barkin RM, Braemn G *et al. Emergency Medicine: Concepts and Clinical Practice*. St Louis; Mosby Year Book.

Gilbert EG, Russell KE, Deskin RW. (1993) Stridor in the infant and child. *AORN Journal*, 58(1), 23–43.

Hay P (1996) Care of the infant with bronchiolitis. *Emergency Nurse*, 4(3), 19–22.

Hazinski M (1992) *Nursing Care of the Critically Ill Child*, 2nd edn. St Louis: Mosby.

Kelnar CJH, Harvey D, Simpson C (1995) *The Sick Newborn Baby*, 3rd edn. London: Baillière Tindall.

Khatib H (1986) Acute gastroenteritis in infants. *Nursing Times*, **82**(17), 31–32.

Kumar PJ, Clark ML (1990) *Clinical Medicine*, 2nd edn. London, Baillière Tindall.

McFarlane K (1992) Caring for the infant with RSV infection. *Paediatric Nursing* **4**(8), 10–12.

Mead D, Sibert J (eds) (1991) *The Injured Child: an Action Plan for Nurses*. London: Scutari Press.

Morcombe J (1998) Reducing anxiety in children in A&E. *Emergency Nurse*, **6**(2), 10–13.

National Meningitis Trust (1992) *Meningitis Factsheet*. London: National Meningitis Trust.

Royal College of Nursing (1990) *Nursing Children in the Accident and Emergency Department*. London: RCN.

Royal College of Nursing and British Association for Accident and Emergency Medicine (1995) *Bereavement Care in A&E Departments*. London: RCN.

Sanchez I, Dekoster J, Powell R (1993) Effect of racemic epinephrine and salbutomol on clinical score and pulmonary mechanics in infants with bronchiolitis. *Journal of Paediatrics*, **122**1, 145–151.

Skuse DH (1997) Emotional abuse and neglect. In: Meadow R, ed. *ABC of Child Abuse*, 3rd edn. Bedford: Jolly and Barber.

Stephenson CA, Seibert JJ, Strain JD, Glasier CM, Leithiser RE Jr, Igbat V (1989) Intussusception: clinical and radiographic factors influencing reducibility. *Pediatric Radiology*, **20**(1–2), 57–60.

Surpure JS (1987) Hyperpyrexia in children: clinical implications. *Paediatric Emergency Care*, **3**, 10–12.

Valman HB (1993) Febrile convulsions. *British Medical Journal*, **306**, 1743–1745.

Wharton BA, Pugh, RE, Taitz LS, Walker-Smith JA, Booth IW (1988) Dietary management of gastroenteritis in Britain. *British Medical Journal*, **296**, 450–452.

Wilson M, Lilley M (1994) Meningitis in childhood. *Paediatric Nursing*, **6**(7), 23–26.

Wolfram PW (1992) Asthma and bronchiolitis. In: Rosen P, Barkin RM, Braen G *et al.*, eds. *Emergency Medicine: Concepts and Clinical Practice*, 3rd edn. St Louis: Mosby Gilbert.

Zukin DD, Grisham JE (1992) The febrile child. In: Rosen P, Barkin RM, Braen G *et al.*, eds. *Emergency Medicine: Concepts and Clinical Practice*. St Louis: Mosby Year Book.

Chapter 16

Pre-school Children

Lynne Poucher & Linda Holt

- Introduction
- Normal development
- The child under stress
- Understanding illness
- Asthma
- Acute laryngotracheobronchitis (viral croup)
- Epiglottitis
- Accidental injury
- Accidental poisoning
- Non-accidental injuries (child abuse)
- Sexual abuse
- Munchausen's syndrome by proxy
- Conclusion

Introduction

Approximately 3 million children attend A&E departments each year. A disproportionate number of these are under 5 years of age (Morton & Phillips 1996). Paediatric admissions have been steadily increasing over the last 20 years, and 90% are admitted via the A&E department (Milner & Hull 1992). This is due, in part, to an increase in the incidence of certain diseases, but also increasingly through the subjective choice of parents to use A&E services in preference to those of primary carers such as general practitioners (GPs).

Between 1 and 4 years, a child's physical and mental development is very rapid. Even during this short time span substantial leaps in the acquisition of language, motor skill and comprehension are made. This rate of development can prove a danger for the unsuspecting parent, who may be unaware of the child's new capabilities, therefore increasing the risk of accident. It can come as a surprise when the child is first able to reach up to a work surface or has the strength to pull over a chair.

Pre-school children usually arrive in the A&E department as a result of accidental injury. The young child, having an insatiable curiosity of his environment, is especially vulnerable; more so as he will be generally unaware of the dangers this environment presents. The challenge of climbing furniture and stairs, the contents of all manner of containers, the sampling of even the most unpalatable of agents, all increase the likelihood of a small child suffering falls, minor injury and poisoning (Mead & Sibert 1991).

With a still developing immune system, the onset of illness is often rapid in pre-school children, leading to a speedy deterioration of the child's general condition. Young children do not have an adult's resilience to withstand heat, fluid and electrolyte loss. They are, however, better able to cope with these metabolic changes than babies. The A&E nurse needs to know what is normal activity and physical development in children of pre-school age, in order to effectively assess their condition and initiate care. This chapter will consider normal childhood development and some of the common reasons for A&E attendance within this age group.

Normal Development

The child in the age range 3 months to 1 year is termed an infant; 1–3 years a toddler; and 3–4 years a pre-school child (Brunner & Suddarth 1991). In the context of this chapter all children above the age of 1 year will be considered pre-school children. The pre-school child, unlike the infant, has begun to develop his own identity. From about the age of 2, the child discovers that he can control what happens around him; motor skills develop rapidly and the child, able to walk, run, climb and jump, uses these new found skills to explore his environment (Valman 1988). The child strives for autonomy and self-esteem. However, he also needs to know the safety limits of behaviour in a given environment. For example, when climbing the stairs with a parent the child may feel good because of the praise for this achievement, but this needs to be tempered so the child is aware that it is not good to climb over a stair gate and attempt to climb the stairs alone.

Pre-school children perceive the world differently from adults. Children of this age begin to demonstrate conceptual intelligence (Lowe 1985). They display various thinking processes which are important to consider when a child is trying to explain the reason for deeds and events. The 2-year-old child is egocentric and will perceive that he is the centre of his world, being unable to identify with anyone else's point of view. The child may well believe that it is he who is responsible for events which we know to be out of his control, such as Mum becoming ill. Children often perceive illness or injury as a punishment for something they did or failed to do (Eiser 1985).

To a young child everything has to exist for a purpose, e.g. aunts and uncles are there to give presents! Children have a tendency to animalistic beliefs: for instance, they may think that inanimate objects can feel pain or that animals and toys can behave like humans; that Teddy really talks and that kittens need dressing up. There is an intuitive, magical quality to their thoughts (Hall *et al.* 1990).

A 3-year-old child's use of language consists of short sentences, each made up of between three to six words. The articulation, vocabulary and grammar of a young child can develop at surprisingly different rates. Often he will repeat words (echolalia) which is a mental replay on sound which often causes confusion. Every answer to a question is immediately followed by

the question 'why?'. A child will also demonstrate over-generalisation, e.g. every fruit is an apple (Hall *et al.* 1990).

The Child Under Stress

The pre-school child is more vulnerable and traumatised when separated from his parents than at any other age. Bowlby (1953), in his famous study *Child Care and the Growth of Love*, showed how a child suffers maternal deprivation when separated from his significant carers, the person (male or female) who supplies love, care, protection and comfort (Lowe 1985). Many reports have confirmed the importance of keeping parent and child together (Ministry of Health 1959, Royal College of Nursing 1994). This is particularly important in A&E attendance, where events leading to attendance will have caused some stress (see Box 16.1).

> **Box 16.1** – *Categories of children's worries (Wolfer & Vistintainer 1975)*
>
> ■ Physical harm or bodily injury in the form of discomfort, pain, mutilation and death
>
> ■ Separation from parent or absence of trusted adult
>
> ■ A strange unknown environment
>
> ■ Uncertainty about limits and expected acceptable behaviour
>
> ■ Loss of control, autonomy and competence

Effective nursing intervention at this early stage can do a lot towards developing a rapport with the child and family, and to alleviate stress and fear. Acknowledging the child's suffering and putting it into context using toys or pictures can be helpful, as is prompt pain relief. Parental input from the outset is essential, not only to reduce stress and induce normality in the child, but also to reduce stress in the parents/carers themselves. Encouraging parents/carers to undress the child and help with the examination, as well as to be there to give reassurance to their child, reinforces the parents' importance in the treatment and helps to allay their fears.

It is easy in circumstances following an accident for parents to feel inadequate or lose confidence in their own abilities. This must be addressed in A&E constructively and without apportioning blame, to enable the parents to support their child. Reassurance, information and what the parents/carers can do to help their child should be clearly communicated. Poor handling of parents in A&E can have a long-term effect on both the child's and the family's recovery (Mead & Sibert 1991).

The environment in which a child is cared for has come under much scrutiny in recent years (Department of Health 1995, Partridge 1997). Facilities for children are best provided in an environment away from adult patients. Children should have separate waiting areas geared towards their needs, with toys or television and videos etc. available. Treatment areas should also be child-oriented, not only in decor and furnishing, but also in equipment, so time is not wasted hunting for appropriate items, such as child-sized BP cuffs etc.

Children should be kept informed in a meaningful manner about their care and about what will happen next. With parental help, boundaries for behaviour can be set, which in turn help the child who feels out of control of what is happening. The A&E nurse's attitude should be family-oriented when dealing with young children. Parents are often under a great deal of stress, feel guilty and are very anxious. These negative emotions can have a profound affect on the child (Wolff 1981). The parents need reassurance and a chance to relay their fears and guilt to the nurse. A critical attitude from nursing and medical staff will only reinforce the guilt and inadequacy the parent is already experiencing. An anxious parent will make the child feel anxious. Keeping the parent informed and building a bond between the family and staff will help the child (Måller et al. 1992).

Understanding Illness

To a young child, illness is remote and viewed as an external process. There is a tendency to believe that it has something to do with magic or is a punishment. A child cannot understand internal body processes. Organs are not seen in the same way as an adult may perceive them; for instance, the head is for thinking and the heart for loving (Eiser 1985). A child will be more concerned about external injury, such as small cuts or marks. The external aspect of his environment, such as lights, equipment, uniforms and noise, will affect the child more than an explanation of what is going on in his body (Jolly 1981).

Play is a very important aspect of the child's care. Through play, a child can express fear and anxiety; hence the child may not tell the nurse where it hurts but will show it on a 'teddy bear'. Watching a child play gives a fair assessment of social and motor skills. Playing with the nurse's pen-torch can often break the ice between child and nurse and lead to the building of a relationship, as will the use of first names (Raikow 1998). When performing a dressing the nurse should allow the child to touch the equipment or dressing material. Apply a dressing to the teddy at the same time. This will help to gain co-operation and dispel misconceptions the child might harbour regarding dressing procedures (Smith et al. 1991).

Communication with the child is important but should be done with care. It is best to gather information before giving it and to listen to what the child has to say first. This enables the nurse to explain what is happening in the appropriate language and at the appropriate level for the child to understand (Jolly 1981).

Asthma

Asthma is one of the most common illnesses affecting young children. It is estimated that there are over 2 million sufferers in the UK and up to 35% of these are children (Burney et al. 1990, Department of Health 1993). Despite technological improvements in asthma management, mortality in children has not decreased and hospital admissions have increased considerably in the under 5s (Morton & Philips 1996). The first attack may occur at any age but about 80% of children will have had the first symptoms before the age of 5 years (Valman 1993). Young children with asthma are particularly vulnerable because they rely on others to detect the severity of their condition and act on their behalf.

When a young child attends A&E with breathing difficulties, it is important that he is not unnecessarily distressed. Practical steps to prevent distress include not separating the child from his parent or carer, behaving in a calm and friendly manner, and assessing the child promptly in an appropriate environment. If a child does become overly upset, the extra energy and oxygen needed when crying can be enough to turn a moderate asthma attack into a severe one.

Assessment

The overall clinical picture is developed from a combination of history, physical assessment and clinical investigations. If the child has obvious breathing difficulty, oxygen and nebulised bronchodilators should be commenced immediately, prior to detailed history-taking from the parents/carers. Questions to be asked in establishing a history of this event and the child's general health are given in Box 16.2.

Physical assessment

Observing the child's respiration is the most reliable indicator of his condition. The respiration rate and depth should be established first. The 'work of

---

Box 16.2 – *Establishing history of asthma attack*

■ How long has this episode lasted?

■ Is the child getting better or worse?

■ What medication has been given prior to A&E attendance and what was the effect?

■ Is there an identifiable trigger to the episode?

■ Is the child on regular medication? If so, what is it?

■ Has the child had previous serious asthma episodes requiring steroids or hospital?

■ How frequent are the asthma symptoms?

■ Does the child have any other illnesses?

---

breathing' correlates to the severity of the asthma (Morton & Philips 1996). An increase in the work of breathing is demonstrated by the use of accessory muscles and by nasal flaring (British Thoracic Association *et al.* 1991). Intercostal and sternal recession is an indication of moderate to severe respiratory difficulty. As the child's ability to speak is an indication of respiratory function, the nurse should note if the child can speak in full sentences, using only a few words or not at all. Parents are invaluable at assessing differences in the child's normal pattern of speech, as ability to converse varies within this age group.

A rise in pulse rate can be indicative of increasing hypoxia, but must be considered within context. If the child is upset, pyrexial or on beta-agonists such as salbutamol, a tachycardia would be expected. Although wheezing is a classic symptom of bronchospasm, it is unreliable in detecting the severity of an episode. At assessment, any audible wheeze or wheeze on auscultation should be recorded and used as a baseline. It is important to remember that if air is not being moved effectively in and out of the lungs, no wheeze will be present. Peak flow measurement is considered an important indication of the severity of an asthma episode; however, in children under 5 years it is unreliable as their ability to use the peak flow meter properly is questionable. Peak flow measurement should therefore only be attempted in children who have previously and regularly used a peak flow meter.

Pulse oximetry is the most useful diagnostic aid in the under-5 age group. It is non-invasive and the monitor can act as a distraction for the child. Pulse oximetry will identify reductions in oxygen saturation which may not be obvious clinically. The lower the oxygen saturation, the more severe the impact of the attack on the child. Oxygen saturations need to be maintained at > 92% (Cardwell 1997). It is important to ensure oximetry reading is accurate; poor contact, excessive movement and temperature of the child's skin can all affect the accuracy of reading. The A&E nurse can check the validity of the oximetry reading by matching the peaks of recording, bleeps or monitored pulse rate to the child's actual pulse rate. These should be about the same if the oxygen saturation level is to be considered accurate. In severe asthma, arterial blood gases should be measured and act as an indication of the level of respiratory distress and possible need for artificial ventilation. If response to treatment is poor, a chest X-ray should be considered to exclude specific localised pathology such as a pneumonthorax.

Management

In cases of *life-threatening* asthma (Box 16.3), these children need immediate high-flow oxygen via a mask, and nebulised beta-agonists such as salbutamol. Preparation should be to establish i.v. access for the administration of medication. Children in this age group both deteriorate and respond to treatment rapidly. The nurse must be vigilant for any changes and equipment should be at hand for intubation and ventilation.

Box 16.3 – *Life-threatening asthma signs*

■ Exhaustion

■ Reduced level of consciousness

■ Reduced respiratory effort with marked use of accessory muscles and severe recession

■ Cyanosis

■ Silent chest on auscultation

■ Oxygen saturation less than 85% on air

Rapid oxygen therapy and nebulised bronchodilators should be commenced in cases of *severe* asthma (Box 16.4). An oxygen saturation of at least 95% should be the aim (Bernardo & Schenkel 1995). It is important not to distress the child unnecessarily as this significantly increases the work of breathing. Intravenous access should be considered, particularly if the child does not respond rapidly to nebuliser therapy.

Compliance with treatment is crucial to the successful management of this group of children. It is important to be calm and to keep the parents/carers informed of treatment plans, to enable them to assist in the care of their child. Initial management involves

---

Box 16.4 – *Severe asthma signs*

- Agitated
- Respiratory rate over 50 breaths/min
- Intercostal recession
- Oxygen saturation less than 90%

Box 16.5 – *Moderate asthma signs*

- Alert and orientated
- Tachypnoea
- Able to speak normally
- Audible wheeze

---

the administration of beta-agonists, such as salbutamol 2.5 mg (British National Formulary 1999), as nebuliser masks can be frightening to children. It is important that the nurse explains what is being done first, and uses toys and play where appropriate. Alternative devices such as mouthpiece nebulisers can be more successful. If the child is very upset, it is sometimes better to get a parent to hold the nebuliser by the child's mouth than to increase the level of distress by attaching the mask to the child. If the child responds well to nebuliser treatment, he should be detained in A&E for at least 1 hour post-nebuliser, to ensure that the response is not transient. If the response is not maintained, the child should be admitted for nebulisers and further observation.

When planning the discharge of a young child from A&E, it is important the parents understand and are happy with the ongoing treatment plan. Although a child may appear well after nebuliser therapy for an acute episode of asthma, the small airways obstruction persists for several days (Morton & Philips 1996). Parents must be able to administer supportive therapy at home. Many devices exists to assist young children in the inhalation of bronchodilators. Spacers are commonly used in children under 5 years (Rees & Price 1989). These create an enclosed space between an aerosol inhaler and the child's mouth, allowing him to work at his own pace, without the need for hand–breathing coordination the aerosol would demand. The child can be taught to take five long exaggerated breaths from the spacer to each actuation of the aerosol into the spacer (McCollum 1993).

A short course of oral steroids can speed up the rate of recovery from an acute episode of small airways obstruction. Prednisolone for 3 days is recommended for children who have not responded to regular home treatment over a period of 24 hours or more prior to A&E attendance (British National Formulary 1996). Children regularly on inhaled steroids may also benefit from this boost. As well as advice on drug therapy, it is important that parents/carers are able to detect their child's worsening condition and know when and where to seek help (see Box 16.5 for moderate asthma signs). Advise parents to return to A&E if:

- respiratory rate increases
- recession becomes apparent
- the child is using accessory muscles to breathe
- breathlessness affects eating/drinking
- the ability to speak deteriorates
- the positive response to inhaled bronchodilators reduces
- the child becomes agitated.

Follow-up should be arranged for all children discharged from A&E. This can usually be done via the child's usual GP or regular asthma clinic.

Acute Laryngotracheobronchitis (Viral Croup)

Croup is a broad term used to describe disease of the upper airway with symptoms which include a cough and stridor. It is most common between 6 months and 3 years of age and is twice as common in boys as it is in girls (Custer 1993). It most commonly occurs in the damper weather of late autumn and winter. Children with croup frequently present in emergency departments in the late evening or at night as symptoms often appear more acute at this time (Morton & Philips 1996).

Physiology

Croup encompasses a range of upper respiratory inflammations, mostly viral in nature. The most common source is acute laryngotracheobronchitis caused by the parainfluenza virus (Custer 1993). It results in tracheal and subglottal swelling. This inflammation spreads to the bronchus and results in increased mucus production. The increase in mucus together with pharyngeal irritation results in the hoarse cough.

Less common symptoms of croup are highlighted in Box 16.6.

Assessment

History

The A&E nurse can quickly put together a picture of a viral croup condition by asking the parents/carers

---

Box 16.6 – *Less common symptoms of croup*

- Inhalation of a foreign body which has become lodged in the laryngeal region. This should be considered in all cases of stridor as inhalation is often witnessed in small children

- Tonsillitis can present with stridor or hoarse cough when there is tonsillar enlargement often associated with glandular fever

- Angioneurotic oedema resulting from an acute anaphylactic reaction

- Bacterial tracheitis is an unusual cause of croup but has a high mortality rate if not treated. These children look toxic, like those with epiglottitis, but are differentiated by their croupy cough. Intubation and antibiotic therapy are required promptly

- Diphtheria is uncommon in the UK but should be considered in children with croup symptoms who have not been immunised against diphtheria

---

about the lead-up to A&E attendance, such as:

- Duration
- Symptoms – are they worse at night?
- Is the child drinking?
- Is the child talking normally?
- Past medical history.

The nurse can expect to find a history of illness worsening over several days. Viral croup usually starts with a coryzal illness (common cold) and is followed after 48–72 hours by a sudden, and often frightening, onset of stridor and a barking cough. At this stage, children are commonly brought to A&E. Unlike epiglottitis, children with croup are able to drink, although they may complain of a sore throat. The A&E nurse should expect these children to be able to talk, but their voices will have varying levels of hoarseness. Significant past medical history is uncommon, but previous airways disease or recurrent croup should be noted. Hyperreactivity of the upper airway may cause recurrent symptoms (Morton & Phillips 1996), but management of each individual episode should still be based on its severity at the time of presentation.

Physical assessment

Assessment of the child in A&E should focus on determining the degree of threat to respiratory function. The work of breathing should be assessed in terms of respiratory rate, use of accessory muscles, nasal flaring and intercostal recession. The degree of stridor is significant: the nurse should note whether

stridor is inspiratory, which usually indicates a supraglottic cause, or expiratory which usually comes from the trachea. In severe cases, inspiratory and expiratory stridor may be present. The loudness of a stridor is not an indication of its severity (Morton & Philips 1996), but loudness of stridor often influences the degree of anxiety. It is important to establish whether stridor is present at rest, or only when the child becomes agitated or exerts him or herself.

Heart rate should be regularly monitored. Tachycardia, particularly if it is coexistent with agitation, restlessness or altered consciousness, is associated with increasing hypoxia. Oxygen saturation should be measured in children with increased respiratory rate, and tachycardia and saturation levels below 95% should be treated with oxygen therapy.

When assessing a child with viral croup, the A&E nurse would expect to find a clinical picture of moderate fever, with the child unwell over a few days with a sudden onset of harsh stridor and a barking cough. The child will usually be active, but irritable and easily upset. The key to successful management lies with accurately assessing and responding to the level of respiratory compromise. Clinical investigations, such as blood tests and chest and neck X-rays, do little to alter the management plan and much to increase the child's distress. For this reason, investigations of this nature should not form part of the initial management.

Management (Box 16.7)

The child should always be nursed in the position that is most comfortable for him. This is usually semi-upright, cradled in the parent's or carer's arms. As anxiety and psychological distress have a detrimental effect on respiratory function, every effort should be

---

Box 16.7 – *Priorities in treatment of croup*

- Rapid and accurate assessment of airway impairment

- Keep the child calm. Nurse in a comfortable position; involve parents/carers

- Give nebulised adrenaline 0.5 mg/kg of 1:1000 preparation up to 5 ml maximum

- Give nebulised steroids – budesonide 2 mg

- Maintain hydration

- Monitor oxygen saturation levels; intubate if child has unresolved, worsening hypoxia

made by the A&E care team to keep the child calm and accommodate his wishes.

Nebulised adrenaline is effective first-line treatment (Goodwin 1996). This is best administered by a parent holding a nebuliser in front of the child, as face masks and mouthpieces can be frightening and considerably increase the child's distress. Adrenaline acts both as a bronchodilator and to suppress histamine, therefore reducing mucous secretions and relieving airway obstruction. The effects of adrenaline nebulisers are relatively short-acting, lasting approximately 2 hours, although the therapy can be repeated. Care should be taken to reassess children carefully as the majority return to their pre-therapeutic state once the effects of adrenaline wear off (Barkin & Rosen 1994).

Longer-term management is aided by the use of corticosteroids. Although oral steroid therapy, such as prednisolone, is the most common current treatment, evidence suggests that nebulised budesonide shows a more rapid and sustained improvement in the child's clinical condition (Doull 1995). This should be augmented with adrenaline nebulisers (Higginson et al. 1996). The early use of inhaled steroids has been proven to lessen the severity and shorten the duration of a croup episode (Husby et al. 1993). Humidification therapy, either in mist tents or with oxygen, has little effect on moderate to severe croup (Morton & Philips 1996) and is not therefore recommended for hospital management of croup.

Children should have oxygen saturation levels monitored, and there should be vigilant observation for clinical signs of hypoxia. In children who are not clinically hypoxic, oxygen therapy is considered unnecessary and sometimes unhelpful if it makes the child distressed. Hypoxia in children with croup is a late sign and should be treated seriously. It usually indicates a need for medical intervention in airway management, and in the case of a fatigued child, intubation is often necessary. All children with clinical hypoxia should be nursed in a high-dependency or resuscitation area, and appropriate airway maintaining equipment should be available.

Hydration is an important and sometimes over-looked area of care in the child with croup. Many are reluctant to drink because of a painful throat, and some, particularly younger children, find it difficult to take fluids because of dyspnoea. Parents should be encouraged to give frequent small amounts of clear fluid wherever possible. This not only prevents dehydration, but also helps to reduce the tenacity of secretions. Milky drinks should be discouraged as they increase tenacity of secretions (Morton & Philips 1996). If a child is too short of breath to take fluids or is clinically dehydrated, intravenous fluid replacement should be considered after initial symptom relief. Antibiotics are not considered useful as croup is predominantly of viral origin.

Criteria for admission

All children with moderate to severe croup should be admitted for nebulisers and observation. This can be determined by poor or transient response to treatment, persistent stridor at rest and any degree of hypoxia. Admission should also be considered for any child who is clinically dehydrated. Social circumstances should be examined when making a decision to admit or discharge the child. If the family live a long distance from health care facilities or have no transport, admission should be considered. If domestic circumstances are not conducive to home management, e.g. a parent/carer smokes or accommodation is damp, or if A&E staff are unsure of the parents' carers' understanding of the needs of a child with croup, short-term hospitalisation should be facilitated. Parental anxiety is also an important consideration, particularly in younger children. Where possible, if parents feel ill-equipped to manage at home, admission may be necessary (Milner & Hull 1992).

Discharge advice

If, after a period of observation, the child is considered well enough to be discharged, the parents/carers should be given clear advice on home care, which should be supported with written information. The advice should include the following:

■ Stay with the child and observe breathing pattern – a worsening obstruction will not always wake the child.
■ If croup returns, look after the child in a warm, humidified environment, such as a steamy bathroom. Cold mist is of no benefit. Maintain this for 10–15 minutes.
■ If there is no improvement, or the child's condition worsens, return to A&E.

Epiglottitis

Aetiology

Epiglottitis is caused by *Haemophilus influenzae*. It is a relatively uncommon but life-threatening condition. Unlike laryngotracheobronchitis, it is has no winter peak of incidence, nor is it more common in the evening or at night (see Table 16.1). It can occur at any time of day, throughout the year. People of all age

Table 16.1 – *Differentiation of croup from epiglottitis*

Symptom	Croup	Epiglottitis
Age	6 months–3 years	2–5 years
Season	Winter	All year
Worst time of day	Evening/night	Anytime
Aetiology	Parainfluenza virus	*Haemophilus influenze* B
Onset	Over days	Over hours
Preceding illness	Yes	No
Fever	<38.5°C	>38.5°C
Sore throat	Sometimes	Yes
Drooling	No	Yes
Cough	Harsh barking	No
Stridor	Inspiratory and expiratory	Soft expiratory
Voice	Hoarse	None
Wheeze	Often present	None
Position	Varied, active	Upright with neck extended

groups are at risk of contracting epiglottitis, but it is most common in 2 to 5-year-olds (Barkin & Rosen 1994).

Anatomy and physiology

Epiglottitis is a serious life-threatening condition because *Haemophilus influenzae* infection causes a rapid inflammatory reaction in the epiglottis, the tissues swell and acute airway obstruction occurs.

Assessment

History

Obtaining an accurate history from parents/carers is imperative as physical examination of the child is restricted when epiglottitis is suspected. Duration of the child's illness is an important factor in determining the likelihood of epiglottitis. Illness is rapid in onset, with respiratory symptoms occurring in a matter of hours. Despite this, other foci of infection are common with epiglottitis, usually otitis media or lymphadenitis. Because of the urgent need for treatment, the A&E nurse should simultaneously perform a physical inspection of the child if epiglottitis is suspected. This should differentiate between inhalation of foreign body and epiglottitis.

Physical assessment

It is vital that the child's throat is *not* examined, because any irritation increases the inflammatory response and increases epiglottic swelling, often resulting in complete airway obstruction. Distressing the child also increases the risk of airway obstruction. For these reasons, assessment is a 'hands-off' visual activity. Children with epiglottitis usually prefer to sit up, often with the neck extended forwards. This allows for maximum use of their compromised airway. Most children will have a soft inspiratory stridor without an associated cough. Most children are reluctant to speak, but those who do usually have a muffled voice. Drooling is a strong indication that the child has epiglottitis. This occurs because swallowing is painful due in part to a severe throat. The child usually has a significant pyrexia, in excess of 38.5°C.

Management

If epiglottitis is suspected, the most important action is to summon specialist help. The child's epiglottis needs to be examined under anaesthetic in theatre and an artificial airway established in a controlled environment. While waiting for this, the A&E nurse should keep the child and parents/carers calm, ensure the child is in the most comfortable position for him, and give oxygen if possible. This is best achieved by sitting the child on a parent's lap and getting the parent to hold the mask near the child. If the child is upset by oxygen therapy it should not be pursued.

As any child with epiglottitis is at risk of airway obstruction at any time, the A&E nurse should always have equipment available to establish artificial ventilation. Because of the position and degree of swelling of the epiglottis, intubation in an emergency can be extremely difficult. It is often necessary to perform a cricothyroidotomy. Once an artificial airway has been successfully established and the child is haemodynamically stable, other investigations and definitive management can take place, usually in ITU. This includes blood screening and culture, the initiation of antibiotics and maintenance of hydration.

Accidental Injury

One of the most common reasons for pre-school children attending the A&E department is accidental injury (Mead & Sibert 1991). In 1991, 688 children died as a result of accidental injury, 44% of whom were under 5 years of age (Towner & Barry 1993). It is estimated that each year in England 10 000 children are left with long-term health problems as a consequence of accidents. The direct cost to the NHS of caring for accident victims is in excess of £200 million (Department of Health 1993).

Most pre-school children suffer accidents in the home environment (Towner & Barry 1993). In recognition of the huge health problem associated with accidents, the government's White Paper *Health of the Nation* (Department of Health 1993) identified accidents as one of the five key areas to be targeted for improvement. The national target is to reduce accidents by one-third by the year 2005. The causes of accidents involving pre-school children are varied. Young children are vulnerable because they rely on their parents to provide a safe environment for them and to keep a careful watch on them while they explore. The role of A&E nurses is not just associated with treatment; they are also in a position to help educate the public and prevent further accidents occurring.

Aetiology of accidental injury

The factors that increase a child's risk of accidental injury are similar to agents that may increase the incidence of non-accidental injury (Sibert *et al.* 1981). A child from a working class background (social class V) is five times more likely to be killed accidentally than those of professional families (Roberts & Power 1996). Environmental stress in the family, such as illness, shortage of money and maternal tension within the family unit, leads to an increase in the incidence of childhood accidents.

The age of the child affects the type of accidents likely to be experienced. Pre-school children are prone to the following accidents (Mead & Sibert, 1991):

- falls
- poisoning
- burns, scalds
- lacerations
- suffocation
- drowning.

In A&E, the main focus of care has traditionally been to diagnose and treat the child's injury. Nurses are very good at providing parents/carers with information about how to look after the child's injury at home, but less good at actively engaging in health promotion. Often, timely intervention by A&E staff can prevent further accidents and ease the impact of family tension or stress. This intervention may be in the form of actual advice on accident prevention or referral to other health professionals. Health visitor liaison services are available to most A&E departments and are able to communicate information to the family's own health visitor (Laidman 1982). The health visitor also has the advantage of knowing the family and can follow up A&E attendance with supportive information and active accident prevention. Parents often respond best to one-to-one advice. By visiting the family at home, the health visitor can identify and discuss specific hazards.

Accidental Poisoning

This most commonly occurs in the age group 1–3 years and accounts for approximately 40 000 A&E attendances per annum in England and Wales (Morton & Philips 1996). This number reflects a marked decrease in incidence since the introduction of child-resistant bottle tops in the mid-1970s (Towner & Berry 1993). Although uncommon, around 10 children per annum die, and others are left with significant physical problems, such as oesophageal stenosis (Mead & Sibert 1991). Accidental poisoning has a higher incidence in families with existing stressors, such as illness, pregnancy or recent birth, absence of one parent, a house move or anxiety/depression in a parent. The most commonly ingested poisons are childhood medicines, such as paracetamol elixir or cough mixture, oral contraceptives and vitamin supplements. Household products, such as detergent, bleach, disinfectant, perfume and cosmetics, are also commonly ingested.

Assessment

History

Establishing a clear history can often prove challenging for the A&E nurse. Both parents and the child are often distressed and information may be scanty. The nurse must try to find out:

- What has been taken – the container is a useful aid to active ingredients.
- How much has been ingested – the container will give useful clues to the amount left, as will the appearance of the child if spillage is possible. Parents/carers should be asked about spillage at home.
- Description of child's behaviour or symptoms since ingestion. Vomiting is of particular significance as it reduces the likelihood of absorption.
- Any pre-existing illness should be noted, as should any medication the child is currently taking.

Unless clear evidence to the contrary exists, the A&E nurse should assume and treat the child as if he has ingested the maximum amount of poison available.

Physical assessment

The majority of children who have ingested the common poisons noted above will show no immediate physical signs. As a baseline, the following should be established:

- respiration rate and depth
- pulse and circulatory status
- conscious level
- pupil size and reaction
- skin condition, evidence of irritation/burns, particularly around or in the mouth.

Management

Specific management of a poison can be aided by gaining specialist advice from a regional poisons unit. Common principles of care exist, however, for most types of ingestion. Gastric lavage has limited effectiveness in children because of the small size of tube used. The insertion of fluid during washout can increase absorption by washing toxins into the duodenum. Gastric lavage also carries a risk of oesophageal or gastric perforation as well as the inherent unpleasantness of the procedure (Valladeres 1996). For this reason it is not recommended except in varying consciousness levels when gastric emptying is considered essential. In those circumstances, intubation and anaesthetic cover are essential before insertion of the gastric tube takes place.

If ingestion has occurred less than 2 hours previously, induced vomiting is considerate appropriate for non-caustic, moderate poisons such as paracetamol. Ipecacuanha is commonly used to induce vomiting and usually takes 15–20 minutes to take effect. Encouraging the child to play and move around decreases the time for the emetic to work. The child should be encouraged to drink clear fluid, such as water or diluted squash, to aid the expulsion of toxins. Milk delays the effect of ipecac. Enforced emesis is only effective in emptying about half of gastric contents (Morton & Philips 1996) and vomiting can persist for some time after ingestion.

In the majority of cases of accidental poisoning, the potential toxicity is low, and therefore enforced emesis is considered unnecessary. In these cases activated charcoal is used as a binding agent to absorb toxins (Greensher *et al*. 1987). Patient compliance is often difficult as the liquid is black and gritty, making it hard to convince children to drink it. Imagination and incorporating the drink into a story or 'adventure' can sometimes be useful in persuading the child to take it.

Non-toxic agents (Box 16.8)

Specific substances should be checked with a poisons centre (Campbell *et al*. 1998). The majority of children who have ingested these substances do not need gastric evacuation or observation and can be safely discharged home. Parents should be constructively

---

Box 16.8 – *Non-toxic agents*

- Most cosmetics – beware of alcohol in perfumes
- Non-leaded paint
- Inks
- Most antibiotics
- Vitamins
- Oral contraceptives

Box 16.9 – *Toxic drugs*

- Paracetamol
- Salicyclates and aspirin
- Tricyclic antidepressants
- Narcotics
- Iron

---

offered advice and support, as many will have found their child's accidental poisoning very distressing.

Toxic drugs (Box 16.9)

Children who have ingested large amounts of paracetamol-based substances or aspirin should have their blood checked 4 hours after ingestion for serum paracetamol or salicylate, both of which demand in-patient treatment. If levels are normal, the child can be discharged home. Ingestion of tricyclic antidepressants is the commonest cause of death in children with accidental poisoning (Morton & Philips 1996). These children should have continuous cardiac monitoring as cardiac dysrhythmia is common and cardiotoxicity is often the reason for mortality. As drowsiness is also common, gastric lavage should be considered for children presenting within 2 hours of ingestion. Activated charcoal has a good absorption rate with tricyclic antidepressants and should therefore be used (Colbridge *et al*. 1997). All children need hospital admission for 24 hours, even if asymptomatic.

Narcotic drugs. Clinical symptoms are similar with all types of opiate drugs, and the nurse should suspect ingestion of narcotics if the child has pinpoint pupils. Sometimes an accurate history can be difficult to obtain, particularly if the drug is an illegal substance. Narcotic drugs cause respiratory depression for several hours after ingestion and have a sudden onset. Induced emesis or gastric lavage should be carried out depending on the child's consciousness level. If the child shows signs of respiratory depression or is

Box 16.10 – *Toxic household products*

- Bleach
- Caustic soda
- Detergent
- Disinfectant
- Antifreeze
- Alcohol

unconscious, intravenous naloxone should be given. Children should be always be admitted following narcotics poisoning.

Iron. Although used as dietary supplement, an excess of iron is extremely toxic. It causes severe gastric haemorrhage. Any symptoms the child may have should be treated on admission; i.v. access should be established at an early stage and fluid resuscitation commenced if necessary. Intramuscular desferrioxamine (30 mg/kg) should be given, and may be necessary over a 24-hour period depending on the severity of symptoms. If the child is drowsy, gastric lavage should be considered.

Toxic household products (Box 16.10)

As a general rule, emetics should not be given. As a first-line treatment, milk can be given. Advice specific to the substance should be sought from the poisons centre. Alcohol is the exception to this rule. Oral fluid of any type is not advised initially. Young children accidentally ingest alcohol in drinks or in perfume/aftershave. Small amounts of alcohol can result in hypoglycaemia in children. A blood sugar level should be established and intravenous dextrose-based fluids given if the child is significantly intoxicated or hypoglycaemic. Drowsy or unconscious children need airway management and close observation. Alcohol needs time to be excreted from the body, and care in A&E revolves around maintaining homeostasis during this time. Gastric lavage and induced vomiting are unhelpful and should not be considered unless other toxins are present. Once the child is alert and aware of his surroundings, he can be discharged. Parents should be advised to increase the fluid intake over the 12 hours after discharge and return if the child shows signs of gastric discomfort.

If the parent/carer offers a history inconsistent with the child's condition, or offers no explanation of poisoning, the possibility of deliberate poisoning by the parent or a third party should be considered. This type of attendance can occur in Munchausen's syndrome by proxy, where the carer is using the child to draw attention to him- or herself (Meadow 1997) (also see later in this chapter). It is often difficult to establish deliberate poisoning conclusively, but a long and vague medical history of the child and frequent hospitalisation may raise suspicions.

Non–accidental Injuries (Child Abuse)

Child abuse presents a difficult situation for A&E staff that requires sensitivity to the needs of both child and family. The definition of child abuse is a non-accidental act committed by a care-giver, usually a family member, that results in physical, sexual or emotional injury or deprivation to an individual less than 18 years old, but most likely less than 5 years old (Dolan 1998). Meadow (1997) also states that child abuse occurs if the child is threatened by an adult in a way that is unacceptable in a given culture at a given time. Child abuse (neglect) is one of the most common causes of death in young children in the UK (Browne 1995). Indeed, child homicide figures for 1992 support this claim, showing that parents and relatives were responsible for three-quarters of the deaths (Central Statistical Office 1994). Twice as many children are left disabled and 10 000 children year are placed on the 'at risk' register.

TYPES OF ABUSE (Box 16.11)

Physical. In 1962, Kempe coined the term 'battered baby syndrome' and did much to focus medical and public attention on this problem. Most commonly, physical abuse is inflicted on the child under the guise of punishment or when an adult loses control. It usually involves violence, often of a short duration but repetitive. Physical abuse includes poisoning and suffocation.

Neglect. Neglect is the persistent and severe failure to provide love, care, food or the physical circumstances to allow for normal development (see Box

Box 16.11 – *Types of child abuse*

- Physical
- Neglect
- Emotional
- Social
- Sexual

Box 16.12 – *Common indicators of child neglect (Sheridan 1995)*

Physical indicators

- Poor hygiene and/or clothing that does not protect a child from weather

- Chronic signs of malnutrition and dehydration

- Poor oral hygiene or untreated dental problems

- Failure to receive immunisations

- Child abandonment

- Delays in seeking prompt medical care for an acute injury or illness

- Failure to give child a prescribed medication, which results in the child developing more severe symptoms

- Failure to thrive in infants

Emotional and behavioural indicators

- Delay or absence of age-appropriate behaviours, especially in infants and young children

- Lethargy in the absence of illness

- Social withdrawal or depression

- Relentless attention-seeking behaviour

- Minimal response to painful medical interventions

- Suicidal ideation or attempts

Box 16.13 – *Common indicators of child abuse (Sheridan 1995)*

Physical indicators
Alterations in skin integrity

- Abrasions to palms, elbows, or knees from being pushed down

- Burns resulting from:
  - cigarettes and cigars
  - curling tongs, clothes irons
  - chemicals
  - friction – being dragged in the ground
  - immersion in hot liquid or 'dunking' injury patterns
  - splashes

- Bite marks – human are crest-shaped

- External genitalia lacerations or abrasions

- Vaginal bleeding, discharge or infections

- Penile bleeding, discharge or infection

- Rectal bleeding, discharge or infections

- Patterned bruises such as from a whip, belt or other implement

- Bruises in various stages of healing

Alterations in musculoskeletal system

- Multiple fractures

- Fractures in various stages of healing

- Spiral or midshaft fractures of long bones

- Fractured ribs – uncommon in young children

- Skull fractures

Neurologic impairment

- Acute onset of paresis

- Post-concussion symptoms

- Intracranial haemorrhage

- Visual impairment resulting from retinal detachment

Non–physical indicators

- Conflicting histories obtained from parent(s) or adult(s) and child regarding the nature of the child's injuries

- Children who are not allowed by the parent(s) or adult(s) to verbalise a history despite the fact that they are developmentally and chronologically old enough to do so

- A history given by the parent(s) or adult(s) that does not fit the nature of the presenting injuries

- Children who display fearful body language, e.g. guarding when a sudden movement is made

- A delay in bringing a child to A&E for treatment of any injury or illness that indicates abuse or neglect

---

16.12). It also includes willfully exposing a child to any kind of danger. Deaths related to neglect outnumber those related to physical abuse (Kempe & Helfer 1983)

Emotional abuse. All abuse involves some emotional ill-treatment. Emotional abuse and neglect refer to hostile or indifferent parental behaviour which damages a child's self-esteem, degrades a sense of achievement, diminishes a sense of belonging and stands in the way of healthy, vigorous and happy development. Iwaniec (1997) argued that parents and carers who persistently criticise, shame, threaten, humiliate, induce fear and anxiety, and who are never satisfied with the child's behaviour and performance (and do so deliberately) are emotionally abusive and cruel.

Sexual abuse. This is discussed in a separate section (p. 246).

Persistent rejection or neglect can lead to the child failing to thrive and can affect the child's stature (Skuse 1989). Common physical and non-physical indicators of child abuse are given in Box 16.13.

Prevalence

One child per 1000 under 4 years of age suffers some form of abuse (Meadow 1997). First-born children are more likely to be affected and it is not uncommon to find one child is abused while other siblings are free from abuse. Young children of pre-school age are more at risk because they cannot seek help. Most children are abused by a parent; particularly common is a cohabitant living in the house who is not the child's biological parent. The younger the parents, the more likely is it that they will abuse their children. Poverty, social isolation, family breakdown and poor parent–child relationships are associated with all forms of child abuse and neglect and have been cited as risk factors for child sexual abuse (Finkelhor 1980). However, child abuse is seen across all layers of society.

The acknowledgement that child abuse exists and is quite common is an important start for A&E staff. While the A&E nurse's main role is suspicion and detection, the nurse needs to keep an open and inquiring mind. Every A&E department should have an agreed procedure for the management of suspected child abuse and the nurse needs to be acquainted with this (Dimond 1993). All such cases need to be reported to senior medical staff and the consultant paediatrician for further investigations and intervention where necessary.

The parents

The vast majority of child abuse involves the child's parents. Approximately one-third of parents who were abused as children are at risk of abusing their own children. As abused children, they may have been subjected to marked negative reinforcement, an inability to get their needs met, little practice in problem-solving, and no basis for trust in others. As a consequence, they may lack empathy with their children as little was directed towards them, and a self-perpetuating cycle then begins (Tercier 1992). The parents may present as hostile and/or exhibit a lack of concern or guilt, or may show a lack of interest or disturbed interaction with the child and seem more interested in their own problems than the child's, e.g. how they are going to get home.

The child

Abused children have a number of characteristics that predispose them to victimisation. They are often the unwanted children of unplanned pregnancies, illegitimate births, the opposite sex from that desired by the parents, born in periods of crisis or from a former relationship. They may have problems that make them difficult to rear: poor feeders, challenging behaviour, abnormal sleep patterns, excessive crying, hyperactivity. They may be children who have experienced poor maternal–child bonding, premature infants, infants separated from their mothers because of illness, stepchildren or foster children (Tercier 1992). The child may be passive, withdrawn and uncomplaining during dressing or can present hyperactive anger and rebelliousness. There may be obvious signs of neglect.

Management of suspected child abuse

The key to management is maintaining a high index of suspicion to permit recognition of actual and potential abuse situations (Barkin & Rosen 1994). This starts at triage: an astute nurse will pick up discrepancies in the history of the incident, incompatibilities between the alleged mechanism of injury and actual injury, and unusual interactions between the child and his carer (Saines 1992). All life-threatening conditions must be given immediate attention; however, while the nursing care and treatment of the child's physical needs remain paramount, the emotional needs of the child and the parent(s) must also be addressed (Sheridan 1995).

The parents need to be informed of a need to notify child protection agencies. Local guidelines for child protection should be followed, and the child and family should be supported and cared for in a private but safe area during their stay in A&E. Some paediatric A&E departments have specific facilities for families during the period of assessment for possible abuse. In general A&E departments, however, it may be preferable to admit the child to a paediatric ward.

The health workers' attitude can have a great impact on the child. It is imperative that the health carer appears non-judgmental and is not disgusted by findings or revelations. These should be handled with diplomacy to prevent a difficult situation from becoming inflamed. It should be acknowledged that abuse cases of any kind can foster feelings among staff of hostility and anger towards alleged perpetrators; however, for nursing to be effective, staff must control these feelings. Team leaders and members should monitor each other's emotional and physical well-being, and provide support for those who appear to be badly affected by the incident (Cudmore 1998).

Careful documentation is critical in cases of suspected child abuse. For the nurse taking a history, the single most important factor is the history of the incident as told by the child. It is appropriate to write verbatim, or as closely as possible, any allegations of abuse or neglect, noting who made them and who was present. It is also appropriate to document specific observed behaviours of the child, siblings and/or parents (Sheridan 1995). Photographs should, if possible, be taken (Dickens 1994) as they may play an important part in subsequent legal proceedings, as well as providing valuable clinical evidence.

No child should be discharged into the custody of parents if staff feel there is a risk to the child's health or welfare. Where parents are unwilling to cooperate, the protection of the Children Act (Department of Health 1989) may need to be applied through an emergency protection order (Oates 1993). In most instances, however, where non-judgmental approaches and open communication prevail, parental agreement will be forthcoming.

Sexual Abuse

This occurs when dependent, developmentally immature children are forced to participate in sexual activity. Although sexual abuse may occur at any age, peaks tend to occur between 2–6 years and 12–16 years (Tercier 1992). Perhaps the most difficult area of abuse to detect in A&E is sexual abuse, primarily because sexually abused children often display no physical signs, (Robinson 1991).

Various degrees and forms of sexual abuse include molestation, touching or fondling of the child's genitalia, masturbation of the perpetrator by the child, combinations of oral–genital contact, attempted or actual anal or vaginal intercourse, exhibitionism, voyeurism and exploitation of children in the preparation of pornographic materials. Sexual abuse differs from other forms of child abuse in that it is not used as a form of punishment. However, while violence is seldom a factor, coercion and threats are common (Tercier 1992).

Sexual abuse may present to A&E staff in a number of different ways:

- *physical complaints*, e.g. abdominal pain, urinary tract infection, per rectum and per vaginal bleeds
- *parental accusation* – this should always be taken seriously, where one parent or carer accuses another
- *request by the child for help* – children do not fabricate stories of sexual activity
- *physical abuse* – children who have been physically abused may present with evidence of sexual abuse; careful examination may reveal trauma or infection
- *emotional or psychological problems* – these may present as bedwetting, night terrors, developmental regression

- *sexually transmitted diseases* – any sexually transmitted disease in a child should be considered evidence of sexual abuse until proven otherwise.

Management

The management of children who are suspected of being sexually abused is similar to that in child abuse. Establishing rapport and trust is critical, using language that is appropriate for the child's age and developmental stage. It is important to stress that children have short attention spans, and therefore a prolonged interview will not be tolerated. Children must be constantly reassured that it is all right to share 'secrets' with the nurse and for this reason it is often best to interview the child away from family members, even those not initially believed to be abusive or neglectful (Sheridan 1995). Once there is significant indication that sexual abuse may have occurred, arrangements should be made for physical examination to be carried out by an experienced paediatrician. It may be appropriate for a forensic doctor to be present to save the child repeated examinations. At this stage the social services and police should be involved. A professional colleague should be present, however, and responses should be recorded verbatim. A number of key facts need to be established in gaining a history of sexual abuse. These are presented in Box 16.14.

All too often A&E staff do not hear the outcomes of particularly difficult cases, such as suspected child sexual abuse. It is good practice to promote interdisciplinary team meetings for period review and updating of such cases to provide feedback, support and opportunities to further improve protocols.

Munchausen's Syndrome by Proxy

Munchausen's syndrome by proxy should be suspected whenever a child develops bizarre signs and symptoms that are not easily explained physiologically and that occur when the parent or carer is alone with the child (Tercier 1992). In over 90% of cases, the perpetrator is the child's natural mother; in 5% it is another female carer; and in less than 5% it is the child's father (Meadow 1997). It is most uncommon for there to be collusion between mother and father; the innocent partner is usually completely unaware and dumbfounded by the deception and subsequent revelations. Munchausen's syndrome by proxy is also classed as abuse of children (Hobbs *et al.* 1993).

The variety of diseases mimicked or produced is

Box 16.14 – *Sexual abuse history*

- Date and time of assault
- Place of assault(s)
- Number of people involved and relationship to abused
- Physical characteristics
- Use of restraints
- Use of sexual aids
- Use of lubricants, powders or other chemicals
- Statements made during assault
- Use of photographs or videotaping
- Removal of locks of hair or other 'artefacts'
- Form of assault, i.e. vaginal, anal or oral intercourse
- Occurrence of ejaculation
- Oral manipulation of breasts or other body parts
- Use of condom
- Bath, douche or clean mouth after assault
- Last bowel movement and last urination
- Last menstrual period, if appropriate
- Use of contraceptive pill or IUD, if appropriate
- Use of tampons or pads, if appropriate

Box 16.15 – *Characteristics of Munchausen's syndrome by proxy (Meadow 1982)*

- Persistent or recurrent illnesses that cannot be explained or are very unusual
- Laboratory results or physical findings that are at variance with the general health of the child
- Symptoms that only occur when the child is in the presence of the caretaker
- A caretaker who appears overly attentive, with prolonged visiting or living in with the child in the hospital
- Standard treatments that are not tolerated, e.g. i.v. lines that always come out, vomiting of medications
- A caretaker who does not seem as concerned about the child's illness as the medical or nursing staff
- A caretaker with previous medical experience or education
- Atypical episodes of seizures, near-miss SIDS or SIDS, apnoeic or cyanotic episodes occurring only in the presence of the caretaker and which do not seem to respond to standard therapy
- A history of multiple resuscitations in a child with no recognisable cardiopulmonary abnormalities
- Siblings with a similar episode or death
- A caretaker with characteristics of Munchausen's syndrome or a hysterical personality disorder
- A caretaker who has had symptoms similar to the victim's within the previous 5 years

startlingly large and limited only by the parent's imagination and ingenuity. The child, who is usually under 5 years, is most commonly presented with problems related to one system, such as recurrent seizures or a story of vomiting and diarrhoea. The illness story is related consistently by the mother, but events relating to the illness start only in her presence. While ideal parenting behaviours may be demonstrated, she may be inappropriately calm in relation to the gravity of the child's problem (see Box 16.15).

Meadow (1997) argued that extreme fabricated illness is very serious and may be life-threatening, requiring immediate liaison with social services and the police to protect the child. The long-term outcome of children who have been abused in this way is worrying as there is a significant incidence of recurrence of abuse of children who remain in maternal care and significant morbidity in the long term. Despite the understandable feelings of anger and frustration of clinical staff in this situation, the need for non-judgmental care remains paramount, as is the need for vigilance to protect these and other children. Support and debriefing should be available for staff, including reception, medical and ambulance personnel, as appropriate, who have been involved in the care of children who have been affected as a consequence of Munchausen's syndrome by proxy (Dolan 1998).

Conclusion

Children of pre-school age are more likely than others to attend the A&E department, because of their vulnerability to accidents and illness. The A&E department can be developed to become more child-oriented, to help reduce these children's anxieties. The A&E nurse must appreciate the importance of supporting and reassuring a child's family, because through helping them the nurse will help the child and increase his cooperation. It is important that all staff working with children have a fundamental knowledge of their normal development and perception, in order to avoid misinterpretation by them of actions taken by the staff.

A&E is usually a young child's first experience of hospital, and he will rely on others to bring him to the A&E department, to explain what is wrong and to explain the treatment being given. As the child's experience in A&E could affect his future attitude to planned admissions, it is the A&E staff's responsibility to ensure that it is a positive experience.

References

Barkin RM, Rosen P (1994) Abuse. In: Barkin RM, Rosen P, eds. *Emergency Pediatrics: a Guide to Ambulatory Care.* 4th edn. St Louis: Mosby.

Bernardo LM, Schenkel KA (1995) Paediatric medical emergencies. In: Kitt S, Selfridge-Thomas J, Proehl JA, Kaiser J, eds. *Emergency Nursing: a Physiologic and Clinical Perspective,* 2nd edn. Philadelphia: WB Saunders.

Bowlby J (1953) *Child Care and the Growth of Love.* London: Penguin.

British National Formulary (1999) London: BMJ.

British Thoracic Society, British Paediatric Association, Research unit of the Royal College of Physicians *et al.* (1993) Guidelines on the management of asthma. *Thorax,* **48**, S1–S24.

Browne K (1995) Child abuse, defining, understanding and intervening. In: Wilson K, James A, eds. *The Child Protection Handbook.* London: Baillière Tindall.

Brunner LS, Suddarth DS (1991) *The Lippincott Manual of Paediatric Nursing,* 3rd edn. London: Harper and Collins.

Burney PGJ, Chinn S, Rona RJ (1990) Has the prevalence of asthma increased in children? Evidence from the national study of health and growth 1973–1986. *British Medical Journal,* **300**, 1306–1310.

Campbell A, Schofield E, McCrea S, Colbridge M, Bates B, Cullen G (1998) Practical advice on managing poisoning from the NPIS (London). *Emergency Nurse,* **5**(8), 16–20.

Cardwell C (1997) Management of acute asthma in children. *Emergency Nurse,* **5**(7), 33–39.

Central Statistical Office (1994) *Social Focus on Children '94.* London: HMSO.

Colbridge M, Bates N, Lawman S, Volans G (1997) Acute poisoning – antidepressants: clinical features and management. *Emergency Nurse,* **5**(5), 13–17.

Cudmore J (1998) Critical incident stress management strategies. *Emergency Nurse,* **6**(3), 22–27.

Custer JR (1993) Croup and related disorders. *Paediatrics in Review,* **14**(1), 19–29.

Department of Health (1989) *The Children Act 1989.* London: HMSO.

Department of Health (1993) *The Health of the Nation: Key Area Handbooks (Accidents).* London: HMSO.

Department of Health (1995) *Children's Charter.* London: Department of Health.

Dickens H (1994) Marks of abuse: recognising child abuse. *Practice Nurse,* **8**(4), 197–198, 200, 202.

Dimond B (1993) Non-accidental injury and the accident and emergency nurse. *Accident and Emergency Nursing,* **1**, 225–228.

Dolan B (1998) The hospital hoppers. *Nursing Times,* **94**(30), 26–27.

Doull I (1995) Corticosteroids in the management of croup.

British Medical Journal, **311**, 1244.

Eiser C (1985) *The Psychology of Childhood Illness.* New York: Springer-Verlag.

Finklehor D (1980) Risk factors in the sexual victimisation of children. *Child Abuse and Neglect,* **4**, 265–273.

Gay J (1991) Caring for Children in A&E. *Paediatric Nursing,* **3**(7), 21–23.

Goodwin N (1996) Respiratory distress. *Practice Nurse,* **15**(11), 562–566.

Greensher J, Mofenson HC, Caroccio TR (1987) Ascendancy of the black bottle. *Paediatrics,* **80**, 949–951.

Hall DMB, Hill P, Elliman D (1990) *The Child Surveillance Handbook.* Oxford: Radcliffe Medical Press.

Higginson I, Montgomery P, Munro P (1996) *What to Do in a Paediatric Emergency.* London: BMJ.

Hobbs CJ, Hanks HGI and Wynne JM (1993) *Child Abuse and Neglect: a Clinician's Handbook.* Edinburgh: Churchill Livingstone.

Husby S, Aggertoff L, Mortenson S (1993) Treatment of croup with nebulised steroid budesonide: a double-blind placebo controlled study. *Archives of Diseases in Children,* **68**, 352–255.

Iwaniec D (1997) *The Emotionally Abused and Neglected Child.* Chichester: John Wiley.

Jolly J (1981) *The Other Side of Paediatrics: a Guide to Everyday Care of Sick Children.* Basingstoke: MacMillan.

Kempe CH, Helfer RE (1983) *The battered child,* 3rd edn. Chicago: University of Chicago Press.

Laidman P (1987) *The Health Visitors' Role in Prevention of Accidents to Children Between Antenatal and Pre-school Age.* London: Health Education Authority.

Lowe GR (1985) *The Growth of Personality from Infancy to Old Age.* Harmondsworth: Penguin.

McCollum J (1993) Asthma patients in the accident and emergency department: a forum for health education. *Accident and Emergency Nursing,* **1**, 139–148.

Måller D, Harris PJ, Wattley L, Taylor J (1992) *Nursing Children: Psychology, Research and Practice,* 2nd edn. London: Chapman and Hall.

Mead D, Sibert J (1991) *The Injured Child: an Action Plan for Nurses.* London: Scutari.

Meadow R (1982) Munchausen syndrome by proxy. *Archives of Diseases of Childhood,* **57**, 92.

Meadow R (1997) *ABC of Child Abuse,* 3rd edn. London: British Medical Association.

Milner A, Hull D (1992) *Hospital Paediatrics,* 2nd edn. Edinburgh: Churchill Livingstone.

Ministry of Health (1959) *The Welfare of Children in Hospital (The Platt Report).* London: HMSO.

Morton R, Phillips B (1996) *Accident and Emergencies in Children,* 2nd edn. Oxford: Oxford University Press.

Oates M (1993) Children Act 1989: the essential issues. *Emergency Nurse*, **1**(1), 21–22.

Partridge J (1997) Environmental provisions for children in A&E. *Emergency Nurse*, **4**(4), 7–9.

Raikow SD (1998) Meeting the emotional needs of the paediatric patient. *Emergency Medical Services*, **27**(4), 28–29.

Rees J, Price J (1989) *ABC of Asthma*, 2nd edn. London: BMJ.

Roberts I, Power C (1996) Does the decline in child mortality injury vary by social class?: a comparison of class-specific mortality in 1981 and 1991. *British Medical Journal*, **313**, 784–786.

Robinson R (1991) Physical signs of sexual abuse in children: skill and experience needed to find and interpret. *British Medical Journal*, **302**, 863–864.

Royal College of Nursing (1994) *The Care of Sick Children: a Review of the Guidelines in the Wake of the Allit Inquiry*. London: RCN.

Saines J (1992) A considered response to an emotional crisis: A&E nurses role in detecting child sexual abuse. *Professional Nurse*, **8**(3), 148–152.

Sheridan DJ (1995) Family violence. In: Kitt S, Selfridge-Thomas J, Proehl JA, Kaiser J, eds. *Emergency Nursing: a Physiologic and Clinical Perspective*, 2nd edn. Philadelphia: WB Saunders.

Sibert J, Maddocks GB, Brown BM (1981) Childhood accidents: an endemic of epidemic proportions. *Archives of Disease in Childhood*, **56**, 225–234.

Skuse (1989) ABC of child abuse: Emotional abuse and delay in growth. *British Medical Journal*, **299**, 113–115.

Smith AL *et al* (1991) *Comprehensive Child and Family Nursing Skills*. St Louis: Mosby Yearbook.

Tercier A (1992) Child abuse. In: Rosen P, Barkin RM, Braen G *et al. Emergency Medicine: Concepts and Clinical Practice*. St Louis: Mosby Year Book.

Towner E, Barry A (1993) Accidental injury in childhood. *Paediatric Nursing*, **5**(10), 10–12.

Valladares P (1996) Comparing clinical management of overdoses. *Emergency Nurse*, **4**(1), 6–8.

Valman HB (1988) *ABC of One to Seven*, 2nd edn. London: British Medical Association.

Valman HB (1993) Bronchial asthma. *British Medical Journal*, **306**, 1676–1681.

Wolfer JA, Vistintainer MA (1975) Paediatric surgical patients' stress response and adjustment as a function of psychological preparation and stress point nursing care. *Nursing Research*, **24**(4), 244–255.

Wolff S (1981) *Children under Stress*, 2nd edn. Harmondsworth: Penguin.

Chapter 17

Age 5 to Puberty

Anita Tyler

■ Introduction
■ Child development
■ Environment
■ Pain relief
■ Fractures
■ Sports injury
■ Abdominal pain
■ Consent
■ Health promotion
■ Conclusion

Introduction

This chapter considers reasons for A&E attendance by children between the ages of 5 and 13 years. While this age range is somewhat arbitrary, especially in the context of the decreasing age of puberty, for the purposes of this chapter it will be used as a chronological benchmark between pre-school children and adolescence. Some of the more common injuries and conditions found in this age group will be considered, with particular reference to a child's development and the need for a suitable environment and a family-centred approach.

Children's school years are proposed as the best years of their lives, but unfortunately they are also a very dangerous time. Each year one in five children attends an A&E (Mead & Sibert 1991) and an unknown number attend their own GP following an injury. In the UK approximately 700 children die each year as a result of an accident, compared with less than 500 who die as a result of malignant disease (Morton & Phillips 1996). Road traffic accidents (RTAs) cause the greatest number of deaths, followed by drowning, suffocation, fire and falls (Mead & Sibert 1991). About 10 000 children are permanently disabled annually as a result of accidents (Morton & Phillips 1996). However, the figures do not show the real impact an accident can have on both the child and the family. The cost can be enormous in both physical and emotional terms.

Child Development

Children are involved in different types of accident according to their stage of development. At 5 years of age children run confidently, although they frequently fall. As they progress from infant to junior school, balance and coordination improve, as does their dexterity. Children in this age group become more aware of their bodies and subsequently may be self-conscious during examinations.

Children aged between 5 and 7 have gained some

independence, both socially and intellectually, but their behaviour is unpredictable at times, and therefore they continue to need supervision, particularly on roads etc. Much of an early schoolgoer's time is spent under adult supervision at school or in the home. Increasingly, as they get older, children spend their time away from home in parks and playgrounds unsupervised. Being unsupervised can lead to children using unsuitable areas to play in, such as derelict buildings or building sites. They can also indulge in dangerous activities, such as playing with fire, increasing the likelihood of injury.

As children approach adolescence they are more likely to attempt to flaunt their independence, resent rules and authority, and take risks. Peer pressure influences children's behaviour in activities which they know to be dangerous but take part in to avoid losing face in front of their friends. Children will often lie about the mechanisms of injury to prevent detection of a banned activity, such as climbing.

Children show a systematic progression in their understanding of illness-related concepts, which is explained by Piaget's theory (1969) of the development of causal reasoning. Despite this acquired understanding, many children regress in behaviour when they become ill, probably as a coping mechanism for the stress associated with hospitalisation (Swanwick 1990). Hospital attendance is stressful at any age and children are not exempt from this. Muller *et al.* (1986) highlighted five areas of concern:

- physical harm
- fear of the unknown
- uncertainty
- separation
- loss of control.

Both the child's and the parent's previous experiences of hospital can have a profound effect on the child's attitude and behaviour.

Environment

The *Children's Charter* (Department of Health 1995) stated that A&E departments caring for children should provide an environment which, as a minimum, has:

- a separate waiting area with play facilities
- a separate treatment area suitably decorated and equipped
- a private room for distressed parents
- at least one registered sick children's' nurse (RSCN) or RN (child)
- a liaison health visitor.

A sick or injured child is usually accompanied to A&E by an adult, and sometimes by numerous family members and friends, including other children. Family-centred care should be the aim throughout the child's stay, and both the child and her family should be involved in decisions about care wherever possible (Cudmore & Lakin 1997, Department of Health 1991). Older children usually benefit from a parent or carer being present during examination/investigation, but pressure should not be put on parents/carers if they feel unable to be with their child during specific treatments. It is important for A&E nurses to reassure parents about their involvement in care if the child requires admission to hospital or needs to go to the operating theatre. In many hospitals, it is common practice for a parent/adult carer to be resident on the ward with the child.

Should a child need critical intervention, such as resuscitation, many parents would wish to stay with their child (Woodward 1994). The needs of parents must be considered, and the provision of a support nurse in the resuscitation area helps to keep them informed and involved with their child's care. Both nurses and medical staff may feel stressed by parental presence in an already tense situation, but in aiming for family-centred care, the parents and the child's wishes should be respected wherever possible.

The majority of children (60–70%) attend the A&E department following trauma. Fortunately, most of them will have relatively minor injuries (Morton & Phillips 1996), although to the child and parents a minor injury may appear catastrophic. An environment which creates a distraction for the child can help to reduce the emotional impact of injury, particularly for younger children. The provision of books, toys and child-friendly surroundings helps to create this environment; however, only 45% of A&E departments provide separate facilities for children (Partridge 1997). Perhaps the most important factor is the attitude of health workers towards children and their families. Children should be approached in a manner which reinstates normality to a threatening situation.

To do this, the nurse must be aware of the developmental stage appropriate to the child's age and attempt to introduce familiarity. This can be done by relating activities and conversation to things included in the child's normal world, such as childhood heroes and school activities. Parents and others, especially other children, can be particularly helpful with this. The younger children in this age group appreciate bravery awards and stickers following their treatment.

Pain Relief

Many children attending A&E will require pain relief in some form. Pain assessment can prove difficult, even in older children, and a long-standing problem in paediatric pain management has been the difficulty of objectively assessing pain (Zacharias & Watts 1998). Nurses can be guided to some extent by the parents' assessment of their child's pain (Whaley & Wong 1990). The impact of anxiety on a child's pain level should not be underestimated and appropriate measures to reduce anxiety are an important part of pain control.

Children require explanation of likely health outcomes, just like adults, as fear of the unknown is a great source of anxiety (Wilson-Barnett 1979). It is imperative that assessment of pain and explanation of procedures are appropriate to the child's understanding, and neither patronising nor beyond comprehension. The use of toys and play demonstration, such as bandaging teddy's leg, can be helpful in reducing anxiety in the younger child. This reinforces the need for the A&E nurse to have an awareness of normal childhood development, so communication is effective and pain assessment accurate. Pain scales, such as numerical continuums for older children and visual analogues for younger children, can be a useful aid to pain assessment, but should not be used in isolation.

For many children, immobilisation and support of an injured area comprise the first step in pain control, but this should not be used as a substitute for analgesia. A&E nurses must not underestimate actual pain, as opposed to the fear of pain and anxiety, as the cause of the child's distress (Morcombe 1998). Even for seemingly minor injuries, analgesia can be administered at an early stage, easing the child's passage through A&E. Simple analgesia such as paracetamol can be very effective and relatively easy to administer in elixir or tablet form, depending on the child's age and preference. Aspirin is not used in children under 12 because of the risk of Reye's syndrome (Nunn 1994). Anti-inflammatory drugs such as ibruprofen are available as elixir and can be useful for soft tissue injuries. Entonox (50% nitrous oxide, 50% oxygen) is a useful and rapid analgesia for children who are able to hold a mask or mouthpiece (Williams 1983). Its restrictions for use are the same as for adults. A safe dose is one which can be self-administered and it should not be used for children with chest and moderate to severe head injury. It is useful for dressings, suturing and prior to the administration of opiates.

Children with burn injuries and displaced fractures often require opiates. Ideally, these should be given intravenously because of faster action times and reduced risk of tissue storage associated with muscular injections following significant trauma (Skinner *et al.* 1991). Intravenous cannulation is not always possible in a distressed child and repeated attempts should be avoided; intramuscular administration could then be considered. Anti-emetics are not routinely used because of a greater risk of extrapyramidal reactions, particularly oculogyric crisis in children under 12 (Hopkins 1992).

Anaesthetic is useful for many procedures. Topical substances containing lignocaine are useful prior to non-urgent cannulation and venepuncture (Smith 1995). Local anaesthetic for suturing and wound cleansing not only provides pain control, but also helps to increase the child's cooperation. Regional nerve blocks are also an effective source of pain relief (Edwards 1994). A femoral block, for example, provides good pain control while X-raying and splinting a fractured femur (Advanced Life Support Group 1993).

Paediatric doses of analgesia should be calculated by the child's weight. It is useful for A&E departments to keep a child's doses book for quick dose/weight references. Good examples of these include the *Alder Hey Book of Childhood Doses* (1990) and *Paediatric Vade Mecum* (Insley 1990).

Fractures

The developmental process of the skeletal system is such that children are prone to greenstick fractures. These are usually a disruption of the bone cortex on one side as opposed to a complete break. A&E nurses must be prudent when assessing limb injuries in children. A child presenting with a greenstick fracture may have no external visible signs, and often the limb is neither swollen nor deformed.

Mechanism of injury is important, as is exact location of pain and extent of movement and pain association. It is often difficult to make this assessment if the child is very distressed and simple immobilisation may be useful until after X-ray. Most greenstick fractures will heal independently; however, it is common practice to immobilise the fracture with plaster for pain control. Occasionally greenstick fractures need surgical reduction because of deformity. Although children most commonly sustain greenstick fractures, they are not exempt from other types of fracture. Treatment for these are similar to that for adults, except that if reduction is necessary in children, it is preferable to carry out the procedure under general anaesthetic. Fractures through a growth plate, the cartilaginous disc between the epiphyses and metaphysis, need close monitoring by orthopaedic specialists (Morton & Phillips 1996).

If a child is discharged with a lower limb cast, her developmental dexterity must be considered. Many 5 to 7-year-olds may be unable to mobilise with crutches partly because of balance and partly because of the weight of the cast. In some cases, a Zimmer frame may be a better aid. Parents and children should be made aware of the risks and side-effects of an immobilised limb and be aware of local facilities for review and advice (see also Ch. 5).

Sports Injury

Children are becoming increasingly competitive, and this creates a potential for serious physical and psychological injury. Psychological problems are difficult to measure, whereas acute physical injury can be seen. There are three main types of musculo-skeletal injury associated with children's sport:

- osteochondritis
- stress fracture
- specific injury.

Osteochondritis refers to a group of conditions affecting the growth plate. The disorder results from the stresses produced at the bone/ligament junction or articular surfaces during physical activity. The most commonly affected areas include:

- metatarsals
- navicular
- lunate
- capitulum
- tibial tuberosity
- calcaneum.

Rest is usually sufficient to cure these injuries, but orthopaedic follow-up should be given (Morton & Philips 1996). Extensive training without a proper build-up period can lead to stress fractures. Runners and gymnasts are the most likely to incur these injuries. Sports injuries can be prevented with careful supervision, a gradual increase in training activity, and correction of poor technique or inappropriate use of equipment.

Abdominal Pain

Children in this age group often attend A&E with acute abdominal pain. Assessment and accurate diagnosis can sometimes be made difficult because of the age and level of cooperation by the child (Box 17.1). The most common reason for A&E attendance is as a result of gastroenteritis (Barkin & Rosen 1994). Urinary tract infection, constipation, appendicitis, pelvic inflammatory disease, menarche, period pain, ectopic pregnancy, inflammatory bowel disease and psychosomatic pain are all reasons for A&E attendance with abdominal pain. The history and development of pain provide many clues for diagnosis. Acute pain of sudden onset is usually due to obstruction, perforation or an ectopic pregnancy. A more insidious onset is indicative of appendicitis, and colicky pain is

---

Box 17.1 – *Assessment of abdominal pain*

The nurse should determine:
- The duration of pain
- The type of pain
- The severity of pain
- The exact location and any radiation
- Factors which worsen or improve pain
- The child's overall posture and level of activity
- Associated symptoms, such as vomiting, nausea, constipation, diarrhoea, dysuria/frequency and vaginal discharge, should be noted
- Any obvious social influences, such as problems at school or family stresses, should not be dismissed

---

usually associated with intestinal disorders such as gastroenteritis or inflammatory bowel disease.

Physical assessment should include pulse, respirations and blood pressure, temperature, skin tone, urinalysis, level of hydration and level of alertness (McGrath 1998). The aim of this is to identify the level of shock or toxicity the child may have. Management of acute abdominal pain should include treatment of shock, pain control and specialist opinion if surgical intervention is considered necessary.

Appendicitis

This condition is common to all age groups (Brunner & Suddarth 1990), and if it cannot be ruled out as the cause of abdominal pain, the child is usually admitted to hospital for observation. The child usually gives a history of moderate pain, commencing centrally and moving down to the right iliac fossa (RIF). These children are often off their food, but continue to drink. They complain of nausea, and may or may not give a history of vomiting. Altered bowel habits including constipation and diarrhoea may be present.

On assessment, children with appendicitis are moderately unwell, not usually shocked or highly toxic. The pulse rate may be raised, and the temperature can be normal or raised. Abdominal examination will reveal guarding and rebound tenderness in the RIF area. If appendicitis is suspected, early surgical intervention is indicated.

Mesenteric adenitis

The physical presentation is similar to appendicitis (Groggins & Higson 1985). The child is moderately unwell, not shocked and may have a pyrexia. It is the history of the child's illness which leads to diagnosis. The child will give a history of several days of mild gastroenteritis and other systemic infection. She will be off her food and drink, and complain of diffuse, intermittent colicky pain initially, then moderate pain settling in the RIF. This is caused by inflammation of the lymph nodes in the mesentery, which subsequently enlarge causing the pain. Depending on the severity of the condition, children with mesenteric ademitis are admitted for antibiotics and pain relief, or can be discharged with oral medication.

Constipation

Children with constipation, particularly in the younger part of this age group, often present to A&E with acute abdominal pain or rectal bleeding. They give a history of infrequent bowel activity, associated with small amounts of hard stools. They complain of several days' history of colicky abdominal pain, anorexia and nausea. Rectal bleeding is not uncommon, particularly in young children. Physical assessment usually reveals no abnormality. Examination of the abdomen reveals a loaded descending colon which can be confirmed on X-ray. Management of constipation includes relief of acute discomfort, either with suppositories or a micro-enema prior to discharge. In the majority of cases, the child can be treated at home with oral stool softeners and dietary advice. Most patients needed to be followed up by their GP or paediatric district nurse/health visitor.

Urinary tract infection

Children with a urinary tract infection (UTI) do not attend A&E with the textbook symptoms demonstrated in adults. A UTI should be considered in all children with undiagnosed malaise or pyrexia of unknown origin. Urinalysis is the most effective way to obtain a definitive diagnosis. It should be performed on any child presenting with dysuria, frequency and suprapubic pain, any child with a pyrexia for which the cause has not been established, children with haematuria, children with pain in the renal area, and any child with sudden onset of enuresis (Morton & Phillips 1996).

Diagnosis can be made by urinalysis, supported by microscopy, but specimens should also be cultured to determine the exact organisms causing infection. Children rarely need admission for UTIs unless they are vomiting and need intravenous rehydration. It is usual to discharge children with antibiotics and advice about increased fluid intake and hygiene. Parents should also be advised that follow-up from their GP is neccesary following a UTI.

Pelvic inflammatory disease and pregnancy

Attendances in A&E with sexually related conditions are not common in this age group. However, A&E staff should be alert to sexual causes of ill health in children with explicit behaviour or 'knowledge beyond their years'. Pregnancy is increasing in young girls, despite better sex education in schools. A&E nurses should sensitively seek to exclude it as a cause of ill health in young girls. The incidence of sexual abuse should not be underestimated as much of it remains undetected (Hobbs *et al.* 1992). This subject is discussed in greater detail in Chapter 16.

Consent

The Children Act (Department of Health 1989) implies that health care staff, including those working within A&E departments, should listen to children, provide them with appropriate information, and take account of their wishes and feelings (Oates 1993). The Act also makes it clear that the child's wishes are paramount and no court direction overrides the child's right of refusal provided he or she has sufficient understanding to make an informed decision.

Examination without consent may be held in law to be an assault and practitioners should take care not to coerce the child. The A&E nurse needs to use professional judgement to decide whether further advice is required if a child refuses to be assessed or to accept prescribed treatment. Oates (1993) suggested that the following questions may be helpful:

- Who has the right of consent?
- Who has parental responsibility?
- What are the child's views?
- Is there an instruction that an examination or assessment should not take place?
- Will the assessment be used in court proceedings?
- Is the child subject to a court order?

Ultimately, it is the doctor who has to decide on the child's ability to understand; however, the A&E nurse, through his understanding of the child's needs, can inform and influence the decision making process.

Health Promotion

Many opportunities exist for health promotion in A&E. The waiting area can be used in a variety of ways to target both parents and children with specific aspects of health promotion and accident prevention.

Attractive displays about the issue of cycle helmets or the prevention of skin cancer provide parents with practical common sense advice. Individual advice supported with written information can help to prevent recurrent accidents, as well as trouble shooting the specific incident. The problem of bullying may also be identified in A&E by a nurse, especially when a child has presented on several occasions with seemingly trivial conditions. The nurse can provide advice and support in the context of health promotion through advising the child and, if appropriate (with the child's permission), the parents of agencies such as Kidscape which offer useful guidance on managing this problem. Any aftercare advice should be directed at both parents and children in order to achieve optimum compliance (see also Ch. 33).

Conclusion

The needs of children between the ages of 5 and 14 vary considerably. The A&E nurse must have an awareness of the developmental stages of children in order to provide appropriate care. The A&E environment is important, as is the attitude of staff to children and their families. Optimum care results from a family-centred approach and involvement in care.

References

Advanced Life Support Group (1993) *Advanced Paediatric Life Support*. London: BMJ.

Alder Hey Book of Childhood Doses, 5th edn. (1990) Cambridge: Alder Hey Books.

Barkin RM, Rosen P (1994) *Abuse in Emergency Pediatrics: a Guide to Ambulatory Care* 4th edn. St Louis: Mosby.

Brunner LS, Suddarth DS (1990) *The Lippincott Manual of Paediatric Nursing*. London: Harper Row.

Cudmore J, Lakin K (1997) Child care in A&E: exploring the issues. *Emergency Nurse* 5(5), 10–11.

Department of Health (1989) *The Children Act 1989*. London: HMSO.

Department of Health (1991) *Welfare of Children and Young People in Hospital* London: HMSO.

Department of Health (1995) *Children's Charter*. London: Department of Health.

Edwards B (1994) Local and regional anaesthesia. *Emergency Nurse* 2(2), 10–15.

Groggins RC, Higson N (1985) *Common Paediatric Emergencies: a Guide for the GP and Casualty Officer*. Bristol: Wright.

Hobbs CJ, Hanks HGI, Wynne JM (1993) *Child Abuse and Neglect: a Clinicians' Handbook*. Edinburgh: Churchill Livingstone.

Hopkins SJ (1992) *Drugs and Pharmacology for Nurses*, 11th edn. Edinburgh: Churchill Livingstone.

Insley J (ed) (1990) *A Paediatric Vade-Mecum*, 12th edn. London: Edward Arnold.

McGrath A (1998) Abdominal examination and assessment in A&E. *Emergency Nurse* 6(4), 15–18.

Mead D, Sibert J (1991) *The Injured Child – an Action Plan for Nurses*. London: Scutari Press.

Morcombe J (1998) Reducing anxiety in children in A&E. *Emergency Nurse* 6(2), 10–13.

Morton RJ, Phillips BM (1996) *Accidents and Emergencies in Children* 2nd edn. Oxford: Oxford University Press.

Muller DJ, Harris PJ, Watley L (1986) *Nursing Children: Psychology, Research and Practice* London: Hodder and Stoughton.

Nunn J (1994) The use of aspirin in children under 12 years old attending a paediatric dentistry department in a dental hospital. *Health Trends* 26(1), 31–32.

Oates M (1993) Children Act 1989: the essential issues. *Emergency Nurse* 1(1), 21–22.

Partridge J (1997) Environmental provisions for children in A&E. *Emergency Nurse* 4(4), 7–9.

Piaget J (1969) *The Theory of Stages in Cognitive Development*. New York: McGraw-Hill.

Royal College of Nursing (1994) *The Care of Sick Children: a Review of the Guidelines in the Wake of the Allit Inquiry*. London: RCN.

Skinner D, Driscoll P, Earlam R (1991) *ABC of Major Trauma*. London: BMJ.

Smith C (1995) IV cannulation: principles and practice. *Emergency Nurse* 2(4), 16–18.

Swanwick M (1990) Knowledge and control. *Paediatric Nursing* 2(5), 18–20.

Whaley LF, Wong DL (1990) *Clinical Manual of Paediatric Nursing*, 3rd edn. St Louis: CV Mosby.

Williams J (1987) Managing paediatric pain. *Nursing Times* 83(36), 36–39.

Wilson-Barnett J (1979) *Stress in Hospitals: Patients' Psychological Reactions to Illness and Healthcare*. Edinburgh: Churchill Livingstone.

Woodward S (1994) A guide to paediatric resuscitation. *Paediatric Nursing* 6(2), 16–18.

Zacharias M, Watts D (1998) Pain relief in children. *British Medical Journal* 316, 1552.

Chapter 18

Adolescence

Lynda Holt

- Introduction
- Adolescent development
- Caring for the adolescent in A&E
- Personal fable
- Risk-taking behaviour
- Substance misuse
- Overdose
- Conclusion

Introduction

Adolescents represent only a small percentage of the total number of patients seen in A&E departments. Their care, however, needs to be specialised and related to their individual stage of development. This chapter will highlight the common areas of adolescent development, such as risk-taking behaviour, and explore them in relation to A&E attendance. Sensation seeking, leading to potentially deviant behaviour such as violent acts, substance misuse and self-harm, will also be considered as will the generic effects of illness and injury on adolescents. The impact of caring for adolescents on A&E nurses will also be examined. Optimum care environments and appropriate nursing skills will be discussed with regard to the quality of service offered to adolescents attending A&E.

Adolescent Development

The research on adolescent development is vast (Bee & Mitchell 1984, Erikson 1965). An understanding of adolescent development is essential for A&E nurses in their daily practice. Adolescence is a period in the life span where the individual, previously dependent on parents and carers for his values and identity, becomes independent, and in this move towards independence, attempts to establish a new and personal identity. The key factors in this process appear to relate to the onset of puberty, i.e. the physical and emotional changes leading to sexual maturity (Hinchliff *et al.* 1996), and the need for independence (Erikson 1965).

Cognitively, adolescents are capable of abstract thought and understand many variables within a situation. They should also be able to understand the consequences of their actions (Bernardo & Schenkel 1995). It is a period where group identity is vital, a time of experimentation with self-image, and a time to question fundamental family values. Adolescents are pushing for independence, testing the boundaries of their existing life and, importantly, hoping to find boundaries which will aid the development of their future identity (Kuykendall 1989).

Caring for the Adolescent in A&E

As a client group, adolescents are considered difficult to care for by the majority of nurses (Blunden 1988). In A&E, many causes of adolescent attendance can be viewed as self-inflicted, e.g. as a result of alcohol or substance testing, which may render A&E nurses less compassionate towards the patient. Caring for adolescents presents a particular challenge, as many nurses are just emerging from adolescence themselves. Kelly (1991) suggested that, to the adolescent, these nurses represent a more realistic role model, enhancing the opportunity for health education. This is particularly pertinent to A&E nurses because there is a greater likelihood of interaction with this age group at a time when they are physically and emotionally vulnerable.

Providing A&E nurses with a better idea of the process of adolescence may equip them more satisfactorily to meet their patients' needs, which will enable them to recognise normal behaviour instead of reacting to it (Holt 1993). Nurses are generally less aware of teenagers needs than those of other age groups (Gilles 1992). In A&E, adult care is the most familiar, and because of the associated anxiety, paediatric care is more often discussed or taught. An understanding of adolescent development (Erikson 1965) could help nurses in A&E to provide holistic care. It would also enable nurses to rationalise behaviour such as rebellion, non-conformity, antagonism and paranoia, which is frequently demonstrated in hospital (Blunden 1988), but is arguably the normal behaviour for an adolescent whose independence has been threatened by illness or injury (Kelly 1991).

Hospital staff, especially in A&E, are quick to meet the physical needs of these patients, such as maintaining a safe environment for the drunk teenager or arresting haemorrhage in a patient with slashed wrists, but often with little regard to their emotional needs (Kuykendall 1989). An understanding of these needs, however, could reduce the risk of confrontation and diminish any perceived power struggle. The question for A&E nurses is how far these needs can be facilitated within an A&E department without compromising the care or well-being of others in the environment.

As with all patients, initial assessment is the key to forming a therapeutic relationship, and the adolescent's response to illness and possible treatment can be quickly gauged, as well as existing coping strategies. Privacy has an important effect on the adolescent because of the significance of self-image; for instance, a wound assessment takes seconds but can cause great embarrassment. Ensuring privacy increases self-esteem and reinforces the adolescent's importance as an individual (Gilles 1992). Independence is often threatened by hospitalisation, even a short period in A&E. Including the patient in the care planning and decision-making reduces non-compliance and aggressive behaviour. Separation is greatly underestimated as a stress for adolescents (Blunden 1988). While they demand peer belonging and demonstrate independence, most need and want parental support (Bernardo & Schenkel 1995). Parents themselves often underestimate the support needed and the fears of adolescents. This may be because of swift medical and nursing intervention (Kelly 1991), aimed at promoting physical well-being. While A&E nurses are quick to include the parents of a sick child, perhaps because of the demonstrated independence of adolescents, this inclusion is often overlooked.

The adolescent patient needs to assert his independence, but is not yet ready to cope with the implications of this. In 'crisis' situations, as a visit to A&E is often perceived, the A&E nurse may be in a position of setting boundaries for the patient. This is not a negative action as it provides the security the adolescent indirectly seeks. All too often, however, on a busy shift, in a packed waiting room, antagonistic behaviour is allowed to escalate into confrontation, often because cues for boundaries have not been recognised by A&E nurses inexperienced in adolescent development. Consistency among staff is essential (Gilles 1997). Boundaries for acceptable behaviour should be decided as a matter of policy, and this should be made clear to patients on admission while respecting their independence and individuality. In addition, Knight & Rush (1998) argue that waiting rooms should be made more 'user-friendly' for adolescents, ideally incorporating separate waiting and treatment areas.

Illness or injury often induces developmental regression, forces the adolescent out of his peer group and imposes a fear of rejection. Even in a short admission to A&E, nurses need to work towards reducing this anxiety. It is paramount for adolescents to be cared for by staff who are comfortable with them, and can behave as adults, listening to them and respecting their needs. Adolescents are not children and, especially at times of high stress, do not respond well to being railroaded by A&E personnel who are threatened or irritated by their behaviour.

Personal Fable

Despite the upheaval and trauma of adolescence during this life phase, mortality is at its lowest, with the top cause of death being accident-related

(Department of Health 1992). An important cause of accident in adolescence is risk-taking behaviour, not just risky sports, but minor law infringement such as failure to wear a safety belt, exceeding speed limits and experimentation with alcohol and illegal substances.

A possible explanation of this is the concept of personal fable (Jack 1989) – a belief that despite risk-taking behaviour they will not be affected by life's difficulties. This has both a positive and a negative function, and represents normal cognitive development. Positively, it allows goals to be believed in and attainable, like dreams of success. Its negative function is that it induces risk-taking behaviour. Normally, consequences of actions are considered, but personal fable gives the security of invulnerability to consequences. This is not unique to adolescents; witness for example, smoking and lung cancer in older people (Winkenstein 1992).

Personal fable affects not only conformity with perceived authority, but also with chronic illnesses, such as diabetes. It is important for A&E nurses to understand this concept in order to intervene in the risk-taking behaviour which can result in an A&E attendance. Personal fable is there to protect the self-concept at the vulnerable time of adolescence. It allows conformity with peers despite negative consequences – for instance, the diabetic patient who presents in A&E with hypoglycaemia because he has been drinking to conform with peers. The patient can 'blot out' the likely hypoglycaemic attack because being the same is more important. Education and support from A&E nurses who understand that this behaviour is not intended to be self-destructive, but is normal adolescent experimentation, can reduce the risk of further occurrence. This perception of invulnerability may contribute to the statistic that the largest cause of adolescent death is from risk-taking – in cars, with fire arms, in water and with toxic substances (Jack 1989). Sensitive questioning helps adolescents expose their personal myth, recognise their irrationality and induce a change in behaviour.

Risk–taking Behaviour

Most common behaviours evolve from experimentation with alcohol, solvents, or drugs, but it can be hard for the busy A&E nurse to accept the drunk who is abusive as 'normal' when his behaviour is disruptive and difficult to contain. The majority of adolescents who attend A&E with drug- or alcohol-related problems are not abusive, and are there because of an injury or illness related to their risk-taking behaviour. These individuals often present with their peer groups and engage in sensation-seeking behaviour, which can appear threatening to A&E nurses. Adequate staffing levels and nurse skill mix, with appropriate back-up such as security officers and an incident alarm, should be available. Sensation-seeking is a normal need for experimentation and new experiences, and adolescents are prepared to take physical and social risks to attain these (Barker 1988). Despite risk-taking and sensation-seeking, most adolescents maintain conventional modes of behaviour and deviants are in the minority. A&E departments frequently treat adolescents as a result of risk-taking behaviour. A non-judgmental attitude is not always easy to foster, and the A&E nurse must be aware of her own vulnerability and biases, as well as understanding adolescent development. This enables the nurse to treat adolescents in an appropriate manner, reduces the risk of confrontation or resentment, and respects the adolescents, rights as individuals.

Not all adolescent risk-taking is because of a low perception of danger. Some revolves around deliberate self-harm. This is usually a cry for help from adolescents who cannot cope with the pressures of growing up. Self-poisoning is the most common reason for hospital treatment (McCallam 1990). Only the minority of adolescents take this route, and of these, the majority are not clinically depressed. This course of behaviour is not just a result of the strains of adolescence, identity confusion, anger and guilt, it is a way of getting back at those seen as responsible for the torment, such as parents, teachers and peers. A study of 100 children after overdose found that only 6% actually wanted to harm themselves, and over 50% had no idea of the risks associated with the pills taken, reinforcing the need for. health education. Those questioned did not consider death a real possibility (Donovan *et al.* 1985). Adolescent patients often demonstrate this by a blasé attitude towards their actions. Despite low suicide intent, the danger of real harm is great because of low risk awareness. Over 100 children and teenagers commit suicide in Britain every year (Lyall 1990).

It is vital that nurses are able to distinguish between normal behaviour and abnormal distress. This can only be achieved by listening to and hearing the adolescent. Nothing should be taken at face value, as the superficial self-confidence, and frequent mood changes common to teenagers can mask real and needy patients, as well as making them difficult to nurse. It is recognised that A&E is not the ideal place for in-depth discussion, but it may be the only opportunity available to the adolescent. An understanding of why the event occurred is essential before discharging the patient. The adolescent practice of 'dumping

Box 18.1 – *Penalties under Misuse of Drugs Act 1971*

Class A, schedule one
- *Simple possession*
  Maximum penalty on indictment is 7 years' imprisonment together with an unlimited fine

- *Possession with intent to supply*
- Possessing a class A, schedule one drug with intent to supply, either by sale or by gift, to another person carries a maximum penalty on indictment of life imprisonment together with an unlimited fine and the seizure of all drug related assets

- *Supplying to another*
  As for possession with intent to supply

- *Examples of class A, schedule one drugs*
  – LSD
  – magic mushrooms

Class A, schedule two
- *Simple possession*
  Maximum penalty on indictment is 14 years together with an unlimited fine

- *Possession with intent to supply*
  Possessing a class A, schedule two drug with intent to supply, either by sale or by gift, to another person carries a maximum penalty on indictment of life imprisonment together with an unlimited fine

- *Supplying to another*
  As for possession with intent to supply

- *Examples of class A, schedule two drugs*
  – cocaine
  – crack and freebase cocaine
  – heroin
  – methadone
  – ecstasy

Class B, schedule one
- *Simple possession*
  Maximum penalty on indictment is 5 years together with an unlimited fine
- *Possession with intent to supply*
  Possessing a class B, schedule one drug with intent to supply, either by sale or by gift, to another person carries a maximum penalty on indictment of 14 years' imprisonment together with an unlimited fine and the seizure of drug-related assets.

- *Supplying to another*
  As for possession with intent to supply

- *Examples of class B, schedule one drugs*
  – cannabis

Class B, schedule two
- *Simple possession*
  Maximum penalty on indictment is 5 years' imprisonment together with an unlimited fine
- *Possession with intent to supply*
  Possessing a class B, schedule two drug with intent to supply, either by sale or by gift, to another person carries a maximum penalty on indictment of 14 years' imprisonment together with an unlimited fine and the seizure of drug-related assets

- *Supplying to another*
  As for possession with intent to supply

Box 18.1 (*Contd*)

- *Examples of class B, schedule two drugs*
  - amphetamines
  - methylamphetamine

Class B, schedule three
- *Simple possession*
  Maximum penalty on indictment is 5 years' imprisonment together with an unlimited fine

- *Possession with intent to supply*
  Possessing a class B, schedule three drug with intent to supply, either by sale or by gift, to another person carries a maximum penalty on indictment of 5 years' imprisonment together with an unlimited fine

- *Supplying to another*
  As for possession with intent to supply

- *Examples of class B, schedule three drugs*
  Tranquillisers

---

distress' on others via self-harm must be controlled and appropriate coping strategies learned in order to prevent further real harm. The A&E nurse has a key role to play, by providing constructive advice and follow-up arrangements where appropriate, not by punitive intervention.

Substance Misuse

Within the past 10–15 years, the worldwide drug culture has evolved dramatically, stemming from two developments. First, the major consumer generation has shifted sharply towards the young, especially adolescent and young adult males; and second, the availability of drugs has become much more widespread (Emmett & Nice 1996). In the UK, around 20–30% of people aged 16–59 years, and about half of those aged 16–29, have taken an illegal substance at some time (Ramsey & Percy 1996). Recent use, which is more likely to reflect regular use, is also highest among people aged 16–29 years, especially if they live in an inner city or are unemployed; up to 18% will have taken one drug, and around 5% will have taken two or more, in the previous month (Ramsey & Percy 1996). In 1994, over 1600 deaths were attributed to misuse of illegal drugs (Home Office 1996). While substance misuse is clearly a problem for young adults as well as adolescents, for convenience the subject will be addressed in this chapter.

In addition, the growth of the rave scene in Britain and designer drugs such as ecstasy, which appear to have become accepted by many as an integral part of relaxation and pleasure, have resulted in a culture in which substance misuse is no longer perceived as an antisocial activity, but where penalties for use and supply are severe (see Box 18.1 and Table 18.1). While the A&E nurse will be aware that alcohol is a major causative factor in attendances, there has been a marked increase in attendances as a consequence of other substance misuse.

The mild, moderate and severe effects of drugs of abuse are outlined in Tables 18.2–18.4.

Alcohol

Alcohol is a central nervous system depressant. It is absorbed into the bloodstream and starts to have an effect within 5–10 minutes of drinking. The rate of absorption is affected by sex, weight, duration of drinking, nature of drink consumed, food in the stomach, physiological factors, genetic variation and rate of elimination. Paton (1994) suggested that there are 4 million heavy drinkers in the UK, of whom 800 000 are problem drinkers and 400 000 are alcohol-dependent. Concomitant misuse of alcohol is common among drug misusers (Anonymous 1997). Signs, symptoms and management of alcohol intoxication are addressed in Chapter 14.

Ecstasy

Ecstasy is a synthetic hallucinogenic form of amphetamine. It was first synthesised in Germany in 1910 and patented as an appetite suppressant. It failed commercially and did not reappear until the late 1980s when it became associated with the 'rave' scene. In its pure form, it is seen as a white powder, but is usually found as tablets or capsules. The colour will depend on any colouring agents that have been added. Ecstasy

Table 18.1 – *Language of substance misuse (Emmet & Nice 1996)*

Word	Meaning
Acid	LSD
Bad trip	A frightening or unpleasant LSD trip
Banging up	To inject drugs
Blow	Herbal cannabis
Buzzing	Feelings after use of ecstasy
Chill out	A period of cooling down to reduce risk of overheating from ecstasy use
Clean	Not using drugs
Coke	Cocaine
Crack	Freebase cocaine
Cut	To mix other substances with a drug to add bulk and weight
Detox	To withdraw from drugs under medical supervision
Dope	Resin and herbal cannabis
Doves	Ecstasy tablets with dove imprint
'E'	Ecstasy
Eggs	Temazepam tablets
Flashback	Tripping out again some time after LSD use. Can be days, months or even years later and is usually a bad trip (q.v.)
GBH	Gamma hydroxybutyrate or sodium oxybate, a liquid hallucinogenic stimulant
Grass	Herbal cannabis
'H'	Heroin
Hash	Cannabis resin
High	The feeling of elation while under the influence of a drug
Hit	To buy or inject drugs
Jack up	To inject drugs
Jellies	Temazepam in capsule form
Joint	A hand-rolled cannabis cigarette
Magic mushrooms	Any of the species of hallucinogenic mushrooms
Main lining	Injecting drugs
Marijuana	Herbal cannabis
Moggies	Mogadon sleeping pills
Poppers	Amyl/alkyl/butyl nitrate
Pot	Cannabis resin
Rock	Freebase cocaine
Score	To purchase drugs
Shoot up	To inject drugs
Smack	Heroin
Snorting	Sniffing cocaine or other drug up the nose
Speed	Amphetamine
Stash	An amount of drugs, usually hidden
Trip	A hallucinogenic experience under LSD
Wacky bacci	Herbal cannabis
Whiz	Amphetamine
Works	Needles and syringes

tablets frequently have images of animals or birds imprinted on them. Ecstasy is generally taken orally and is very rarely injected or smoked (Milroy 1999).

For most users, ecstasy provides a feeling of euphoria, together with an increase in confidence, serenity and empathy towards other people. As an amphetamine derivative, it is also provides users with feelings of energy and freedom from hunger. While adverse reactions are rare, Cook (1995) and Preston (1992) described the presenting signs of severe reaction as convulsion and collapse, dilated pupils, hypotension, tachycardia, hyperpyrexia and death from disseminated intravascular coagulation. Walsh (1996) suggested that signs which should alert an A&E nurse

Table 18.2 – *Mild clinical effects of drugs of abuse (Schofield et al. 1997)*

Clinical effects	MDMA	Amphetamine	Cocaine	Cannabis	LSD
Gastrointestinal effects	✓	✓	✓	✓	✓ (i.v.)
Dilated pupils	✓	✓	✓	✓ (child)	✓
Dry mouth	✓	✓		✓	
Slurred speech			✓	✓ (high dose)	
Salivation					✓
Appetite stimulation				✓	
Chest discomfort		✓	✓		
Agitation	✓	✓	✓	✓ (high dose)	✓
Relaxation				✓	
Tremor	✓	✓	✓	✓ (child)	✓
Ataxia			✓	✓ (child)	✓
Sweating	✓	✓	✓	✓ (child)	
Mild increase in body temperature	✓	✓	✓		
Trismus (jaw clenching)	✓	✓	✓		
Bruxism (teeth grinding)	✓	✓	✓		

Table 18.3 – *Moderate clinical effects of drugs of abuse (Schofield et al. 1997)*

Clinical effects	MDMA	Amphetamine	Cocaine	Cannabis	LSD
Headache	✓	✓	✓	✓	✓ (i.v.)
Hypertonia	✓		✓		✓
Hypotonia				✓	
Hyperreflexia	✓	✓	✓		✓
Hyperventilation	✓	✓	✓		✓ (i.v.)
Incontinence			✓		
Extrapyramidal symptoms	✓		✓		
Tachycardia	✓	✓	✓	✓ (high dose)	✓
Hypertension	✓	✓	✓	✓	
Hallucinations	✓	✓	✓	✓ (high dose)	✓
Paranoia	✓		✓	✓ (high dose)	
Palpitations	✓	✓	✓	✓	
Dehydration	✓	✓			
Hypothermia				✓ (child)	
Drowsiness			✓	✓	

to an ecstasy-induced collapse include admission from a late night party or rave of a previously fit young person who has collapsed for no apparent reason. Some deaths have been related to cerebral oedema secondary to excess water ingestion, because the drug has an antidiuretic effect on the kidney.

The control of the patient's temperature is key to survival, as temperatures of up to 42°C are not uncommon. Cool replacement fluids should be given at as fast a rate as the patient can tolerate and unnecessary clothing should be removed. A brisk fluid-led diuresis should be encouraged; however, if this does not control the rise in temperature then endotracheal intubation, sedation and paralysis will be instituted (Henry *et al.* 1992). If the temperature continues to rise, dantrolene may be used. This has muscle-relaxant properties and is used in the treatment of malignant hyperthermia following anaesthetic hypersensitivity (Jones 1993).

A central venous catheter should be inserted to measure and guide the rapid dehydration of the patient, and a urinary catheter to monitor renal function. The colour of the urine should be observed for an orange tinge which is suggestive of rhabdomyolysis, the breakdown of skeletal muscle, due to the toxic effects of released globins. Blood tests

Table 18.4 – *Severe clinical effects of drugs of abuse (Schofield et al. 1997)*

Clinical effects	MDMA	Amphetamine	Cocaine	Cannabis	LSD
Pyrexia	✓	✓	✓	✓	✓ (mild)
Delirium	✓	✓	✓		✓
Hypotension	✓	✓	✓	✓ (high dose)	
Convulsions	✓	✓	✓		✓ (i.v.)
Hypoxia	✓		✓		
Coma	✓	✓	✓	✓ (child)	✓ (i.v.)
Arrhythmias/dysrhythmias	✓	✓	✓		
Myocardial infarction			✓		
Rhabdomyolysis	✓	✓	✓		✓ (i.v.)
Renal failure	✓	✓	✓		✓ (i.v.)
Disseminated intravascular coagulation (DIC)	✓	✓	✓		✓ (i.v.)
Pulmonary oedema			✓		✓ (i.v.)
Adult respiratory distress syndrome (ARDS)	✓				
Subarachnoid/intrac erebral haemorrhage	✓	✓	✓		

for creatinine kinase may be ordered to measure this process. Other blood tests may include regular clotting tests, and the patient should be closely observed for clinical signs of coagulation problems. The picture of disseminated intravascular coagulation, falling platelet and fibrinogen count, raised PT and KCCT is an ominous sign (Jones 1993).

Cannabis

Cannabis is the most commonly used illegal drug in the world. It is the collective term for all psychoactive substances derived from the dried leaves and flowers of the plant *Cannaibis sativa* (Schofield *et al*. 1997). It may be smoked or eaten in food. If smoked, its effects appear within 10–30 minutes and the effects have a duration of 4–8 hours. If eaten, it takes approximately 1 hour to produce its effects. Cannabis comes in three forms:

- **herbal** – a dried plant material, similar to coarse cut tobacco and sometimes compressed into blocks
- **resin** – dried and compressed sap, found in blocks of various sizes, shapes and colours
- **oil** – this is rare, it is extracted from the resin by the use of a chemical solvent and ranges in colour from dark green or dark brown to jet black with a distinctive smell like rotting vegetation.

After use, cannabis has the effect of creating feelings of relaxation, happiness, increased powers of concentration, sexual arousal, loss of inhibitions, increased appetite and talkativeness. There is little evidence that smoking cannabis is harmful in the short term, but users will develop a strong psychological habituation with continued use. Withdrawal effects include disturbed sleep patterns, anxiety, panic and restlessness. It is with these effects that patients may present to the A&E department and they should be managed symptomatically.

Amphetamine

Amphetamines are central nervous system stimulants whose action resembles those of adrenaline. They produce a sensation of euphoria and exhilaration as well as increased energy, stamina and strength. They may be injected intravenously, ingested or smoked. Absorbed by the gastrointestinal tract they may have an effect within 20 minutes of ingestion; however, the effects are immediate if injected and last 4–6 hours. They are most commonly seen in the form of a coarse off-white/pink crystalline powder with an average purity of less than 5%.

Signs and symptoms of intoxication include tachypnoea, tachycardia, dilation of pupils, dry mouth, pyrexia, blurring of vision, dizziness and loss of coordination. The after-effects of lethargy and fatigue can last for several days. Since tolerance develops rapidly, individual response varies greatly, and toxicity correlates poorly with dose. Fatalities are rarely reported but predominantly result from convulsions and intracranial haemorrhage. Sedatives, such as chlorpromazine, and antihypertensives may be used for management of the patient.

Cocaine

Cocaine is derived from the leaves of the coca bush, *Erythoxylon coca*, or may be synthesised artificially. It is commonly seen as a white crystalline powder with a sparkling appearance. It is a central nervous system stimulant and is commonly sniffed through the nose or taken by intravenous injection. Effects are felt within a few minutes and last up to half an hour. It may also be neutralised to produce 'crack', which is a potent form of cocaine made by mixing it with baking soda, heating it and then smoking it in cigarettes or a pipe. If smoked or injected, the effects are immediate and last 10–15 minutes. 'Speedballing' or 'snowballing' is a technique particularly prone to fatality and involves mixing cocaine and heroin and injecting the mixture.

The effects of use include feelings of energy, strength, exhilaration, euphoria, confidence and well-being. Users often become very talkative. Adverse effects include agitation, panic and feelings of persecution or threat. Regular use can damage nasal passages and cause exhaustion and weight loss. Tolerance rapidly develops with continued use, and marked physical and psychological addiction occurs. Fatalities may rapidly occur secondary to convulsion, intracranial haemorrhage, intestinal ischaemia, respiratory arrest or cardiac arrhythmias. Sedatives, such as haloperidol, diazepam for convulsions and antihypertensives may be required as part of the management regime in A&E.

Heroin

Opiates such as heroin are analgesics that depress the central nervous system through suppression of noradrenaline. In its pure pharmaceutical form, heroin is a pure white, fine-grained powder. Medicinally, it is known as diamorphine and is used for severe pain, including chest pain. In its street forms it is coarser and varies in colour from a pinkish cream to dark brown. Heroin can be smoked, sniffed or injected. Intravenous injection (mainlining) results in an almost instantaneous effect ('rush'). It generates feelings of euphoria and inner peace, freedom from fear, worry, pain, hunger and cold, and can last 2–6 hours.

Its adverse effects include depressed breathing, severe constipation, nausea and vomiting. In acute intoxication, symptoms include pinpoint pupils, depression of heart rate and respiration, and suppression of the cough reflex. Severe physical and psychological dependence can occur with continued use. Heroin use carries a high risk of overdose, as the street strength of the drug, which is usually around 20% can range from 10% to over 60%. In cases of overdose, naloxone is a specific opioid antagonist and is given in a dose of 0.4 mg which can be repeated at intervals of 2–3 minutes up to a maximum of 10 mg.

Methadone

Methadone is a synthetic opiate analgesic which is frequently prescribed by specific medical practitioners, usually GPs or drug clinic physicians. It is used in the treatment of heroin addiction to control withdrawal symptoms. It can be used orally or by injection and generates similar feelings to heroin use, with similar signs, symptoms and management as heroin overdose.

Overdose

The incidence of self-harm, of which 90% of cases involve self-poisoning, now accounts for around 20% of admissions to general medical wards and is the most frequent reason for admission to hospital in young female patients (Merson & Baldwin 1995). Poisonings can be categorised into three groups: accidental, intentional and iatrogenic. Accidental poisoning most commonly occurs among young children, although death is relatively uncommon. Intentional ingestion includes recreational drug use and suicide attempts. Iatrogenic poisoning usually results from unanticipated drug interactions (Zull 1995). In cases of intentional poisoning the A&E nurses should ascertain which drugs have been taken by asking the patient or attending friends or relatives (see Box 18.2).

Harding-Price (1993) noted, however, that the Children Act gives children under the age of 16 the right to refuse consent to treatment. Castledine (1994) stressed the importance of establishing a good relationship with the patient, but in all cases a patient must consent if care is to be given or he can sue for assault and battery. Castledine suggested that if a patient is mentally confused due the physical effects of illness or as a consequence of mind-altering drugs, the A&E nurse could proceed to treat on the basis of urgency and necessity. Careful recording of the patient's details, and the nursing and medical staffs' actions are important in such cases.

Conclusion

Adolescent attendance patterns highlight the need for A&E nurses to understand the normal processes through which adolescents pass. Nurses can appear judgmental and less sympathetic towards a patient

Box 18.2 – *Information to be determined when interviewing a patient following drug overdose*

- What was ingested? Was anyone present at the time to verify the history? Are there any empty or partially filled bottles at home or elsewhere?

- How much was taken? If pill bottles are available, calculate the number of missing tablets from the initial amount prescribed, taking into account the date on the prescription

- What was time of the ingestion? The nurse must take into account the time at which the person was last seen and when symptoms of intoxication began if the timing is not clear

- What was the route of the poisoning, i.e. oral, intravenous, smoked, inhaled, snorted, subcutaneous?

- Does the patient have a history of substance misuse, depression or schizophrenia?

- What is the patient's medical history, past and present prescription drugs, and allergies?

perceived as being responsible for his own illness (Lyall 1990). A&E nurses can be affected by the apparent lack of compliance from adolescent patients. This can lead to paternalisms or confrontational behaviour which destroys the therapeutic relationship and exacerbates conflict. Adolescents cannot be treated wholly as adults as they lack the emotional maturity to cope with independence and still need the emotional support of parents and other carers (Kelly 1991). A&E attendance is often a result of normal adolescent behaviour and A&E nurses should be equipped with the knowledge necessary to provide appropriate support and education. An environment which provides boundaries, privacy and protected independence, with support, and peer support if appropriate, should be developed.

It is important to remember that psychological distress can be just as great as physical illness or trauma. A&E nurses have a responsibility to consider the needs of young people as individuals. Perhaps an alteration of attitude is more important than a vast financial outlay in the improvement of adolescent care.

Further reading

Stark M, Payne-James J (1996) *Symptoms and Signs of Substance Misuse*. London: Greenwich Medical Media.

References

Anonymous (1997) Helping patients who misuse drugs. *Drugs and Therapeutics Bulletin* **35**(3), 18–22.

Barker P (1988) *Basic Child Psychiatry*. Oxford: Blackwell.

Bee H, Mitchell S (1984) *The Developing Person*. New York: Harper & Row.

Bernardo LM, Schenkel KA (1995) Pediatric medical emergencies. In: Kitt S, Selfridge-Thomas J, Proehl JA, Kaiser J, eds. *Emergency Nursing: a Physiologic and Clinical Perspective*. Philadelphia: WB Saunders.

Blunden R (1988) An artificial state. *Paediatric Nursing*, **3**, 12–13.

Castledine G (1994) Ethics and law in A&E. *Emergency Nurse*, **2**(1), 25.

Cook A (1995) Ecstasy (MDMA): alerting users to the dangers. *Nursing Times*, **91**(16), 32–33.

Department of Health (1992) *Health of the Nation*. London: HMSO.

Donovan DM, Queiser HR, Salzberg PM *et al.* (1985) Intoxicated and bad drivers: subgroups within same population of high risk drivers. *Journal of Studies in Alcohol*, **46**(5), 375–382.

Emmett D, Nice G (1996) *Understanding Drugs: a Handbook for Parents, Teachers and other Professionals*. London: Jessica Kingsley.

Erikson E (1965) *Childhood and Society*. Harmondsworth: Penguin.

Gilles M (1992) Teenage traumas. *Nursing Times*, **88**(27), 58.

Harding-Price D (1993) A sensitive response without discrimi-

nation: drug misuse in children and adolescents. *Professional Nurse*, **April**, 419–422.

Henry J, Jeffreys KJ, Dawling S (1992) Toxicity and deaths from 3, 4 methylenedioxymethamphetamine ('ecstasy'). *Lancet*, **340**, 384–387.

Hinchliff SM, Montague SE, Watson R (1996) *Physiology for Nursing Practice*, 2nd edn. London: Baillière Tindall.

Holt L (1993) The adolescent in accident & emergency. *Nursing Standard*, **8**(8), 30–34.

Home Office (1996) Statistics of drug addicts notified to the Home Office. *Issue 15/96*. London: Home Office.

Jack M (1989) Personal fable. *Journal of Pediatric Nursing*, **4**(5), 334–338.

Jones C (1993) MDMA: the doubts surrounding ecstasy and the response of the emergency nurse. *Accident & Emergency Nursing*, **1**, 193–198.

Kelly J (1991) Caring for adolescents. *Professional Nurse*, **6**(9), 498–501.

Knight S, Rush H (1998) Providing facilities for adolescents in A&E. *Emergency Nurse*, **6**(4), 22–26.

Kuykendall J (1989) Teenage traumas. *Nursing Times*, **85**(27), 26–28.

Lyall J (1990) A time to listen. *Nursing Times*, **86**(14), 16–17.

McCallam I (1990) Growing pains. *Nursing Times*, **86**(34), 62–64.

Merson S, Baldwin D (1995) *Psychiatric Emergencies*. Oxford: Oxford University Press.

Milroy CM (1999) Ten years of 'ecstasy'. *Journal of the Royal Society of Medicine*, **92**, 68–72.

Paton A (1994) *ABC of Alcohol Abuse*. London: BMJ.

Preston A (1992) Pointing out the risk. *Nursing Times*, **88**, 24–26.

Ramsey M, Percy A (1996) Drug misuse declared: results of the 1994 British Crime Survey. *Home Office Research Study 151*. London: Home Office.

Schofield E, Lawman S, Volans G, Henry J (1997) Drugs of abuse: clinical features and management. *Emergency Nurse*, **5**(6), 17–22.

Walsh M (1996) *Accident & Emergency Nursing: a New Approach*, 3rd edn. Oxford: Butterworth-Heinemann.

Winkenstien M (1992) Adolescent Smoking. *Journal of Pediatric Nursing*, **7**(2), 120–127.

Zull DN (1995) Poisoning and drug overdose. In: Kitts, Selfridge-Thomas J, Prochl JA, Kaiser J, eds. *Emergency Nursing: a Physiologic and Clinical Perspective*, 2nd edn. Philadelphia: WB Saunders.

Chapter 19

Young Adults

Judy Davies

■ Introduction
■ Sporting injuries
■ Road traffic accidents
■ Alcohol-related attendances
■ Accidents related to sexual activity
■ Psychological illnesses in young adults
■ Conclusion

Introduction

Young adults attending A&E are at the peak of life's activity cycle, both physically and sexually. The age group 18–39 years is not, however, homogeneous in its characteristics as it encompasses the period of time in the life cycle from experimentation to full maturity.

As young adults mature from adolescence and settle down, the pattern changes. They have families, face financial burdens, have challenges at work or out of work, and may lack traditional family support. Partnership, pregnancy and parenthood may bring a sense of stability and responsibility, although these also carry the risk of stress-related illnesses. For many, the fun of youth is lost too quickly and the responsibilities of adult life come too soon. This chapter will consider the range of physical and psychological ailments that affect young adults.

Sporting Injuries

Many people's leisure activities involve some kind of sport and this is especially so in the young adult male. Women are less likely to take part in sports activities, and with age there is a decreasing participation among both sexes in all sports except bowls. (Department of Health 1992). It was probably not envisaged that a campaign to encourage people to take more exercise and to be involved in health education programmes, such as 'Look after your heart', would have the direct consequence of increasing the numbers of personal injuries.

The range of injuries seen in the A&E department will vary with the sports location and season as well as the mechanism of injury (Renstrom 1994) (Table 19.1). Overuse injuries come from repetitive activity and are common in sports in which endurance is a factor, e.g. long distance running, swimming and aerobics (Sperryn 1994). Overload injuries are more common and may be the result of overloading one's own tissues, such as an Achilles rupture, or by an outside force, as in contact sports such as football, rugby or vehicular sports.

Table 19.1 – *Sports-related injuries*

Sport	Potential injuries
Boxing	Cumulative brain damage, ocular injuries, lacerations, nasal fractures
Football/rugby	Spinal cord injuries, head injuries, knee strains, fractures, groin strains, lacerations
Running	Lower extremity injuries, strains, sprains
Skiing	Head injuries, lower extremity fractures, exposure to elements
Horse riding	Head injuries, crush injuries, spinal injuries

In the young adult the muscles are the greatest points of weakness. The knee is the most vulnerable point in children under 15; after this and up to the age of 19 the pelvis is the weakest, with avulsion fractures commonly occurring. From 19 to 30 years of age the hamstring and quadriceps muscles are especially vulnerable. After the age of 30 the tendons start to degenerate and become weaker than the muscles (Noble 1990). A study funded by the Sports Council suggested that annually between 1 and 1.5 million injuries caused by sport resulted in A&E attendance and a further 4–5 million injuries resulted in temporary incapacity (Nicholl *et al.* 1991).

Eighty-two per cent of all patients with sporting injuries are not detained in hospital and are treated in the A&E department with possible subsequent referral to orthopaedic or physiotherapy clinics. Attendances at these clinics can be greatly reduced by employing a full-time physiotherapist to work in A&E (Bakewell 1993). Sporting injuries benefit from quick physiotherapy: haematomas are prevented from fibrosing and long-term injuries avoided (Wardrope & English 1998). The educational value of employing a physiotherapist could be enormous for junior medical staff, for the A&E nurse and, most importantly, for the patient.

Although most sports injuries are minor, vigilant triage is essential to identify and prioritise the more serious sports injuries. Head, chest and long bone injuries sometimes result from sports activities; 18% of patients in spinal injury units have sustained their injury as a result of a sporting activity (Grundy *et al.* 1991), particularly rugby, horse riding and motor sports. These serious injuries can have long-term implications for a young person. Paralysis, brain damage or serious reduction in mobility will almost certainly lead to loss of earnings, relationship and sexual problems, depression and a very altered lifestyle.

Road Traffic Accidents

Young adults are the largest accident risk group (Department of Health 1992). In the under 35 age group, injury is the commonest cause of death and has been described as 'the last great plague of the young' (Skinner *et al.* 1991).

Many of the more serious injuries of adulthood result from road traffic accidents (RTAs). Most of the pedestrian deaths seen in the A&E department will be children and elderly people, but those dying in cars are predominantly young adults. In addition, for each fatality on the roads there are 12.6 serious injuries and 50.2 minor injuries (Office of Population Census and Surveys 1991). The number of pedestrian deaths have remained more or less consistent since 1953, but fatalities from motor vehicles, motorcycles and push bikes have dropped by about one-third. This reduction has been largely attributed to changing legislation. The imposition of speed restrictions and attention to safer road design by the Ministry of Transport have contributed to falling road deaths. These dropped by 14% when severe petrol shortages in 1973–1975 forced the government to impose a national speed limit of 50 mph.

A disproportionately high number of people involved in RTAs have consumed alcohol, and these people are the most likely to sustain serious injuries; 20% of all fatalities are alcohol-related and at night this figure rises to 60% (Department of Health 1992). Legislation limiting the engine capacity of motorcycles that learners can ride and the introduction of a two-part test have led to a 40% reduction in those killed or seriously injured on motorbikes since 1983 (Department of Transport 1989). The mandatory use of seat belts, introduced in 1981, has considerably reduced motor vehicle deaths; however, while the number of fatal head injuries has declined, a pattern of blunt abdominal trauma has emerged (Cope & Stebbings 1996). The introduction of the mountain bike has led to a huge surge in the popularity of cycling, with off-road cycling and safety helmets helping to lessen the number of accidents.

The Transport Road Research Laboratory has estimated that, while 28% of accidents involve environmental factors and 8.5% vehicular factors, human error is clearly responsible for most accidents, although this may be a direct result of inexperience (Sabey & Staughton 1975). The number of road accidents in the over 25s declines quickly as experience and social maturity develop (see Tables 19.2 and 19.3). Although

Table 19.2 – *Deaths from motor vehicle accidents in England (1991)*

Age (years)	Male No.	Male %	Female No.	Female %
< 5	41	1.4	25	2.0
5–14	146	5.1	71	5.7
15–24	893	31.5	236	18.9
25–34	537	18.9	108	8.7
35–44	300	10.6	89	7.1
45–54	239	8.4	88	7.1
55–64	180	6.3	110	8.8
65–74	223	7.9	188	15.1
75–84	227	8.0	253	20.3
> 85	49	1.7	80	6.4
Total	**2835**		**1248**	

Table 19.3 – *Deaths from motorcycle accidents in England (1991)*

Age (years)	Drivers Male	Drivers Female	Passengers Male	Passengers Female
< 14	0	0	1	0
15–24	232	9	11	15
25–34	130	2	4	6
35–44	59	2	1	1
45–54	22	1	1	1
55–64	9	0	0	0
65–74	9	3	0	0
> 75	2	0	0	0
Total	**463**	**17**	**18**	**23**

legislation and attention to environmental issues have reduced the number of road deaths, the problems of inexperience, immaturity, impetuosity and sometimes lack of control are harder to address.

Alcohol–related Attendances

Only 17% of the population admits to total abstinence, while the remaining 83% have very different drinking habits. Occupations, genetic and parental influences, life events, peer pressure and personality all have an effect on alcohol consumption. Alcohol-related attendances in the A&E department may be prompted by injuries, intoxication, medical problems or antisocial behaviour. The former two reasons are most common in the young adult who has had a single episode of heavy drinking, while the latter two are common in the older, habitual heavy drinker.

The intoxicated patient brought to A&E needs a thorough initial assessment. It is tempting at triage to assess these patients as 'drunk', do an alcometer reading and put them to the back of the queue. However, Ellis *et al.* (1992) advise that, due to the high incidence of trauma in patients with alcohol intoxication, A&E staff should be aware of the possibility of non-obvious physical injury, including cervical spine and head injury, when assessing an intoxicated patient.

Alcoholic coma

Alcoholic coma can be a serious medical emergency requiring admission to hospital. The A&E nurse should be aware that a patient's condition can move from mild to life-threatening as previously ingested alcohol and/or drugs are absorbed (Taylor & Ryrie 1996). Most deaths occur because of respiratory depression or aspiration. Deep alcoholic coma should be treated aggressively with a cuffed endotracheal tube, oxygen and ventilation. If low blood sugar levels necessitate glucose, it should be accompanied by intravenous thiamine. Otherwise, when carbohydrate metabolism begins again, low levels of B_1 (thiamine) will precipitate Wernicke's encephalopathy, which consists of ocular muscle palsies, nystagmus, ataxic gait and progressive mental impairment. A patient in alcohol withdrawal is generally dehydrated and orthostatic. Hypoglycaemia, acidosis, hypovolaemia and electrolyte disturbance need treatment with intravenous fluids, CVP line, blood gases, glucose and thiamine.

Zull (1995) noted that, in addition to correction of dehydration and electrolyte abnormalities, the patient may require sedative therapy. Minimal tremulousness in a patient with normal mental status may not require any tranquilliser therapy. However, the patient who is agitated, hallucinating or having seizures, or who has evidence of autonomic hyperactivity, such as fever and tachycardia, should be calmed rapidly. The benzodiazepine sedatives are the preferred agents and diazepam can be given at 15–30 minute intervals, after which the dose and frequency should be decreased or a switch to an oral route made. Drugs such as haloperidol and chlorpromazine are generally avoided because they may increase the risk of seizures. If seizures occur, i.v. diazepam is the treatment of choice.

Many young adults are ill informed about safe drinking patterns. Alcohol education continues to receive a low priority in both policy and resources and it is believed that isolated campaigns to educate the public are ineffective (King's Fund 1991). Increased alcohol consumption is always followed by increased deaths from cirrhosis, public drunkenness, drink driving offences and psychiatric admissions (Central Policy Review Staff 1982), so education of the young is essential. All A&E departments will have their own regular patients who are heavy drinkers, many of whom will be in their 20s or 30s. Apart from acute intoxication, they may present with other medical and psychological problems. The most common medical problems are gastritis, haematemesis, oesophageal varices, fits and trauma. Psychological problems include parasuicide, depression and acute anxiety attacks, which will be considered elsewhere in this book.

Accidents Related to Sexual Activity

The peak of life's sexual activity occurs in young adulthood. Many young men and women come to the accident department because of their sexually related activities. This may be due to accidents, because the GP is unable to obtain a more appropriate referral or because of embarrassment and distress. All of these patients need to be treated with tact and confidentiality by an experienced nurse. It is not the A&E nurse's role to question patients' sexual activities and preferences and it is essential that problems are discussed in a private place, preferably with staff of the same sex. Patients should not be interrogated in depth at the reception desk. A history of rape, buggery, incest, transsexualism or transvestism may be reasons for a patient refusing to remove clothing or declining to see a doctor of a particular sex.

Genital trauma may bring an acutely embarrassed patient to the A&E department. Sexual intercourse can cause lacerations to the vagina and penis, which can bleed profusely. Human bites to the penis can pose a serious problem and are associated with a 50% infection rate (Wolfe *et al.* 1992). Suturing, with the additional help of ice packs and pressure to the penis, will usually stop the bleeding. The young uncircumcised male may also come to A&E with a paraphimosis after his first sexual encounter. This can normally be reduced using lignocaine and ice packs, followed by manipulation of the retracted foreskin. For entrapment of the foreskin in a zip, similar treatment can be used. Usually, this can be accomplished by slowly and methodically unzipping the zipper. The application of mineral oil to the zip and entrapped foreskin may ease and prevent the use of invasive techniques (Kanegaye & Schonfield 1993). Tetanus prophylaxis should be considered.

Both male and female patients come to the A&E department with foreign bodies in their rectum, vagina or urethra, although they may initially complain of abdominal pain, constipation or rectal bleeding. Many of these patients can be treated without admission, but the sexual use of vibrators or other objects may cause serious injury and perforation of the bowel. Presenting complaints include gross haematuria, lower abdominal pain and possible urinary retention. Fever may also be present if the foreign body has been in situ for a while. Physical examination may reveal the foreign body palpable in, or protruding from, the urethra. There may be a discharge, mass or genital oedema. Urine and urethral discharge cultures should be obtained. A broad-spectrum antibiotic may also be prescribed (Kidd 1995).

The most common foreign body is a lost tampon which can occur because of a broken string, because of the insertion of two tampons for heavy loss or as a result of having sexual intercourse with a tampon in situ. The tampon can easily be removed with the aid of a good light and Cusco's speculum.

Weekends are a common time for young women to ask for postcoital contraception when GP surgeries and family planning clinics are closed. Unprotected intercourse, split condoms or rape may be the reasons for this request. The 'morning-after pill' can be given within 72 hours and is 99% effective.

For various reasons, young men and women often prefer to come to A&E with these problems and other sexually related diseases. The principal reason may be a desire for anonymity. Patients may be reluctant to go to a general practitioner who is well known both to them and their families. They feel, unjustly, that there will be a greater degree of confidentiality in a place where they are not known and to which they will not have to return. Appointments do not have to be made and a decision to seek immediate treatment for an embarrassing problem can be acted upon.

Psychological Illnesses in Young Adults

The young adult is particularly likely to present in A&E with a psychological illness. Many find the transition from adolescence to adulthood extremely difficult and stress-related illnesses are common. Those without a strong support network may feel overwhelmed by the problems confronting them (Broadhead *et al.* 1983).

Young adulthood is a time when specific mental illnesses can develop. The one which is probably best known as a disorder of the young is schizophrenia. It occurs in 0.8% of the population and is commoner in males than in females (Lyttle 1986). It usually develops in adolescence and reaches a peak between 20 and 39 years of age. It is at this time that the A&E nurse first meets the patient whose symptoms are of disordered thoughts, inappropriate moods, auditory hallucinations or persecutory delusions. These patients can be frightening and difficult to contain in A&E if psychiatric referral takes time. The care and nursing management of patients with a psychiatric crisis, including schizophrenia, are considered in detail in Chapter 14.

Several illnesses affect young women in particular. In women under 40, anorexia nervosa and bulimia may be seen as causes of collapse, bradycardia or electrolyte imbalance. Postnatal depression or psychosis may also be seen in the A&E department when young women may overdose, present with acute delusions or be involved in episodes of harm to their children.

Certain types of individual who are confronted by stress develop anxiety states. These are classified according to their severity: mild, moderate, severe and panic (Stuart & Sundeen 1991). They are often a feature of young adult life and symptoms usually persist for an average of 5 years before treatment is sought (Marks 1981). Symptoms include palpitations, tachycardia and chest pain. It is important to get a full history to rule out organic causes such as pneumothorax, infection or myocardial infarct. Individual stress counselling and relaxation groups run by a community psychiatric nurse can be very beneficial to these patients. Life events such as bereavement, divorce, unemployment, marriage, retirement, parenthood and physical illness can precipitate these illnesses.

The young adult is at greater risk of death from suicide than any other age group. Deaths in the young adult are four times higher among men than among women and the person most at risk is the young male city dweller with a history of psychiatric illness. Since 1920, the months of April, May and June have consistently been the peak months for suicides (Gelder *et al.* 1983). Successful suicides are rarely the business of the A&E department, but parasuicide attempts should never be taken lightly; 10–16% of survivors go on to subsequent successful suicides (Lindars 1991). For every suicide there are 30 other cases of self-harm (Evans 1993).

The difference between the two groups, suicide and self-harm, is not always clear-cut. Those who commit suicide are a small group who plan the act, take precautions against being discovered, use dangerous methods and, in one-sixth of cases, leave a suicide note. The majority of these people have given a warning of suicidal intent.

Conclusion

Young adults use A&E in a different way from children, the middle-aged or the elderly. They may have moved away from the influence and environment of the family and may not be registered with a GP. They rarely have long-term health care needs and so tend to use the accident department as a 'drop-in' centre not requiring organised planned appointments.

The commonest reason for attendance is accidental injury. Young people may have a lamentable lack of knowledge of their own bodies and become aggressive or depressed if they have to confront personal injury or disease (Furnham & Stacey 1991). They have high levels of anxiety about their body image and a visit to hospital can be an emotionally traumatic time when they become impatient and frightened if they are not treated quickly. This means that the A&E nurse needs to be aware that reassurance and explanations are necessary and not be surprised that young people, even in their 20s, want their parents with them. Young adults in the 18–39 year age range are a diverse group and good communication skills are essential to ensure that all patients receive the appropriate treatments for their specific needs. As with every group of patients, the young adult needs tolerance, flexibility and, that vital ingredient, time.

References

Bakewell P (1993) *A Physiotherapy Research Post in Accident and Emergency*. Norwich: Norfolk and Norwich Hospital.

Broadhead WE, Kaplan BH, James SA *et al.* (1983) The epidemiological evidence for a relationship between social support and health. *Journal of Epidemiology* **117**, 521–535.

Central Policy Review Staff (1982) *Alcohol Policies in the UK*. Sweden: University of Stockholm.

Cope A, Stebbings W (1996) Abdomen. In: Skinner D, Driscoll P, Earlam R, eds. *ABC of Major Trauma*, 2nd edn. London: BMJ.

Department of Health (1992) *Health of the Nation*. London: HMSO.

Department of Transport (1989) *Road Casualties in Great Britain: 1988*. London: HMSO.

Ellis JI, Whiting M, Roper M (1992) Alcohol-related emergencies. In: Schwartz GR, Cayten CG, Mangelsen MA *et al.* eds. *Principles and Practice of Emergency Medicine*. Philadelphia: Lea & Febiger.

Evans M (1993) Suicide: a target for health. *RCN Nursing Update Nursing Standard* **7**(18), 9–14.

Furnham A, Stacey B (1991) *Young People's Understanding of Society*. London: Routledge.

Gelder M, Gath L, Mayou R (1983) *Oxford Book of Psychiatry*. Oxford: Oxford University Press.

Grundy D, Russell J, Swain A (1991) *ABC of Spinal Cord Injury*. London: BMJ.

Kanegaye J, Schonfield N. (1993) Penile zipper entrapment: a simple and less threatening approach using mineral oil. *Paediatric Emergency Care* **9**(2), 90–91.

Kidd PS (1995) Genitourinary emergencies. In: Kitt S, Selfridge-Thomas J, Proehl JA, Kaiser J, eds. *Emergency Nursing: a Physiologic and Clinical Perspective*. Philadelphia: WB Saunders.

King's Fund (1991) *Health of the Nation: Strategy for the 1990s*. London: King Edward Hospital Fund.

Lindars J (1991) Holistic care in parasuicide. *Nursing Times* **87**(15), 30–31.

Lyttle J (1986) *Mental Disorder*. London: Baillière Tindall.

Marks I (1981) *Cure and Care of Neuroses*. Chichester: John Wiley.

Nicholl JP, Coleman P, Williams RT (1991) Pilot study of the epidemiology of sports injuries and exercise-related injuries. *British Journal of Sports Medicine* **25**(1), 61–66.

Noble C (1990) *The Invicta Manual of Sports Injuries*. Sandton, South Africa: Pfizer Laboratories.

Office of Population Census and Surveys (1991) *Mortality Statistics: 1991*. Fareham, Hants: OPCS.

Renstrom PAFH (1994) *Clinical Practice of Sports Injury Prevention and Management*. Oxford: Blackwell Scientific.

Sabey BE, Staughton GC (1975) Interacting roles of environment, vehicle and road user. Crowthorne: Transport and Road Research Laboratory.

Skinner D, Driscoll P, Earlham R (1991) *ABC of Major Trauma*. London: BMJ.

Sperryn N (1994) ABC of sports injuries: overdose injuries in sport. *British Medical Journal* **208**, 1430–1432.

Stuart GW, Sundeen SJ (1991) *Principles and Practice of Psychiatric Nursing*, 4th edn. St Louis: Mosby.

Taylor R, Ryrie I (1996) Chronic alcohol abusers in A&E. *Emergency Nurse* **4**(3), 6–8.

Wardrope J, English B (1998) *Musculo-skeletal Problems in Emergency Medicine*. Oxford: Oxford University Press.

Wolfe JS, Gomez R, McAninch JW (1992) Human bites to the penis. *The Journal of Urology* **147**, 1265–1267.

Zull DN (1995) Poisoning and drug overdose. In: Kitt S, Selfridge-Thomas J, Proehl JA, Kaiser J eds. *Emergency Nursing: a Physiologic and Clinical Perspective*. Philadelphia: WB Saunders.

Chapter 20

Middle Years

Grant Williams

- Introduction
- Chest pain
- Pancreatitis
- Epigastric pain
- Homelessness
- Conclusion

Introduction

The life continuum represents a sequence of physical, psychological and social attributes that an individual may experience, and will have an influence on how individuals develop within a changing society and cope with the associated demands and crises (Erickson 1963, Roper *et al.* 1990). Ill health cannot be attributed to any single cause and may be viewed as a multifaceted effect of modern society and increasing age. In the person who has attained middle adulthood, which for the purposes of this chapter is arbitrarily defined as 35–64 years of age, it is reasonable to suppose that the majority of individuals have experienced many life events and that their psychosocial make-up influences their level of health. It is at this time of life that the onset of chronic disease can be ascribed to environmental and social factors.

This chapter will consider conditions most commonly associated with middle age: health problems due to lifestyle, stress-related conditions and degenerative and age-related diseases. In addition, the presentation of homeless people to A&E will also be considered. Those who are homeless are most commonly middle-aged and have high physical and social needs which will be considered here.

Chest Pain

The estimated prevalence of coronary heart disease in asymptomatic, middle-aged men is 4% and is one of the commonest reasons for hospital admission (Jowett & Thompson 1995). Chest pain can occur at rest or with exercise and may result from a sudden decrease in coronary blood flow, due to coronary thrombosis or spasm, or from an inability to increase coronary blood flow sufficiently to meet myocardial oxygen demands, e.g. during exercise (Tueller Steuble 1991).

The patient presenting to A&E complaining of chest pain requires careful assessment to determine the symptoms and subtle features which differentiate chest pain that is cardiac in origin from that which is

---

Box 20.1 – *Causes of chest pain*

Cardiovascular
- Myocardial ischaemia (angina)
- Myocardial infarction
- Coronary artery spasm
- Pericarditis
- Dissecting aortic aneurysm
- Mitral valve prolapse

Non-cardiac causes
- Pleurisy
- Pneumothorax
- Malignancy
- Rib fracture
- Peptic ulceration
- Pneumonia
- Hiatus hernia
- Musculoskeletal pain
- Gall bladder disease
- Anxiety/cardiac neurosis

Box 20.2 – *Characteristic descriptions of chest pain*

- **Stable angina**
  Typically constricting, retrosternal pain, radiating to the arms (predominantly the left), neck or jaw. It often occurs in response to stimuli that increase the oxygen demand of the heart, such as physical exertion or emotion, and is relieved by rest

- **Unstable angina**
  As in stable angina, but the periods of pain are prolonged and may occur at rest and have no precipitating factors

- **Myocardial infarction**
  Typically severe, crushing, retrosternal pain which may extend to the arms, jaw or back and which often lasts >30 minutes. It is accompanied by nausea, vomiting and sweating. The onset of pain is not always associated with exertion and is not relieved by rest. Some patients, however, have little or no pain, especially the elderly and diabetics

- **Pericarditis**
  The pain is usually sharp and retrosternal and may be more apparent on inspiration. It is often worse when lying flat but is relieved when sitting up and leaning forwards

- **Pleuritic pain**
  This is usually a sharp, localised pain, which is worse on inspiration and coughing

- **Pulmonary embolism**
  The pain is pleuritic in nature and may be associated with haemoptysis and breathlessness

- **Oesophageal pain**
  Oesophageal pain is usually associated with, or eased by, food and is typically worse when lying flat. Oesophageal rupture is usually preceded by vomiting

- **Aortic dissection**
  The patient experiences a 'tearing' pain, as opposed to the crushing pain of myocardial infarction. This pain is typically felt in the back

- **Musculoskeletal pain**
  Pain due to the spinal or muscular disorders can usually be identified by the effect of movement and position. Unlike the other conditions, the chest wall is tender to touch at the specific locations (Adam & Osborne 1997)

- **Stress–related**
  The patient will appear flushed and distressed and may be hyperventilating, which will lead to a sensation of central chest pain

---

non-cardiac (see Box 20.1). Chest pain can be very frightening for the patient, especially if it the first episode, and A&E staff need to assess and determine the likely signs of such pain. A number of key characteristics may help the assessing nurse to distinguish cardiac pain from that of other causes:

- *Location*. Cardiac pain is typically centrally located. Chest pain that is peripheral to the sternum is rarely cardiac in origin.
- *Radiation*. Ischaemic pain, especially when severe, may radiate to the neck, jaw and arms. Pain situated over the left anterior chest and radiating laterally may have various causes, such as pleurisy, chest wall injury and anxiety.
- *Provocation*. Anginal pain is precipitated by exertion, rather than occurring after it. It disappears a few minutes after the cessation of activity when blood flow can again match the oxygen requirements of the muscle. In contrast, pain associated with a specific movement, such as bending, stretching or turning, is likely to be musculoskeletal in origin.
- *Character of the pain*. Cardiac pain is frequently described as 'heavy', dull or 'like a tight band around the chest'. It may be appreciated more as discomfort than pain. Pleural pain, for instance, may be described as 'sharp' or 'catching' (see Box 20.2).
- *Pattern of onset*. The pain of aortic dissection, massive pulmonary embolism or pneumothorax is usually very sudden in onset (within seconds). Myocardial infarction may build up over several

Table 20.1 – *Oxygen masks, flow rates and approximate concentrations of delivered oxygen. (From Jowett & Thompson 1995)*

Mask oxygen flow L/min	Edinburgh (%)	MC(%)	Nasal cannulae	Hudson (%)
1	25–30	–	25–30	–
2	30–35	30–50	30–35	25–38
4	35–40	40–70	32–40	35–45
6	–	55–75	–	50–60
8	–	60–75	–	55–65
10	–	65–80	–	60–75

minutes or longer, whereas angina builds in proportion to the intensity of the exertion.

■ *Associated features.* The severe pain of myocardial infarct, massive pulmonary embolus or aortic dissection is often accompanied by autonomic disturbance, including sweating, nausea and vomiting. If the patient is flushed, it may reflect a pyrexia or it may be stress-related. Pallor may be indicative of inadequate cardiac function or shock. Breathlessness is associated with raised pulmonary capillary pressure or pulmonary oedema in myocardial infarction and may accompany any of the respiratory causes of chest pain. Associated gastrointestinal symptoms may provide the clue to non-cardiac chest pain, such as heartburn, peptic ulceration, diarrhoea and vomiting.

The classic pain of angina pectoris is diffuse and retrosternal and will often diminish after rest. In the case of myocardial infarct, it is localised in the centre of the chest, is usually severe in nature, radiating to the left arm and jaw, and is not relieved by rest. Myocardial infarction and its management will be addressed in Chapter 26.

It is vitally important to take a careful history from the patient who presents complaining of chest pain. The patient should be encouraged to describe the pain – its intensity, location, duration, what brought it on and whether there is any relevant history (Walsh 1996). Assessing whether the patient can talk in sentences or whether there is pain on movement can indicate whether the chest pain is respiratory or musculoskeletal in origin. Note also that the fear and anxiety brought on by chest pain can exacerbate symptoms in the patient.

Recording of temperature, pulse and blood pressure and a 12-lead ECG can offer an indication of the likelihood of cardiac-related chest pain. A raised temperature may be a result of the breakdown of cardiac enzymes in response to a myocardial infarct that has happened within the previous few hours or may be a result of underlying infection. Recording of pulse

oximetry, which measures arterial oxyhaemoglobin saturation (S_pO_2), gives important information about the supply of oxygen to the tissues (Moyle 1994). Patients whose oxygen saturation levels are under 95% on air are regarded as hypoxic and should be given oxygen via a mask or nasal cannula (Table 20.1). Supplementary oxygen intake to increase oxygen saturation levels helps to relieve tachycardia induced by hypoxia, thereby reducing cardiac workload.

In the absence of pain and with the patient at rest, the 12-lead ECG may be normal; therefore the ECG should also be performed during an episode of chest pain. ST-segment and T-wave changes, which occur during spontaneous chest pain and disappear with relief of the pain, are significant. Even without changes, the ECG should be repeated after 1 hour as the absence of abnormality does not rule out disease. Following myocardial infarction, the levels of some of the myocardial enzymes will rise, and estimation of their serum levels is often of diagnostic importance. In addition, the degree of their elevation may give some indication of the size of the infarct (Jowett & Thompson 1995). The measured cardiac enzymes are creatine kinase (CK), lactate dehydrogenase (LDH) and serum glutamic oxaloacetic transaminase (SGOT or AST) and they are released in the first 24 hours after the onset of a myocardial infarct. These enzymes may provide retrospective confirmation of infarction rather than a guide to immediate management (analgesia, aspirin, thrombolysis). If the clinical picture suggests myocardial infarct, the patient should be treated as such.

Pain relief may be achieved by administering sublingual GTN tablet or spray, repeated as necessary. Nitrates relax smooth muscle, mainly in the venous system, to increase capacitance and thus reduce cardiac preload. Arteriolar relaxation also occurs, with a fall in peripheral resistance (afterload). The resulting reduction in blood pressure leads to a reduction in chest pain. For patients suspected of having non-cardiac-related chest pain, magnesium trisilicate may relieve symptoms, suggesting an oesophageal or gastric origin of the pain. The use of antacids to differentiate epigastric pain from cardiac pain is common in A&E; however, consideration must be given to the patient's history, cardiac risk factors and ECG as well as the patient's response to therapy (Novotny-Dinsdale & Andrews 1995).

Pancreatitis

The pancreas plays a major role in the neutralisation of gastric contents, digestion and glucose homeostasis. Acute pancreatitis is an inflammatory condition of the pancreas and is most frequently associated with biliary tract disease, trauma, infectious disease and alcoholism, and has a higher incidence in middle-aged individuals. Pancreatitis is considered to be the result of some factor or change within the pancreas that affects activation of the proteinases and lipase of the exocrine secretion, with subsequent breakdown of the ducts, parenchymal tissue and blood vessels. The causative factor may be an obstruction to the flow of the pancreatic secretion within the ducts. Continued secretion produces dilatation and back pressure, resulting in duct disruption and the escape of enzymes into the parenchyma (Topping 1992).

Acute pancreatitis is a serious and potentially life-threatening condition. In the mild form, the pancreas become swollen and oedematous and, with treatment, the patient is likely to recover within a few days. If the process is severe it can lead to haemorrhagic pancreatitis with parenchymal necrosis. Necrosis results from the intrapancreatic activation of the proteinases and lipase, initiating autodigestion of the pancreatic tissue and blood vessels. Enzymes and blood may escape into the surrounding tissue and peritoneal cavity; peritonitis, paralytic ileus or ascites may then develop.

The patient will usually present following the onset of sudden, severe pain in the epigastrium or right hypochondrium penetrating through to the back. The pain may be described by the patient as penetrating or boring. It often occurs within 12–24 hours following a large meal and alcohol. The pain is usually associated with nausea and vomiting. Abdominal distension and rigidity can appear as a result of the development of peritonitis. This is caused by chemical irritation of the viscera and peritoneum by the enzymes that escape from the pancreas.

Shock is attributed to the severity of the constant pain, the exudation of plasma into the peritoneal cavity, and the loss of blood resulting from the erosion of vessels within the pancreas associated with necrotising and haemorrhagic pancreatitis (Topping 1992). The patient can present in moderate to severe distress with tachycardia and tachypnoea as a result of volume depletion. The patient's temperature may be elevated in the early stages but may become subnormal if peritonitis and shock develop. The pulse is rapid and the blood pressure falls with the decrease in the intravascular volume. The patient is flushed at first, and then usually becomes pale. If peritonitis develops, a dusky or cyanotic colour is possible. A deficiency of insulin may develop when the islets of Langerhans are involved in the pathological process, and hyperglycaemia and glucosuria may be present.

The patient with acute pancreatitis is critically ill, and care is directed towards the reduction of pancreatic secretion to a minimum, relief of pain, prevention of shock (or correction if it has developed), correction of electrolyte and fluid imbalances and prevention of infection. As the disease process continues, mortality rises; overall it is 10–20%. In haemorrhagic pancreatitis, mortality is greater than 50% (Novotny-Dinsdale & Andrews 1995). Intravenous saline, plasma, plasma expanders and whole blood may be required as determined by the clinical response, urinary output and central venous pressure.

Early interventions include administration of oxygen and positioning the patient for comfort, which may be obtained by crouching or leaning forward. Food and fluids should be withheld to rest the gastrointestinal tract, decrease pancreatic activity and thus help to alleviate pain. A nasogastric tube should be passed and regularly aspirated to relieve vomiting and distension and to prevent acid gastric secretion from entering the duodenum and further stimulating the pancreas. Analgesia, usually i.v. pethidine, should be prescribed, as it depresses the central nervous system and relaxes smooth muscle. Opiates such as morphine should be avoided as they can induce spasm of the pancreatic and biliary ducts, thereby increasing pain.

The release of vasoactive substances following auto-digestion of pancreatic tissues causes alterations in permeability of the capillary membrane. This leads to large losses of fluid into the extravascular space and particularly into the peritoneal cavity. Fluid losses lead to a low circulating blood volume with reactive constriction of the abdominal blood vessels resulting in poor perfusion of the pancreas, further damage to pancreatic tissue and continued downward spiral in the patient's condition (Adam & Osborne 1997). The patient's condition may change rapidly, so frequent observation of vital signs and general appearance is essential. A weak, rapid pulse, pallor, fall in blood pressure and increasing weakness may manifest haemorrhage or shock. If these signs of hypovolaemic shock are present, two large-bore i.v. lines of a crystalloid solution should be started as a rapid fluid infusion. In haemorrhagic pancreatitis, administration of blood products may be necessary.

Metabolic complications, such as hypocalcaemia and hypoglycaemia, are negative prognostic indicators. Hypocalcaemia is suspected if the patient develops muscle spasms, twitching or tetany. Magnesium, phosphate and potassium are also related to alterations in capillary permeability and nasogastric losses. Continuous ECG monitoring is useful for signs of arrhythmias associated with hypokalaemia and hypomagnesaemia. Electrolyte levels should be monitored and corrected as required. In addition, careful monitoring of fluid intake and output should be undertaken, with patients catheterised to monitor hourly urinary output.

Antibiotics are prescribed since inflammation and necrosis make the pancreas very vulnerable to infection. The aims of care should include stable vital signs, adequate fluid resuscitation and alleviation of pain. Psychological support for the patient and his family is especially important at this stressful time.

Epigastric Pain

Gastritis is a common condition which relates to an inflammation of the stomach lining and involves the symptoms of vomiting. The term gastroenteritis refers to an inflammation of both the gastric and intestinal mucosa. Gastritis is usually associated with dietary indiscretions due to overindulgence of alcohol or food, but it may also be a result of stress, non-steroidal antiinflammatory drugs (NSAIDs) or uraemia.

The inflammation is usually self-limiting and without sequelae, but patients presenting with gastritis may require antacids to alleviate vomiting and nausea. Advice to patients includes taking clear liquids only until 8–12 hours have passed without vomiting, and then starting with bland foods before gradually resuming a normal diet.

The term 'peptic ulcer' refers to an ulcer in the lower oesophagus, the stomach, the duodenum or the jejunum after surgical anastomosis to the stomach. It is a common condition and has its highest incidence in males aged 40–55 years, with perforation occurring in approximately 5–10% of affected individuals. While epigastric pain resolves with antacids and is self-limiting and short-lived, ulcers are repetitive and are worse after specific foods or drinks.

Ulceration of the gastric mucosa leads to excoriation and mucous membrane sloughing. An imbalance between pepsin, hydrochloric acid secretion and bicarbonate causes gastric erosion. Bacterial invasion from *Helicobacter pylori* has been implicated as an important aetiological factor in peptic ulcer disease, accounting for 90% of duodenal ulcers and 70% of gastric ulcers (Shearman 1995). *H. pylori* causes acute inflammation of the mucosa by causing degeneration, detachment and necrosis of the epithelial cells. Chronic ingestion of medications that irritate the gastric mucosa, such as aspirin or NSAIDs can also lead to the development of ulcers (Selfridge-Thomas 1997). While duodenal and gastric ulcers are different conditions, they share common symptoms and will be considered together.

The most common presentation is that of recent abdominal pain which has three notable characteristics: localisation to the epigastrium, relationship to food and episodic occurrence. The pain is probably caused by acid coming into contact with the ulcer. Occasional vomiting may occur in about 40% of patients with peptic ulcer. In some patients the ulcer is completely 'silent', presenting for the first time with anaemia from chronic undetected blood loss, or as an abrupt haematemesis or acute perforation; in others there is recurrent acute bleeding without ulcer pain between attacks.

A peptic ulcer may progressively erode the submucosal, muscular and serous layers of the gastrointestinal wall. When perforation occurs, the contents of the stomach escape into the peritoneal cavity; this occurs more commonly in duodenal than in gastric ulcers. The most striking symptom is sudden, severe pain; its distribution follows the spread of gastric contents over the peritoneum. Initially, the pain may be referred to the upper abdomen, but it quickly becomes generalised; shoulder tip pain may occur as a result of irritation of the diaphragm. The pain is accompanied by shallow respirations due to epigastric pain and limitation of diaphragmatic movements. A rapid pulse and reduction in blood pressure indicate shock. Pyrexia may also be present as a result of peritonitis. Pallor, a cold clammy skin, nausea and vomiting may be also evident. The abdomen is held immobile and has 'board-like' rigidity.

Non-operative treatment includes i.v. morphine for pain relief, aspiration of the stomach contents using a nasogastric tube and continuous gastric suctioning, i.v. electrolytes and fluids, and antibiotic therapy. After initial treatment for shock, emergency surgery may be performed to close the perforation or resect the affected area; however, perforation carries a mortality of approximately 10%. The nurse should monitor the patient's vital signs closely for signs of deterioration and offer reassurance to the patient and his family.

Where there is no indication of perforation, the patient is usually managed with a range of anti-ulcer medications such as ranitidine and/or metronidazole, which have antibacterial effects on *H. pylori*, and referred back to his GP.

Homelessness

Few would need convincing that the extreme conditions of homelessness, of sleeping rough, are bound to affect health (Best 1995). The homeless are disproportionately white, male and middle-aged (Anderson *et al.* 1993), although there are increasing numbers of young men and women and black and Asian people (Pleace & Quilgars 1996). In a study of the records of 1873 homeless users of an A&E department compared with 28 420 housed people, a disturbing health profile emerged (North *et al.* 1996):

- Homeless people's accidents and injuries were four times more likely to be the result of an assault than those of housed people.
- Homeless people had twice the rate of infected wounds than housed people. These infections were twice as likely to be severe enough to warrant an admission to hospital for further treatment.
- A substantial proportion (10%) of homeless people attending A&E did so for mental health reasons. This was the second largest presenting category for homeless people to A&E, but only ranked 10th for housed attenders.
- Homeless people were five times more likely to attend A&E due to deliberate self-harm than were housed people. Depression was very common among people of no fixed abode and hostel residents.
- Asthma was twice as common among homeless than among housed attenders.
- Epilepsy was four times as common among homeless than among housed users of the A&E department.

The literature on homelessness reveals the almost universal acceptance that there is a close link between ill health and homelessness (Fisher & Collins 1993, Marren-Bell 1993, Moore *et al.* 1997). Difficulties in obtaining access to primary health care services have meant that A&E departments have been an important source of health care provision for some homeless men and women. Minor, acute illnesses pose particular problems for homeless people who lack the facilities to look after themselves when well, and who are at risk of particular infections and infestations precisely because of their circumstances. Respiratory illness has been found to be a major health problem associated with being homeless (Balazs 1993). Other common conditions are chronic obstructive airways disease, tuberculosis, foot problems, infestations and epilepsy. Homeless people attending A&E also exhibit a disproportionate prevalence of infections, scabies and lice (Scott 1993). Emergency admission rates are also higher (Scheur *et al.* 1991). Low temperature is an important cause of morbidity and mortality among the homeless. In Britain, for each degree Celsius that the winter is colder than average, there are an extra 8000 deaths (Balazs 1993).

A&E nurses may offer the only social contact for some homeless people. A novel Canadian study found that compassionate care of homeless people who present to A&E departments significantly lowered their repeat visits. The researchers identified 133 consecutive homeless adults visiting one inner city emergency department who were not acutely psychotic, extremely intoxicated, unable to speak English or medically unstable. Half were randomly assigned to receive compassionate care from trained volunteers. All patients otherwise had usual care and were followed for repeat visits to A&E departments. The researchers found that the attendance by homeless people who received compassionate care was significantly lower. While acknowledging that compassionate care is not necessarily cost-effective if staff costs are taken into account, the authors argued that the basic justification for compassion is decency not economics (Redelmeier *et al.* 1995).

Conclusion

This chapter has considered a number of conditions which tend to present in the middle years of the life span. For the A&E nurse, identification and management represent a challenge of psychological as well as physical care, because many of these patients may present with these conditions for the first time. The support and guidance of the nurse can have a significant effect on the patient and his family in their subsequent adaptation to these conditions.

References

Adam SK, Osborne S (1997) *Critical Care Nursing: Science & Practice*. Oxford: Oxford Medical.

Anderson I, Kemp P, Quilgars D (1993) *Single Homeless People*. London: HMSO.

Balazs J (1993) Health care for single homeless people. In: Fisher K, Collins J, eds. *Homelessness, Health Care and Welfare Provision*. London: Routledge.

Best R (1995) The housing dimension. In: Benzeval M, Judge K, Whitehead M, eds. *Tackling Inequalities in Health: an Agenda for Action*. London: King's Fund.

Erickson EH (1963) *Childhood and Society*. New York: WW Norton.

Fisher K, Collins J (1993) *Homelessness, Health Care and Welfare Provision*. London: Routledge.

Jowett NI, Thompson D (1995) *Comprehensive Coronary Care*, 2nd edn. London: Scutari.

Marren-Bell U (1993) Homelessness: the A&E response. *Emergency Nurse*, **1**(1), 4–6.

Moore H, North C, Owens C (1997) Health and healthcare for homeless people. *Emergency Nurse*, **5**(1), 25–29

Moyle JTM (1994) *Pulse Oximetry*. London: BMJ.

North C, Moore H, Owens C (1996) *Go Home and Rest?: The Use of an Accident and Emergency Department by Homeless People*. London: Shelter.

Novotny-Dinsdale V, Andrews LS (1995) Gastrointestinal emergencies. In: Kitt S, Selfridge-Thomas J, Proeh JA, Kaiser J. eds. *Emergency Nursing: A Physiologic and Clinical Perspective*, 2nd edn. Philadelphia: Saunders.

Pleace N, Quilgars D (1996) *Health and Homelessness in London: a Review*. London: King's Fund.

Redelmeier DA, Molin JP, Tibshini RJ (1995) A randomised trial of compassionate care for the homeless in an emergency department. *The Lancet*, **345**, 1131–1134.

Roper N, Logan WW, Tierney AJ (1990) *The Elements of Nursng: a Model for Nursing Based on a Model of Living*. Edinburgh: Churchill Livingstone.

Scheur MA, Black M, Voctor C, Benzeval M, Gill M, Judge K (1991) *Homelessness and the Utilisation of Acute Hospital Services in London*. London: King's Fund Institute.

Scott J (1993) Homelessness and mental health. *British Journal of Psychiatry*, **162**, 314–324.

Selfridge-Thomas J (1997) *Emergency Nursing: an Essential Guide for Patient Care*. Philadelphia: WB Saunders.

Shearman DJC (1995) Diseases of the alimentary tract and pancreas. In: Edwards CRW, Bouchier IAD, Haslett C, Chilvers ER, eds. *Davidson's Principles and Practice of Medicine*, 17th edn. Edinburgh: Churchill Livingstone.

Topping EA (1992) Caring for the patient with disorders of liver, biliary tract and exocrine pancreas. In: Royle JA, Walsh M, eds. *Watson's Medical-Surgical Nursing and Related Physiology*, 4th edn. London: Baillière Tindall.

Tueller Steuble B (1991) Acute chest pain. In: Swearingen PL, Hicks Keen J, eds. *Manual of Critical Care*, 2nd edn. St Louis: Mosby.

Walsh M (1996) *Accident & Emergency Nursing: a New Approach*, 3rd edn. Oxford: Butterworth Heinemann.

Chapter 21

The Elderly

*Brian Dolan**

- Introduction
- Physiology of old age
- Assessing the elderly person in A&E
- Hypothermia
- Elder abuse
- Confusion
- Falls
- Conclusion

Introduction

The elderly constitute a growing proportion of attendances to A&E departments. This chapter will consider the needs of elderly people in A&E. It will consider the demography and physiology of old age before considering assessment and presentations, such as hypothermia, elder abuse, confusion and falls, and dehydration and infection. Information on discharge will also be addressed in this chapter.

Britain, in demographic terms, is an ageing society. In 1971, just 2.3% of the UK population were 80 years or over; by 1991 this figure had reached 3.7% (Central Statistics Office 1993). This translates to 2.2 million people, with a further 6.9 million aged 65–79. By 2001, it is predicted that the very elderly, i.e. those aged 80 or over, will have risen to 2.5 million, while the 65–79 year age group will have fallen slightly to 6.5 million.

Generally, the elderly are perceived as a burden on society, using up resources and performing no useful function. Johnson (1976) suggested that the state, and by extension the health service, devalues the human status of the elderly by making them, as a whole, appear dependent and in need of welfare, reinforcing society's negative view of old age. However, elderly people are not a homogenous group and nurses can do much to challenge stereotypical responses to old age while maintaining the dignity and independence of the patient in their care.

Physiology of Old Age

As people age there is a general deterioration of bodily function. Most changes in bodily functions with ageing tend to emphasise the negative nature of these changes (Brookbank 1990). Hinchliff *et al.* (1996) suggested that some of these negative changes may be due not simply to age alone, but also to pathological states existing within the individual or to a lack of use

*The author would like to thank Michael Fanning and Jenny Hilton for their contributions to earlier drafts of this chapter.

Table 21.1 – *Physiological changes in the elderly (from Greaves et al. 1997)*

Change	Clinical consequences
Brain – shrinkage and loss of neurones (cerebral atrophy)	Increasing forgetfulness Dementia Vulnerability to toxic confusional states
Peripheral and autonomic nervous system – reduced awareness of touch, temperature, pain; impaired proprioception; impaired control of posture and balance	Hypothermia Postural urine incontinence Constipation
Eye – Cataracts, macular degeneration	Impaired eyesight Stiffening of lens Presbyopia (failure to accommodate to near and distant vision)
Ear	Deafness
Bones, joints and muscles Osteoporosis	Fractures of femoral neck, wrist and vertebrae Increased curvature of spine (kyphosis)
Osteoarthritis Loss of muscle, strength and bulk capacity to respond to displacement	Stiffening of knees, hips and fingers Immobility, falls

of the particular system. Although the rates of ageing are considered to be inevitable, the reality is that the rate of deterioration in organ function can be reduced by factors such as regular exercise and accelerated by habits such as cigarette smoking and heavy alcohol consumption. There is considerable variability in individuals' susceptibility to ageing. For instance, a marathon runner aged 80 will have muscle that is virtually indistinguishable physiologically from that of a 20-year-old. Table 21.1 outlines some of the organ and tissue changes associated with ageing.

Assessing the Elderly Person in A&E

An elderly person presenting to A&E requires a thorough assessment of her physical and psychological needs. The nurse should introduce himself when first meeting the patient, both as a courtesy and as an opportunity to establish a rapport. If the patient has walked into the department, the nurse should accompany her to the cubicle and observe features such as gait, balance and pace.

If the patient needs to get undressed, she should do this herself, if she is able. It is important for the patient to feel in control as far as is possible. Offering the patient a seat while undressing will allow her to remove her clothes more easily, if, for instance, trousers are being worn. It also enables the nurse to assess the patient's balance and ability to self-care. Providing steps for the patient to climb onto the trolley where she is able to do so is preferable to lifting her up with the aid of other colleagues. It is not essential for patients to remove all their clothing when getting undressed and undergarments should only be removed if necessary. If the patient is wearing pyjamas or a nightdress on presentation there is rarely a need to change into a hospital gown.

Careful attention should be paid to the patient's skin condition – are there old wounds, unhealed ulcers or bruises? The latter may give an indication of elder abuse (considered later in this chapter). While nutritional intake is difficult to assess in A&E due to the transient nature of patients, it is possible to determine whether a patient is obese or emaciated and therefore at greater risk of development of pressure sores (Wickham 1997a,b).

Physiological observations of an elderly patient should be included in the assessment. Taking a blood pressure, pulse or respirations immediately after the patient has climbed onto a hospital trolley is likely to provide inaccurate baseline readings, due to the additional strain this effort places on the cardiovascular system of the older person. The heart rate of the elderly person is likely to be slower, with arrhythmias being relatively common in otherwise asymptomatic patients. This seldom requires evaluation or treatment. Similarly, the older person's blood pressure is likely to be elevated, usually as a consequence of atherosclerosis, predisposing the patient to the development of cardiovascular diseases, such as congestive cardiac failure, stroke, transient ischaemic attacks and dementia.

An accurate baseline temperature should be recorded. In elderly people, the temperature is usually recorded at 36.5°C or above, due to the reduction in basal metabolic rate. The patient's respiration rate may be increased due to underlying conditions such as chronic obstructive airways disease. It is not unknown for patients who have recently been A&E attenders or in-patients to have ECG adhesive tabs or patient identification bracelets still attached. This can assist the nurse in establishing reasons for recent visits and assessing the patient's personal hygiene. Poor personal hygiene may reflect difficult socioeconomic circumstances rather than an inability on the part of the patient to cope, and the nurse should take this into account when assessing the patient. The patient's pre-existing medical history, as well as medication, should be assessed and recorded during the examination.

The nurse should also use language the patient will understand and provide frequent orientating information about the time, place and person, including explanations of equipment, procedures and routines. Because elderly adults process information more slowly, the nurse should develop comfortable and natural ways of talking to the patient, bearing in mind normal deterioration in hearing and other faculties which are associated with ageing. Others involved in the care of the patient, such as relatives or ambulance crew, should be consulted about the patient's condition. However, the patient's view should be sought as much as possible with others used to supplement the information provided by her.

Hypothermia

The existence of hypothermia in elderly people can be identified by the measurement, rectally, of a persistently low body core temperature of below 35°C (Watson 1996). Of the 1057 people who died from hypothermia in the UK in 1985, almost all were over the age of 65. It is estimated that for each 1°C below the average winter temperature, there are an additional 8000 deaths per year (Stoyle 1991).

Physiology

Normally when the body temperature falls, shivering occurs. This is a protective mechanism which functions to raise core temperature. The ability to shiver, however, gradually decreases as the core temperature falls below 34°C. Muscle weakness then occurs, as the core temperature drops further. Activity becomes difficult as muscular movements become uncoordinated, and dulling of mental faculties becomes evident. Consciousness is lost at a body temperature of 30–32°C. At 22–28°C cardiac arrhythmia occurs, and at 18–22°C the heart stops (Hinchliff et al. 1996).

The heat regulating centres are situated in the anterior hypothalamus. In cold weather, when the body's need is to conserve heat, the hypothalamic heat production centre responds to impulses from the thermoreceptors by causing peripheral vasoconstriction via the sympathetic nervous system. When the superficial vessels are constricted, blood flows via the deeper vessels and thus heat loss via the skin is minimised. The skin may appear white or cyanosed; the latter occurs when blood is trapped in vasoconstricted vessels and loses oxygen to the tissues (Hinchliff et al. 1996).

The ability of people to respond appropriately to changes in the ambient temperature decreases with age. Old people may not realise how cold they are, and therefore fail to act to increase their body temperature. The peripheral blood vessels of elderly people are not so responsive to sympathetic stimulation, in many cases due to atheromatous deposits. The ability to spontaneously bring about the cessation of heat loss and to initiate heat production is lost at 28°C (Hinchliff et al. 1996). When the core temperature falls below 30°C, mortality is 70%, compared with 33% above this temperature (see Box 21.1).

Assessment

Recording of accurate observations is essential. The heart rate will usually be bradycardic due to the reduction in basal metabolic rate. Similarly the respiration rate will be slower and will be deep or shallow depending on the degree of hypothermia. A rectal temperature should always be taken, using a low-reading thermometer. Some patients may not feel cold to touch, despite a low core temperature. This may be especially true for older persons who may be less able to vasoconstrict peripherally as an initial response to hypothermia (Manning & Stolerman 1993). If possible, temperature should be continuously monitored and the pulse and blood pressure should be obtained every half-hour. The patient is often hypotensive due to the increased blood viscosity which is a consequence of hypothermia.

As hypothermia progresses, all body systems begin

Box 21.1 – *Factors that predispose elderly people to hypothermia (Wanich Bradway 1996)*

- Age-associated physiological changes
  - impaired sensitivity to temperature
  - chronic low temperature
  - sweat gland atrophy
  - less intense/decreased shivering

- Decreased heat production
  - hypopituitarism
  - hypoglycaemia
  - starvation and malnutrition
  - immobility and decreased activity

- Increased heat loss
  - decreased subcutaneous fat
  - cold exposure

- Thermoregulatory impairment secondary to:
  - tumours
  - trauma
  - cerebrovascular disease

- Sepsis

- Drug-induced
  - alcohol-induced vasodilation
  - barbiturates
  - phenothiazines
  - benzodiazepines
  - anaesthetic agents
  - narcotics

- Environmental
  - lack of insulation, heating
  - improper clothing
  - inability to recognise cold and use blankets

Table 21.2 – *Signs and symptoms of hypothermia*

Rectal temperature	Signs and symptoms
36.5–35°C	Usually non-specific May feel cold to touch Lethargic Possible shivering with tachycardia Pale
35–32°C	Cold skin Pallor/waxy appearance Lose shiver response at 34°C Bradypnoea Confusion
32–30°C	Loss of consciousness Rigid muscle tone Bradycardia Dilated pupils Hypotension
30–28°C	Flaccid muscle tone Fixed dilated pupils Cardiac arrythmias, particularly atrial fibrillation
28–22°C	Cyanosis Severe respiratory depression Barely detectable pulse Cardiac arrhythmias and ventricular fibrillation
Below 22°C	Cessation of cardiac function

to function in an increasingly sluggish manner: the level of consciousness and mental speed reduce; reflexes are slowed, including pupillary responses; muscles stiffen; and the skin becomes cold and pale, cyanotic or waxy depending on the degree of hypothermia. All these changes help to confirm the diagnosis (Wanich Bradway 1996).

An elderly person who presents to A&E with hypothermia may look grey, due to pallor and cyanosis, with skin which is cold to the touch in both exposed and unexposed areas. The voice becomes husky and mental processes slow down. The more severe the hypothermia, the more serious the signs which are manifested (see Table 21.2).

It is important for the nurse to establish the risk factors, potential complications and reasons for hypothermia. Mobility tends to decrease with age and muscle atrophy takes place, reducing the elderly person's ability to generate heat through muscular activity. Depression and loss of self-esteem may lead older people to look after themselves less well, while depressed socioeconomic circumstances may lead them to live in poor housing and to reduce the amount they spend on heating. Lloyd (1990) suggested that a leading factor associated with hypothermia is malnutrition, since if an elderly person is malnourished, hypothermia can develop even if the surrounding environment is relatively warm.

Assessment should include a 12-lead ECG and cardiac monitoring because of the risk if dysrhythmia or ischaemic changes. Common ECG abnormalities include prolongation of the PR interval, QRS complex and the ST segment. A J wave, found between the QRS complex and the ST complex, is a specific finding in hypothermia that disappears when the temperature begins to return to normal (Manning & Stolerman 1993).

Blood screens for metabolic causes, such as hypoglycaemia or hypothyroidism, should be undertaken.

Arterial blood gas values and serum electrolytes are useful in determining respiratory status and acid–base balance. Both hyponatraemia and hypokalaemia are frequently found in hypothermia; however, elderly persons who are severely dehydrated or volume-depleted may present with hypernatraemia.

Management

Management will depend on the level of the core temperature. In mild cases it is sufficient to wrap the patient up warmly, provide hot drinks and warm up the environment. In all cases of hypothermia the removal of wet/soiled clothing should be undertaken as soon as possible, and the patient should be dried and covered with top and bottom blankets.

In more severe cases, when the body core temperature is below 34°C, it is necessary to monitor body temperature and to rewarm the patient slowly. Rewarming should be carried out with caution and only at a rate of 0.5°C/hour. Ideally, the patient should be nursed in a room where the room temperature can be maintained at between 25 and 30°C (Herbert & Howell 1991). This slow rewarming is carried out to prevent a catastrophic drop in blood pressure, effectively precipitating hypovolaemic shock in the patient because of peripheral vasodilation. Special blankets with reflective inner surfaces ('space blankets') should not be used as they reduce the impact of other warming measures by keeping out heat from an already cold patient (Herbert & Howell 1991). The patient's head should also be covered as up to 40% of body heat is lost through the scalp.

Below 30°C, active core rewarming should be attempted. This involves supported ventilation with warmed, humidified oxygen (Toulson 1993), warmed intravenous fluid (at 38°C) and possibly warmed peritoneal lavage. This is a risky intervention in elderly patients because of possible pulmonary oedema, renal failure or cardiac arrhythmia. Patients should be handled gently as the cold myocardium is extremely irritable and minimal physical stimulation can lead to ventricular fibrillation or asystole.

Care must be exercised in pronouncing hypothermic individuals dead. No certification of death should be issued until patients have been rewarmed to 36°C and have been unresponsive at that temperature. After an episode of hypothermia, it will be essential to prevent a recurrence. An in-depth nursing assessment of the elderly person, including state of nutrition, ability to carry out activities of daily living, and details of social circumstances, is crucial (Watson 1996). Only patients who have had a mild case of hypothermia, i.e. above 34°C, may be discharged following preventative advice. Those with lower core temperatures will usually require admission to intensive care units for further management.

Elder Abuse

Elder abuse is a subject that has attracted growing attention in the last 20 years. However, there remains a relative paucity of British research and few known policies or guidelines on how to deal with a potentially abused or at-risk elderly patient attending the A&E department (Decalmer & Glendenning 1993). The Royal College of Nursing (1991) has defined elder abuse as 'the ongoing inability of an informal carer to respond adequately to meet the needs of a dependent older person'. It is estimated that one in 20 older people have suffered some kind of abuse, with one in 50 reporting physical abuse (Ogg & Bennet 1992).

The picture of abuse may be clouded by acute or chronic illness, and therefore careful consideration should be given to the clarity of the history and to whether presenting features are secondary to ill health or abuse.

Howell & Hopwood (1995) identified five major categories of abuse:

Physical abuse. The most commonly reported type of physical abuse is violence (Stewart 1991). Indicators of physical abuse may include:

■ lacerations and/or bruises in various stages of healing
■ scalds and/or burns with demarcation lines and without splash marks
■ scalds and/or burns involving the buttocks and/or genitals
■ fractures in usually mobile patients.

Psychological abuse. Mental mistreatment is secondary in frequency to physical abuse (Bennet 1990). Examples include threats of punishment, name calling and/or intimidation. Psychological abuse is difficult to measure in the elderly patient, particularly if mental impairment is evident. Indicators of abuse may present as:

■ behavioural signs, such as shame, passivity and anxiety
■ cowering in the presence of the care-giver
■ referral of attention to care-giver when questioned.

It is worth noting, however, that the elderly patient may be anxious due to the confines of the A&E department and may display many of these characteristics for this reason.

Financial/material abuse. This involves improper use of finances and resources of the elderly person for the gain of the carer/relative. Examples of this include:

■ theft of money and possessions
■ sudden or gradual transfer of assets to the care-giver.

While this type of abuse is unlikely to become an issue in the A&E department, it is critically important that health professionals are aware of its occurrence and the devastating effects it may have on the elderly person.

Sexual abuse. Although relatively rare, this form of abuse usually occurs as a result of an incestuous relationship between mother and son. As the elder begins to dement, consent is less easily achieved and violence may occur. Indicators may include:

■ perineal bruising or lacerations
■ recurrent sexually transmitted diseases
■ unexplained vaginal discharge.

Intentional or unintentional neglect. Neglect includes the willful or non-wilful deprivation of care-taking, as regards the activities of daily living. With intentional neglect, the abuser is aware of the effect the neglect is having on the victim. Examples include:

■ withholding spectacles, hearing aids and walking aids
■ refusing adequate food and/or beverages
■ refusing assistance with personal hygiene.

Unintentional neglect may occur when the caretaker is incapable of providing an adequate standard of care due to a mental or physical incapacity. This may include refusal of interventional services by district nurses and social services for fear of being seen as unable to cope (see Boxes 21.2 and 21.3).

Numerous professionals and carers may be involved in the assessment and ongoing care process of elder abuse (Tonks & Bennet 1999). Bennet (1995) believes the physical and psychological manifestations of abuse/neglect will gradually become incorporated into health professionals' knowledge base, as happened with child abuse (see Ch. 16), and that greater diagnostic expertise will develop. In the meantime, the possibility of abuse should be borne in mind by A&E nurses and health care staff when dealing with elderly people.

Confusion

Confusion in the elderly is a catch-all term that covers both dementia and delirium, but may also be a consequence of depression. They are, however, quite

---

Box 21.2 – *Manifestations of inadequate care (Fulmer & O'Malley 1987)*

■ Abrasions	■ Dehydration
■ Lacerations	■ Malnutrition
■ Contusions	■ Inappropriate clothing
■ Burns	■ Poor hygiene
■ Freezing	■ Oversedation
■ Depression	■ Over/undermedication
■ Fractures	■ Untreated medical problems
■ Sprains	■ Failure to meet legal obligations
■ Pressure sores	■ Behaviour that endangers
■ Dislocations	patient or others

Box 21.3 – *Physical indicators of abuse not shared with neglect (Fulmer & O'Malley 1987)*

Unexplained bruises and welts
■ Face, lips and mouth, torso, back, buttocks, thighs – in various stages of healing
■ Clustered, forming regular patterns reflecting the shape of the article used (cord, buckle, hand)
■ On several different surface areas
■ Lesions which regularly appear after absence, weekend or holiday

Unexplained burns
■ Cigar, cigarette – especially on soles, palms, back or buttocks
■ Immersion burns – sock-like on feet, glove-like on hands, doughnut-shaped on buttocks or genitalia
■ Patterned, like electric burner, iron etc.
■ Rope burns on arms, legs, neck or torso

Unexplained fractures
■ To skull, nose, facial structure – in various stages of healing
■ Multiple or spiral fractures

Unexplained lacerations or abrasions
■ To mouth, lips, gums or eye
■ To external genitalia

Sexual abuse
■ Difficulty in walking or sitting
■ Torn, stained or bloody underclothing
■ Pain or itching in the genital area; bruises or bleeding in the external genitalia, vaginal or anal areas
■ Venereal disease

---

different (see Table 21.3). Dementia is a long-term, non-reversible loss of both short-and long-term memory. Delirium is an acute confusional state, which usually has a physical cause. Delirium can also be superimposed on dementia (Birkland & Dyck 1993).

Table 21.3 – *A comparison of clinical features of delirium, dementia and depression. (From Foreman 1986)*

Feature	Delirium	Dementia	Depression
Onset	Acute/subacute; depends on cause; often at twilight	Chronic; generally insidious; depends on cause	Coincides with life changes; often abrupt
Course	Short; diurnal fluctuations in symptoms: worse at night, in the dark and on waking	Long; no diurnal symptoms; progressive yet relatively stable over time	Diurnal effects: typically worse in the morning. Situational fluctuations, but less than with acute confusion
Progression	Abrupt	Slow but even	Variable, rapid–slow, uneven
Duration	Hours to less than 1 month, seldom longer	Months to years	At least 2 weeks; can last several months to years
Awareness	Reduced	Clear	Clear
Alertness	Fluctuates; lethargic or hypervigilant	Generally normal	Normal
Attention	Impaired; fluctuates	Generally normal	Minimal impairment; is distractible
Orientation	Fluctuates in severity; generally impaired	May be impaired	Selective disorientation
Memory	Recent and immediate impaired	Recent and remote impaired	Selective or patchy 'islands' of intact memory
Thinking	Disorganised, distorted, fragmented; slow or accelerated incoherent speech	Difficulty in abstraction; thoughts impoverished; judgement impaired; words difficult to find	Intact but with themes of hopelessness, helplessness or self-deprecation
Perception	Distorted; illusions, delusions and hallucinations	Misperceptions often absent	Intact; delusions and hallucinations absent except in severe cases
Psychomotor	Variable; hypokinetic, hyperkinetic or mixed	Normal or may have apraxia	Variable; psychomotor retardation or agitation
Sleep–wake	Disturbed, cycle reversed	Fragmented	Disturbed, often early waking
Associated	Variable affective changes; symptoms of hyperarousal, exaggeration of personality type; associated with physical illness	Affect tends to be superficial, inappropriate and labile; attempts to conceal deficits in intellect; personality changes; lack of insight	Affect depressed; exaggerated and detailed complaints; preoccupied with personal thoughts; insight present; verbal elaboration

In the A&E setting, the nurse may play an important role in the detection and management of patients with delirium. Foreman (1986) noted that the characteristics of elderly patients that make them vulnerable to delirium are also those that make caring for elderly patients a challenge. These include altered physiological functioning associated with ageing, changes in the sensory organs, changes in cognitive functioning that accompany ageing and illness, malnutrition, and the presence of multiple chronic illnesses and the concomitant treatments. Foreman (1996) noted that the great majority of delirium escapes detection as a result of:

■ the fluctuating nature of the condition
■ the variable presentation between and within individuals
■ the similarity of clinical features of delirium, depression and dementia

- the frequent coexistence of delirium, depression and dementia
- the failure to use routinely standardised methods of detection.

Assessment

The time-frame for the development of delirium is highly significant. Important information can be gleaned unobtrusively from observing and interacting with the patient. The nurse should note the following:

- Is the patient alert?
- Does the patient respond appropriately to questions?
- How is the patient groomed?
- Are the patient's clothes soiled?
- Orientation to time, place and person and situation should also be assessed.

Getting information from the ambulance crew, relatives, home wardens and neighbours can also be crucial in determining the onset and degree of delirium in the patient. This information will be helpful in determining the patient's health and mental status before arrival in the A&E department. It may also explain whether the patient is there because she realises that something is wrong or because someone else has noticed a problem.

A recent onset of confusion is the hallmark of an acute confusional state and requires medical rather than psychiatric management. 'Recent' is usually understood to be less than 1 month. The nurse should look for a fluctuating level of consciousness, another hallmark symptom of delirium. During the assessment, the nurse may observe the following behaviour: the patient appears alert and attentive one moment and falls asleep the next. The history provider may also describe a similar history.

The patient's physical condition will provide clues as to the cause of the confusional state. Temperature, blood pressure, pulse and respirations should be taken to assess for signs of infection. Infections, such as urinary tract and chest infections, are causes of delirium in elderly patients. Simple diagnostic tests such as urinalysis will help to identify potential causes. Evidence of dehydration will often be present in the confused, elderly patient. The nurse should observe mucous membranes, skin turgor and vital signs, as significant dehydration may be the cause of the confusional state. In addition, hypoxia, hypothermia, CVA and metabolic disorders such as diabetes may also present as acute confusion.

Any of these disorders may lead to delirium and all will require medical management. A history of psychiatric illness should alert the nurse to the possibility of a concurrent mental illness which could potentiate the confusion. This confusion could be a result of the illness itself or a side-effect of medication the patient is receiving.

Blood screening for infections or metabolic causes should also be undertaken. A chest X-ray may reveal a chest infection, especially if accompanied by pyrexia.

Management

There are two key elements to the management of delirium:

- eliminate or correct the underlying aetiological disturbance
- provide symptomatic and supportive care.

Assessment should identify or rule out physical causes of confusion. Intravenous therapy may be required to correct fluid and electrolyte imbalances. Sedative drugs should not be given unless the patient's behaviour is overly disruptive. Where possible, frequent changes of nurses should be avoided, to enable a rapport to be built up with the patient and to facilitate orientation. Effective communication includes ensuring that the patient's hearing aids and spectacles are present and working as necessary.

Falls

Downton (1993) noted that 28–35% of elderly people living at home have at least one fall per year, while Greaves et al. (1997) noted that only about 3% of elderly people who fall sustain an injury that requires medical attention. It is the most common cause of emergency admission to an acute elderly care ward, often after a prolonged period lying on the floor unable to get up.

Problems in mobility caused by joint stiffness, muscle wasting and bone disease are compounded by delay in neuromuscular coordination, cardiovascular function, environmental factors and drugs (Walsh 1996). As a consequence, elderly people are more likely to sustain falls than younger individuals. Precipitating causes include changes of posture; for example, getting out of a chair, which is an unstable situation requiring strength and coordination, is a typical cause of falls. In falls due to extended movement, the person reaches out or up, dislocating her centre of gravity, and owing to a slowing of postural reflex movements she is unable to compensate by moving her feet quickly enough to prevent a fall. Illnesses such as cardiac disease, diabetes and poor vision also contribute to the incidence of falls in older people, as do medications such as diuretics, hypnotics and antihypertensive drugs, due to their hypotensive side-effects (Greaves *et al.* 1997).

The commonest injuries sustained following a fall are fractures of the femur, wrist (Colles' fracture) and upper humerus. Pretibial lacerations, minor head injuries and facial lacerations are also common. Neck of femur fractures are sustained by 57 000 people each year – about one a day per hospital, a figure that could double by 2015 (Audit Commission 1996). Holt *et al.* (1994) noted that the mortality rate for patients with neck of femur fractures is 12%, with a female: male ratio of 6:1, probably due to the increased incidence of osteoporosis in women and their greater longevity compared with men. Fox *et al.* (1994) showed that the mean hospital stay was 31 days, but that those patients with dementia averaged 56 days and those with pressure sore averaged 53 days. Holt *et al.* (1994) suggested that the best predictors of discharge mobility and postoperative complications were age and mobility pre-injury. Fractures are considered in detail in Chapter 5.

Perhaps the greatest impact of falls among elderly people is the subsequent loss of self-confidence it creates. The prognosis in these instances is poor. In the very old, about a quarter will die within a year of their initial fall. If they have lain for more than an hour, half will be dead within 6 months (Greaves *et al.* 1997). Redfern (1991) believes that falls may lead the elderly person to become house-bound, chair-bound and then bed-bound, consequently becoming more immobile and dependent.

A study by Runciman *et al.* (1996) suggested that prompt follow-up by health visitors following an elderly person's attendance to A&E may be the key to preventing readmission in those elderly people who have severe physical illness with multiple pathology and functional disability. The A&E nurse has a crucial role in coordinating these services as well as supporting the patient during her stay in the department. An occupational therapist's assessment of the patient's home circumstances may reduce the incidence of falls in the home (Hann 1997) and the nurse should ensure that the patient is aware of the services available. Discharge planning requires special consideration for elderly patients who have fallen. Before patients are discharged, it is important to see whether they can walk either unaided or with the use of aids. Further falls or lack of stability may indicate the need for further intervention, especially if there is no professional or family support at home.

Particular attention should be paid when providing information about prescribed medications. As loss of short-term memory may affect retention of information, patients should be encouraged to coordinate medication time with activities of daily living, such as mealtimes. Medication bottle tops should be easy to open, as elderly people may have difficulty with them because of the loss of manual dexterity.

Kingston & Hopwood (1994) believe that a thorough and uniform assessment of the elderly and their problems in A&E departments should subsequently lead on to a planned and successful discharge with relevant referrals made to the appropriate members of the primary care team.

Risk assessment of the elderly patient prior to discharge should include:

- *Medical condition* – the patient's medical condition must be stable before discharge is contemplated.
- *Mobility* – the ability to walk unaided, with a stick or zimmer frame, but without carer support, is an important determinant of fitness for discharge.
- *Social support* – it is important to establish whether the elderly person lives alone or has formal or informal support available.
- *Lifestyle* – a patient who is currently bed bound is more likely to require readmission than one who is normally outgoing.
- *External influences* – those living alone in a tower block without working lifts will find it more difficult to mobilise than someone living in sheltered accommodation. The handover ambulance crew can often provide useful information about the environment to which the patient may be returning.

The A&E nurse should also offer dietary advice, where appropriate. For example, patients with a predisposition to constipation should be encouraged to eat foods which are high in fibre, while those who are predisposed to osteoporosis or penicious anaemia should be encouraged to eat dairy products.

Conclusion

The care of older people in A&E is going to become an increasingly important part of the A&E nurse's role as demographic changes in the population take hold. The assessment of elderly people, because of their social, psychological and physical vulnerability, is a critically important dimension of care in A&E; however, older people should not be seen as a homogenous group who are all victims or who are automatically infirm because of their age. The A&E nurse has the opportunity to challenge stereotypes, provide health promotion and offer guidance on services available to older patients, as well as acting as an advocate for those unable to speak up for themselves. It presents a challenge which A&E nurses should embrace as part of their role as health providers.

Further reading

Bennet GCJ, Ebrahim S (1995) *Health Care in Old Age*, 2nd edn. London: Edward Arnold.

Kingston P, Bennet G (1993) *Elder Abuse: Concepts, Theories and Interventions*. London: Chapman & Hall

Kingston P, Penhale B (eds) (1995) *Family Violence and Caring Professions*. Basingstoke: Macmillan.

Wade L, Water K (1996) *A Textbook of Gerontological Nursing: Perspectives on Practice*. London: Baillière Tindall.

Wanich Bradway C (ed.) (1996) *Nursing Care of Geriatric Emergencies*. New York: Springer.

Wolf RS, Pillemer KA (1989) *Helping Elderly Victims: the Reality of Elder Abuse*. New York: Columbia University Press.

References

Audit Commission (1996) *United they Stand: Co-ordinating Care for Elderly Patients with Hip Fracture*. London: HMSO.

Bennet G (1990) Assessing abuse in the elderly. *Geriatric Medicine*, **20**(7), 49–51.

Bennet GCJ (1995) Health perspectives and elder abuse. In: Kingston P, Penhale B, eds. *Family Violence and Caring Professions*. Basingstoke: Macmillan.

Birkland P, Dyck E (1993) 'Psychiatric' or 'medical'?: assessing confusion in the elderly patient. *Journal of Emergency Nursing*, **19**, 408–411.

Brookbank JW (1990) *The Biology of Ageing*. New York: Harper Collins.

Central Statistics Office (1993) *Key Data*. London: Government Statistical Service.

Decalmer P, Glendenning F (eds) (1993) *The Mistreatment of Elderly People*. London: Sage.

Downton J (1993) *Falls in the Elderly*. London: Edward Arnold.

Foreman MD (1996) Delirium in the emergency department. In: Wanich Bradway C, ed. *Nursing Care of Geriatric Emergencies*. New York: Springer.

Foreman MD (1986) Acute confusional states in the hospitalised elderly: a research dilemma. *Nursing Research*, **35**, 34–38.

Fox H, Pooler J, Prothero D, Bannister GC (1994) Factors affecting the outcome after proximal femoral fractures. *Injury*, **25**, 297–300.

Fulmer T, O'Malley T (1987) *Inadequate Care of the Elderly: a Health Care Perspective on Abuse and Neglect*. New York: Springer.

Greaves I, Hodgetts T, Porter K (1997) Care of the elderly. In: Greaves I, Hodgetts T, Porter K, eds. *Emergency Care: a Textbook for Paramedics*. London: Baillière Tindall.

Hann (1997) Use of Occupational therapists in A&E. *Emergency Nurse*, **5**(6), 26–30.

Herbert R, Howell S (1991) Maintaining body temperature. In: Redfern S, ed. *Nursing Elderly People*, 2nd edn. Edinburgh: Churchill Livingstone.

Hinchliff S, Montagne SE, Watson R (1996) *Physiology for Nursing Practice*, 2nd edn. London: Baillière Tindall.

Holt E, Evans RA, Hinadley CJ, Metcalf JW (1994) 1000 femoral neck fractures: the effect of pre-injury mobility and surgical experience on outcome. *Injury*, **25**, 91–95.

Howell F, Hopwood A (1995) Identifying abuse of elderly people. *Emergency Nurse*, **3**(1), 7–9.

Johnson ML (1976) That was your life: a biological approach to later life. In Munnichs JMA, Van Den Heuval WJA, eds. *Dependency or Interdependency in Old Age*. The Hague: Martinus Nijhoff.

Kingston P, Hopwood A (1994) The elderly person in A and E. In: Sbaih L, ed. *Issues in Accident and Emergency Nursing*. London: Chapman & Hall.

Lloyd EL (1990) Temperature recommendations for elderly people: are we wrong? *Age & Ageing*, **19**, 267–267.

Manning B, Stolerman DF (1993) Hypothermia in the elderly. *Hospital Practice*, **28**(5), 53–70.

Ogg J, Bennet G (1992) Elder abuse in Britain. *British Medical Journal*, **305**, 998–999.

Redfern S (1991) *Nursing Elderly People*. Edinburgh: Churchill Livingstone.

Runciman P, Currie CT, Nicol M, Green L, Mikam V (1996) Discharge of elderly people from an accident and emergency department: evaluation of health visitor follow-up. *Journal of Advanced Nursing*, **24**, 711–718.

Royal College of Nursing (1991) *Guidelines for Nurses: Abuse and Older People*. London: RCN.

Stewart C (1991) Emergency Medicine Reports. *The Practical Journal for Emergency Physicians*, **12**(20), 179–186.

Stoyle J (1991) *Caring for Older People: a Multi-cultural Approach*. Cheltenham: Thornes.

Tonks A, Bennet (1999) Elder abuse. *British Medical Journal*, **318**(7179), 278.

Toulson S (1993) Treatment and prevention of hypothermia. *British Journal of Nursing*, **12**, 662–666.

Walsh M (1996) *Accident & Emergency Care: a New Approach*, 3rd edn. Oxford: Butterworth-Heinemann

Wanich Bradway C (1996) Thermoregulatory disorders. In: Wanich Bradway C, ed. *Nursing Care of Geriatric Emergencies*, New York: Springer.

Watson R (1996) Hypothermia. *Emergency Nurse*, **3**(4), 10–15.

Wickham N (1997a) Pressure area care in A&E: Part one. *Emergency Nurse*, **5**(3), 26–31.

Wickham N (1997b) Pressure area care in A&E: Part two. *Emergency Nurse*, **5**(4), 25–29.

Part 5

Physiology for A&E Practice

22. Physiology for Practice 295

23. Wound Care 307

24. Pain Management 325

25. Local and Regional Anaesthesia 333

Chapter 22

Physiology for Practice

Marion Richardson

- Introduction
- Homeostasis
- Oxygen transport
- Carbon dioxide transport
- Oxygen/carbon dioxide homeostasis
- Oxygen therapy
- Flight physiology
- Temperature control
- Fluid and electrolyte balance
- Haemostasis
- Shock
- Conclusion

Introduction

This chapter looks at some of the physiological mechanisms which support normal body function, the failure of which may necessitate nursing intervention in the A&E patient. The basic physiological concepts of homeostasis are examined and a number of homeostatic mechanisms throughout the body are described to show how levels of oxygen and carbon dioxide, fluids and electrolytes are maintained. The mechanisms of oxygen and carbon dioxide transport to and from the cells and the importance of temperature regulation are discussed. Finally, the breakdown of homeostatic mechanisms is considered in a discussion of physiological shock.

Homeostasis

The term 'homeostasis' was first used by an American physiologist, Walter Cannon, in 1932. The word comes from the Greek and means 'standing the same', something of a misnomer since physiological function is never static but rather maintains an equilibrium despite constant fluctuations. Homeostasis is essential if the metabolic activities which occur constantly in all cells are to continue. The body must be able to sense alterations in the level of required nutrients and be able to correct the deficit or excess. Throughout the body there are many self-regulating homeostatic mechanisms which aim to maintain an internal 'steady state' for optimal physiological functioning. The cells must receive adequate oxygen and other nutrients, and a constant cellular pressure and temperature must be maintained.

Most homeostatic mechanisms within the body work by 'negative feedback', where a deviation from the normal steady state will cause a response to restore the steady state – thus too little of something will cause more to be produced, too much of something will trigger mechanisms to reduce the amount. Once steady state is reached, the homeostatic mechanisms are switched off. An example of a see-saw is commonly

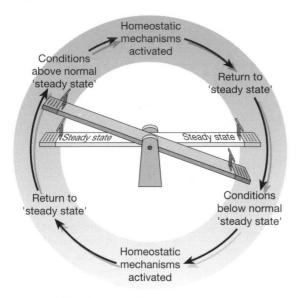

Figure 22.1 – *Homeostasis: maintaining a steady state.*

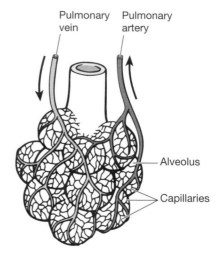

Figure 22.2 – *Capillary network surrounding the alveolus.*

used to illustrate this concept (Fig. 22.1). Examples of homeostatic mechanisms are seen in temperature regulation and in the regulation of oxygen and carbon dioxide levels within the body and these will be described in more detail later.

Oxygen Transport

The atmosphere comprises of a mixture of gases of which the most important physiologically is oxygen. Inspired air consists of approximately 21% oxygen, 79% nitrogen and small amounts of carbon dioxide (0.04%) and other rarer gases including water vapour. Each gas within this mixture exerts its own pressure, known as the *partial pressure*, and the total pressure of the mixture is equal to the sum of the pressures of all the gases within it (Dalton's law of partial pressures). Atmospheric air pressure at sea level is known to be 101.3 kPa or 760 mmHg, and since oxygen comprises 21% of the mixture, its partial pressure, usually written as PO_2, can be calculated thus:

$$\frac{21}{100} \times 101.3 = 21.2 \text{ kPa}$$

The PN_2 can be similarly calculated as 79.6 kPa.

As atmospheric air passes through the respiratory tract, it becomes humidified with more water vapour, which reduces the partial pressure of the other gases as the pressure exerted by the water accounts for a larger proportion of the total pressure. The partial pressures are further modified as the gases combine with the air in the physiological 'dead space' in the

respiratory tract before finally meeting and mixing with gases in the alveoli. As a result, the alveolar PO_2 is considerably less than atmospheric PO_2, and alveolar PCO_2 and water vapour pressure are measurably higher, although the total pressure remains the same as atmospheric pressure. Alveolar PO_2 is 13.3 kPa and alveolar PCO_2 is 5.3 kPa, and it is these amounts of gas that are available at the alveolar capillary membrane in the lungs where gaseous exchange takes place.

In the alveoli, gaseous exchange is possible because of the very thin pulmonary membrane between the alveoli and capillaries and the vast network of capillaries surrounding them (Fig. 22.2). The rate at which a gas will diffuse across a membrane is affected by several factors:

- the surface area available for diffusion
- the thinness of the membrane across which diffusion occurs
- the ease with which the gas will enter a solution – its solubility
- the existence of a pressure gradient, i.e. different pressures on either side of the membrane.

Within the lungs, all of these factors combine to allow rapid and efficient transfer of oxygen into the blood and carbon dioxide out of the blood and into the alveoli ready to be expired.

Blood within the alveolar capillaries contains less oxygen and more carbon dioxide than alveolar air as a result of cellular metabolism which removes oxygen from arterial blood and replaces it with carbon dioxide produced as a result of metabolic activity. Blood arriving at the lungs has a PO_2 of 5.3 kPa and a PCO_2 of 6.1 kPa. When alveolar air and this blood are in close

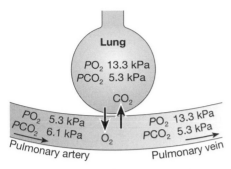

Figure 22.3 – *Gaseous exchange across the alveolar–capillary membrane.*

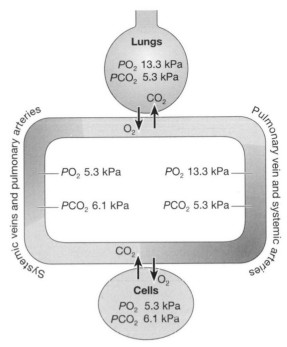

Figure 22.4 – *Oxygen and carbon dioxide exchange throughout the body.*

proximity at the alveolar membrane, gases rapidly diffuse across the membrane until their pressures are equal on either side. Blood leaving the lungs contains oxygen and carbon dioxide at virtually the same partial pressures as those contained within the alveoli, so that the pulmonary vein and systemic arterial partial pressure of oxygen (P_AO_2) is 13.3 kPa and P_ACO_2 is 5.3 kPa (Fig. 22.3); these quantities of gas are carried *in solution* within the blood to the tissues.

At the tissues, gases diffuse in the opposite direction across pressure gradients and thin membranes. Oxygen is given up to the tissues and replaced with dissolved carbon dioxide produced by the tissues. Partial pressures of oxygen and carbon dioxide within the cells are the same as those in blood arriving at the lungs (Fig. 22.4) since the gases cannot cross the thicker membranes of blood vessels in the rest of the circulation.

Oxygen carried in simple solution is not an efficient means of transporting blood around the circulation, as a vast blood volume would be required to supply the 250 ml of oxygen required every minute, even when the body is at rest. Oxygen carried by this means accounts for only 1% of the total oxygen transported in the blood, but it is an important 1% as this is the only oxygen that exerts a pressure: not only does it maintain the pressure gradients necessary for diffusion, but it is this that is recorded when arterial blood gases are measured. Normal P_AO_2 and P_ACO_2 are the same as the pressures within alveolar air, i.e. 13.3 and 5.3 kPa, respectively. This Po_2 governs the far greater amount of oxygen that can be transported bound to haemoglobin. Normally, 99% of oxygen is carried in the blood bound to haemoglobin and, once bound, is no longer free to exert a pressure.

Haemoglobin (Hb) is a conjugated protein found in red blood cells and consists of four haem groups containing iron and four polypeptide chains. Each of these haem groups can combine with one molecule of oxygen to form oxyhaemoglobin, which is bright red and gives arterial blood its distinctive colour. This process is known as oxygenation. Normal Hb is approximately 15 g/dl and each gram of Hb can carry 1.34 ml O_2, so that the total oxygen capacity of the blood, i.e. the total amount that could be carried, is 15 × 1.34 = 20.1 ml/dl. This equation is simpler if SI units are used – normal Hb is 2.2 mmol/L blood and each molecule of Hb can combine with four molecules of O_2, so the oxygen capacity is 8.8 mmol/L (1 mmol O_2 = 22.4 ml). Amounts of oxygen carried bound to Hb can thus be far in excess of the normal requirements of the body.

The amount of O_2 that actually binds to Hb is called the oxygen content and the percentage of available Hb carrying O_2 is the oxygen saturation. It is this oxygen saturation that is recorded by pulse oximetry and it is dependent on both the Hb levels in the blood and on the Po_2 of the blood.

Oxygen does not bind to each haem molecule with the same ease and a graph plotting Hb saturation against Po_2 is not linear. The first haem group combines with O_2 with relative difficulty, the second and third groups combine more readily and the fourth combines with the greatest difficulty of all. It will be seen from Figure 22.5 that at a Po_2 of 5.3 kPa, as in blood arriving at the lungs, almost 70% of the Hb sites are bound with oxygen and exposure to a Po_2 of 13.3 kPa at the alveoli

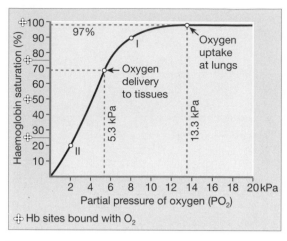

Figure 22.5 – *The oxygen dissociation curve.*

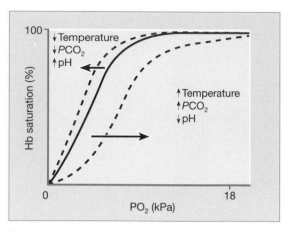

Figure 22.6 – *Factors influencing a shift in the dissociation curve.*

will allow up to 97% of the Hb to become saturated with O_2. At the tissues, O_2 is unloaded from the haem molecules in response to the fall in PO_2, so that a tissue PO_2 of 5.3 kPa will mean that oxygen from the 70–97% range can be removed for use. In normal circumstances, Hb saturation of 100% is rarely achieved and normal oxygen saturation as recorded by a pulse oximeter will be in the region of 97–98%.

The 's' shape of the oxygen–haemoglobin dissociation curve is important physiologically for a number of reasons. Normal physiological function occurs over only a small part of this curve (Fig. 22.5) and a large reserve is available in the event of a fall in arterial PO_2, such as in lung disease, during exercise or at altitude. Even at a PO_2 of only 8 kPa, 90% saturation of Hb with oxygen will be achieved in blood leaving the lungs (point I in Fig. 22.5). During strenuous exercise, it is possible to achieve a PO_2 at the tissues of as little as 2 kPa and this will allow 80% of the bound oxygen to be released (point II in Fig. 22.5), thus supplying the increased amount of oxygen required by the tissues.

Several factors affect the ease with which O_2 binds with Hb and will influence the position of the oxygen–haemoglobin dissociation curve. The factors influencing 'shifts' in the curve are summarised in Figure 22.6. The result of a shift to the left is that loading of Hb with O_2 occurs more readily, i.e. at a lower PO_2, while a shift to the right facilitates unloading of the O_2 at the tissues.

Carbon Dioxide Transport

Carbon dioxide is transported around the body in three ways:

- – 5% in simple solution
- – 5% bound to haemoglobin, at different sites from those for O_2
- – 90% as bicarbonate (hydrogen carbonate) ions.

Tissue cells constantly produce CO_2 and this diffuses across a pressure gradient into the capillaries supplying the tissue. Some remains dissolved in the plasma but most crosses into the red blood cells (erythrocytes), where the presence of an enzyme, carbonic anhydrase, promotes the conversion of CO_2 and water within the cells to carbonic acid. The carbonic acid then dissociates into hydrogen and hydrogen carbonate according to the equation

$$H_2O + CO_2 \Leftrightarrow H_2CO_3 \Leftrightarrow H^+ + HCO_3^-$$

HCO_3^- is then removed to the plasma where it is transported combined with sodium found in the plasma.

CO_2 carried in this way does not exert a pressure within the blood and the equation reverses readily when blood arrives at the lungs so that CO_2 is readily released to be blown off.

Oxygen/Carbon Dioxide Homeostasis

Variations in arterial PO_2 and PCO_2 are sensed by chemoreceptors. Peripheral chemoreceptors in the aortic arch and at the bifurcation of the common carotid artery are sensitive to falls in P_AO_2, and rises in P_ACO_2. Once altered levels are sensed, the respiratory centre in the medulla of the brain is stimulated, via the vagal and glossopharyngeal nerves, to increase the rate and depth of respiration by stimulating the diaphragm and intercostal muscles via the phrenic and

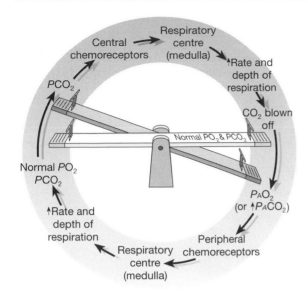

Figure 22.7 – *Respiratory homeostasis.*

intercostal nerves. Once levels O_2 are restored to normal, the mechanism is switched off.

Central chemoreceptors in the ventral surface of the medulla are bathed in cerebrospinal fluid, which is particularly sensitive to rises in P_ACO_2. Inspiratory neurones in the respiratory centre of the medulla are again stimulated to increase both the rate and depth of respiration until the CO_2 is removed at the lungs and levels within the blood return to normal. The homeostatic mechanism is then switched off.

These homeostatic mechanisms are diagrammatically represented in Figure 22.7.

Oxygen Therapy

The aim of oxygen therapy is to raise the Po_2 in the lungs, thus increasing the pressure gradient across the alveolar capillary membrane and allowing more oxygen to enter the blood for transport to the tissues. There are, however, potential hazards which should be considered when oxygen therapy is indicated:

■ Patients with long-term respiratory disease may rely on low Po_2 levels to stimulate the respiratory centre (anoxic drive) rather than rises in Pco_2 levels. High levels of oxygen administered to these patients will cause respiratory depression and possibly apnoea.
■ High concentrations of O_2 over prolonged periods may cause lung damage with oedema. Concentrations of administered O_2 should be kept as low as possible whilst maintaining adequate blood gas levels.

■ Compressed O_2 is very drying and should be humidified prior to administration. Patients receiving O_2 will require regular mouth rinses.
■ In neonates, particularly premature infants, blindness caused by retrolental fibroplasia, i.e. fibrosis behind the lens of the eye, may develop as a result of high-level O_2 administration.

Flight Physiology

With the increase in the transportation of the ill and injured by air, it has become increasingly important that nurses familiarise themselves with altitude physiology, particularly with respect to available oxygen and hypoxia.

As altitude increases, during flight or when ascending mountains, barometric pressure falls and the gases within the atmosphere expand. While the percentage of oxygen within the atmosphere remains the same, the Po_2 will fall. At 10 000 feet (300 metres) atmospheric pressure is 70 kPa or 523 mmHg and the Po_2 will be 21% of this, i.e. 15 kPa. Alveolar Po_2 at this height will be reduced to approximately 9 kPa, causing a marked reduction in the pressure gradient across the alveolar capillary membrane. Hypoxic hypoxia may become apparent in anyone above 10 000 feet unless supplementary oxygen is administered. Blood oxygen saturation of 98% at sea level will be reduced to 87% at 10 000 feet and to only 60% at 20 000 feet. In pressurised cabins, pressure is usually maintained at about 8000 feet and the fit adult can readily adjust to cope with the resultant physiological alterations.

The symptoms of hypoxia include increases in heart and respiratory rate, headache, fatigue, nausea and dizziness. Perhaps the most threatening factor is that the onset is insidious and may occur in the carer as well as the patient. Prevention of hypoxia should always be the primary concern.

Pressures within body cavities alter with changes in barometric pressure. At altitude, gases within the cavities expand and then contract again during descent. These effects are particularly noticeable in the smaller body cavities, such as the middle ear and sinuses. Normally expanding and contracting gases will pass through the Eustachian tubes or the sinus cavities so that the pressure changes are equalised. In individuals with allergies, a cold or sinus infection, this movement of gases is limited or obstructed and painful otitis media or sinusitis may result. Those patients in whom respiration is compromised require careful monitoring and any pneumothorax must be treated prior to air transport as it will be likely to collapse further at altitude. Endotracheal tube balloons, intravenous fluid bags, anti-shock trousers and pneumatic splints are also subject to pressure changes and need close observation to ensure accurate functioning.

Temperature Control

Humans are homeothermic and maintain a constant core temperature, i.e. the temperature within the internal organs, of 37°C, regardless of the external temperature. The skin temperature may be several degrees different from the core temperature and will vary between areas of the body, as those who always seem to have cold feet will know.

Body temperature is usually lower, by about 0.5°C at night (the circadian rhythm) and is 0.5–1°C higher in women during the second half of the menstrual cycle. Children have higher core temperatures than neonates and the elderly, and core temperature can rise by up to 2°C during strenuous exercise. Despite these normal variations, maintenance of a constant body temperature is essential for optimal functioning of cellular enzymes. The body must maintain a careful balance between heat gained and heat lost. A summary of factors influencing heat gain and loss are given in Box 22.1.

Box 22.1 – *Factors influencing heat gain and loss*

Heat gain	Heat loss
■ External temperature	■ External temperature
■ Metabolism	■ Evaporation
■ Food and drink	■ Conduction
■ Shivering	■ Convection
■ Hormones	■ Radiation
■ Behaviour (put on clothes)	■ Body excretions — air — urine — faeces
	■ Behaviour (take off clothes)

Temperature homeostasis

Temperature-sensitive receptors, thermoreceptors, are found peripherally in the skin, sensitive to external temperature changes, and centrally in the hypothalamus, sensitive to changes in temperature of blood bathing them and thus to core temperature. When stimulated, the thermoreceptors initiate impulses via afferent nerves to the temperature-regulating centres in the anterior hypothalamus.

When core temperature falls below normal, the hypothalamus acts to conserve heat in the following ways:

■ Peripheral vasoconstriction mediated via the sympathetic nervous system closes down the surface blood vessels, ensuring that blood is kept closer to the warm core and heat loss through the skin is minimised.

■ Shivering is initiated by the posterior hypothalamus and results in uncoordinated muscle activity which generates heat.

■ The thyroid gland is stimulated to produce the hormone thyroxin which raises the basal metabolic rate of cells, thus increasing heat production. Once temperature reaches normal levels, the mechanism is switched off.

A rise in core temperature above 37°C will stimulate responses aimed at losing heat:

■ Peripheral blood vessels are dilated under the influence of the sympathetic nervous system and heat is lost through the skin by radiation, conduction and convection.

■ Sweat glands are stimulated, again via the sympathetic nervous system, to increase secretion, and heat is lost by evaporation. Evaporation of sweat is reduced when humidity is high and this is consequently a less effective means of reducing temperature.

A diagrammatic representation of thermoregulatory mechanisms is given in Figure 22.8.

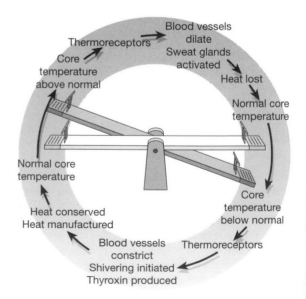

Figure 22.8 – *Thermoregulation.*

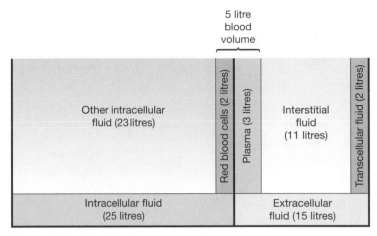

Figure 22.9 – *Body fluid compartments.*

Hypothermia

A core temperature below 35°C is termed hypothermia and, if not treated, the negative feedback mechanisms which maintain temperature homeostasis will fail, and damage or death may ensue. The ability to shiver decreases when the core temperature falls below 34°C and consequently the core temperature will fall further. Hypothermia slows the chemical reactions of metabolism and reduces blood flow to all organs. The resultant hypoxia will cause drowsiness and loss of consciousness as a result of cerebral ischaemia. Cardiac arrhythmias will occur at about 25°C and the heart will cease to beat at about 20°C.

The O_2 requirements of the tissues are substantially reduced at low temperatures and gradual warming of the patient combined with controlled oxygen therapy may result in full recovery provided no physiological damage has occurred. The elderly and neonates are particularly prone to hypothermia because of less efficient thermoregulatory mechanisms, as are those who misuse drugs and alcohol or who live 'rough' and who are not always able to take voluntary measures to regain heat.

Pyrexia

Pyrexia or fever occurs when body temperature rises above normal as a result of pyrogens produced by bacteria, viruses or necrotic tissue, which affect the temperature-regulating centre. Head injury and brain damage may have a similar effect. The temperature-regulating centre is 'reset' at a higher level by the pyrogens and the body will continue to produce heat to maintain the higher level until the pyrogens are removed from the body.

Hyperpyrexia, i.e. a core temperature above 40.5°C, is a dangerous condition. Cellular metabolism is greatly increased and the body is unable to lose the heat produced sufficiently to reduce the temperature. Cells throughout the body are destroyed by literally burning themselves out and irreversible brain damage will occur at about 42°C.

Fluid and Electrolyte Balance

Water is the basis of all body fluids, e.g. plasma, tissue fluids and lymph, and accounts for approximately 60% of total body weight. Body water contains many electrolytes, substances which dissolve and dissociate into ions (develop electrical charges). The main electrolytes in the body are sodium (Na^+), potassium (K^+), calcium (Ca^{2+}) and magnesium (Mg^{2+}), all of which are positively charged *anions*, and the negatively charged *cations* chloride (Cl^-), hydrogen bicarbonate (HCO_3^-), protein (Pr^-) and phosphate (PO_4^{2-}).

Fluid is either inside the cells (intracellular) or outside the cells (extracellular). Extracellular fluid includes blood plasma, interstitial or tissue fluid which bathes the cells, and transcellular fluid, i.e. fluid in body cavities such as intraocular, peritoneal and pleural fluid, cerebrospinal fluid and digestive juices. Figure 22.9 shows how these fluid compartments compare.

Intracellular fluid contains positively charged potassium and magnesium and negatively charged protein and phosphate. Extracellular fluid contains positively charged sodium ions and negatively charged chloride ions (Fig. 22.10). The ions are prevented from diffusing into other compartments by the selective permeability of the cell membranes and by the presence of a sodium pump within cell walls which

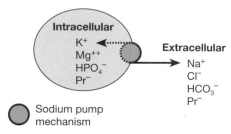

Figure 22.10 – *Electrolytes in fluid compartments.*

actively pumps out sodium and exchanges it for potassium.

The interstitial fluid which bathes cells throughout the body must be maintained in a stable state as it provides the cells with the chemicals and maintains the correct temperature for them to function effectively. Disturbances in the electrolyte content and the concentration, osmolality and osmolarity of the extracellular fluid will affect the intracellular fluid and will impair cell and body function as a result. Normal cell function relies on fluid and electrolyte homeostasis.

Fluids normally enter the body only through the mouth in response to thirst, i.e. when osmoreceptors in the hypothalamus are stimulated by a fall in the osmotic pressure of plasma passing over them. Fluid balance by intake alone would be inefficient since either too much or too little may be ingested for any number of reasons. Similarly, oral regulation of electrolyte balance is inefficient. The body regulates levels of both water and electrolytes at the point of exit, mainly by the action of hormones on the distal tubules of the kidney.

Water balance is coordinated by the thirst centre in the hypothalamus which controls the release of antidiuretic hormone (ADH). When the concentration of extracellular fluid falls as a result of a fluid intake below body requirements, osmoreceptors in the anterior hypothalamus sense the change and trigger impulses to allow the release of ADH from the posterior pituitary gland. ADH acts on the distal tubules of the kidney so that water is reabsorbed into the circulation. The mechanism is switched off once extracellular osmolarity returns to normal.

The hormone aldosterone, secreted from the adrenal cortex, is responsible for maintaining sodium levels in the body. A fall in blood sodium levels, or a rise in serum potassium, increases the release of aldosterone which acts to reabsorb sodium from the renal tubules and to reduce its excretion in saliva, gastric juices and the skin. Aldosterone production is also stimulated by a fall in the extracellular fluid volume via the renin–angiotensin system. Potassium balance is closely linked with sodium and when sodium

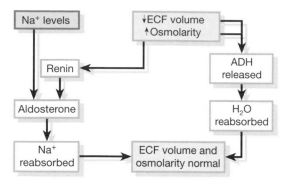

Figure 22.11 – *Water and sodium balance.*

is reabsorbed, potassium is generally excreted. The body is inefficient at conserving potassium and blood levels are not indicative of total body potassium as most of this electrolyte is intracellular.

Fluid and sodium balance are closely linked and hormonal responses are triggered by both changes in extracellular fluid (ECF) volumes and changes in plasma osmolality. A diagrammatic representation is given in Figure 22.11.

Calcium and phosphate levels in the body are regulated by the secretion of parathyroid hormone from the four parathyroid glands. The hormone is released directly in response to extracellular fluid concentrations of calcium and acts on bone and the kidney tubules to return calcium to the fluid. When calcium is reabsorbed, phosphate is lost.

Haemostasis

Haemostasis is the term used to describe the arrest of bleeding, a homeostatic process designed to maintain the body's blood volume. Haemostasis will normally control bleeding in all but large arteries and veins, although intervention will be needed if bleeding is to be arrested in these large vessels.

The process of haemostasis can be divided into stages, although physiologically it occurs as a continuous process:

1. Myogenic reflex. Damaged vessels will normally dilate immediately after injury under the influence of histamine released by mast cells in response to the trauma. Within seconds the vessels constrict and the cut ends retract as platelets within the vessels begin to clump together and release powerful vasoconstrictors, serotonin and thromboxane A. This so-called 'myogenic reflex' occurs even in large vessels and lasts for approximately 20 minutes, enough time for stages two and three to commence.

2. Platelet plug formation. When blood vessels

are cut, filaments of collagen and elastin are exposed and attract passing platelets which adhere to them. This adherence causes the release of adenosine diphosphate (ADP) from the platelets, red blood cells and vessel walls. ADP triggers a change in the shape of the platelets which encourages them to clump together. Other substances, including serotonin, also encourage platelet clumping until a plug of platelets is formed which is large enough to close the wounded vessel. A platelet plug is formed within a few seconds of injury and is sufficiently strong to stop bleeding in smaller vessels. The plug must then be stabilised by fibrin fibres or it will break down after about 20 minutes and bleeding will start again.

3. Fibrin clot. Fibrin is an insoluble protein that is laid down as a mesh of fine threads which adhere to one another and to blood cells and platelets. They become entangled in the platelet plug, attract more cells to plug the damaged area and gradually make the clot firmer and more stable. Fibrin is formed by a complex process initiated when tissues are damaged. The complexity of the process is important since clotting within undamaged vessels would be undesirable.

The early stages of fibrin formation also trigger the complicated clotting cascade involving 13 different factors, mostly blood constituents, which ultimately result in a blood clot. Blood is prevented from clotting, or the process is prolonged, if any of the factors is absent (as in haemophilia) or by the use of anti-coagulants (such as heparin), which prevent their production.

4. Fibrinolysis. During this stage fibrin is broken down and removed by phagocytes. The enzyme plasmin, which is responsible for this process, may be activated by streptokinase and other fibrinolytic agents.

Shock

Shock is a clinical syndrome characterised by a lack of adequate tissue perfusion needed to meet the oxygen and nutritional needs of the cells. Cells and organs throughout the body are unable to function adequately and, as shock progresses, may fail and ultimately cause death if left untreated. Shock is commonly classified according to its pathophysiological cause, but any condition, physical or psychological, which reduces the heart's ability to pump or reduces venous return is a potential cause of shock.

Classification of shock

Hypovolaemic shock

The causes of hypovolaemia are:

- loss of blood as in haemorrhage
- loss of plasma as in severe burns and peritonitis
- loss of body fluids through diarrhoea, vomiting or sweating.

Fifteen per cent or more of total blood volume may be lost before signs of hypovolaemic shock are noted in an adult.

Cardiogenic shock ('pump failure')

Events which reduce the ability of the heart to pump efficiently result in cardiogenic shock. These include:

- myocardial infarction
- cardiac arrhythmias
- cardiac tamponade.
- disorders in the lungs, e.g. tension pneumothorax.

Neurogenic shock

In neurogenic shock, sympathetic and parasympathetic nervous control is lost. The venous 'tone' essential to the maintenance of normal blood pressure and venous return is lost and blood pools in the venules and capillaries. Common causes include:

- severe head injury
- spinal injury
- drug reaction and anaesthetics
- neurological illness, e.g. Guillain–Barré syndrome.
- severe fright may also result in neurogenic shock.

Septic shock

Damage is caused by overwhelming bacterial infection usually by Gram-negative bacilli such as *Escherichia coli* and *Klebsiella*. The bacteria cause damage by invading cells and histamines, and other proteolytic enzymes are released which cause vasodilation and increased capillary permeability.

Fluid leaks out of the capillaries causing hypotension and ultimately hypovolaemia. Septic shock often has an insidious rather than a sudden onset and is some-times referred to as 'hot shock' because sufferers are pyrexial as a result of the precipitating infection. Toxic shock is a type of septic shock and is generally associated with menstruating and prolonged use of tampons. The causative organism in this instance is *Staphylococcus aureus*.

Anaphylactic shock

Anaphylaxis occurs as the result of an antigen–antibody response in sensitive individuals. Mast cells degranulate and release histamines and kinins into the circulation. The result is widespread oedema, including laryngeal oedema, which can rapidly cause death if not treated with adrenaline. Causes include:

- insect bites and stings
- drug allergy, especially to penicillin
- food allergies
- mismatched blood transfusion.

Physiology of shock

Whatever the initial cause of shock, the pathophysiological response is the same (Fig. 22.12). Cells throughout the body are deprived of oxygen, resulting in cell membrane damage. Histamines and kinins are released in response to the damage and cause vasodilation and increased capillary permeability. White blood cells leak out of the capillaries and proteins pass into the extracellular fluid. Oedema occurs within the cells and the interstitial fluid volume increases as the fluid compartments break down. The result is a decrease in the circulating blood volume and a consequent reduction in venous return, in the amount of blood available for oxygenation and in cardiac output (CO). Metabolism continues within the cells despite the lack of oxygen, and lactic acid, produced as a result of cellular metabolism, builds up causing metabolic acidosis.

Compensatory mechanisms

In the initial stages of shock, the body's homeostatic mechanisms are triggered and attempt to return the body to steady state. Sympathetic nerves are stimulated by the fall in arterial blood pressure and a fall in P_{O_2}. They act to preserve blood supply to the vital organs, i.e. the heart and the brain, by vasoconstriction and by increasing heart rate, although stroke volume, the volume pumped by each contraction, diminishes. This may be felt as a rapid, weak pulse. The skin becomes cold as blood is diverted to the vital organs and patients may become confused and disorientated as blood supply to the brain is reduced. The fall in P_{O_2} levels triggers deep and rapid breathing ('air hunger') but this will only rectify the situation if sufficient blood is passing through the system for adequate oxygenation to occur. The fall in P_{O_2} at the tissues means that more O_2 can be unloaded from Hb, but demand will exceed supply unless intervention occurs. Administered O_2 will only partially rectify the situation.

In the early stages of shock, interstitial fluid is returned to the circulation through the capillary walls in an attempt to raise the circulating blood volume, but once cell damage begins this mechanism also fails. Sodium and water are preserved in the body by the production of ADH and aldosterone and this further helps to raise blood volume. Urine output falls as a result.

Without intervention, these compensatory mechanisms ultimately fail. Hyperventilation occurs in response to metabolic acidosis and causes respiratory acidosis in addition. P_{CO_2} falls, causing a reduction in blood flow to the brain and a reduced level of consciousness. Adrenaline and noradrenaline are pro-

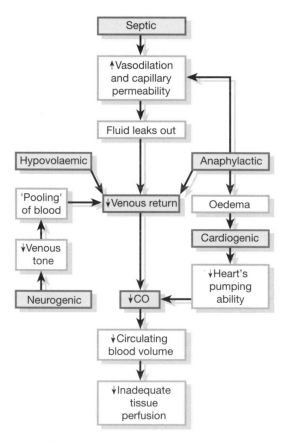

Figure 22.12 – *The causative mechanisms of shock.*

duced in response to sympathetic nervous stimulation and cause vasoconstriction, which causes further hypoxia by decreasing blood flow through the lungs. Reduced blood volume and flow result in poor renal perfusion with resultant oliguria. Disseminated intravascular coagulation occurs when the clotting system is activated by enzymes released from the breakdown of cells and this further reduces blood flow. This vicious circle is illustrated in Figure 22.13. Once shock progresses to this stage, it is irreversible and death will ensue despite intervention.

Conclusion

A basic understanding of physiological mechanisms employed to maintain homeostasis is vital if the A&E nurse is competently to manage the complex assaults on normal body systems that are regularly witnessed in patients attending A&E.

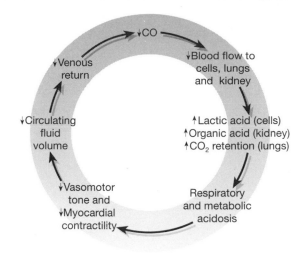

Figure 22.13 – *The vicious circle of irreversible shock.*

Further reading

Hinchliff SM, Montague SE, Watson R (1996) *Physiology for Nursing Practice*, 2nd edn. London: Baillière Tindall.

Hartshorn JC, Sole ML, Lamborn ML (1997) *Introduction to Critical Care Nursing*. Philadelphia: WB Saunders.

Chapter 23

Wound Care

Lynda Holt

- Introduction
- Anatomy of the skin
- Wound healing
- Wound assessment
- Wound cleansing
- Wound closure
- Wound infection
- Managing bite wounds
- Tetanus prophylaxis
- Discharge information
- Conclusion

Introduction

Wound management forms a large percentage of the A&E nurse's workload, and with changes in working patterns, the A&E nurse may be the only health professional involved in a patient's care. It is important that traumatic wound care in A&E is seen as more than the best way to achieve technical closure. Wound care is about an extensive knowledge of skin anatomy, the physiological processes of healing, the causes and impact of wound infection and empowerment of patients to manage their own wounds. This chapter aims to provide the knowledge base needed for safe and effective wound management.

Anatomy of the Skin

The skin represents up to 15% of body weight (Flanagan & Fletcher 1997). Its thickness varies around the body, with areas of greatest friction, such as the soles of the feet, being thickest and areas of low friction, like eyelids, being the thinnest. The skin has five primary functions (Box 23.1):

- protection
- sensation
- thermoregulation
- vitamin D synthesis
- excretion and reserve.

The skin is made up of two main parts, the epidermis and the dermis, which cover the subcutaneous fat layer and deep structures (see Fig. 23.1).

Epidermis

This is subdivided into five distinct layers. Working from the surface these are as follows:

Stratum corneum. This outer layer consists of dead cells. They contain keratin, which absorbs water making the skin susceptible to maceration if constantly exposed to water. These cells shed continuously at a rate of 1,500,000 per hour. The whole layer is replaced

Box 23.1 – *Functions of the skin*

■ **Protection from:**
  - bacteria and viruses
  - heat and cold
  - dehydration
  - some chemical substances
  - mechanical damage

■ **Sensation**
  - largest sensory organ
  - contains nerve endings – most concentrated in fingertips and lips
  - sensitive to touch, pain, heat, cold, vibration and pressure
  - skin hairs are also sensitive to touch, reducing risk of injury to the skin

■ **Thermoregulation**
The skin is responsible for maintaining the body's core temperature. It is controlled by the hypthothalamus. The skin stabilises heat generated by metabolism. This is done by heat conduction, convection and radiation from the skin surface. Heat loss is also influenced by vasodilation and constriction, varying the amount of blood flowing beneath the skin surface. This mechanism also prevents excessive heat loss in cold weather. Sweat production and evaporation have a cooling effect. The body is insulated from the environment by a layer of subcutaneous fatty adipose tissue

■ **Vitamin D synthesis**
Vitamin D is synthesised from ultraviolet light falling on the skin. Vitamin D is necessary for calcium absorption. Vitamin D can also be synthesised from dietary intake

■ **Excretion and reserve**
Some gaseous exchange takes place through skin. Sodium and urea are excreted via sweat. The skin provides a water reserve which is drawn into the circulating blood volume in cases of sudden fluid loss, such as haemorrhage or chronic dehydration. The fat layer can also be converted into energy

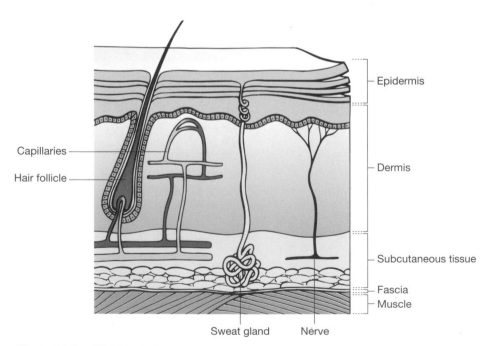

Figure 23.1 – *Skin structure.*

every 24 hours (Collier 1996). The primary function of this layer is to act as a barrier.

Stratum lucidum. This layer of dead cells is found in areas needing extra protection, such as the soles of the feet and the palms of the hands.

Stratum granulosum. These cells are dead granular cells, not yet flattened, and contain cytoplasmic granules which are the precursor to keratin.

Stratum spinosum. These form a layer of living cells which act as intracellular bridges preventing cell separation.

Stratum basale. This layer lies next to the dermis. These cells are responsible for germination of new epithelial cells and are reliant on the dermis for nutrients from the blood supply.

Dermis

This is made up of two primary layers of connective tissue, ground substance and cells. The ground substance supports fibres and cells of the dermis. It forms a jelly-like matrix which is susceptible to some microorganisms, e.g. *Clostridium* and *Streptococcus pyogenes*. These dissolve the matrix, creating a tract for deep infection. The fibres contained include collagen. This gives strength to the jelly-like matrix tissue and the water-holding element of the skin, with reticular formation surrounding the collagen bundles and elastin. Cells in the dermis include:

■ Fibroblast – used in wound healing. These lie between bundles of collagen and act to synthesise elastin and collagen.
■ Tissue macrophages – these phagocytic cells engulf debris and matter during healing.
■ Tissue mast cells – found near hair follicles and blood vessels, these cells produce histamine and heparin.
■ Transient cells – these move between dermis and blood vessels. They include neutrophils, lymphocytes and monocytes. Quantities vary at different stages of healing.

The dermis is formed of two distinct layers. The papillary layer lies next to the basal layer of the epidermis. It is composed of connective tissue, and houses capillary vessels, nerve endings, temperature and touch sensors, and lymph vessels. The root of sebaceous glands, sweat glands and hair follicles are also found in the dermis. This layer is largely responsible for the tensile strength of skin. The reticular layer is at the base of the dermis; blood vessels and collagen fibres increase in size in this layer. There is no real physiological separation between the papillary and reticular layers, more a gradual change from one to the other.

Table 23.1 – *Phases of wound healing*

Duration	Phase	Signs
First hour	Haemostasis	Initial vasoconstriction Coagulation of wound
10 minutes–5 days	Inflammatory	Vasodilation, pain, heat, swelling
3 days–1 month	Proliferation	Wound size diminishing Surrounding skin of normal colour Less pain
3 weeks–1 year	Maturation	Wound healed Scarring fades

Wound Healing

Terminology and the number of stages in the healing process vary between texts (Collier 1996, Desai 1997). The general consensus is that four phases of healing occur; they usually follow a set pattern, but can occur concurrently, and different parts of the same wound can heal at different rates (see Table 23.1).

Haemostasis

The body's initial response to a cut in the skin is bleeding. This extravasation initiates platelet activity and coagulation of blood. It also results in vasoconstriction and release of histamines and ATP, which also attract leucocytes. Platelets begin to aggregate and the coagulation cascade results in the development of a fibrin mesh, or beginnings of a scab, which temporarily seals the wound (Hinchliff *et al.* 1996) (see also Ch. 22).

Inflammatory

As well as a haemostatic response, the body also responds to tissue trauma by releasing prostaglandins and activated proteins which initiate vasodilation in the area. This has two main functions: firstly, it increases blood supply to the area, and secondly it increases capillary permeability. This is to enable plasma to leak into tissues around the area of injury. This creates wound exudate. Neutrophils leak into the area of the wound and offer initial protection from infection by engulfing and digesting bacteria. Neutrophils have a short life span, and so are replaced by monocytes which are capable of phagocytosis. Thus, not only do they promote new tissue formation and angiogenesis, but they also continue to engulf and destroy bacteria and debris from the wound including old neutrophils (Whitby 1995).

The signs of an inflammatory response are often confused with infection, so it is important to establish a clear history of the duration since injury. Inflammatory responses occur before infection has had time to develop. The signs of the inflammatory response include:

■ redness – because of local vasodilation
■ heat – because of increased blood supply and metabolic activity
■ oedema – because increased capillary permeability allows fluid to leak into the extracellular space
■ pain – due to pressure of fluid in tissues and chemical irritation from enzymes such as prostaglandin.

This inflammation is vital to the natural healing. If it is suppressed by drugs or illness, healing will be delayed. For this reason non-steroidal anti-inflammatory drugs (NSAIDs) are not recommended in the initial management of wounds. Macrophages are essential for transition into the proliferation stage of healing, as they begin to produce transforming growth factor (TGF) which promotes angiogenesis and the formation of new tissues. Macrophages also produce fibroblast growth factor (FGF) which stimulates fibroblast production.

Proliferation

This starts 3–5 days post-injury. As its name suggests, this part of the healing process is about growth and reproduction of tissue to replace that lost in injury. In order to produce new tissue, the wound needs a good oxygen supply and essential nutrients like vitamin C. As angiogenesis occurs in response to wound hypoxia and TGF, new capillary loops develop and the wound is oxygenated. Three distinct processes occur during the proliferation phase:

Granulation. This is the formation of new tissue up from the base and in from the sides of a wound. It is dependent on the division of endothelial cells forming new capillary loops, until eventually they meet up with existing undamaged blood vessels. At the same time, fibroblasts begin to produce a network of collagen and ground substance which fills tissue spaces and begins to bind fibres together. Collagen synthesis depends on adequate nutrients, i.e. vitamin C, copper and iron (Flanagan 1997). This can usually be obtained from a healthy diet. Collagen forms in a haphazard and jelly-like structure, and with adequate

vitamin C matures into a strong cross-linked structure which gives the tissue its tensile strength.

Contraction. This occurs at the same time as epithelialisation. In wounds where tissue loss has occurred, once the wound bed has filled with healthy granulation tissue, myofibroblasts develop which contract and pull the wound edges together, therefore decreasing the overall size of the wound.

Epithelialisation. This is the resurfacing of the wound by regeneration of epithelial cells. This will only occur where basal cells are in contact with the dermal layer, and therefore in deep wounds regeneration will only occur around wound margins until granulation has taken place. In wounds of varying depth, small islands of epithelialisation will occur in superficial parts of the wound. This gradually migrates across wound surfaces until epithelialisation is complete. The attachment of this layer to dermal connective tissue is fragile and easily displaced. Regeneration therefore continues until the epidermis has regained its usual thickness. Epithelial regeneration requires a warm, moist environment. If a wound surface has dry scabs or necrotic areas, these will form a barrier to migration of new cells. Cells eventually burrow under scabs.

As the wound cavity is filled with granulation tissue and the surface is regenerated with epithelial cells, the proliferation stops. If this does not happen, e.g. if over-granulation occurs due to continued hypoxic stimulation, perhaps as a result of local ischaemia, then excessive scar tissue is formed (Flanagan & Fletcher 1997).

Maturation

This begins around 3 weeks after injury, and is a process of returning the area to its usual functional structure. The process is twofold: firstly collagen is remodelled, sometimes over a period of years. The aim of this is to gradually replace newly formed type III collagen, laid down in the proliferation phase, with stronger more organised collagen fibres. The amount of collagen does not change; its bundles become thicker and shorter and hold the wound together more tightly. Although the skin and wound scar become stronger, the area only usually regains about 80% of the pre-injury tensile strength (Brown 1988). This takes a long time; at 3 months post-injury 50% of tensile strength is considered good healing (Morrison 1992).

The second part of the process is the rationalisation of blood vessels bringing extra nutrients to the area. This process occurs gradually, and its progression can be monitored by the gradual fading of the scar. It will become paler and flatter as blood vessels diminish. Once maturation is achieved the scar will appear white;

it is avascular, has no sebaceous glands and no hairs (Flanagan 1997).

Scarring

Dermal damage results in an abnormal formation of connective tissue. This is permanent and manifests as a scar on the skin surface. Scarring follows three phases, although the time span increases with age, skin pigmentation and as a result of poor general health (Table 23.2).

Keloid scarring results from the formation of large amounts of scar tissue in the proliferation phase of healing. It results from an increase in collagen synthesis and lysis to an extent where tissue formation exceeds cell breakdown (Bryant 1992). Keloid scarring is also considered to be related to the melanocyte-stimulating hormone as it is much more common in people with heavily pigmented skin (Bales & Jones 1997).

Tissue growth is persistent, with scarring often being much larger than the original wound. Hypertrophic scarring forms in a similar fashion to tissue growth, but follows the line of incision. This type of scarring is more common in the young. Generally, scars which lie parallel to the body's natural tension lines have a better cosmetic prognosis. Tattoo scarring results from gravel or foreign bodies being left in a wound. It forms unsightly purple or blue blotches in the scar and is difficult to remedy after initial wound healing.

Factors affecting wound healing

Although patients with sudden traumatic wounds do not have the same physiological and educational preparation as patients undergoing surgery, many of the influences on wound healing can be optimised by effective education and empowerment during their initial visit to A&E for wound management. Medical factors affecting healing potential can also be identified at this early stage, and the patient care plan designed to accommodate them. The main influences on wound healing are listed in Box 23.2.

Nutrition deserves more elaborate exploration, as it is fundamental to adequate healing and is often overlooked both in discharge information and in promoting well-being in hospital in-patients. Malnutrition affects healing in several ways:

■ poor healing with reduced tensile strength and an increased risk of wound dehiscence (McLaren 1992)
■ an increased likelihood of infection (Dickson 1995)
■ poor quality scarring.

Protein and calorie intake need to be above normal recommended levels to support additional collagen synthesis and metabolic activity (see Table 23.3).

Vitamin deficiency

Vitamin C is essential for the synthesis of collagen; a deficiency reduces wound tensile strength, increases the fragility of capillaries and impairs angiogenesis. Vitamin A supplement improves healing in patients on corticosteroids (Pinchofsky-Devin 1994). It can help to restore inflammatory response and reduces the risk of wound infection. Similarly, a vitamin A deficiency increases infection risk. Vitamin B complex is necessary for wound strength as it contributes to cross-linking of collagen fibres. Vitamin K is essential for the clotting process in early wound healing.

Trace element deficiency

Iron deficiency has two significant impacts on wound healing: firstly, in patients with anaemia, oxygen transportation is reduced and therefore tissue perfusion is inhibited; and second, iron is a necessary co-factor in collagen synthesis. Copper deficiency is rare but where it occurs, enzyme activity is restricted and collagen cross-linkage is impaired. Zinc deficiency delays wound healing because it slows collagen synthesis, reduces wound strength and decreases speed of epithelialisation.

Wound pain

Wound pain is initiated by the inflammatory response and is a normal part of the healing process. It is caused by a combination of noxious stimuli including histamine and peptides, such as substance P (a pain transmitter) and prostaglandin (a chemical stimulus

Table 23.2 – *Scar formation*

No. of weeks post-injury	Scar characteristics
0–4 weeks	Soft, weak scarline
4–12 weeks	Scar contracts, becomes harder and stronger
12–52 weeks	Scarline flattens and becomes soft and supple, moving easily with surrounding skin. Gradually, whitens as vascularity decreases. Skin does not regain pre-injury elasticity

Box 23.2 – *Factors affecting wound healing*

■ **Age**
With age, all metabolic processes slow down and collagen production is lower; therefore wounds heal more slowly and have less tensile strength

■ **Tissue perfusion**
Many diseases cause hypoxia and reduced tissue perfusion. Those with a significant effect on wound healing include:
— anaemia
— peripheral vascular disease
— respiratory disease
— arteriosclerosis
— dehydration.
The result of this is reduced fibroblast activity and collagen synthesis, reduced epithelial regeneration and greater susceptibility to infection because of decreased leucocyte activity

■ **Other diseases**
These include diabetes, immune disorders and cancer, because of dampened inflammatory response and susceptibility to infection. Also, inflammatory conditions, liver failure and uraemia

■ **Psychological factors and body image**
Stress and anxiety supress the immune system and are linked with sleep disturbance. This has been shown to delay healing (Pediani 1992). Anabolic healing is enhanced by sleep. Altered body image can occur from seemingly minor wounds and this can adversely affect healing in terms of stress and compliance with wound care strategies

■ **Poor wound care**
Inadequate wound cleansing or inappropriate wound dressing is an avoidable factor in healing

■ **Nutrition**
Protein, vitamins and trace elements are vital for prompt, adequate wound healing. These include:
— iron
— copper
— zinc
— vitamin A
— vitamin C
Vitamins B, E and K also influence healing, and adequate protein and calorie intake is also necessary

■ **Hydration**
To maintain metabolism, between 2 and 2.5 L of fluid in 24 hours is needed. Less than this will result in fluid being drawn from interstitial spaces. Patients who are already clinically dehydrated will have delayed healing

■ **Smoking**
Both carbon monoxide and nicotine, as end-products of smoking, have an adverse effect on peripheral tissue perfusion, therefore increasing hypoxia risk. There is also an increased risk of thrombus formation in smokers (Sianna *et al.* 1992)

■ **Drug therapy**
Anti-inflammatory agents, immunosuppressive drugs, cytotoxics and corticosteroids all impinge on the healing process

Table 23.3 – *Calorie and protein intake in wound healing*

	Energy (kcal)	Protein (g)
Men	2150–2510	54–63
Women	1680–2150	42–45

for pain). Part of the response is to protect the wound from further injury. The impact of wound pain should not be underestimated and analgesia suitable for the stage of wound healing should be used. NSAIDs are not ideal during the initial post-injury phase as they dampen the inflammatory response needed for healing. Non-pharmacological methods of pain relief should

Table 23.4 – *Mechanism of injury related to wound type*

Mechanism of injury	Type of wound	Appearance
Stanley knife, broken glass, surgical wound	Incision	Straight, clean cut
Tear on jagged edge or barbed wire, from direct blow, sudden contact with solid mass	Laceration	Irregular break of skin
Fall off moving object, such as bicycle, friction of skin against hard surface	Abrasion	Superficial skin loss, friction burn
Blunt trauma, repeated blows	Contusion/ bruising	Damage to vessels beneath surface with or without laceration
Stab wound, gunshot injury	Penetrating injury	Deep wound, not necessarily large at skin surface
Scald, chemical splash, contact burn	Burn	Erythema, skin loss or blistering
Fingertips caught in doors/machinery, mechanical saw	Avulsion or amputation	Skin pulled off. Underlying tissue with or without involvement. Complete or partial digit loss
Trapped between shearing forces	Degloving injury	Full-thickness skin loss with underlying structures intact

also be considered. Box 23.3 highlights some of the pain triggers.

If ongoing wound care will be needed, e.g. in management of burns, patients should be prescribed analgesia to take prior to dressing changes. Appropriate explanations of interventions and psychological support will help to alleviate pain (see also Ch. 24).

Wound Assessment

As with all patients attending A&E, the immediate history of events leading up to A&E attendance is imperative. It should consider when, where and how the injury occurred. Most wounds treated in A&E are of a traumatic nature, and as a result patients are often anxious or distressed by the sudden and unexpected interruption to their normal activity. The mechanism of injury gives important clues to the type of wound being dealt with. Table 23.4 relates the mechanism of injury to wound type. Figure 23.2 highlights the mechanism of injury and skin damage.

Wound examination

All traumatic wounds should be considered contaminated; some of these will appear clean on initial examination, while others will be obviously contaminated. The distinction between 'clean' and 'dirty' wounds lies with how contaminants are removed. In clean wounds, simple wound cleansing is adequate, whereas dirty wounds require surgical cleaning, removal of contaminants or excision of devitalised tissue (Dimick 1988). It is important to assess the degree of contamination carefully before a management plan is decided upon, as a direct correlation exists between the degree of contamination and the incidence of infection (Edlich *et al.* 1988). The size, shape, wound depth and anatomical site of the wound should be assessed and documented. Diagrams in the patient's notes, or a photograph with a measurement

scale, are useful if the wound is likely to need follow-on care.

Neurovascular integrity should be examined. Assessment of vascular integrity should include the patient's estimation of blood loss, together with objective evidence of haemorrhage. The wound should be carefully inspected for continuous oozing of blood

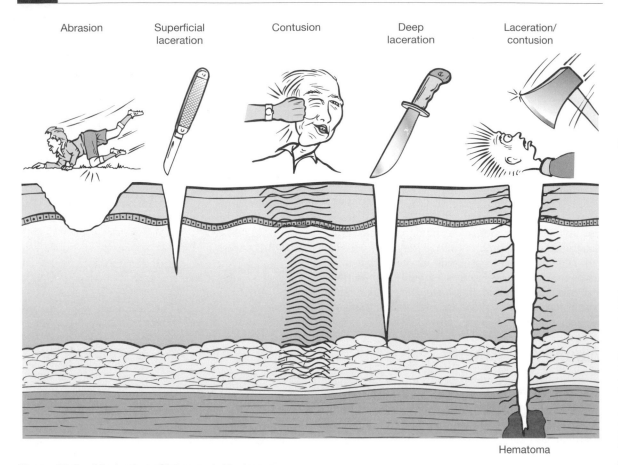

Figure 23.2 – *Mechanism of injury and skin damage.*

(suggestive of venous bleeding), spurting of bright red blood (indicative of arterial injury) and haematoma formation, which could pose a risk to healing in the form of potential infection. If bleeding is uncontrolled, direct pressure should be applied and the injured area elevated if possible. Vascular integrity distal to the wound can be assessed by observing skin colour distally to the wound, feeling skin temperature, and checking distal pulses and the speed of capillary refill.

Nerve function should be assessed in terms of sensation by gentle pinprick tests distal to the wound. Motor nerve function should also be performed in hand or wrist injuries. Gross neurological integrity can be assumed if the patient can grasp a pencil using all fingers of the affected hand (McGuire 1982).

Tendon injury should also be identified and eliminated as part of the assessment stage of wound management. This is particularly important in hand injuries. Extensor tendon injury is most common, e.g. mallet finger, which results in an inability to fully extend the digit. Flexor tendon injuries following injury to the palmar aspect of the hand are less common, but have a high incidence of disability when missed, as they leave the patient unable to bend the injured digit. Flexor tendon injury is difficult to detect as tendons contract when cut and are therefore not always visible at the wound edges. If the mechanism of injury and initial examination suggest tendon injury, the wound should be explored until tendon edges or an intact tendon are visualised. Findings of neurovascular examination should always be documented, even if normal.

As part of both the examination and cleansing aspects of wound care, the potential for foreign bodies should be assessed and the wound examined to exclude or remove them. If the history suggests glass may be present in the wound, an X-ray is a useful way of locating or excluding this (Miller 1995).

Wound Cleansing

There are two important considerations in wound cleansing: firstly the way it is carried out, and secondly the solution used. Wound cleansing is essential for the prevention of infection, tattoo scarring and exclusion of foreign bodies. The nurse carrying out this cleansing prior to wound closure has a responsibility to ensure that the wound is decontaminated and if any doubt exists the wound should not be closed.

The use of local anaesthetic may be necessary to achieve thorough wound cleansing. Thomlinson (1987) found the use of cotton wool or gauze swabs to clean wounds to be ineffective. While large debris such as grit was removed, bacteria were simply moved around the wound surface. Gentle irrigation with warm fluid is the most effective and least painful method of wound cleansing (Edlich *et al.* 1988). Highly contaminated wounds demand a high-pressure irrigation using an 18 g needle and syringe (Stevenson 1976). Wound irrigation should continue until all obvious contamination has been removed.

In some cases, such as dirty abrasions and gritty wounds of varying depths, surgical scrubbing of the wound is indicated. The patient should be given appropriate anaesthesia and/or analgesia. Local infiltration of lignocaine or topical application of gel is usually adequate. The procedure should be carried out in a gentle manner so that further tissue damage is avoided; small circular movements are more effective than scrubbing across the wound (Trott 1991).

Wound cleansing solutions have been the subject of much debate over recent years. Recent research suggests that tap water is as effective for initial cleansing of wounds as other commercial products (Dealey 1994, Riyat & Quinton 1997). Riyat & Quinton cultured tap water from various outlets in an A&E department and grew no bacteria. Patients whose wounds were cleansed with tap water had no higher incidence of wound infection. In many A&E departments, normal saline is the cleanser of choice. This is a safe, isotonic solution and an adequate cleaning agent for most wounds. Like tap water, it is most effective when warmed to body temperature. A range of other solutions is used for wound cleansing in A&E, most of which have some degree of tissue toxicity.

Antiseptic solutions include cetrimide, Savlon and chlorhexidine. They generally claim to destroy bacteria and have a detergent component for wound cleansing. Most, however, need to be in contact with bacteria for 20 minutes to have any effect (Russell *et al.* 1992). Povidone-iodine is a broad-spectrum antiseptic agent. It has a slow release capacity where povidone acts as a carrier gradually releasing iodine into the tissues. It has been suggested that this reduces tissue toxicity and irritation but preserves antibacterial properties (Trott 1991). However, its value has been persistently questioned, because it is cytotoxic to fibroblasts

(Dealey 1994) and therefore reduces the tensile strength of the wound and slows the epithelialisation process. To overcome this, the iodine solution should be no more concentrated than 0.001%. Commercial preparations start at 0.75% – this is a 7.5% povidone-iodine solution; however, Brennan & Leger (1985) found that povidone-iodine was toxic to wound healing in a 5% solution. Iodine is more effective than other antibacterial agents, particularly against Gram-negative bacteria (Trott 1991). Therefore, if the wound is infected and antibiotics are not appropriate, providone-iodine could be used as a short-term cleaning solution if diluted to 5%, but is not recommended for routine wound cleansing or prophylaxis.

Desloughing solutions like hydrogen peroxide are not effective as a routine treatment. Their ability to destroy bacteria is considerably reduced once in contact with blood or pus. While the oxidising activity does remove slough, it also breaks down granulating wound tissue. If diluted to a strength which is non-toxic to tissues, the hydrogen peroxide is no longer effective on bacteria. Hydrogen peroxide should only be used as a one-off treatment for extremely sloughy wounds and the area should be irrigated with saline afterwards. This makes its use in traumatic wound management very limited.

Eusol (Edinburgh University solution of lime) type preparations are rarely used and there is no clinical indication for their use in *any* circumstances. Considerable evidence exists to highlight the limited antibacterial effects of sodium hypochlorite and their devastating degree of tissue damage is well documented (Brennan & Leger 1985, Dealey 1994). Table 23.5 lists cleaning solutions and their properties.

Wound Closure

Wound closure can be divided into three separate methods:

- Primary closure – where edges of wounds are brought together
- Secondary closure – where the wound heals by granulation and epithelialisation
- Tertiary closure – where delayed wound closure is indicated.

The first two methods are both commonly used for traumatic wound closure in A&E.

Primary wound closure

This is the best method of wound closure, but it is not suitable for all wound types. Primary closure occurs when the wound has been artificially closed by

Table 23.5 – *Properties of cleaning solutions*

Solution	Antibacterial activity	Tissue toxicity	Advantages	Disadvantages
Tap water	None	None	Cheap Easily accessible Large volumes	Potential for environmental contamination
Normal saline	None	None	Isotonic Gentle	Cost (compared with tap water)
Povidone iodine	Gram –ve Gram +ve	Toxic at >5% (sold in 7.5 and 10% solutions only)	Highly antibacterial	Potentially delays healing at strengths commonly used
Chlorhexidine	Strong Gram-positive, slight Gram-negative	Low toxicity	No clinical advantages	Antibacterial action reduced when in contact with blood or pus
Cetrimide	Low activity	Irritant	Good detergent	Antibacterial properties inactivated by blood and pus Easily contaminated by infection
Hydrogen peroxide	Weak action on anaerobic surface	Very toxic to cells	No clinical advantages	Inactivated by pus

suturing, surgical glue, staples or adhesive strips. This should take place immediately following injury. Primary closure entails aligning skin layers and underlying structures, eliminating any dead space. This prevents haematoma formation or fluid build-up, which could pose an infection risk and delay healing (Dimick 1988) (see Fig. 23.3).

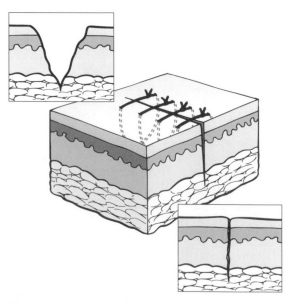

Figure 23.3 – *Primary closure.*

The dermal layer gives the skin its tensile strength, and although full-strength recovery and scar minimisation can be capitalised upon by careful approximation of the dermal layer, the time elapsed since initial injury must be considered when undertaking primary closure. The greater the duration since injury, the higher the risk of infection (Trott 1991). As a general rule, up to 6–8 hours post-injury is considered safe for primary closure; however this time varies between anatomical sites. The face, for example, should be considered for primary closure up to 24 hours post-injury. Similarly, if a wound is heavily contaminated or in an anatomical site prone to infection, such as the hand, safe primary closure times are considerably shorter. Primary closure should only be carried out once the wound is thoroughly cleaned, foreign bodies have been eliminated and there is minimal or no tissue loss.

Suturing

Wounds suitable for suturing should be clean, with no devitalised tissue and minimal tissue loss (Castille 1998). The wound depth is partial or full dermal depth, and neurovascular damage should be excluded before wound closure. Healing occurs across wound layers, so it is important to accurately match each skin layer. Wound edges should be everted to prevent haematoma formation due to continued bleeding (Larsen & Wischman 1993). In addition, because scars contract

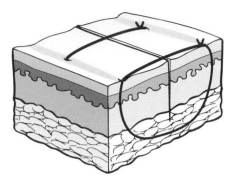

Figure 23.4 – *Everting wound edges with square sutures.*

during the maturation phase of healing, everted wound lines will flatten to the normal plane of the skin. Achieving proper wound edge eversion lies with suturing technique. The most commonly used technique in A&E is an interrupted box suture (Jay 1999). This is basically a square suture, with width and depth of suture equal. This helps to evert wound edges. If suture width is greater than its depth then the wound edges will roll or invert (see Fig. 23.4). Suture products vary greatly, but general principles for use can be adapted. Sutures are designed to be absorbed or removed (see Table 23.6).

Absorbable sutures, such as catgut or synthetic polymers, are broken down by protein synthesis over about 3–4 weeks and therefore dissolve. Catgut is organic material which absorbs more rapidly but has a lower tensile strength than synthetic sutures. It has largely been superseded by synthetic suture materials.

Polyglycolic acid makes up some of the most popular braided synthetic polymers. It has a lower rate of skin reaction and is less susceptible to infection than catgut (Trott 1991) Monofilament sutures are made up of a single fibre, and braided sutures are made from numerous fibres twisted together. For this reason braided sutures create easier access for infection unless coated to replicate a monofilament.

Monofilament polyglyconate polymers are becoming increasingly popular as they are strong and have a lower infection potential. Absorbable sutures should be used for deep tissue repair and in areas such as the mouth or perineum. Their use for skin wounds in children because the sutures do not have to be removed is arguable. This is because dissolvable sutures stay in the wound longer, even in children whose protein synthesis is quicker. Because sutures are present, wound discomfort is greater, which negates the benefits of not putting the child through suture removal.

Non-absorbable sutures are used for dermis and epidermal skin closure. Monofilament nylons and polypropylene are the most commonly used because they carry a low infection risk and are of a high tensile strength. Because they are synthetic, they are far less likely to cause an inflammatory response, which is common with silk and other organic sutures. Silk sutures are considered easier to use because they knot more easily and do not slip in handling, like nylon. However, long-standing evidence (Alexander *et al.* 1967) makes it difficult to justify the use of organic sutures because of the potential risk of infection and inflammation. Non-absorbable sutures are removed 5–14 days post-insertion, depending on anatomical site and the patient's age. Table 23.7 gives guidance for the suture removal times.

Table 23.6 – *Suture material*

Type	Description	Ease of use	Tensile strength	Inflammatory reaction risk	Infection risk
Silk	Organic, non-absorbable	Easy	Low	High	High
Nylon	Synthetic, non-absorbable monofilament	Moderate	High	Low	High
Polypropylene	Synthetic, non-absorbable monofilament	Difficult	High	Low	High
Catgut (plain or chrome)	Organic from sheep, absorbable	Moderate	Moderate	High	High
Polyglycolic acid	Synthetic braided, absorbable	Moderate	High	Low	Medium
Polydioxanone	Synthetic monofilament, absorbable	Easy	High	Low	Low

Table 23.7 – *Guidance for removal of suture times*

Anatomical site	Removal of sutures*
Face	3–5 days
Scalp	7 days
Trunk	7–10 days
Hands and feet	7–10 days
Arms and legs	7–10 days
Over a joint	10–14 days

*Where time span exists, the longer duration is needed for elderly people and those with identified healing problems.

Insertion of sutures is a practical skill which requires a good deal of regular practice both to acquire an adequate competence level to work on patients and to remain competent. The information in this text is given to provide theoretical support to practical learning. In order to facilitate good wound edge apposition, the suture needles should be inserted separately into each side of the wound, starting at the centre of straight laceration or at strategic points along the wound, such as the point of a flap or irregularities in a linear wound (Castille 1998). Stitches should be placed loosely as the wound swells during the inflammatory phase. Stitches will become snug over the first few days. Common errors in suturing are shown in Box 23.4.

Box 23.4 – *Common errors in suturing. (After Castille 1998)*

- **Sutures too tight.** This inhibits normal wound healing and can create vascular compromise at wound edges. This delays healing and can result in increased scarring. Stitch hold and criss-cross scarring can also occur from tight sutures

- **Sutures too loose.** This is less problematic than sutures which are too tight, but can result in the wound gaping, therefore delaying healing because wound edges are not together. It also increases the possibility of stitches falling out

- **Sutures too near the wound edge.** These are likely to tear out if the wound comes under any pressure, causing further tissue trauma

- **Wound edges overlapping or inverted.** This interferes with wound healing; the overlap creates a potential for wound dehiscence and leads to more obvious scarring

---

Sutured wounds do not need a dressing unless there is associated skin loss or the sutures are in need of protection, e.g. where the patient is a young child or a person working in a dirty environment. Dressings should provide a warm environment and be permeable to allow the wound to breathe. Some patients prefer sutured wounds to be dressed, and this should also be taken into consideration.

Adhesive strips

The use of adhesive strips has several advantages over suturing. It is usually less traumatic and painful for the patient, tissue trauma is decreased, there is little risk of reaction to the material being used, and there is a lower risk of induced wound infection (Herman & Newberry 1998). Adhesive tapes are useful for superficial wounds, where skin edges can be aligned and there is minimal wound tension. They also give a better cosmetic result than suturing. Adhesive strips should be applied to clean, dry skin. Debate exists around the use of tincture of benzoid on adjacent skin to increase adherence of paper strips, but this carries a risk of skin irritation or toxicity, so if used, it should be applied sparingly (Edlich *et al.* 1988).

Depending on the size of the wound and its tension, it may be appropriate to apply strategic anchoring tapes before working across the wound from one end to the other, particularly for jagged wounds or pretibial lacerations (see Fig. 23.5). Tapes should be placed at about 3 mm intervals, and care is necessary not to invert wound edges. Reinforcing tapes can be applied parallel to the wound to prevent adhesive strips from curling up. A dressing is not strictly necessary over these wounds, but may be used if the wound needs extra protection. Adhesive strips should be removed after 3–4 days from the face, and 5–7 days in most other areas. Patients with friable skin or pretibial lacerations should have adhesive strips in place for at least 10 days.

Wound staples

These have the same tensile strength as sutures and can be used for linear wounds of moderate tension. They provide a fast and economical method of wound closure. Staples cause little tissue reaction and have a low susceptibility to infection (Herman & Newberry 1998). The disadvantage of wound staples as a skin closure technique is the difficulty in obtaining accurate wound edge approximation. This results in more obvious scarring. Wound stapling is not therefore recommended for areas of high cosmetic importance. Staples should be removed after 7–10 days.

Tissue adhesive

This works by gluing the wound and is appropriate for

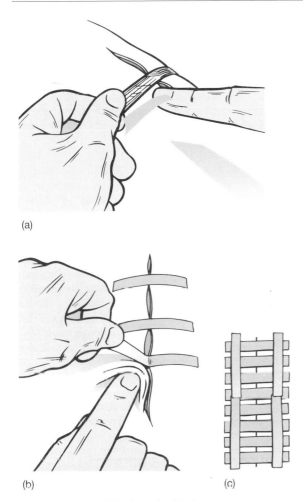

(a)

(b)   (c)

Figure 23.5 – *Application of adhesive tapes*

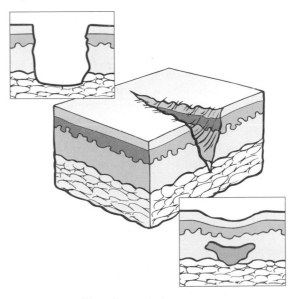

Figure 23.6 – *Wound granulation.*

> **Box 23.5** – *The optimum wound dressing. (After Dealey 1994)*
>
> - High humidity between wound surface and dressing
> - Allows gaseous exchange
> - Provides thermal insulation
> - Impermeable to bacteria
> - Removes excess exudate
> - Free of particles and toxic wound contaminants
> - Can be removed without causing further tissue trauma

small wounds with minimal tension. The wound edges should be manually apposed, then the adhesive dropped onto the wound surface at 3 mm intervals. The wound should be manually held together for 30 seconds after the adhesive is applied (Davis & Cordeaux 1996). Tissue adhesive is quick to use and less painful than suturing or staples. It does, however, demand practice and skilful handling to correctly appose the wound edges as it is difficult to correct after application. When used correctly, the infection rate from this type of wound closure is low (Morton *et al.* 1988) and a good cosmetic effect can be achieved. The application of tissue adhesive does cause considerable discomfort to patients as its bonding reaction generates heat which in some cases is sufficient to cause thermal damage (Trott 1991).

Secondary closure

This occurs by granulation when skin loss excludes primary closure (see Fig. 23.6). Wound dressings are fundamental to the healing of these wounds. The dressing should be able to create an optimal healing environment (see Box 23.5).

Dressing characteristics

Wound humidity. Epithelialisation of a wound is 40% faster when the wound surface is covered with a film dressing (Collier 1996). This is because the moist wound surface allows epithelial cells to slide across it as they regenerate. Wound pain is also reduced in a moist healing environment (Eaglestein 1985).

Gaseous exchange. The benefit of wound oxygenation depends on the depth and stage of healing.

For superficial wounds involving the epidermis, gas-permeable dressings are advantageous. For wounds which heal by granulation, some degree of tissue hypoxia is necessary to stimulate angiogenesis and fibroblastic activity (Knighton *et al.* 1981). Where healing is by granulation, hydrocolloid dressings are effective. Cherry & Ryan (1985) suggested that the low Po_2 produced under the dressing stimulates the formation of vascular tissue and therefore speeds up wound healing. Gaseous exchange from the wound surface is inhibited by exudate, making atmospheric oxygen through permeable dressings an unreliable source of oxygenation. With the exception of superficial regenerating wounds, gas-permeable dressings appear to offer little benefit (Dealey 1994).

Thermal insulation. A constant wound temperature of 37°C promotes mitotic and macrophage activity (Collier 1996). If the thermal environment is kept stable under a dressing, this cellular activity is further enhanced. If that wound becomes exposed, perhaps for a dressing change, its surface temperature drops and cellular activity is inhibited. It can take up to 3 hours for this activity to return to normal (Myers 1982). This supports the need for wound dressings and highlights the impact of removing dressings for cleaning or observation on the speed of healing.

Permeability to bacteria. Dressings should provide the wound with protection from microorganisms. They should also contain any existing bacteria within the dressing. Certain types of dressing, such as gauze and some tulle dressings, allow tracts to be created, therefore increasing the infection rate. Any dressing which becomes wet, or where wound exudate soaks through, becomes a passage for infection both into the wound and out from it. Dressings that become wet should therefore be padded over or changed.

Removal of excess exudate. Although the wound surface should be moist, excessive exudate causes skin maceration around the wound. For this reason, the dressing chosen should be of an absorbency level suitable for the amount of exudate. Many commercial dressings are made in a variety of absorbencies, so layers of gamgee are not necessarily the only option for heavily exudating wounds. The dressings should not shed particles or toxins. Many wound care products, e.g. cotton wool, gauze and gamgee, shed fibres into the wound, creating a potential for infection. More commonly, these particles increase or renew the inflammatory response to the injury, therefore delaying healing. The dressing fibres can also cause granulomas to form, damaging the strength of the wound and increasing its susceptibility to infection. The use of these products has been somewhat superseded.

Removal without causing tissue trauma.

Dressings which stick to the wound surface should be avoided, particularly dry dressings on open wounds. Exudate can also cause a dressing to stick if it dries, which is why dressings with adequate absorbency are essential. New granulation tissue is fragile and easily destroyed in dressing removal, so the A&E nurse should remove dressings slowly while supporting the wound surface in order to reduce the risk of tissue trauma.

Types of dressing

Many wound dressing products are available for hospital use, either for general use or by medical prescription. These can be broadly grouped into seven categories (see Table 23.8).

Wound dressings most commonly used in A&E warrant further consideration. Dressings which promote regeneration are used for grazes, abrasions, minor burns and other superficial wounds involving the epidermis. The most effective dressings for this are vapour-permeable films or membranes. They provide the moist environments needed and some thermal protection; however, membranes have limited absorbency for light exudate. Neither should be used on infected wounds. Non-adherent dressings also tend to be used for superficial wounds; however, not only do they have little absorbency, but they cannot provide a moist environment for regeneration and are therefore not recommended.

Tulle dressings are often used for minor burns or other wounds with superficial skin loss. These are woven mesh dressings impregnated with soft paraffin to reduce adherence. As they have no absorbency capacity and cannot maintain a moist healing environment, a secondary dressing is also needed. These tulles are particularly detrimental to multi-thickness wounds as granulating tissue rapidly grows into the tulle mesh and is then damaged when the dressing is removed. Impregnated tulle, such as Inadine, can be useful for treating superficial wounds with moderate infection.

Dressings which promote granulation are used for wounds involving the dermal layer where tissue loss has occurred. Occlusive hydrocolloid dressings provide a warm, moist environment and promote granulation. They are designed to absorb moderate amounts of exudate and can be left in place for several days. As exudate is absorbed into the dressing, a distinctive odour is produced, which although it is not offensive can cause some concern for patients if it is not expected. Hydrocolloid dressings should not be used on infected wounds. Absorbent gauze or gamgee dressings are often used for granulating wounds; however, clinical evidence suggests their only benefit is as a secondary dressing away from the wound

Table 23.8 – *Types of wound dressing*

Type	Examples	Uses	Contraindications
Low adherent	Melolin NA Release	Dry wounds to provide protection	Regenerating wounds
Absorbent dressings	Gauze Gamgee	Secondary dressing	Use next to wound surface
Gas-permeable film and membrane	Opsite Tegaderm Spyroflex	Epithelialising wounds Sites of primary wound closure Minor burns	Wounds with moderate to heavy exudate Infected wounds
Hydrocolloids	Granuflex Intrasite	Granulating wounds Light to moderate exudate	Infected wounds Dry wounds
Alginates	Kaltostat Sorbsan	Heavily exudating wounds and cavity packing	Dry wounds Necrotic wounds
Medicated low adherent dressing	Inadine Actisorb	Superficial infected wounds	Sensitivity to drug
Foams	Allervyn Lyofoam	Heavily exudating wounds Debriding wounds Cavity wounds	Dry wounds

surface, to soak up heavy exudate. When placed close to the wound, e.g. over tulle in a minor burn, absorbent pads will rapidly dehydrate the wound, may stick and have the potential to shed fibres into the wound. Alginates have proved beneficial for heavy exudating wounds as they are an interactive dressing, altering as they absorb wound exudate.

Tertiary closure

This is essentially delayed primary healing. The wound is left until oedema has settled, there is no infection present and all foreign bodies have been removed. Scar formation is good with tertiary healing, far better than primary healing which results in infection. For this reason, it is worth considering delayed wound closure for heavily contaminated wounds.

Wound Infection

Most traumatic wounds occur in unsterile conditions, and therefore all carry a risk of infection. But just because contaminants can get in does not mean that all wounds become infected. A number of factors affect infection potential. This infection potential can be increased by the following:

Wound characteristics. These include the duration from injury to wound cleansing and closure – the longer the delay, the greater the infection risk. The mechanism of injury and the degree of tissue devitalisation affect the infection rate; crush injuries with high tissue damage have a correlating high infection rate (Cardany 1976). Wounds in different anatomical areas have varying infection rates: those occurring below the knee have the highest infection rate, those on upper limbs follow, with facial and scalp lacerations having the lowest rates (Rutherford & Spence 1980).

Wound management. Wound cleansing is a key feature of wound care. Proper cleansing with appropriate lotions, such as saline or tap water, prevents further tissue damage and reduces infection potential. Careful tissue handling also helps to prevent infection. Wound closure is important as improper wound apposition can result in haematoma formation which provides an excellent medium for bacteria growth. If the wound is sutured, the choice of material influences infection potential, with organic or braided sutures carrying a greater infection risk (Edlich *et al.* 1988).

Patient's condition. Patients who suffer unexpected traumatic wounds are at greater risk of infection if they are malnourished, immunosuppressed or taking steroids.

Recognising wound infection

Most traumatic injuries present in A&E before infection has had time to develop; therefore the nurse's

Box 23.6 – *Signs of wound infection*

- Localised pain
- Erythema
- Skin warm to touch
- Local oedema
- Excess exudate
- Pus
- Offensive odour
- Systemic symptoms
  - pyrexia
  - tachycardia
  - tachypnoea

job for these patients is to identify the potential for infection. In patients who present to A&E later, perhaps following a bite or with a wound initially managed at home, the nurse should look for signs of infection (see Box 23.6).

Patients with wound infection should have a wound swab taken for culture and sensitivity prior to starting antibiotic therapy. The wound should be thoroughly cleaned and dressed, and follow-up arrangements made.

Managing Bite Wounds

Bite wounds warrant special consideration because of their potential for infection. Table 23.9 shows a breakdown of the sources of bite wounds.

Bite wounds most commonly occur on the hands and are potentially high risk for infection. The reasons for this are twofold: firstly, because of the number of pathogens found in the perpetrator's mouth, both human and animal; and secondly, because of how the pathogens are transferred – usually by deep, penetrating puncture wounds. Wound management can go some way to reducing the infection risk, with thorough

Table 23.9 – *The sources of wound bites*

Source	Percentage of total
Dogs	80%
Cats	10%
Humans	5%
Other	5%

wound cleansing debridement of devitalised tissue and wound closure using adhesive strips – *not* sutures (Kizer & Callahan 1984).

Wounds to hands or feet, cat bites and bites in patients with a high infection risk should not be closed; they should be dressed and allowed to heal by secondary closure or by tertiary closure once infection is controllable. Prophylactic antibiotics are not necessary in all cases (Larsen & Wischman 1993). Proper wound management is much more effective in preventing infection (Trott 1991). Patients with a high risk of infection or with deep penetrating wounds, particularly on the limbs, should be considered for prophylactic antibiotics.

Tetanus Prophylaxis

Tetanus is caused by *Clostridium tetani*, a Gram-positive anaerobic bacteria. It is a systemic infection which, once activated, is difficult to control as it is resistant to antibiotic therapy. *Clostridium tetani* spores are found in human and animal excrement, garden moss and soil. The effects of the bacteria on humans are largely controlled by immunisation. This starts in childhood vaccination programmes and should be repeated at 10-yearly intervals, although the Department of Health (1990) states that a total of five vaccinations with tetanus toxoid is 'probably' sufficient to provide life-long immunity. The need for tetanus prophylaxis following injury depends on the patient's pre-existing tetanus immunisation status and the type of injury sustained. Table 23.10 shows the type of tetanus prophylaxis required.

Table 23.10 – *Tetanus prophylaxis*

Type of wound	Not immunised/part immunised	≥ 10 years since last vaccination	5–10 years since last vaccination
Clean	Start and complete immunisation with tetanus toxoid	Tetanus toxoid booster	None
Dirty, tetanus prone	Human tetanus immuno-globulin and tetanus immunisation course	Human tetanus immuno-globulin and tetanus toxoid booster	Tetanus toxoid booster

Tetanus toxoid provides active immunisation, and therefore its action is not instantaneous as antibodies need to develop. Tetanus immunoglobulin provides passive immunity and is therefore immediately effective. It is for this reason that it is used for patients with no immunisation and for those who have sustained particularly dirty wounds. Tetanus prone wounds are those which are contaminated with soil, faeces, saliva or dirt, and those sustained by crush injury. Wounds over 6 hours old, those with extensive devitalised tissue and with obvious signs of infection should also be considered high risk (Beales 1997).

Discharge Information

It is important that patients fully understand the wound healing process and know that they are expected to manage the wound at home or until follow-up care is due. Flanagan (1997) highlighted the importance of a number of factors influencing a patient's ability to manage an injury at home (see Box 23.7). Patients should have access to wound care materials if appropriate, and access to advice and support from A&E staff.

Conclusion

Wound care is an important part of the A&E nurse's work and is an area of care where the nurse has a great deal of influence. As a result, it is imperative that, in addition to good practice and wound care skills, the nurse also has an in-depth knowledge of wound healing, the threats to healing and the range of wound management methods available. This way, A&E nurses can continue to deliver informed, high-quality care to their patients.

> **Box 23.7** – *Personal influences on wound healing*
>
> ■ **Knowledge and understanding** – the patient's and carer's level of knowledge will affect their ability to promote wound healing. The nurse needs to ensure the patient understands wound care guidance and any dieting changes necessary
>
> ■ **Compliance** – this is complex and is influenced by the success of treatment so far, the duration of injury, previous experience and the degree of trust in the health care professional
>
> ■ **Motivation** – this may be influenced by the carer's fear, guilt and how the patient sees the injury in relation to the rest of her life
>
> ■ **Attitude** – a positive attitude to recovery will enhance motivation and compliance, particularly if supported with appropriate education
>
> ■ **Body image** – this may impact on how the patient cares for the wound
>
> ■ **Financial status** – this affects the patient's ability to comply with health care advice

---

References

Alexander J, Kaplan J, Altemeier W (1967) The role of suture materials in the development of wound infection. *Annals of Surgery*, **165**, 192–195.

Bales S, Jones V (1997) *Wound Care Nursing: a Patient Centred Approach*. London: Baillière Tindall.

Beales J (1997) Tetanus immunisation: its implications in A&E. *Emergency Nurse*, **5**(5), 21–23.

Brennan SS, Leger DJ (1985) The effect of antiseptics on healing wounds: a study using the rabbit ear chamber. *British Journal of Surgery*, **72**(10), 780–782.

Brown G (1988) Acceleration of tensile strength of incisions treated with EGF and TGF. *Annals of Surgery*, **208**, 788–794.

Bryant RA (ed.) (1992) *Acute and Chronic Wounds*. St Louis: Mosby Year Book.

Cardany C (1976) The crush injury: a high risk wound. *Journal of American College of Emergency Physicians*, **5**, 965–970.

Castille K (1998) Suturing. *Nursing Standard*, **12**(41), 41–48.

Cherry G, Ryan T (1985) Enhanced wound angiogenesis with a new hydrocolloid dressing. In: Ryan T, ed. *An Environment for Healing: the Role of Occlusion*. London: Royal Society of Medicine.

Collier M (1996) The principles of optimum wound management. *Nursing Standard*, **10**(43), 47–53.

Davis J, Cordeaux S (1994) Tissue adhesive: use and application. *Emergency Nurse*, **2**(2), 16–18.

Dealey C (1994) *The Care of Wounds*. Oxford: Blackwell Scientific.

Department of Health (1990) Joint Committee on Vaccination and Immunisation: tetanus. *Immunisation against Infectious Disease*. London: HMSO.

Desai H (1997) Aging and wounds. *Journal of Wound Care*, **6**(4), 192–196.

Dickson J (1995) The problem of hospital induced malnutrition. *Nursing Times*, **92**(4), 44–45.

Dimick A (1998) Delayed wound closure: indications and techniques. *Annals of Emergency Medicine*, **17**(12), 1303–1304.

Eaglestein W (1985) Experiences with biosynthetic dressings. *Journal of the American Academy of Dermatology*, **12**, 434–440.

Edlich R, Rodeheaver G, Morgan R (1988) Principles of emergency wound management. *Annals of Emergency Medicine*, **17**(12), 1284–1302.

Flanagan M (1997) *Wound Healing*. Edinburgh: Churchill Livingstone.

Flanagan M, Fletcher J (1997) Wound care: the healing process. *RCN Nursing Update (Nursing Standard*, suppl.), **11**(40), 5–17.

Herman M, Newberry L (1998) Wound management. In: Newberry L, ed. *Sheehy's Emergency Nursing: Principles and Practice*. St Louis: Mosby.

Hinchliff S, Montague S, Watson R (1996) *Physiology for Nursing Practice*. 2nd edn. London: Baillière Tindall.

Jay R (1999) Suturing in A&E. *Professional Nurse*, **14**(6), 412–415.

Kizer K, Callahan M (1984) A new look at managing mammalian bites. *Emergency Medicine Reports*, **5**(8), 53–58.

Knighton D, Silver I, Hunt T (1981) Regulation of wound healing angiogenesis: effect of oxygen gradients and inspired O_2 concentration. *Surgery*, **90**, 262–270.

Larsen J, Wischman J (1993) Tissue integrity – surface wounds. In: Kidd P, Neff J, eds. *Trauma Nursing: Art and Science*. St Louis: Mosby.

McGuire M (1982) A minor hand injury. *Registered Nurse*, **1**, 28–32.

McLaren SMG (1992) Nutrition and wound healing. *Journal of Wound Care*, **1**(3), 45–55.

Miller M (1995) Principles of wound assessment. *Emergency Nurse*, **3**(1), 16–18.

Morrison MJ (1992) *A Colour Guide to the Nursing Management of Wounds*. London: Mosby.

Morton R, Gibson M, Sloan J (1988) The use of tissue adhesive for the primary closure of scalp wounds. *Archives of Emergency Medicine*, **5**, 110–112.

Myers J (1982) Modern plastic surgical dressing. *Health and Social Services Journal*, **92**, 336–337.

Pediani R (1992) Preparing to heal. *Nursing Times*, **88**(27), 68–70.

Pinchofsky-Devin G (1994) Nutritional wound healing. *Journal of Wound Care*, **3**(5), 231–234.

Riyat MS, Quinton DN (1997) Tap water as a wound cleansing agent in A&E. *Journal of Accident and Emergency Medicine*, **14**, 165–166.

Russell A, Hugo W, Ayliffe G (1992) *Principles and Practice of Disinfection. Preservation and Sterilisation*. Oxford: Blackwell Scientific.

Rutherford W, Spence R (1980) Infection in wounds sutured in the A&E department. *Annals of Emergency Medicine*, **9**, 350–352.

Sianna J, Franklin B, Grottup F (1992) The effect of smoking on tissue function. *Journal of Wound Care*, **1**(2), 37–41.

Stevenson T (1976) Cleansing the traumatic wound by high pressure syringe irrigation. *Journal of American College of Surgeons*, **5**, 17–21.

Thomlinson D (1987) To clean or not to clean. *Nursing Times*, **83**(9), 71–75.

Trott A (1991) *Wounds and Lacerations: Emergency Care and Closure*. St Louis: Mosby Year Book.

Whitby D (1995) The biology of wound healing. *Surgery*, **13**(2), 25–28.

Chapter 24

Pain Management

Brian Dolan

- Introduction
- Physiology of pain
- Pain theories
- Assessing pain
- Pharmacological pain management
- Non-pharmacological pain management
- Conclusion

Introduction

Pain is a complex phenomenon which has physiological, psychological and emotional components and is a unique experience for each individual (Sofaer 1993). The International Association for the Study of Pain Subcommittee on Taxonomy (1979) have described pain as 'an unpleasant sensory and emotional experience associated with actual or potential damage or described in terms of such damage'. O'Hara (1996) suggested that pain is a valuable and necessary part of the body's mechanism which usually indicates that something is wrong, e.g. tissue damage or disease.

This chapter will consider the physiological and psychological elements of pain and will identify assessment tools that may be used in the A&E department. Pharmacological and non-pharmacological methods of pain management will be considered and the nurse's role in relieving pain and suffering will be explored.

Physiology of Pain

Pain is felt when a stimulus is sufficiently strong to exceed the pain threshold. The stimulus activates specialised pain receptors in free nerve endings, known as nociceptors, which are found in large numbers in the skin, arterial walls, periostium and joint surfaces and in smaller numbers in deep tissues (Halliday *et al.* 1992). Stimuli which activate nociceptors may be:

- *mechanical*, when nociceptors are stretched or compressed
- *thermal*, by heat or cold
- *chemical*, when substances such as histamines, bradykinins and serotonin are released by damaged tissues.

Sensory, or afferent, nerve fibres carry impulses to the central nervous system (CNS). Motor, or efferent, nerve fibres transmit impulses away from the CNS via the ventral nerve roots to the effector organs such as muscles. The afferent nerve fibres are divided into three groups, A-delta, A-beta and C fibres, and are classified according to the diameter and conduction velocity of the axon, or nerve cell. The A-beta fibres are large in diameter and surrounded by a fatty sheath (myelin). They transmit impulses at speeds of 30–100 metres/second (m/s) and are 'low threshold fibres' because minimal stimulation is required to generate an impulse. They respond to light touch. A-delta fibres are small-diameter, lightly myelinated fibres, which have a conduction velocity of between 6 and 30 m/s. They respond to pressure (at any intensity), heat over 45°C (considered the noxious range), chemicals and cooling. C fibres are small-diameter, unmyelinated fibres which carry impulses relatively slowly, at speeds of 1–2.5 m/s. They also respond to light pressure and warmth and account for 60–70% of all sensory nerve fibres (Bentley 1998).

Pain relay systems

Once nociceptors are stimulated, the sensory information is relayed to the brain via the spinal cord. There are two types of pain relay system; the fast pain system and the slow pain system.

Fast pain system

The initial, sharp pain felt when trauma occurs is carried by A-delta fibres, which transmit the impulses very quickly. The nerve fibres terminate on neurones in the dorsal horn of the spinal cord from where long fibres cross to the other side of the cord and ascend to the thalamus and the sensory areas of the cerebral cortex. The cortex is responsible for the ability to localise fast pain. Opiates have little effect on this system.

Slow pain system

Slow pain may take more than a second to be perceived and may increase in intensity over seconds or minutes. The pain is burning, throbbing or aching, may be felt in superficial or deep structures and is generally poorly localised. The stimulus may be mechanical, thermal or chemical.

Nerve fibres of the slow pain system are fine, unmyelinated type C fibres which conduct more slowly than A-delta fibres. These fibres also terminate in the dorsal horn of the spinal cord, in the substantia gelatinosa. There is a short connecting fibre to a point deeper within the dorsal horn before connecting fibres cross the spinal cord and ascend to the brain. Slow pain fibres terminate in the reticular area of the brain stem and are then connected by further short fibres to the thalamus. There is no connection to the cerebral cortex and this pain is difficult to localise. Opiate drugs exert a blocking action on the slow pain system.

Pain transmitters

Hinchliff *et al.* (1996) noted that a major recent development in the study of pain has been the discovery of various peptides which have been implicated in pain transmission and pain relief. Substance P is a neurostransmitter which has been identified in various parts of the nervous system, including the substantia gelatinosa of the dorsal horn. Noxious stimulation causes the release of substance P from dorsal root afferents and consequently it has been suggested that substance P acts, at least partly, as a transmitter for pain.

While substance P has been implicated in the transmission of pain, other neurochemicals have been discovered which appear to possess analgesic properties. These include endorphins and encephalins, which have an analgesic action similar to that of morphine. While further research is required, the existence and action of encephalins and endorphins go some way to explain phenomena such as the placebo response, where an individual perceives pain relief even though no analgesic agent has been given. It may be that in such cases, the mere expectation of pain relief is sufficient to release psychogenically the endogenous opiates, which would then cause a genuine analgesia even without the administration of an analgesic drug (Hinchliff *et al.* 1996).

Effects of pain

Physiological effects

The physiological responses that occur when the nociceptors are stimulated are similar to those of the stress ('fight or flight') response. The sympathetic nervous system is activated and results in tachycardia, tachypnoea, hypertension, sweating and pallor. The sympathetic system causes general vasoconstriction, but dilates the arteries supplying vital organs such as the muscles (O'Hara 1996). Tidal volume and alveolar ventilation may be reduced, as is gastric motility. Skeletal muscle spasm may occur and hormonal changes may cause electrolyte imbalances and hyperglycaemia (Sutcliffe 1993).

Non-physiological effects

An individual's perception of and response to pain will be affected by a number of factors other than those described above. Culture appears to play a part in the tolerance of pain, due to differences in pain thresholds. There are, however, several thresholds and these are identified in Box 24.1 identifies each.

There is evidence that all people, regardless of cultural background, have a uniform threshold. Sternback

Box 24.1 – *Pain thresholds*

■ **Sensation threshold** – the lowest stimulus value at which a sensation, such as tingling or warmth, is first reported

■ **Pain perception threshold** – the lowest stimulus value at which the person reports that the stimulation feels painful

■ **Pain tolerance (or upper threshold)** – the lowest stimulus level at which the subject withdraws or asks to have the stimulation stopped

■ **Encouraged threshold** – the highest stimulus level the subject will tolerate after being encouraged to tolerate higher levels than identified in the pain tolerance threshold

& Tursky (1965) found that there was no difference among four different ethnic groups in the level of electric shock that was first reported as producing a detectable sensation. The sensory conducting apparatus, in other words, appears to be essentially similar in all people so that a given level of input always elicits a sensation.

Cultural background, however, does have a powerful effect on the pain perception threshold. For instance, levels of radiant heat that are reported as painful in people of Mediterranean origin are described only as warm by northern Europeans (Hardy *et al.* 1952). The most notable effect of cultural background, however, is on pain tolerance levels. Sternback & Tursky (1965) reported that the levels at which subjects refused to tolerate electric shocks, even when they were encouraged experimenters, depended in part on the ethnic origin of the subject. For the A&E nurse, this may explain the differing reactions.

Anxiety and the perception of pain have been also been linked (Cave 1994, Hayward 1975). Walsh (1993), in a study of patients with relatively minor problems, found that 90% had pain and many were also anxious. Walsh (1993) suggested this may be due to a variety of reasons, such as:

■ the sudden and unexpected disruption of the illness or injury
■ fear of treatment
■ fear of the possible long-term effects of the illness or injury
■ fear of the unknown hospital treatment.

As McCaffery (1983) noted, 'pain is always a subjective experience and pain is what the patient says it is and exists when the patient says it does'.

Pain Theories

A number of theories have been proposed and developed in order to understand and explain the process of pain. Two will be considered here: specificity theory and gate control theory.

Specificity theory

The traditional specificity theory was first proposed by Descartes in 1664. It suggests that pain is a specific sensation and that the intensity of pain is proportional to the extent of the tissue damage (Watt-Watson & Ivers Donavon 1992). According to this theory, pain associated with a minor cut gives minimal discomfort, whereas pain associated with major trauma hurts a lot.

It is now known that pain is not simply a function of the amount of bodily damage, but is influenced by attention, anxiety, suggestion, experience and other psychological variables (Melzack & Wall 1982). However, while current research indicates that conduction of pain impulses is more complex than originally proposed, the recognition of the specific pain pathways inherent in the specificity theory provides the basis for surgery in intractable pain. The procedure interrupts the pain pathway and impulses do not reach conscious level (Hallet 1992).

Gate control theory

The gate control theory of pain proposed by Melzack & Wall (1965) revolutionised the understanding of pain. Their theory states that within the spinal cord, there are factors that may block or close the 'gate' to pain messages, but equally there are factors that open up the gate and make individuals more aware of pain. It suggests that there is a relationship between the inputs from touch receptors and pain receptors at the level of the spinal cord. In particular, it suggests that interneurones in the substantia gelatinosa of the dorsal horn can regulate the conduction of ascending fibre afferent input (Hinchliff *et al.* 1996). The substantia gelatinosa is an area of special neurones located close to each posterior column of grey matter and extending the length of the spinal cord (see Fig. 24.1).

The theory suggests that large-fibre inputs close the gate and small-fibre inputs open the gate; however, the activity of the gating mechanism is also affected by emotion and impulses from descending tracts from areas of the brain (brain stem, thalamus and cerebral cortex).

Melzack & Wall (1965) felt that this theory explains why the relationship between pain and injury is so variable and why the location of pain can differ from

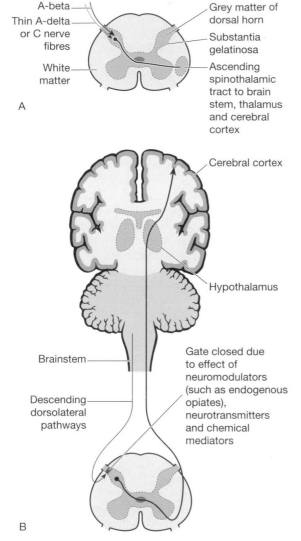

Figure 24.1 – *The gate control theory. A: Diagrammatic cross-section of the spinal cord. B: Internal in fluences on the gate mechanism. (After Davis 1993.)*

the site of injury. It also explains how pain can persist in the absence of injury or after healing and why the nature and location of pain can change over time. Hallet (1992) suggested that the gate control theory expands the role of the spinal cord: it is not just a relay station, but a centre for filtering and integrating incoming sensory information. The theory also establishes a basis for the following procedures in alleviating pain and suffering, many of which can be used in A&E:

■ use of sensory input, such as distraction and guided imagery

■ reducing fear and lowering the level of anxiety
■ patient education about the cause and relief of pain
■ local counter-irritants, massage and heat applications
■ electrical stimulations
■ acupuncture.

Assessing Pain

Individuals not only feel and react differently to pain, but describe it differently as well (Sofaer 1998). It is difficult to measure as it is a subjective phenomenon, and this is further complicated where patients are unable to describe their pain because of the location or severity of their injury or because they are unconscious or intubated.

The use of pain assessment tools by health professionals helps to provide objective data which can be used to plan relevant pain-relieving measures and measure their effect. In some situations it will be immediately obvious that the patient is profoundly distressed and requires urgent intervention, e.g. the patient suddenly presenting to A&E with severe crushing chest pain. Intervention in these circumstances should be immediate and only a brief assessment of the situation is required. In other circumstances, however, a more thorough assessment is required and should be ongoing in light of the patient's clinical condition. Hallett (1992) identified the range of information that should be included when making pain assessments (see Box 24.2).

Pain assessment tools

A number of pain assessment tools are used in A&E (Longstaff 1997, O'Hara 1996). Visual analogue scales (VAS) can be used to measure pain and treatment effectiveness and satisfaction (see Fig. 24.2). The VAS consists of a 10 cm line that ranges from 'no pain' to 'worst possible pain'. The advantages of a VAS are as follows:

■ it is sensitive to small changes
■ it can be used to measure pain intensity
■ it can be used to measure pain relief
■ it is easy for the patient to use.

The disadvantages of VAS are that:

■ pain is scored on a single dimension only
■ some patient groups, such as the visually impaired or the elderly, may find it difficult to use.

For children over the age of 3 years and those unable to grasp the concept of linear scales, pain rating scales using pictures of faces have become popular. The faces, which are in increasing degrees of distress,

---

Box 24.2 – *Detailed pain assessment* (After Hallet 1992)

Location
The location should be identified as specifically as possible. For instance, abdominal pain may be localised to the lower or upper left or right quadrant, epigastrium or mid-abdomen. The site may be well defined or diffuse or the pain may radiate, involving a wide area. Observing the pain's location(s) on the patient's body can help to localise the sites of pain, as well as identifying physical changes at the site, such as swelling or discoloration.

Intensity
The intensity or severity of pain experienced should be translated into words or numbers that can provide objective data for ongoing assessment. Visual analogue scales and numerical scales, with or without written descriptions, are often used.

Quality
A description of pain, using the patient's own words, is helpful in determining the origin of pain, its cause and possible pain relief measures. For instance, patients with cardiac-related chest pain may describe it as 'crushing', whereas patients with non-cardiac-related chest pain may described a 'sharp' pain, usually related to inspiration. Other words used to describe pain are throbbing, stabbing, cramping, hot-burning and aching.

Onset and duration
When the pain first began and how the pain has changed over time should be determined. If the pain varies over the course of a day, this variation and the circumstances surrounding the variation should be noted. The pattern may be constant, intermittent, variable etc.

Relief measures
The efficacy of measures used by the patient to relieve pain should be identified. Any medications, including analgesia, taken by the patient prior to attendance at A&E should be recorded.

Exacerbating factors
Often patients may be comfortable at rest, but have difficulty moving due to pain. For instance, patients with abdominal pain may be more comfortable sitting upright than lying flat on the A&E trolley. In most instances, the A&E nurse should support patients by making them as comfortable as possible, except where this may compromise their safety such as lying over the end of the trolley.

Associated symptoms
Associated symptoms can include nausea and vomiting, profuse perspiration, fainting, inability to perform usual functions, dulling of senses, apathy, clouding of consciousness, disorientation and inability to rest and sleep.

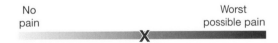

Figure 24.2 – *Visual analogue scale.*

are shown to patients, who are then asked to point to the one which depicts the amount of pain they are feeling. A numerical interpretation may be attached by the nurse in order to facilitate documentation.

However, concern about pain scales has been expressed by Mather & Mackie (1983), who noted that children played down their pain because they did not want to be given an injection. In this instance, the children were capable of evaluating their pain and using the visual analogue scale available to do this. However, the consequences of pain reporting were unpleasant, i.e. administration of an injection, and so the pain report was inaccurate.

Similarly, adult patients, particularly those who are elderly, may minimise their pain reports and will suffer in silence because they do not want to be seen as a 'nuisance' to nursing staff or to their families. The A&E nurse should therefore reassure patients that their needs are being taken seriously and evaluate pain requirements and relief at regular intervals. As none of these assessment tools is of use in the semi-conscious patient or in infants, the A&E nurse must use her observational skills and knowledge of physiological responses to pain to estimate its severity. The most important observations include facial expression, grimacing, movement, posture and interaction with others. In severe pain, the patient's blood pressure and pulse rate may rise, and respirations may increase and therefore should be recorded.

Pharmacological Pain Management

Most acute pain is managed solely with drugs. In England during 1995 there were 32 million prescriptions for non-opioid drugs (mainly paracetamol and its combinations), 17 million for non-steroidal anti-inflammatory drugs (NSAIDS) and 4 million for opioids (McQuay *et al.* 1997). Drugs that are used to relieve pain work in several ways: by altering the pain sensation, depressing pain perception or modifying the patient's response to pain. As a general principle, drugs are used most effectively if their selection is based on the cause and intensity of pain. They can be delivered in a variety of ways, including:

- orally
- intramuscularly
- intravenously
- subcutaneously
- rectally
- epidurally
- topically
- by inhalation.

Analgesics act in the brain, spinal cord, nerve endings and at the site of tissue damage to reduce the amount of pain being felt. Analgesics are selective as they are able to diminish pain without affecting other sensations (O'Hara 1996). Analgesics can be divided into two groups: opiates and non-opiates.

Opiates

Opiates are used in the treatment of moderate to severe pain and work by binding to the opiate receptors in the CNS. When bound in the CNS, these receptors block the transmission of the painful (nociceptive) message. Opiate analgesics may initially produce sedation, reduce fear and anxiety and promote sleep. Opiates stimulate the chemoreceptor trigger zone (CTZ) in the brain stem, causing nausea and vomiting in about 30% of patients. Opiates can also produce respiratory depression by acting on respiratory centres in the brain. The antidote naloxone can reverse this effect.

Morphine

Morphine is a derivative of the opium poppy and is an extremely effective analgesic agent. In A&E, it is usually administered intravenously. It alleviates pain and anxiety, however the nurse should note the following (Trounce 1997):

- The pupils of the eye are constricted due to an effect on the nucleus of the third facial nerve.
- Morphine stimulates the vagus nerve which may present difficulties when morphine is used for the pain of coronary thrombosis as it may further slow the pulse and lower the blood pressure.
- Morphine causes spasm of the sphincters, including the sphincter of Oddi, and therefore should be not be used in pancreatitis.

In trauma cases, oral or intramuscular morphine should not be given as the shocked patient will have poor perfusion. This leads to limited absorption of the drug initially and bolus absorption following resuscitation (Driscoll *et al.* 1994).

Diamorphine

The actions of diamorphine are similar to those of morphine, but it is 2.5 times more potent as an analgesic agent (Thompson & Webster 1992) and is the drug of choice in the management of severe central chest pain. Intravenous administration should be accompanied with anti-emetics, and the depressant effects on the respiratory centre need to be borne in mind, particularly in patients with chronic chest disease. Diamorphine is usually administered in dose of 2.5–5 mg i.v., repeated as necessary. Diamorphine, a class A controlled drug, is also known as heroin and the antidote naloxone 0.4 mg i.v. should always be available.

Pethidine

Pethidine is a synthetically derived analgesic which has similar actions to diamorphine and is chemically related to atropine. It is less powerful than morphine but has a lower risk of respiratory depression and does not cause constriction of the pupils; it is therefore is used in head injuries where observation of the pupil size may be important (Trounce 1997). Unlike morphine, it does not cause spasms of the sphincters and is the analgesic of choice in pancreatitis.

Non-opiates

Effective relief can be achieved with oral non-opioids and NSAIDs. These drugs are appropriate for treating much pain after minor surgery, such as incision and drainage, or on discharge home, for instance, following musculo skeletal injury. Two examples of non-opiates are entonox and NSAIDs.

Entonox

This gaseous mixture of 50% oxygen and 50% nitrous oxide can be effective as a short-term analgesic agent. Its primary use is to provide pain relief to conscious patients who are able to use the demand valve system of delivery for analgesia during unpleasant procedures, e.g. during splinting (Adam & Osborne 1997). It is contraindicated when there is a pneumothorax or a fracture to the base of the skull (Driscoll *et al.* 1994).

NSAIDs

These are the most widely used analgesics. Commonly used NSAIDs include aspirin, indomethacin and ibuprofen. They are effective particularly in relieving pain associated with inflammation, such as musculoskeletal disorders, trauma to peripheral tissues and headache. NSAIDs also act on the hypothalamus to reset the body's thermostat during febrile episodes, reducing the temperature.

NSAIDs inhibit the production of prostaglandins, which cause pain and inflammation. However, prostaglandins are also responsible for maintaining the mucous lining of the gastric mucosa. As a consequence, the use of NSAIDs can lead to gastric damage, which may range from nausea or 'heartburn' to gastrointestinal bleeding. This can be ameliorated by recommending the patient take the NSAIDs with meals and/or milk. NSAIDs can also trigger asthmatic reactions and patients should be asked if they suffer from asthma before NSAIDs are prescribed or dispensed.

Non–Pharmacological Pain Management

In addition to pharmacological interventions, there is a wide range of pain-relieving strategies that can be employed by the A&E nurse to relieve patient pain and suffering. McCaffery (1990) has suggested that a combination of pharmacological and non-pharmacological methods probably yields the most effective relief for the patient.

Information

Attention to factors identified by the patient and, for example, to his level of anxiety regarding pain is essential. Hayward's (1975) classic study showed that patients who were kept informed about the level of discomfort and pain they could expect reported lower levels of pain. It is both unwise and unethical for the A&E nurse to state that a patient will not feel pain before a painful procedure. This is especially true for children who may subsequently lose trust in their health carers. Honesty with reassurance can do much to alleviate the mental suffering associated with current or impending pain from nursing and medical procedures.

Immobilisation and elevation

This simple but effective measure can do much to alleviate pain and suffering and is particularly useful for patients who have sustained musculoskeletal injuries. The A&E nurse can use slings, splints, pillows or blankets to place the injured limb in a comfortable position and should advise the patient to move it as little as possible. Swelling and pain, particularly when associated with soft tissue injury, can also be reduced by elevation of an injured limb (Walsh 1996).

Warm and/or cold compresses

For patients who have sustained musculoskeletal injuries, superficial burns or other injuries, the use of cold compresses can reduce swelling and alleviate pain. They act by reducing the release of pain-causing chemicals, such as lactic acid, potassium ions, serotonin and histamine (Lee & Warren 1978). The nurse should ensure that the cold compress does not cause further injury, such as frostbite, and therefore ice should be placed in a plastic bag and covered with a paper or cloth towel. The use of gel packs which can be kept cool in the fridge or warmed in hot water can reduce this risk.

Warm compresses may also be used to reduce pain by triggering pain-inhibiting reflexes through temperature receptors. They are particularly effective for muscle and joint pain. However, because warmth increases swelling and the tendency to bleed, it is contraindicated after trauma. Because heat can burn, it should be used with particular caution over areas with impaired sensation or in patients with limited or no ability to communicate.

Distraction

McCaffery (1990) defined distraction as simply focusing attention on stimuli other than the pain sensation. One of the most frequently used distraction techniques in A&E involves breathing exercises. Patients are directed to focus their breathing by concentrating on inhalations and exhalations. Appropriate use of humour is also a successful distraction strategy that has been shown to improve the release of the body's natural endorphins (Watt-Watson & Ivers Donovan 1992).

Conclusion

The A&E nurse has a key role in the assessment and management of pain. This chapter has outlined the physiological and psychological effects of pain as well as a number of assessment tools the nurse may employ in A&E. Pharmacological and non-pharmacological means of delivering pain relief have also been considered. Non-pharmacological methods in particular are usually effective, simple to apply and easy to learn.

The A&E nurse has a responsibility to obtain a working knowledge of the range of strategies available to decrease pain and to use them to alleviate patient suffering and improve the quality of care.

References

Adam SK, Osborne S (1997) *Critical Care Nursing: Science and Practice*. Oxford: Oxford Medical.

Bentley J (1998) The science of pain: an update. In Sofaer B, ed. *Pain – Principles, Practice and Patients*. Cheltenham: Stanley Thorne.

Cave I (1994) Pain in A&E: the patient's view. *Emergency Nurse*, **2**(2), 19–20.

Davis P (1993) Opening up the gate control theory. *Nursing Standard*, **7**, 25–26.

Driscoll P, Gwinnutt C, Brook S (1994) Extremity trauma. In: Driscoll PA, Gwinnutt CL, LeDuc Jimmerson C, Goodall A, eds. *Trauma Resuscitation: the Team Approach*. Basingstoke: Macmillan.

Hallet N (1992) Pain: prevention and cure. In: Royle JA, Walsh M, eds. *Watson's Medical-Surgical Nursing and Related Physiology*. London: Baillière Tindall.

Halliday T, Robinson D, Stirling V *et al.* (1992) Book 3, the senses and communication. In: *Biology: Brain and Behaviour*. Milton Keynes: Open University.

Hardy JD, Wolff HG, Goodell H (1952) *Pain Sensations and Reactions*. Baltimore: Williams & Wilkins.

Hayward J (1975) *Information: a Prescription against Pain*. London: RCN.

Hinchliff S, Montague S, Watson R (1996) *Physiology for Nursing Practice*, 2nd edn. London: Baillière Tindall.

International Association for the Study of Pain Subcommittee on Taxonomy (1979) Pain terms: a list with definitions and notes on usage. *Pain*, **6**, 249–252.

Lee JM, Warren MP (1978) Clinical applications of cold for the musculoskeletal system. *Cold Therapy in Rehabilitation*. London: Bell and Hyman.

Longstaff M (1997) Methods: pain measurement in A&E. *Emergency Nurse*, **4**(4), 20–22.

McCaffery M (1983) *Nursing the Patient in Pain*, 2nd edn. London: Chapman & Hall.

McCaffery M (1990) Nursing approaches to non-pharmacological pain control. *International Journal of Nursing Studies*, **27**, 1–5.

McQuay H, Moore A, Justins D (1997) Treating acute pain in hospital. *British Medical Journal*, **314**, 1531–1315.

Mather L, Mackie J (1983) The incidence of postoperative pain in children. *Pain*, **15**, 271–282.

Melzack R, Wall PD (1965) Pain mechanisms: a new theory. *Science*, **150**, 971–979.

Melzack R, Wall PD (1982) *The Challenge of Pain*. New York: Basic Books.

O'Hara P (1996) *Pain Management for Health Professionals*. London: Chapman & Hall.

Sofaer B (1993) *Pain – a Handbook for Nurses*, 2nd edn. London: Chapman & Hall.

Sofaer B (1998) *Pain – Principles, Practice and Patients*. Cheltenham: Stanley Thorne.

Sternback RA, Tursky B (1965) Ethnic differences among housewives in psychophysical and skin potential responses to electric shock. *Psychophysiology*, **1**, 73.

Sutcliffe AJ (1993) Pain relief for acutely ill and injured patients. *Care of the Critically Ill*, **9**(6), 266–269.

Thompson DR, Webster R (1992) *Caring for the Coronary Patient*. Oxford: Butterworth-Heinemann.

Trounce J (1997) *Clinical Pharmacology for Nurses*, 15th edn. Edinburgh: Churchill Livingstone.

Walsh M (1993) Pain and anxiety in A&E attenders. *Nursing Standard*, **17**(7), 40–42.

Walsh M (1996) *Accident & Emergency Nursing: a New Approach*, 3rd edn. Oxford: Butterworth-Heinemann.

Watt-Watson JH, Ivers Donovan M (1992) *Pain Management: Nursing Perspective*. St Louis: Mosby Year Book.

Chapter 25

Local and Regional Anaesthesia

Bernie Edwards

- Introduction
- Pharmacology of local anaesthetics
- Classification of local anaesthetics
- Benefits of local anaesthetics
- Disadvantages and limitations of local anaesthetics
- Types and uses of local anaesthesia
- Nursing implications of procedures involving local anaesthetics
- Conclusion

Introduction

The first recorded use of a local anaesthetic was the application of cocaine to the cornea by Freud and Koller in 1884 (Yertis *et al.* 1993). The development of other agents, notably procaine in 1904 and lignocaine in 1947, along with the pioneering of sophisticated techniques, has led to a growth in the use of local anaesthetics to achieve a pain-free operative field. This chapter will describe the pharmacology of local anaesthetics, discuss the advantages and disadvantages associated with their use, and outline the principles of managing patients undergoing procedures involving local anaesthetics in the A&E department.

Pharmacology of Local Anaesthetics

Local anaesthesia is a method of rendering surgical operations painless to a conscious patient. It stops impulse conduction when applied locally to nerve fibres or nerve trunks conveying impulses from the affected area. The action is reversible and is followed by complete recovery of function. The passage of an impulse along a nerve axon is dependent upon the interchange of sodium and, to a lesser extent, potassium ions across the nerve cell membrane. During the resting phase the cell membrane is largely impermeable to sodium ions. This, in combination with the sodium pump, raises the concentration of sodium in the extracellular fluid to 10 times that inside the cell. This contrasts with that of potassium ions, the concentration of which is 30 times greater inside the nerve cell compared with the outside. This ratio of sodium to potassium gives rise to an electrical potential difference across the cell membrane of -70 mV (inside negative) (Hinchliff & Montague 1988).

When stimulus energy is applied to the cell membrane it becomes permeable to sodium ions, leading to an influx into the cell where there is an exchange with potassium ions. This interchange of ions reverses the electrical potential difference, the inside of the cell transiently becoming positive with respect to the outside to about +40 mV. The depolarisation travels the length of the nerve fibre, causing the impulse to be experienced as a conscious sensation, in this case pain (Hinchliff & Montague 1988). For this to occur, a critical level of depolarisation of the cell membrane must be reached, the threshold potential. Local anaesthetics work by binding to the sodium channels in the membrane, thereby preventing changes to sodium permeability. Local anaesthetics can, therefore, be considered as having a membrane-stabilising effect (Yertis *et al.* 1993) (see also Ch. 22).

The smaller the diameter of nerve fibre, the more sensitive it is to the effects of local anaesthetic. The clinical sequelae following injection are initial loss of autonomic function, followed by loss of pain sensation, then touch and pressure sensation and finally motor function. Recovery proceeds in the reverse order (Henderson & Nimmo 1983). The interference with autonomic function means that all local anaesthetics, with the exception of cocaine, cause local or regional vasodilation depending on the technique used. Local vasodilation can lead to rapid dispersal, thereby minimising the duration of the local anaesthetic. The addition of a vasoconstrictor such as adrenaline can delay absorption, thereby prolonging anaesthesia and preventing flooding of the circulation. If used, the total dose should not exceed 0.5 mg or the concentration 1:200 000 (Trounce 1990).

The duration of action is dependent upon:

- the drug used
- the concentration and dose of local anaesthetic
- the rate of diffusion from the injection site to the axon.

This latter point is important as it emphasises the need to allow sufficient time for the local anaesthetics to work before commencing the procedure.

Classification of Local Anaesthetics

The ideal should possess the following characteristics:

- non-irritant
- rapid onset of effect
- non-toxic
- have a duration of action appropriate to the operation
- leave no local after-effects.

Local anaesthetics can be divided into two chemical groupings: amides and esters. Amides are metabolised by the liver and can therefore only be used in those patients whose liver function is uncompromised. Esters are broken down in the plasma by pseudocholinesterase, and then by the liver to para-aminobenzoic acid (Yertis *et al.* 1993). This compound can produce allergic reactions in some people. The properties of four commonly used local anaesthetics are outlined in Table 25.1.

Benefits of Local Anaesthetics

The major benefit is the absence of those complications which may arise from the use of general anaesthetics and intubation. The laryngeal and cough reflexes remain, reducing the risk of respiratory obstruction. Local anaesthetics do not automatically depress respiratory function, making them ideal for patients with poor lung function. The patient will not experience the discomforts associated with general anaesthesia, such as nausea and vomiting, dizziness and sore throat. The associated shorter recovery time will facilitate earlier discharge. In addition, many, though not all, minor procedures can still be performed even if the patient has eaten.

The numbing effect of local anaesthetics on the surgical site usually lasts beyond the operative period,

Table 25.1 – *The pharmacology of four common local anaesthetics (Rivellini 1993, Trounce 1990, Wellington et al. 1987)*

Agent	Group	Percentage	Concentration	Potency	Onset	Duration
Cocaine	Ester	4–20	N/A	High	Slow	30–45 mins
Lignocaine/lidocaine	Amide	1–4	0.5–2	Moderate	Slow	1–2 hours
Prilocaine	Amide	N/A	0.5–1	Moderate	Slow	1–2 hours
Bupivacaine	Amide	N/A	0.25–0.75 (Used in epidurals)	High	Slow	4–8 hours

providing highly specific, temporary postoperative pain relief. Also, because patients remain conscious, they are able to cooperate, if required, and report any abnormalities, making the early detection of complications more likely (Rivellini 1993).

Disadvantages and Limitations of Local Anaesthesia

The first major disadvantage with local anaesthesia is that, while patients may not feel pain, they will often experience other sensations associated with the procedure, such as pressure and movement. Because they are conscious they will also be able to see, hear and smell all that is going on. There will be many patients who simply do not wish to be awake because they would rather not know anything.

Many patients also find the feelings of numbness, paraesthesia, paralysis and the sense of being detached from the affected part of body disconcerting (Rivellini 1993). The use of local anaesthetic requires the active cooperation of the patient and so may not suitable for confused, aggressive and agitated people. Patients with learning difficulties may pose particular problems for the nurse but should by no means automatically be excluded.

The use of local anaesthetic is limited by the suitability of the surgical site. In addition, many of the procedures involved are technically difficult and require a high level of expertise beyond that of the majority of A&E staff. It is important to remember that whilst the term 'local' is used, local anaesthetics are only minimally metabolised at the site of injection; most pass ultimately into the bloodstream and, potentially, may produce systemic toxic effects. These result from the membrane-stabilising effects on other cells, notably those of the cardiovascular and central nervous systems. These are listed in Box 25.1.

Other potential toxic effects include hypotension due to loss of vascular tone, respiratory depression and allergic reactions, although the latter two are uncommon (Rivellini 1993; Trounce 1990).

Types and Uses of Local Anaesthesia

The types of local anaesthesia are categorised according to the method of administration or site of injection and are broadly divided into local or regional (Rivellini 1993):

■ **Local**
 — topical
 — infiltration

Box 25.1 – *Potential toxic effects of local anaesthetics on the cardiovascular and central nervous systems*

Central nervous system
■ Tinnitus

■ Paraesthesia of mouth and tongue

■ Metallic taste in the mouth

■ Dizziness and light-headedness

■ Talkativeness

■ Feelings of confusion and disorientation

■ Agitation and tremor

■ Drowsiness

■ Convulsion

■ Coma

Cardiovascular system
■ Myocardial conduction

■ PR interval

■ Sinus bradycardia

■ AV block

■ Cardiac output

■ Hypotension

■ Resistant ventricular arrhythmias

■ Cardiac arrest

■ **Regional**
 — nerve block
 — intravenous regional (Bier's block)
 — epidural (extradural) block
 — spinal (subarachnoid) block.

Local anaesthesia is used for relatively minor procedures whereas regional anaesthesia is reserved for these that are more complex. The last two techniques are not usually seen in A&E and are therefore beyond the scope of this chapter.

Surface or topical application

This involves direct application of the local anaesthetic to mucous membranes or open wounds, such as grazes. Suitable sites include the cornea, conjunctiva, upper airway and urethra. Local anaesthetics for this purpose come in the form of sprays, solutions, jellies and ointments. One local anaesthetic used as a topical agent is cocaine. Unlike other local anaesthetics, cocaine potentiates the action of the sympathetic nervous system thus causing local vasoconstriction. It is highly effective on very vascular areas, such as the nasal membranes. It also causes dilation of the pupil when used on the cornea. Cocaine, however, has powerful central effects making it too dangerous to inject (Trounce 1990).

Creams containing a combination of lignocaine and prilocaine can be used prior to venepuncture in children. A thick layer is applied under an occlusive dressing and left for 60–120 minutes. This time lag sometimes makes it impractical for use in A&E (Smith 1995). Chronic long-term use of topical preparations can lead to sensitisation and local allergic reactions.

Local infiltration

This involves subcutaneous injection of a local anaesthetic solution into the area surrounding the operation or wound site. This is ideal for the suturing and extensive cleansing of minor wounds and the drainage of superficial wound abscesses. While this provides excellent levels of pain relief, infiltration itself can be painful. Care needs to be exercised to avoid injection of large volumes of local anaesthetic as this can lead to localised oedema, causing distortion of wound edges and tissue hypoxia. This makes apposition and healing of the wound edges difficult.

Lignocaine is the drug of choice due to its rapid onset. Toxicity can be avoided if the dose does not exceed 3 mg/kg body weight, approximately 20 ml of a 1% solution in an adult. Care should be taken to avoid introducing lignocaine directly into a vein. Lignocaine can also be used both topically as a 4% solution or 1–2% jelly and in peripheral nerve blocks. The normal duration of 15–45 minutes can be increased to 2 hours by the addition of adrenaline (Trounce 1990).

Peripheral nerve blocks

These are achieved by injecting local anaesthetic around nerve trunks supplying the injury/operation site. The main advantage is it requires fewer injections and avoids the pain involved of injection directly into already sensitive tissue. However, some of the techniques involved are difficult.

The most frequent use of a nerve block is the ring block to achieve anaesthesia of a digit. This involves injection into the base of the finger via the interdigital web. Both sides of the finger are infiltrated to ensure blockage of all four digital nerves. *It is imperative that adrenaline is not added to the local anaesthetic solution as this will lead to vasoconstriction and occlusion of the digital arteries.*

Brachial plexus or axillary blocks can be used to achieve anaesthesia of the forearm and hand. They also act as muscle relaxants as the motor fibres are also blocked. The local anaesthetic is injected into the neurovascular sheath surrounding the axillary artery and the median, radial and ulnar nerves. Potential complications, as with all nerve blocks, relate to the possibility of damage to surrounding structures (Rivellini 1993).

Intravenous regional anaesthesia (Bier's block)

This technique is used primarily to achieve anaesthesia below the elbow, although it can also be used for procedures below the knee. The main uses of this technique are for the manipulation of Colles' and Smith fractures.

Following insertion of an intravenous cannula, the arm is elevated for about 2 minutes to drain some of the blood from the veins in order to reduce the dilation of the local anaesthetic. A cuffed tourniquet, underlaid by wool, is placed around the upper arm and inflated to a pressure at least 100 mmHg above that of the patient's systolic blood pressure.

The local anaesthetic, e.g. 40 ml prilocaine 0.5%, is injected into the collapsed veins of the limb; this will cause the limb to develop a blue, mottled appearance. The maximum length of time for which the cuff can remain inflated is 1.5 hours. However, pain from the direct compression of nerve and muscle tissue will be evident after 30 minutes and may be unbearable after an hour. This discomfort may be eased by the use of a double-cuff. When this is used, the proximal cuff is inflated prior to infiltration. Following infiltration the distal cuff is inflated and the proximal cuff let down. Thus, the tourniquet effect is maintained by the distal cuff which is located over an area of the limb that has been anaesthetised (Rivellini 1993).

It is imperative that the pressure in the cuff is maintained constantly for at least 30 minutes to permit fixation of the local anaesthetic to the tissues of the limb (Rivellini 1993). Release or leakage of the anaesthetic into the systemic circulation prior to this time can lead to cardiovascular and CNS depression. The presence of resuscitation facilities and circulatory access are mandatory.

The use of intravenous regional anaesthesia is contraindicated in cases of:

■ patient refusal

- sickle cell disease
- Raynaud's disease
- severe atheroma
- epilepsy
- heart failure
- liver disease
- anticoagulant therapy.

Nursing Implications of Procedures Involving Local Anaesthetics

Preoperatively

The patient's past and current medical history should be assessed and factors that might contraindicate the use of local anaesthetics should be noted, in particular previous allergic reactions. A baseline of the current neurovascular status of the proposed surgical site should be established. The nurse needs to be familiar with the technique to be used, the length of time the block will last and whether any vasoconstrictive agent has been added (Rivellini 1993).

Thorough preparation of the patient includes the provision of information about both the nature of the procedure and the feelings the patient may experience during it. Explanation of sights and sensations which may result from the procedure needs to be given before they occur, e.g. the change of limb colour associated with the infiltration of local anaesthetic during intravenous regional anaesthesia.

Informed consent will need to be obtained. For minor procedures such as suturing this can be obtained verbally, but for techniques involving intravenous regional anaesthesia formal written consent will be required, as will baseline observations and the patient's weight.

Intraoperatively

Special consideration should be given to the fact that patients are awake. Careless remarks should be avoided and technical terms, when used, even between staff, need to be explained. The focus of conversation should be the patient rather than the procedure. Where conscious awareness of the procedure causes distress, social conversation can be used to distract the patient (Edwards 1994).

Constant vigilance is required to assess for signs of toxicity and allergic reaction. The neurovascular function of the affected area should be continuously observed and compared with that of equivalent unaffected areas. This is particularly pertinent with procedures involving manipulation of a limb or the application of a plaster cast, as the complications of either are mimicked by the action of local anaesthetic. Tourniquet time, where appropriate, should be noted (Rivellini 1993). The patient should be specifically encouraged to report any discomfort experienced.

Postoperatively and advice for discharge

Pain provides a protective function both as an initiator of reflex mechanisms and by alerting the person when a body part has sustained trauma. In eliminating pain, local anaesthetics eliminate these protective mechanisms. Nurses will need to consider measures to ensure the safety of the patient and the body part. Limbs should not be allowed to rest on or become trapped in cot sides.

Transient loss of motor function necessitates that affected extremities will need to be supported in anatomically neutral positions. A sling will serve both to protect and to support the weight of an arm. Any attempt at using the affected area until full sensation has returned should be discouraged. The post-anaesthesia levels of sensory and motor function should be continually assessed and delays in expected dissipation times reported. It is vital that care is taken to differentiate between paraesthesiae related to dissipation of the block and those of neurovascular compromise (Rivellini 1993). These observations should be documented at least once prior to discharge.

The residual effect of the local anaesthetic will provide immediate pain relief. However, as this is only temporary, postoperative analgesia will need to be prescribed and administered before the effect dissipates. As far as possible, it is helpful to give some indication as to the possible levels of discomfort the patient may experience once the local anaesthetic has worn off. This will help the patient to determine whether this is normal or an indicator of residual or developing complications.

Conclusion

This chapter has highlighted both the rationale for the use of local anaesthetics and the nursing implications. Local anaesthetics are a valuable weapon in the armoury of A&E care. Used with vigilance they can provide an alternative to the torture of the 'one quick pull' and the fear of 'being put to sleep'.

References

Edwards B (1994) Local and regional anaesthesia. *Emergency Nurse*, **2**(2), 10–15.

Henderson J, Nimmo W (1983) *Practical Regional Anaesthesia*. Oxford: Blackwell Scientific.

Hinchliff S, Montague (1988) *Physiology for Nursing Practice*. London: Baillière Tindall.

Rivellini D (1993) Local and regional anaesthesia. *Nursing Clinics of North America*, **28**(3), 547–572.

Smith C (1995) IV cannulation: principles and practice. *Emergency Nurse*, **2**(4), 16–18.

Trounce J (1990) *Clinical Pharmacology for Nurses*, 13th edn. Edinburgh: Churchill Livingstone.

Wellington F *et al* (1987) *Baillière's Pharmacology and Drug Information for Nurses*, 2nd edn. London: Baillière Tindall.

Yertis S, Hirsch N, Smith G (1993) *Anaesthesia A-Z: an Encyclopaedia of Principles and Practice*. Oxford: Butterworth-Heinemann.

Part 6

Emergency Care

26. Cardiac Emergencies   341

27. Medical Emergencies   371

28. Surgical Emergencies   393

29. Gynaecological and Obstetric   411
    Emergencies

30. Ophthalmic Emergencies   429

31. Ear, Nose and Throat Emergencies   447

Chapter 26

Cardiac Emergencies

Jamie Walthall

- Introduction
- Related anatomy and physiology
- The cardiac cycle
- Assessment
- Basic ECG interpretation
- Cardiac arrest
- Rhythm disturbances
- Heart block
- Pacing
- Acute chest pain
- Acute cardiac failure
- Viral/inflammatory conditions
- Conclusion

Introduction

In 1992 the government released a White Paper, *Health of the Nation*, which set out to target key health care aspects. One of the main priorities was to reduce the mortality and morbidity rate of coronary heart disease. Statistics show that in the UK there is a death every 16 minutes in these under 65 years from coronary heart disease (CHD) (Office of Health Economics 1990). The overall mortality rate for CHD was 26% of all deaths in England and Wales in 1990 (Office of Population Census and Surveys 1990). A&E departments will see a high proportion of patients suffering from a cardiovascular disorder.

The aim of this chapter is to give a systematic approach to the multiple problems that may be encountered by cardiac patients. A general overview of anatomy and physiology has been included to enable the disease process to be more accurately defined. The management of the particular cardiac problems described in this chapter is set out as a suggested guideline and is not a definitive directive for all cardiac patients, as each problem should be judged on an individual basis.

Related Anatomy and Physiology

The heart can be described as a muscular pump containing four chambers, situated at an oblique angle in the mediastinal cavity (Tortora & Grabowski 1996) (Figs 26.1 and 26.2).

As the heart beats it expels blood into two closed circuits. The first circuit is fed from the left side of the heart. This supplies oxygenated blood from the lungs to the systemic circulation. The second circuit is the pulmonary circuit. This enables the right side of the heart to receive deoxygenated blood which is then pumped back to the lungs via the pulmonary artery (Marieb 1995).

The heart is composed of a triple layer, which enables the protection of the inner components (Tortora & Grabowski 1996):

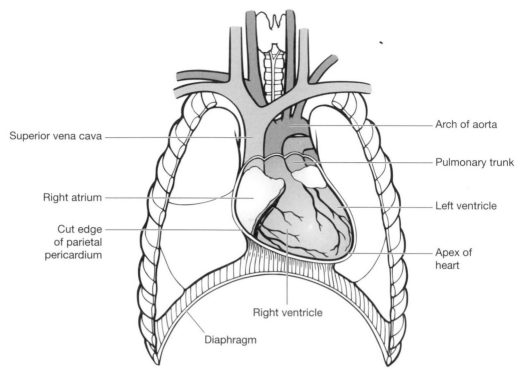

Figure 26.1 – *Anterior view of the chest.*

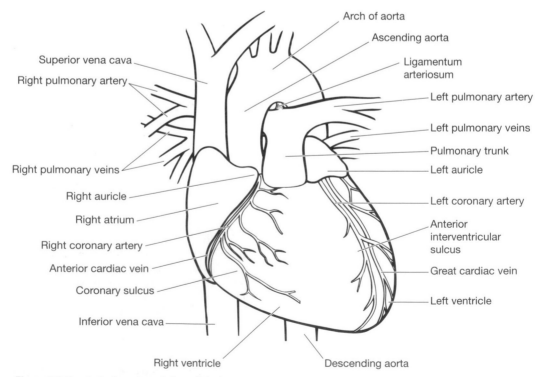

Figure 26.2 – *Anterior external view of the heart.*

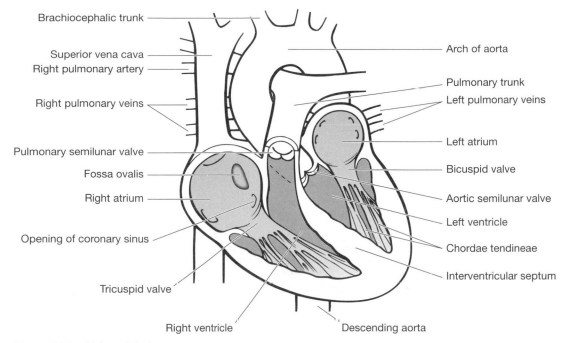

Figure 26.3 – *Valves of the heart.*

■ *The pericardium* – the outer layer is composed of thick fibrous tissue that surrounds and protects the heart.
■ *The myocardium* – this is the muscular layer that forms the basis of the pumping action of the heart. It is present within both the atria and the ventricles, with the ventricles having the greater ratio of muscle.
■ *The endocardium* – this is composed of a thin layer of endothelial and connective tissue covering the inside of the heart, including the valves, which enables a smooth flow of blood through the heart, with little resistance.

Cardiac valves (Fig. 26.3)

The atrioventricular (AV) valves refer to the mitral and tricuspid valves, which lie between the atria and the ventricles, the mitral on the left and the tricuspid on the right. The valves are supported by a network of strands called chordae tendineae. The passive movement of blood from the atria to the ventricles, across the AV valves, occurs in the cardiac cycle in the phase known as ventricular filling. As the pressure in the ventricles increases, the valves are forced to close, preventing a back-flow of blood.

At the origin of the aorta and the pulmonary artery sit the semilunar valves. These consist of three cusps, and prevent the back-flow of blood into the heart. During ventricular diastole (relaxation), these valves are closed, but as ventricular systole (contraction) occurs the valves are forced to open and blood is ejected out into either the aorta or the pulmonary artery. Should these valves be diseased or damaged, stenosis or regurgitation may occur. More often than not this precludes the need for the surgical intervention.

Coronary circulation

To maintain oxygenation and the supply of nutrients, the heart derives its own blood supply via the coronary arteries (see Fig. 26.4). The left and right coronary arteries originate from the aorta. As suggested, they branch into a network of arteries supplying both the right and left sides of the heart.

The Cardiac Cycle

The cardiac cycle is divided into three main phases (Tortora & Grabowski 1996):

■ ventricular relaxation (diastole)
■ ventricular filling
■ ventricular contraction (systole).

For simplification only the left side of the heart will be explained.

Ventricular relaxation. This follows ventricular contraction (systole). The ventricles relax, resulting in

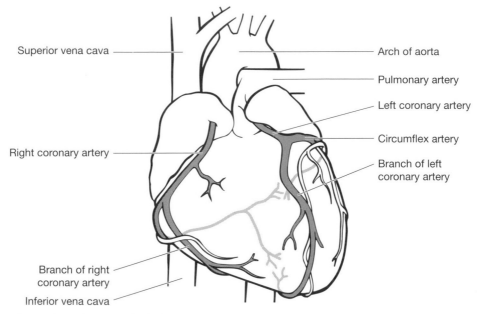

Figure 26.4 – *Coronary circulation.*

pressure within the left ventricle falling below that of the aorta, and thus the aortic valve closes. As Tortora & Grabowski (1996) stated all valves within the heart are now closed. At the same time, blood is passively flowing into the left atrium via the pulmonary system. As pressure and volume within the left atrium increases, the mitral valve opens and the second phase of the cardiac cycle is now entered.

Ventricular filling. Tortora & Grabowski (1996) identified that the ventricular filling phase of the cardiac cycle is divided into three stages. The first stage is referred to as rapid ventricular filling and involves passive filling of the left ventricle from the left atrium. The second stage of ventricular filling is known as diastasis and refers to slow ventricular filling. At the end of diastasis, the pressures in the left atrium and the left ventricle are now equal. The third stage of ventricular filling is due to the contraction of the atrium, with blood being forced into the left ventricle.

Ventricular contraction. As the left ventricle starts to contract the mitral valve closes. The left ventricle is now a closed chamber. The muscles within the left ventricle start to contract and there is a resultant increase in pressure. Once the pressure in the left ventricle is greater than that of the aorta, the aortic valve opens and blood is ejected out (the stroke volume). As the pressure in the left ventricle drops with the expulsion of blood, the aortic valve closes and the cardiac cycle starts again.

Assessment

When a patient attends the A&E department with a cardiac event, one of the most important factors relied upon is the presenting history (Barrett 1983). The history provides subjective information about the presenting complaint, symptoms, past medical history and any other relevant information (Alexander *et al.* 1994). During initial assessment, the patient's need for immediate care must be paramount. Hence, the use of the ABC principle should be initiated automatically (Box 26.1).

Box 26.1 – *ABCs*
A Check the patency of the **airway**
B Check the adequacy of the **breathing**
C **Circulation**: signs of shock, pallor etc.

The remainder of the assessment should include:

■ *Assessment of patient's appearance.* – this should include pallor, posture and any non-verbal signs.
■ *Pain assessment.* – location, type, site and severity of pain, including any measures taken to relieve the pain.
■ *Baseline observations.* – these should include blood pressure, pulse, temperature, respiration and oxygen saturation. Often temperature is forgotten,

but the incidence of a mild pyrexia is a common response to muscle damage (Alexander *et al.* 1994).

■ *Electrocardiograph (ECG)* – note any arrhythmia and use of cardiac monitor.

Clinical investigations

Clinical investigations to support assessment should include blood analysis (see Box 26.2) and chest X-ray to determine heart size and detect oedema (Jowett & Thompson 1995).

Basic ECG Interpretation

It is important for A&E nurses to accurately record and interpret an ECG of a patient presenting with a cardiac condition. An inherent and rhythmical electrical activity is the reason for the heart's continuous beating (Tortora & Grabowski 1996). The cardiac cells (myocardial cells) located within the myocardium undergo chemical changes, which in turn trigger electrical impulses (action potentials) and result in myocardial contraction.

The normal heartbeat is known as sinus rhythm. In essence, this means that the impulses have been generated by the normal heart conductive system (Fig. 26.5). The detection of these electrical impulses can be recorded via an ECG. To obtain a 12-lead ECG, electrodes are placed across the chest and each limb (see Fig. 26.6).

> **Box 26.2** – *Blood analysis in cardiac patients*
>
> ■ **Cardiac enzymes** – these indicate muscular damage which may suggest cardiac ischaemia (Julian 1988)
>
> ■ **White cell count** – a raised white cell count in the cardiac patient is usually indicative of myocardial damage
>
> ■ **Erythrocyte sedimentation rate (ESR)** – a raised ESR may indicate an increase in fibrinogen due to myocardial necrosis
>
> ■ **Urea and electrolytes (U&E)** – any change in the sodium or potassium should be noted as these ions are related to cardiac cells and their function
>
> ■ **Glucose** – the appearance of hyperglycaemia can be stress-related and linked to any acute changes in the myocardium, e.g. myocardial infarction (Woods *et al.* 1995)
>
> ■ **Lipids** – these will give an indication as to the risk factors incorporated with ischaemic heart disease; they include cholesterol and triglycerides
>
> ■ **Clotting screen** – this is useful when the patient may be anticoagulated

Having positioned the ECG electrodes, it is important to understand the representation being made by each electrode. The heart's electrical

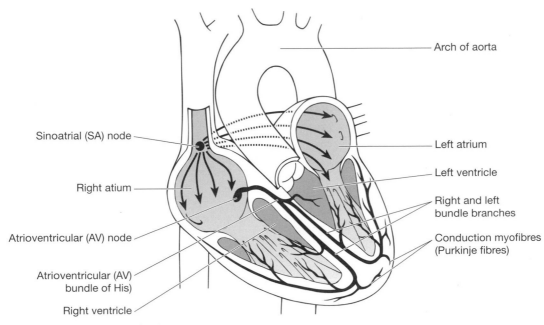

Figure 26.5 – *Cardiac conduction.*

Arch of aorta

Sinoatrial (SA) node

Left atrium

Left ventricle

Right atium

Right and left bundle branches

Atrioventricular (AV) node

Conduction myofibres (Purkinje fibres)

Atrioventricular (AV) bundle of His)

Right ventricle

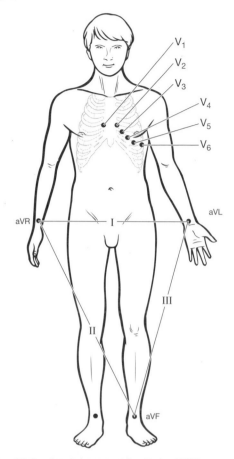

Figure 26.6 – *Lead placement for 12-lead ECG.*

impulses start at the SA node and depolarise down the conductive system as far as the apex of the heart. This directional flow is known as the cardiac vector. The four limb leads attached as shown in Figure 26.7 form what is known as the Einthoven triangle. The fourth lead not shown within the triangle acts as an earth and helps to standardise recordings. Leads I, II and III are

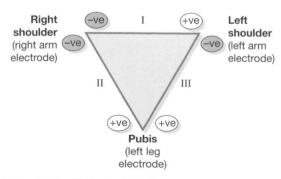

Figure 26.7 – *Einthoven triangle.*

known as bipolar leads, because each lead represents the electrical activity between two poles:

- Lead I represents electrical activity from the right arm to the left arm.
- Lead II represents electrical activity from the right arm to the left leg.
- Lead III represents electrical activity from the left arm to the left leg.

Leads AVR, AVL and AVF are known as unipolar leads. They read electrical impulses from one electrode, with the ECG machine calculating the effect of the other limb leads to give an average reading between the points of the triangle formed by the bipolar leads.

The abbreviations for the unipolar leads are as follows:

- A – augmented (amplified)
- V – vector (force of direction of impulse)
- R, L, F – the direction being viewed, i.e. right, left or foot.

Thus, AVR looks at the right atrium (although in practice this is of little consequence), AVL looks at the lateral aspect of the heart, and AVF looks at the inferior aspect (see also Box 26.3). The chest leads are a much more simplified version for looking at the frontal plane of the heart. These are unipolar leads which pick up electrical activity from the point at which they are placed (Box 26.3):

Box 26.3 – *Areas of heart shown in specific leads*	
I	Left lateral surface
II	Left lateral and inferior surface
III	Inferior surface
AVR	Right atrium
AVL	Left lateral surface
AVF	Inferior surface
V_1	Right anterior
V_2	Right anterior surface and some of left anterior surface
V_3	Septal area
V_4	Anterior surface of left ventricle
V_5	Left anterior/lateral surfaces
V_6	Lateral aspect of left ventricle

- V_1 is placed over the 4th intercostal space to the right of the sternum.

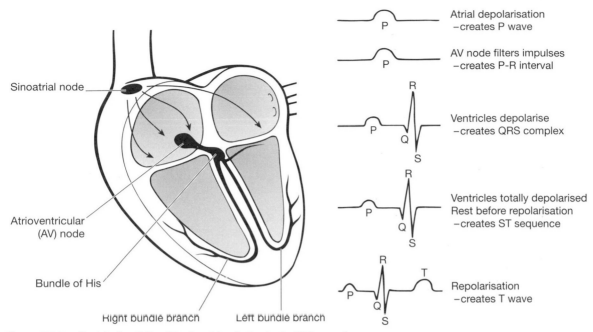

Figure 26.8 – *Electrical activity of the heart in relation to the ECG recording.*

- V_2 is placed over the 4th intercostal space to the left of the sternum.
- V_1 and V_2 thus view the anterior surfaces of the right and part of the left ventricles.
- V_3 is placed on the chest midway between V_2 and V_4; hence it is useful to apply V_4 before V_3. V_3 looks at the septum.
- V_4 is placed on the 5th intercostal space, midway along the clavicular line, and views the septum and the anterior wall of the left ventricle.
- V_5 is placed along the same line as V_4, but anteriorly to the midaxillary line.
- V_6 is again placed along the same line as V_4 and V_5, but rests on the midaxillary line.
- V_5 and V_6 view predominately the lateral wall of the left ventricles.

Components of a normal ECG

The ECG complex is made up of a sequence of electrical events occurring in the heart. The activity starts with impulses being transmitted from the sinoatrial node across the atria. As the atria depolarise, the P wave is created. The AV node filters and holds atrial impulses to allow significant ventricular filling time prior to contraction. This is represented as a straight line (isoelectric line) on the ECG and is called the P–R interval. As depolarisation occurs through the

bundle branches, and a wave of depolarisation spreads across, the QRS complex is created on the ECG. This is followed by a short resting period, depicted again as an isoelectric line called the ST segment, before the T wave is created by ventricular repolarisation (Fig. 26.8).

When this is all put together, a single heartbeat is represented in the ECG trace as shown in Figure 26.9.

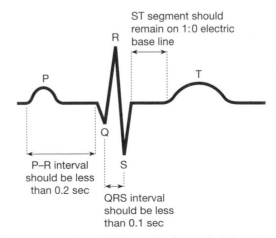

Figure 26.9 – *Normal ECG complex from a single heartbeat.*

Basic rhythm recognition

To make an accurate analysis of cardiac activity it is necessary to obtain a 12-lead ECG trace as opposed to a rhythm strip. The rhythm strip only shows one view of the heart which is dependent on the electrode positioning. As a result, myocardial damage or stress can easily be missed.

Once the 12-lead ECG has been obtained (see Fig. 26.10), it is necessary to work through each lead methodically, looking at each waveform to ensure that any changes/abnormalities are recognised. To interpret an ECG, the A&E nurse should start by looking at the rhythm strip to determine whether a basic rhythm is present. If a rhythm exists, complexes will be repetitive and components of those complexes will form the same pattern. It is also necessary to determine whether this pattern is occurring at regular intervals or not. Once an underlying rhythm is established, the rate of the rhythm should be determined.

ECG tracings are standardised so that heart rate can be calculated from the tracing. Most ECG machines are set to pass paper through at 25 mm/s. As graph paper is standardised, one small square represents 0.04 s (1 mm of paper), one large square represents 0.2 s (5 mm of paper) and five large squares represent 1 s (25 mm of paper). Therefore, if there is one QRS complex per five large squares, the heart rate would be approximately 60 beats/min. Once an approximate rate is established, the nurse should look at the make of the repetitive complexes, checking whether the P waves are followed by the right length of interval and the QRS complex is followed by a T wave (see Box 26.4).

Once a basic rhythm has been established from the rhythm strip, attention should be focused on the various leads to determine whether any area of the

heart is damaged or ischaemic. It is important that ECG interpretation does not take precedence over the patient's clinical condition. The clinical picture and condition of the patient are by far the best indicators of overall well-being. For this reason there is no substitute for the A&E nurse's fundamental assessment skills.

Cardiac Arrest

Cardiorespiratory arrest is defined as the sudden cessation of spontaneous respiration and circulation (Jowett & Thompson 1995). The three main causes of cardiac arrest are:

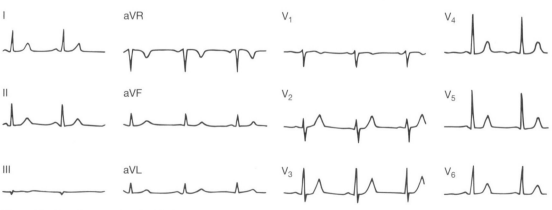

Figure 26.10 – *A normal 12-lead ECG trace.*

- ventricular fibrillation (VF)/pulseless ventricular tachycardia (VT)
- asystole
- electro-mechanical dissociation (EMD)

It is identified by:

- sudden loss of consciousness
- absence of a central pulse (carotid/femoral)
- absence of respiration.

Systemic management

In A&E departments, cardiac arrests in most instances are anticipated. Therefore, the A&E nurse is responsible for (Alexander *et al.* 1994):

- recognising cardiac arrest
- correct procedure for summoning help
- commencing basic life support (Fig. 26.11).

Ventricular fibrillation (VF)

The most common cause of cardiac arrest is usually VF or pulseless ventricular tachycardia (VT), which has an 80–90% mortality rate for patients outside of the hospital environment (Colquhoun *et al.* 1995). In VF, the cardiac cycle is disrupted and the cardiac cells behave chaotically, depolarising in a disorientated and disorderly fashion or fibrillation (Fig. 26.12). As a result, cardiac output is compromised to the extent that blood circulation stops. This results in hypoxia, loss of consciousness and absence of respiration. The physiology of VT is discussed later in this chapter. Simply put, the ventricular contractions occur at such a rate that ventricular filling time is inadequate and cardiac output is compromised. In severe cases, circulation ceases as in VF.

Immediate management

Cardiac arrest management has been standardised by the development of advanced life support (ALS)

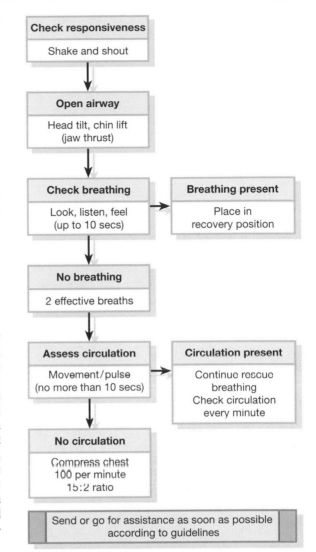

Figure 26.11 – *Adult basic life support.*

protocols (Advanced Life Support Working Party 1997). If the VF arrest is witnessed and monitored, a

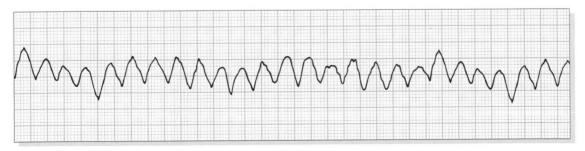

Figure 26.12 – *Ventricular fibrillation.*

precordial thump may be of benefit in an attempt to 'shock' the heart and restore normal electrical activity. Opinion is divided over the benefit versus risk of this action (Advanced Life Support Working Party 1997). The optimum first-line treatment for VF and pulseless VT is early defibrillation. The aim of defibrillation is to depolarise the myocardium simultaneously, to allow normal cardiac cell function to resume (Colquhoun *et al.* 1995).

A key factor in reducing mortality lies with the speed of defibrillation, which should be given without delay (Advanced Life Support Working Group of the European Resuscitation Council 1998). For this reason, A&E nurses should be appropriately skilled in performing defibrillation as they are likely to be the first personnel in attendance.

Defibrillation

The paddles of the defibrillator are positioned to enclose as much myocardium as possible (Skinner & Vincent 1997) (see Fig. 26.13). A conductive medium, such as jelly pads, should always be used, both to enhance contact and to reduce skin damage. Good contact with the chest is vital to maximise conduction and prevent 'arcing' of electrical current. The paddles should be placed firmly over jelly pads and perpendicular pressure should be applied. One paddle should be placed below the right clavicle in the midclavicular line and the other over the lower left ribs in the mid-anterior line (just outside the position of the normal cardiac apex) (Advanced Life Support Working Group of the European Resuscitation Council 1998). In female patients the second pad or paddle should be placed firmly on the chest wall just outside the position of the normal cardiac apex, avoiding the breast tissue.

Prior to defibrillation, GTN patches and external pacing generators should be removed. Internal pacers or defibrillating systems do not preclude the need for external DC shock in the case of VF or pulseless VT. The defibrillation regime should follow the algorithm shown in Figure 26.14.

Once the initial pulse check is done and found to be absent in VF, pulse checks between shocks are not necessary as the rhythm is not compatible with a cardiac output. The Resuscitation Council state that in pulseless ventricular tachycardia, pulse checks should be performed if there is a change in morphology which may result in a cardiac output (Advanced Life Support Working Group of the European Resuscitation Council 1998). The safety of the resuscitation team is paramount and it is the responsibility of the person administering DC shocks to ensure that other team members are clear of the patient. This should be ascertained verbally and visually before proceeding

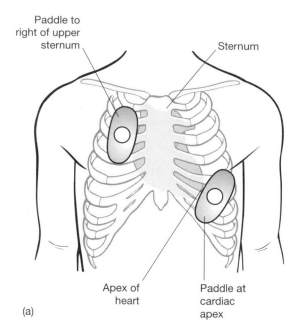

(a)

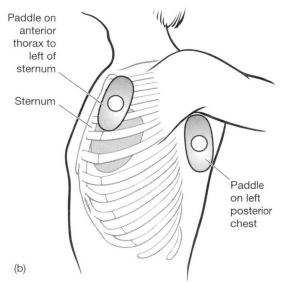

(b)

Figure 26.13 – *Positioning of defibrillator paddles.*

with defibrillation. ALS courses provide a standardised approach to training for all team members and should be a priority for A&E nurses.

Asystole

This is total cessation of circulation, brought about by the lack of cardiac pacemaker activity, either natural or artificial (Colquhoun *et al.* 1995) (Fig. 26.15). Asystole

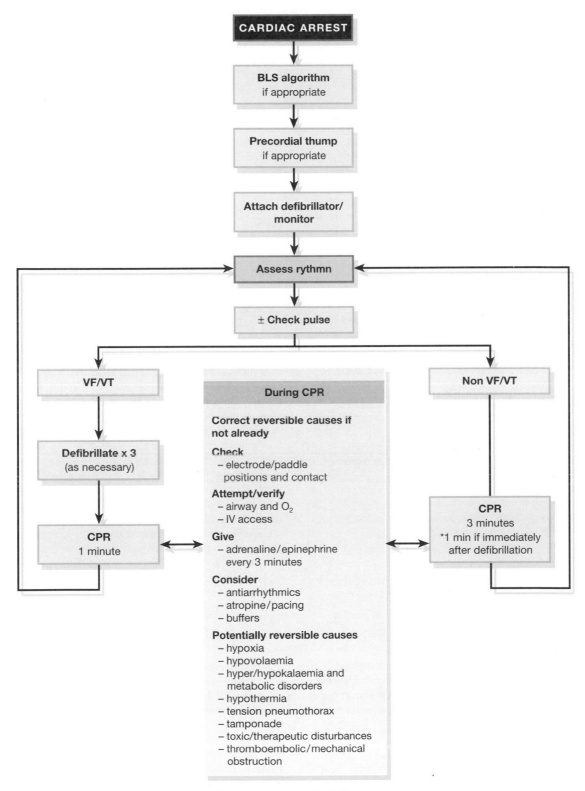

Figure 26.14 – *The universal algorhythm (after Robertson et al. 1998).*

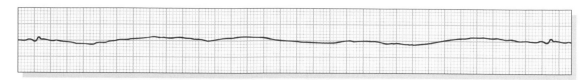

Figure 26.15 – *Asystole.*

accounts for 25% of all cardiac arrests within the hospital environment (Jowett & Thompson 1995). The treatment is continued cardiac compression with ventilation. Adrenaline (epinephrine) and atropine are used to stimulate cardiac activity, but the prognosis for a successful resuscitation remains poor, with the overall survival rate being about 10–15% of the survival rate with VF/VT rhythms.

Electromechanical disassociation (EMD)

This presents as a full QRS complex on the heart trace, but with the absence of any central pulse, hence the lack of systemic circulation. The causes are divided into the categories primary and secondary (see Box 26.5).

Box 26.5 – *Causes of electromechanical disassociation*

Primary causes
■ Myocardial infarction (particularly inferior wall)
■ Drugs (beta-blockers or calcium antagonists) or toxins
■ Electrolyte abnormalities (such as hypocalcaemia, hyperkalaemia)
■ Atrial thrombus or tumour (myxoma)

Secondary causes
■ Tension pneumothorax
■ Pericardial tamponade
■ Cardiac rupture
■ Pulmonary embolism
■ Prosthetic heart valve occlusion
■ Hypovolaemia

For the resuscitation attempt to be of any success, the cause must be isolated and the appropriate treatment initiated. Once again, the prognosis remains poor, with less than 10% of long-term attempts succeeding (Peatfield *et al.* 1977).

Drug therapy

Pharmacological intervention may be used during cardiac arrest to (Jowett & Thompson 1995):

■ correct hypoxia and acidosis
■ accelerate or reduce the heart rate
■ suppress ectopic activity
■ stimulate the strength of myocardial contraction.

Adrenaline. Adrenaline is the first drug used in cardiac arrest. Its therapeutic action is to improve coronary and cerebral perfusion. To date, clinical evidence that adrenaline improves survival or neurological recovery in humans is absent (Advanced Life Support Working Group of the European Resuscitation Council 1998). Adrenaline is an alpha- and beta-agonist and acts upon receptor sites to increase circulation to vital sites (Handley 1992). Its action in cardiac arrest is to cause vasoconstriction increasing cerebral and coronary perfusion.

Atropine. Atropine is used to block the action of the vagus nerve, thereby increasing sinoatrial node activity. However, the efficacy of this drug has been questioned, as repeated doses reduce electrical stability of the heart, increasing the risk of VF (Cooper & Abinader 1979). The dose in asystole is 3 mg once only.

Lignocaine. Predominately used as a local anaesthetic, lignocaine possesses class 1B anti-arrhythmic activity thus suppressing ventricular ectopic activity (Chamberlain 1991; Handley 1992).

Calcium salts. In cardiac cell activity, calcium ions play a vital role in contraction, as well as during the cell's action potential. Calcium is usually administered when the patient is hypocalcaemic, hyperkalaemic or suffering from EMD (Handley 1992) and when the patient is known to be taking calcium channel blockers.

Sodium bicarbonate. Controversy continues as to the efficacy of this drug. It is predominately used for the reversal of metabolic acidosis, but recent trials show that it is only effective in severe cases of acidosis when the pH is greater than 7.1 and it is a metabolic acidosis (Advanced Life Support Working Party 1997).

Whether the resuscitation is successful or not, thought and consideration for family or relatives must be a priority. Clear lines of communication must exist between medical and nursing staff and any family/ friends. If the need to break bad news arises, ideally the doctor and the A&E nurse should perform this, with one or the other actually breaking the news. More often than not these simple communication skills are forgotten (see Box 26.6). A detailed discussion of this subject is given in Chapter 13.

> **Box 26.6** – *Communicating with relatives/friends*
>
> ■ Prepare yourself. Compose your thoughts
>
> ■ Enter the room/area with another person, e.g., a doctor or nurse
>
> ■ Confirm that you are talking to the correct relatives/friends
>
> ■ Spend time with the relatives. Avoid appearing harassed or impatient
>
> ■ Maintain eye contact when talking
>
> ■ Be prepared to emphasise and repeat any information
>
> ■ Avoid using the wrong terms, i.e. 'slipped away' or 'passed on'. Be honest, say the person has died
>
> ■ Don't be afraid of silences
>
> ■ Be prepared for wide variety of reactions

Ethical considerations

Occasionally the subject of 'do not resuscitate' orders will present itself. This decision should involve the medical staff, the patient (if possible) and the family and must be clearly documented (Alexander *et al.* 1995). This subject is also addressed in detail in Chapter 38.

Rhythm disturbances

It is important when caring for a patient with a presenting cardiac condition that the recognition of any abnormalities is accurate and prompt. Rhythm disturbances can be divided into two groups: ventricular and atrial arrythmias. Those commonly treated in A&E are discussed below.

Ventricular ectopics (VEs)

This is due to premature discharge of an ectopic ventricular focus (Schamroth 1990) (Fig. 26.16). The impulse avoids travelling through conducting tissue, but travels through ordinary muscle structure. Causes of VEs include:

■ hypoxia
■ myocardial ischaemia
■ hypokalaemia
■ hypercalcaemia
■ acidosis
■ caffeine
■ digoxin toxicity.

Assessment

The aim of assessment is to determine both causative factors and level of systemic compromise. This should include pulse speed, regularity and pressure, respiration and blood pressure. Repeated VEs reduce ventricular filling time and can result in a reduction of circulatory volume. A 12-lead ECG should be obtained to confirm diagnosis. ECG characteristics are shown in Table 26.1.

Management

The patient may present with palpitations or shortness of breath. Immediate treatment of ventricular ectopics can include the use of anti-arrhythmic drugs, such as intravenous lignocaine, bretylium or amiodarone. For

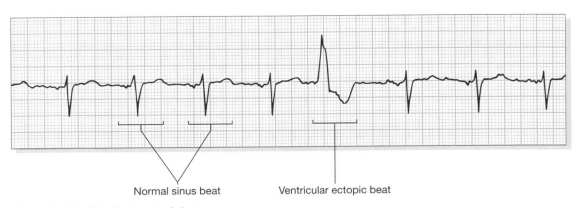

Normal sinus beat   Ventricular ectopic beat

Figure 26.16 – *Ventricular ectopic beat.*

Table 26.1 – *ECG characteristics of ventricular ectopics*

Component	Finding
Rhythm	Irregular, due to premature beats
Rate	60–100 beats/min
P wave	Not related to QRS complex of the VE
QRS	Wide and bizarre complex of a VE

Table 26.2 – *ECG characteristics of ventricular tachycardia*

Component	Finding
Rhythm	Either regular or slightly irregular
Rate	Faster than 100 beats/min
P waves	Dissociated from QRS complexes
QRS	Wide and bizarre

long-term control, oral preparations such as beta-blockers, calcium channel blockers or disopyramide can be used. Correction of the urea and electrolyte imbalance can lead to the resolution of VEs.

Ventricular tachycardia (VT)

Ventricular contraction is stimulated from within as ventricular myocardium and does not follow normal electrical conductivity (see Fig. 26.17). The causes of VT are the same as these of VEs, but it is considered more dangerous due to its capacity to significantly decrease cardiac output. The cardiac output is compromised due to the shortening of the cardiac cycle, and thus there is a reduced amount of blood available for ejection (Woods *et al.* 1995). The ventricular myocardium is not able to sustain rapid contraction over prolonged periods of time and there is therefore a tendency for VF to follow untreated VT.

Assessment

This is the same as assessing a patient with multiple VEs. The important factor is determining the degree of systemic compromise through levels of consciousness, pulse, respirations and blood pressure. ECG characteristics are shown Table 26.2.

Management

Presenting symptoms may include shortness of breath, palpitations, dizziness and diaphoresis. Treatment may incorporate the use of lignocaine, bretylium or magnesium sulphate. If initial drug therapy is not successful and the patient is showing signs of cardiovascular compromise, cardioversion with synchronised DC shock should be carried out. The patient should be sedated for this procedure, unless his clinical condition is deteriorating too rapidly to facilitate this. If VT becomes pulseless at any time, emergency defibrillation should be carried out, and the algorithm in Figure 26.14 followed.

Supraventricular tachycardia (SVT)

This does not always stem from atrial activity, but it does originate from above the ventricles and is difficult to pinpoint the exact causative factor from the ECG (Fig. 26.18). The atria can depolarise in a retrograde fashion or a circular fashion depending on the causative factors.

Causes include:

- atrial tachycardia
- atrial flutter/fibrillation
- stimulants, e.g. caffeine or nicotine
- idiopathic.

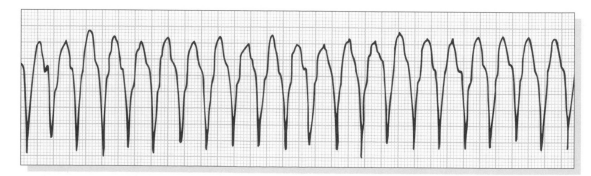

Figure 26.17 – *Ventricular tachycardia.*

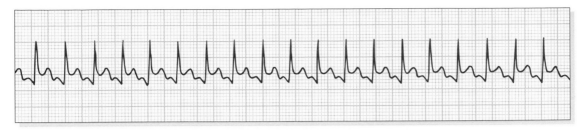

Figure 26.18 – *Supraventricular tachycardia.*

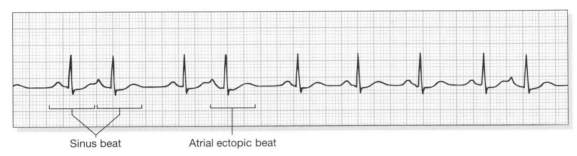

Sinus beat   Atrial ectopic beat

Figure 26.19 – *Atrial ectopic beats.*

Assessment

This should concentrate on determining the patient's capacity to compensate for the rapid heart rate. Pulse, respirations and blood pressure are vital indicators. The patient will probably be aware of palpitations or 'pounding' in his chest and may complain of pain, dizziness and shortness of breath. The ECG characteristics are shown in Table 26.3.

Management

Depending on the patient's tolerance of the SVT, vagal stimulation can be attempted to slow down the heart rate. This can be achieved by carotid sinus massage and is sometimes sufficient to control SVT, but over-zealous treatment can result in profound bradycardia or VF (Skinner & Vincent 1997). Drug therapy of choice is adenosine given intravenously in incremental doses of 3 mg, 6 mg and 12 mg every 1–2 minutes.

Table 26.3 – *ECG characteristics of supraventricular tachycardia*

Component	Finding
Rhythm	Regular
Rate	>100 and up to 280 beats/min
P wave	Not usually visible
QRS	Usually narrow

Adenosine works by depressing AV node conduction and therefore prevents re-entry rhythms from sustaining SVT, allowing sinus rhythm to return. Side-effects of adenosine are common, and the nurse should expect the patient to be flushed, nauseous and have some chest discomfort. These effects are short-lived and should have passed in a matter of minutes (Opie 1995). If the patient's condition continues to deteriorate, a synchronised DC shock is indicated.

Atrial ectopics

This is a premature discharge of an ectopic atrial focus from a point other than the sinoatrial node (Julian 1988) (Fig. 26.19). Causes include:

- alcohol
- mitral valve disease
- coronary artery disease
- hyperthyroidism
- heart failure
- viral infections.

It can also occur in healthy individuals.

Assessment

Diagnosis is made on ECG tracing as the patient is usually unaware of the occurrence of atrial ectopics. Pulse rate should be checked for irregularity and respiration may be slightly increased. ECG findings are shown in Table 26.4.

Table 26.4 – *ECG characteristics of atrial ectopic beats*

Component	Finding
Rhythm	Slightly irregular
Rate	Usually within normal limits
P wave	Precede every QRS
QRS	Normally no change is seen

Table 26.5 – *ECG characteristics of atrial fibrillation*

Component	Finding
Rhythm	Irregular
Rate	Variable, but usually >100 beats/min
P waves	Not present
QRS	Normal

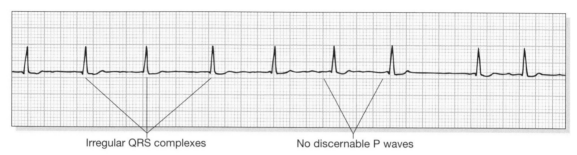

Irregular QRS complexes   No discernable P waves

Figure 26.20 – *Atrial fibrillation.*

Management

The patient is usually unaware, but can present with shortness of breath. The treatment of atrial ectopics is not usually required unless the patient shows signs of compromisation. Drugs used include disopyramide.

Atrial fibrillation

Atrial fibrillation (AF) is a rapid and disorganised depolarisation of the atria (Jacobson 1995). Much of the electrical activity is filtered by the AV node, so the ventricular rate is not necessarily increased (Fig. 26.20). Causes include:

- rheumatic heart disease
- heart failure
- myocardial infarction
- congenital heart disease
- mitral valve disease.

Assessment

This should detect any systemic compromise resulting from AF. Respirations, pulse and blood pressure should be ascertained. The patient may complain of weakness, dizziness or shortness of breath. ECG changes are listed in Table 26.5.

Management

The treatment of AF is usually to eliminate the cause.

Common drugs used include digoxin, verapamil, diltiazem and beta-blockers. If the patient is severely compromised, cardioversion may be necessary. Other symptoms can include an increased risk of thrombus formation, and hence the need for anticoagulants.

Atrial flutter

Atrial flutter occurs when there is rapid atrial excitement (Lange 1994, O'Connor 1995). The term flutter is used as the P waves appear 'saw-toothed' (O'Connor 1995) (Fig. 26.21). The atrial rate can be anything between 250 and 350 beats/min, but the ventricular rate is much lower because of AV filter. The causes include:

- heart failure
- valvular disease
- acute MI
- hypertension.

Assessment

Assessment is the same as for AF (see Table 26.6).

Management

Treatment comprises digoxin or verapamil, or in severe cases cardioversion may be required. Other drugs which may aid treatment include amiodorone, beta-blockers or disopyramide.

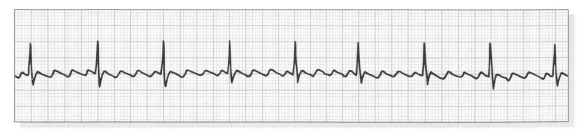

Figure 26.21 – *Atrial flutter.*

Table 26.6 – *ECG characteristics of atrial flutter*

Component	Finding
Rhythm	Usually regular
Rate	Variable, but usually >100 beats/min
P waves	Usually obscured by flutter waves
QRS	Normal, may be widened by bundle branch block

Table 26.7 – *ECG characteristics of first degree heart block*

Component	Finding
Rhythm	Regular
Rate	Sinus, between 60 and 100 beats/min
P wave	Normal
P–R interval	Prolonged, i.e. >0.20 s
QRS	Normal

Heart Block

Heart block occurs when the impulses from the atria to the ventricles are delayed at the AV node (Hampton 1992). There are, for the purpose of this chapter, three types of heart block:

- first degree heart block
- second degree heart block
- third degree (complete) heart block.

These can be a complication of a myocardial infarction.

First degree heart block (Fig. 26.22)

As can be seen from the rhythm strip, the P–R interval is prolonged. This is due to the delay at the AV node, where impulses conduct to the ventricles but with delayed conduction times (Jacobson 1995, Jowett &

Thompson 1995). The ECG characteristics are given in Table 26.7.

Management

In most instances the patient remains asymptomatic and does not require any further treatment, but for the reasons of safety should be re-evaluated at regular intervals.

Second degree heart block (Fig. 26.23)

There are two types of second degree block: type I (Wenckebach) and type II (see Table 26.8 for ECG characteristics). In type I, second degree AV block a gradual lengthening of the P–R interval occurs because of lengthening AV conduction time, until an atrial pulse is non-conducted, so a P wave is not followed by a QRS. Then the sequence begins again. The blocked P wave may occur occasionally or

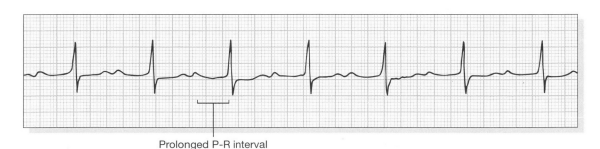

Prolonged P-R interval

Figure 26.22 – *First degree heart block.*

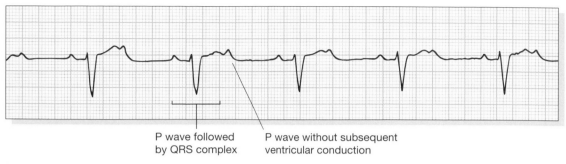

P wave followed
by QRS complex

P wave without subsequent
ventricular conduction

Figure 26.23 – *Second degree heart block A: Wenckebach type. B: Mobitz type II.*

frequently, regularly or irregularly. Of the second degree heart blocks, type I is the most common, is usually transitory and rarely progresses to complete heart block. It produces little or no clinical symptoms. In type II second degree AV heart block, a P wave is blocked without progressive antecedent P–R elongation and occurs almost always in a setting of bundle branch block. Type II second degree block frequently progresses to complete heart block. Clinical symptoms such as dizziness or faintness may occur with frequent non-conducted P waves (Erickson 1991, Wyatt *et al.* 1999).

Management

Depending on the patient's tolerance to the rhythm, there may or may not be a need for treatment. If the patient is compromised, atropine is the first-time drug for bradycardias. Then consider isoprenaline and seek expert help. The patient may need temporary pacing.

Third degree (complete) heart block (Fig. 26.24)

This type of heart block is characterised by the unrelated impulses sent between the atria and the ventricles. When this occurs there is no correlation of the electrical activity and a disassociation develops

between the atria and ventricles. This in turn means that the cardiac output is reduced to the point where the patient usually becomes symptomatic.

Assessment

The patient will often present with current bradycardia of 30–40 bpm, as only ventricular contraction rate will be felt by pulse. It is important to assess the level of circulatory compromise as a treatment guideline. Some patients will present profoundly, with a history of collapse. This is due to severe circulatory collapse as a result of poor cardiac output due to decreased atrial and ventricular synchronicity. The ECG characteristics are given in Table 26.9.

Management

Treatment ultimately depends on the symptoms encountered. Drug therapy includes atropine and isoprenaline, but in most instances requires the insertion of either a temporary or a permanent pacing system to maintain the patient's cardiac equilibrium. In cases of profound collapse, external pacing is necessary to maintain circulatory volume.

Table 26.8 – *ECG characteristics of second degree heart block*

Component	Finding
Rhythm	Regular
Rate	Sinus or atrial beats
P waves	Normal
P–R Interval	Can lengthen or can be normal
QRS	Normal

Table 26.9 – *ECG characteristics of third degree heart block*

Component	Finding
Rhythm	Regular
Rate	Normal atrial rate, but the ventricular rate can be less than 45 beats/min
P wave	Normal, but shows no relation to the QRS complexes
P–R interval	No consistent P–R interval exists
QRS	Normal, although sometimes wide

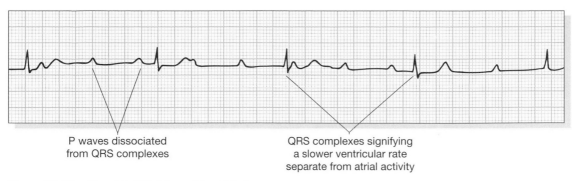

P waves dissociated
from QRS complexes

QRS complexes signifying
a slower ventricular rate
separate from atrial activity

Figure 26.24 – *Complete (third degree) heart block.*

Pacing

It is sometimes necessary to support a patient's conductive system by means of a pacing system. The purpose of pacemakers is to control the electrical activity of the heart (Julian 1988). Both temporary and permanent pacing systems contain two components:

■ pulse generator (pacing box) – this forms the electrical supply source for pacing; the box usually contains batteries as its power source
■ pacing catheter – this conductive wire has either one or two electrodes to provide an electrical stimulus to the heart, once the pacing catheter electrodes are in direct contact with the myocardium.

There are currently three types of pacemaker available:

• non-invasive temporary pacing
• temporary (transvenous) pacing
• permanent pacing.

Non-invasive temporary pacing (NTP)

This system of pacing is used predominately by A&E departments to treat symptomatic bradycardias and ventricular asystole. Most A&E departments in the UK have access to a defibrillator with pacing facilities, e.g. the Physio Control Lifepak 9P. The advantages of NTP include its ability to be initiated rapidly, its ease of use and the fact that CPR can be continued without risk to the user (Beeler 1993). To use NTP, two large electrodes are placed on the chest as shown in Figure 26.25.

Once NTP has been commenced it is important to look for signs of electrical and mechanical capture. When looking for signs of electrical capture, a heart trace can provide the evidence required. A pacing spike should be followed by a wide QRS and a tall broad T wave (Fig. 26.26). Mechanical capture is seen by the improvements in the patient's condition. Compared with other forms of pacing, NTP is, on the surface, a more favourable approach to emergency pacing.

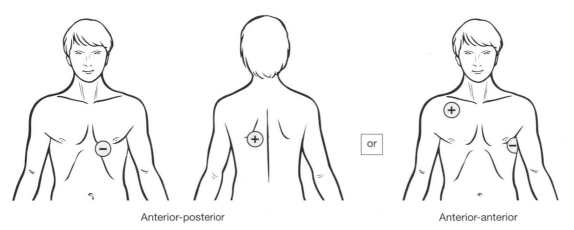

Anterior-posterior

or

Anterior-anterior

Figure 26.25 – *Positioning of pacing pads for non-invasive temporary pacing.*

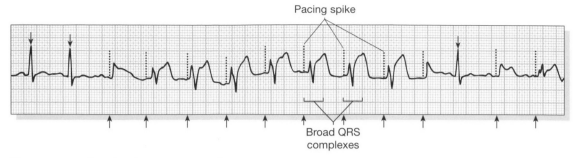

Figure 26.26 – *Non-invasive temporary pacing.*

Temporary pacing (transvenous)

The indications for the insertion of a temporary transvenous pacing wire include (Timmis & Nathan 1993):

- extreme bradycardia
- complete heart block
- asystole
- very occasionally for tachycardias.

A bipolar pacing catheter is inserted through a central or peripheral vein (subclavian, external jugular or antecubital fossa) under sterile conditions, using ECG monitoring and fluoroscopy equipment. A local anaesthetic is used prior to insertion. Once the pacing catheter has been sited, the electrodes are then connected to the external pulse generator (pacing box). Complications include:

- pneumothorax
- infection
- cardiac perforation
- arrhythmias.

Permanent pacing

The decision to use an implantable pacing system remains dependent on the patient's symptoms. Symptomatic patients are fitted with a permanent pacemaker by inserting the power source (lithium-driven) with a subcutaneous pocket under the clavicle or axilla. The procedure is performed under a local anaesthetic. The majority of permanent pacemakers fitted today have an approximate life span of 15 years.

Acute Chest Pain

Angina (angina pectoris)

Angina is a symptom, not a disease, brought on by inadequate coronary blood flow to the myocardium (Jowett & Thompson 1995, Woods *et al.* 1995). Pain is usually caused by a lack of oxygen reaching myocardial cells. It usually presents as central chest pain with either a rapid or gradual onset, with possible radiation to the jaw, back and arms. It can occur at rest or on exertion. It rarely has a duration of more than 30 minutes (Smith 1988). Other associated symptoms include indigestion, dizziness, belching and epigastric discomfort after eating.

Assessment

When a patient presents to the A&E department with chest pain secondary to angina it is usually because previous attempts to relieve the pain have failed. When assessing the patient it is important to gain a detailed history. This should include the type and duration of the pain, what the patient was doing when the pain started, and whether anything has been taken to relieve it. Any radiation of pain should be noted because it helps to confirm a clinical picture of cardiac pain. Any symptoms associated with the onset of pain or still present are also important as they act as an indication of the level of systemic compromise resulting from myocardial hypoxia. The patient's medical and drug history should also be noted.

Physical assessment should include baseline observations of pulse rate, regularity and pressure, respirations and blood pressure. These should enable the A&E nurse to determine the impact of the angina on the patient's overall condition. Temperature should also be checked as a rise in temperature can be indicative of tissue breakdown, consistent with a myocardial infarction. Cardiac monitoring and a 12-lead ECG recording complete the clinical picture. The ECG will show any associated rhythm disturbance and most importantly any ischaemic changes to the myocardium as a result of hypoxia. ECG changes show as ST-segment depression in the area affected by hypoxia (see Fig. 26.27).

Clinical investigations include blood analysis to detect electrolyte imbalance, or cardiac enzymes

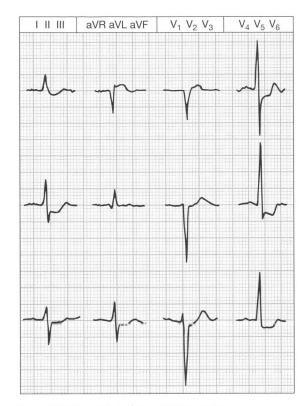

| I II III | aVR aVL aVF | V₁ V₂ V₃ | V₄ V₅ V₆ |

Figure 26.27 – *Inferior/lateral ST depression.*

consistent with myocardial infarction. Blood should be taken for full blood count, urea and electrolyte levels, glucose (which can rise after acute infection) and cardiac enzymes. A chest X-ray is useful to detect any cardiac failure or enlargement. Isoenzymes may also be useful if other trauma, such as cardiac massage, has taken place.

Management

It is useful to obtain i.v. access early in the patient's management in order to administer pain relief or supportive drugs if necessary. The aim is to restore a normal blood flow through the coronary arteries, so that myocardial oxygen supply and demand are met. It is important that oxygen therapy is commenced at the earliest opportunity. This both acts as a pain-relieving agent and reduces the likelihood of tissue damage. It is necessary to reduce the workload of the heart, which relieves the symptoms experienced by the patient.

Sublingual glyceryl trinitrate (GTN) is an effective first-line treatment. It works by causing venous and coronary artery dilatation. This in turn causes a reduction in preload and consequently a reduction in afterload (Khan 1988), therefore allowing blood to flow

with less effort from the myocardium, increasing the amount of oxygen to the heart and subsequently decreasing chest pain. If sublingual GTN is not effective, opiate pain relief should be given intravenously until pain relief is established. GTN substances should also be given as an i.v. infusion titrated to the patient's pain blood pressure, to ensure that vasodilation is not excessive.

Other drugs that can be used include:

- beta-blockers
- aspirin
- calcium antagonists.

Other aspects in the management of angina include a reduction in activity and adjustments in lifestyle, if risks to the patient's health have been noted. If symptoms do not settle with GTN, or if ECG changes persist after pain subsides, the patient should be admitted for observation and specialist management. If angina is considered unstable, intractable or crescendo in nature, the patient should be admitted (see Table 26.10).

Myocardial infarction

Myocardial infarction (MI) is defined as the death or

Table 26.10 – *Classification of angina*

Classification	Characteristics
Stable angina	Condition in which the frequency and severity of angina remain well controlled and unchanged over months
Angina decubitus	Pain occurring when lying down
Unstable angina	Condition in which the pain is increasing in frequency, severity and duration. Occurs with less activity or at rest
Printzmetal's angina	Unusual form where pain occurs at rest or long after activity has ceased. Accompanied by transient ST-segment elevation. Coronary artery spasm without underlying disease is often the cause
Crescendo angina	Form of angina where chance of an MI occurring within a few days is high
Intractable angina	Continued pain with increasing frequency, despite treatment

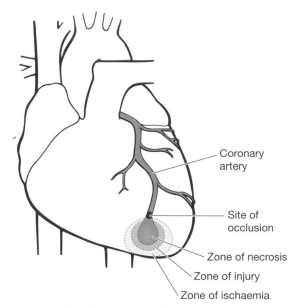

Figure 26.28 – *Post-myocardial infarction damage.*

necrosis of part of the myocardium due to the reduction or cessation of blood flow (Alexander *et al.* 1995, Hendrick 1994). The treatment of acute MI remains a major medical challenge, with over 250 000 patients presenting annually in the UK (Hillis 1998). Acute infarction is caused by the rupture of atheromatous deposits within the artery and the subsequent formation of a clot (thrombus), which in turn occludes the artery, denying blood (and thus oxygen and nutrients) to the myocardium (Quinn 1996). The site of the infarction is dependent upon which coronary artery has become occluded and where in that artery the blockage has occurred.

There are three stages in the classification of tissue damage (Quinn 1996) (Fig. 26.28):

■ Ischaemia – tissue damaged caused by a lack of oxygen. Early oxygenation can salvage the damage.
■ Injury – greater degree of damage, but still salvageable.
■ Infarction – necrosed or dead tissue.

The crucial aspect in the management of MIs is rapid commencement of treatment as soon as possible after the onset of symptoms. Mortality from MIs is approximately 17%, with 60% of these deaths occurring within the first hour (Office of Population Census and Surveys 1990). In A&E, rapid treatment relies on accurate and thorough assessment by A&E nurses.

Assessment

Assessment of patients having an MI should follow the same structure as a patient with angina. In addition, the patient is likely to appear:

■ pale
■ sweating or clammy
■ short of breath
■ possibly cyanositic
■ nauseous and vomiting
■ anxious.

The 12-lead ECG is an important tool in the diagnosis of an MI, but should be taken in context with the overall clinical picture. The ECG usually demonstrates specific changes in the areas of myocardial damage. These are linked to the time span of injury and duration of pain. During the first hour of pain there is little change to the ECG, however, T waves may flatten. After this, the ST segment may elevate and during the next 12–24 hours Q waves begin to develop as myocardium becomes necrotic and electrical conduction ceases. T waves become inverted because repolarisation changes. In some instances, the ECG trace will remain with Q waves and inverted T waves in damaged areas. In other instances, T waves will turn upright after a period of time (see Fig. 26.29).

In addition to the progress of the MI, the ECG will also depict the areas of the myocardium affected by the infarct (see Box 26.3, p. 346).

Blood pressure. In the majority of cases the blood pressure appears low. This is due to poor ventricular function and a reduced cardiac output. The frequency of BP recordings should be of an optimum level to detect any further changes in the patient's condition.

Pulse. Predominately the patient will be tachycardic as a response to the decreased cardiac output, but the anxiety levels should also be taken into account as these can also induce a tachycardia due to the sympathetic response. Specific side-effects of infarction should also be considered. Bradycardia is frequently associated with inferior infarction.

Respiration. Tachypnoea or dyspnoea will usually be evident. These can indicate levels of hypoxia and the onset of pulmonary oedema. Oxygen therapy is vital in MIs to ensure the myocardium is receiving as much oxygen as possible.

Temperature is sometimes forgotten, but in the instance of an MI, a mild pyrexia can be indicative of muscle damage due to an inflammatory response (Woods *et al.* 1995)

Blood analysis. Similar to chest pain from angina, blood analysis should include *cardiac enzymes.* Following an MI there is a rise in the levels of myocardial enzymes present. It is these enzymes that aid in the diagnosis of an MI (Jowett & Thompson 1995) and they include (see also Table 26.11):

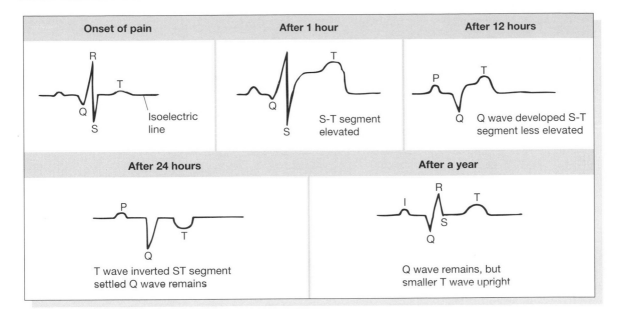

Figure 26.29 – *ECG changes following myocardial infarction.*

- creatinine kinase (CK)
- lactic dehydrogenase (LDH)
- aspartate aminotransferase (AST).

Changes to other levels are as follows:

- *Full blood count.* A rise in both the white blood count and ESR is indicative of muscle necrosis.
- *Urea and electrolytes.* Sodium and potassium ions are important in cardiac function due to their involvement within the action potential. This analysis is also important as it helps to determine if there is any renal function impairment present.
- *Glucose.* As previously stated, a rise in the blood glucose can be indicative of stress-related hyperglycaemia. However, 5% of cardiac patients admitted to hospital have previously undiagnosed diabetes (Alexander *et al.* 1995).
- *Lipids.* Raised cholesterol and triglycerides are common in ischaemic heart disease.

Chest X-ray may show fluid levels associated with oedema or an enlarged heart.

Management

The aim of care is to (Alexander *et al.* 1995):

- limit the infarction size
- re-establish an optimal cardiac output
- relieve pain
- detect and prevent any life-threatening complications.

Oxygen therapy should be commenced as early as possible in an attempt to limit myocardial damage and relieve pain. Pain control in patients with an MI should be achieved by using i.v. opiates, such as diamorphine or cyclomorph. These provide pain relief but also have a mild diuretic effect, hence enabling a better ventricular function (Opie 1994). An anti-emetic, such as cyclizine or metoclopramide, is also indicated as it

Table 26.11 – *Cardiac enzyme changes following a myocardial infarction*

Enzyme	Released into circulation		Range (normal)
	Initially	Peaks	
Creatinine phosphokinase (CPK)	6 h	18–36 h	200–1000 u/ml (100 u/ml)
Serum aspartate transferase (formerly glutamic oxalo-acetic transaminase, SGOT)	12–24 h	36–48 h	>100 u/ml (50 u/ml)
Lactic dehydrogenase (LDH)	2–3 days	7 days	

reduces any previous nausea and counteracts the nauseated feelings associated with opiates.

Thrombolytic therapy

Thrombolytic therapy is vital if the integrity of the myocardium is to be preserved. Rapid administration of thrombolytic therapy reverses the effects of ischaemia and injury before necrosis can occur, therefore dramatically changing the outcome for the patient (Quinn & Thompson 1995). For this to be most effective, the Department of Health (1992) recommends drug therapy within 30 minutes of the patient arriving at hospital. This has implications both for patients treated in A&E and for those 'fast-tracked' to coronary care areas. It is essential that pre-determined protocols exist for the treatment of these patients and that criteria are set down to facilitate the administration of thrombolytic drugs at an early stage (see Fig. 26.30).

Thrombolytic therapy dissolves the thrombus/clot occluding a coronary artery and restores blood flow to the myocardium, therefore limiting damage. Therapy is administered via an intravenous route, usually prepared as an infusion, although some thrombolytes, e.g. anistrephase, are given as a bolus administration.

The thrombolytic drug used most commonly is strepokinase, which is a bacterial protein that reduces circulatory fibrinogen and clotting factors V and VIII (Alexander *et al.* 1996). Recombinant tissue-type plasminogen activator (tPA) is fibrin-specific and works mainly on the clot, therefore reducing the risk

of systemic effects. It is, however, very expensive and therefore is normally used only if streptokinase is unsuitable (see Box 26.7). Anistreplase (ASPAC) is similar to tPA, but can be given as a bolus over a few minutes. Unfortunately, like tPA, its cost prohibits its general use.

During therapy, the A&E nurse should be vigilant for signs of reperfusion (see Box 26.8) and complications. Blood pressure and ECG monitoring should be frequent, and the patient should not be left unattended. Complications include reperfusion arrythmias, including VF, allergic reactions and hypotension. The patient may feel flushed, generally unwell and have a headache. Bleeding episodes can also occur.

Other drugs of benefit include aspirin, which inhibits platelet aggregation and reduces blood viscosity, therefore reducing the risks of further

---

Box 26.7 – *Contraindications of streptokinase thrombolytic therapy*

- Known/suspected aortic aneurysm
- Severe hypertension
- Active bleeding
- CVA in the last 12 months
- Major surgery in the last 6 months
- Recent laser treatment for diabetic retinopathy
- *Allergy to streptokinase
- *Prior administration of streptokinase within the last 12 months
- *Severe hypotension not responsive to fluid/drug therapy

*Seek senior medical opinion as anistreplase may be used.

Box 26.8 – *Signs of reperfusion*

- Abrupt end to chest pain
- ECG change to ST segment – ST elevation rapidly returns to normal and Q waves do not develop
- Improved left ventricular function
- Early peak in cardiac enzyme excretion because of renewed blood flow
- Reperfusion arrythmias or conduction defects

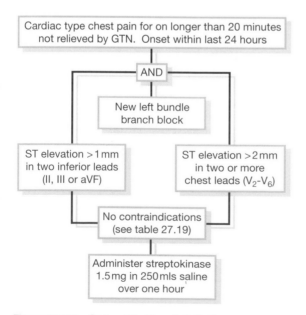

Figure 26.30 – *Protocol for thrombolytic therapy.*

thrombus activity. For the appropriate management of patients suffering from an MI, A&E staff must be aware of current trends and treatments in cardiac care in order to understand more fully, and care more competently, for this group of patients (Hendrick 1994). For optimal care, patients with an acute MI should be 'fast-tracked' to coronary care units at the earliest opportunity.

Acute Cardiac Failure

In 1995 the New York Heart Association renamed and reclassified all types of heart failure under the heading of 'heart failure'. There are now four classifications of heart failure, but for the purposes of this chapter the term is used to depict the clinical manifestations that relate to this condition. Heart failure is characterised as the heart's inability to provide an adequate cardiac output for the body's metabolic requirements (Alexander *et al.* 1995).

Acute left ventricular failure (LVF)

Left ventricular failure often presents suddenly and is usually associated with pulmonary oedema. LVF is also a frequent complication of MI. Common causes include:

- myocardial infarction
- coronary artery disease
- diabetes
- hypertension
- cardiomyopathy
- valvular disease
- arrhythmias.

The mechanics of LVF mean that the heart is regarded as a failing pump, with more blood remaining in the ventricle at the end of each cardiac cycle (Tortora & Grabowski 1996). Often, this build-up of pressure results in blood being forced to seep back into the lungs, causing an increase in pressure and resulting in pulmonary oedema. In response to the pump mechanism failing, blood can also back up from the right ventricle into the systemic circulation, causing peripheral oedema due to the increase in capillary pressure causing fluid to seep into the tissues. This is most noticeable in the ankles and feet.

Assessment

Typically, LVF and pulmonary oedema occur in the night or early hours of the morning due to an increase in venous return when lying down (O'Connor 1995). The usual presentation in A&E includes:

- cold/clammy appearance
- severe dyspnoea
- cyanotic appearance
- tachycardia
- raised jugular venous pressure (JVP).

The assessment findings are summarised in Box 26.9.

Box 26.9 – *Assessment findings in left ventricular failure*

- **Respirations.** Airway is of paramount importance, as the presence of pulmonary oedema exacerbates any shortness of breath and causes hypoxia. Depending on the severity of the hypoxia, airway adjuncts such as oropharyngeal or nasopharyngeal airways may be required. Extreme cases may require intubation and ventilation.

- **Pulse.** Tachycardias are prominent in LVF with the heart beating faster in an attempt to compensate for the reduced cardiac output

- **Blood pressure.** Hypotension is usually present due to the failure of the pumping mechanism and hence a reduced cardiac output

- **Temperature.** Possible occurrence of pyrexias

- **Urine output.** With the use of diuretics, it is vital to keep an accurate hourly record of the output to monitor the effectiveness of the diuretics

- **Cardiac monitoring.** This should be maintained throughout the stay in the A&E department and on transfer. Rhythm changes, such as increasing ventricular ectopics, or left bundle branch block should be considered. Profuse sweating may make electrode placement difficult to achieve

- **Central venous pressure monitoring.** This measurement is important in monitoring and maintaining the haemodynamic status of the patient

---

Immediate priorities for care

- Airway assessment
- Oxygen therapy
- Baseline observations
- Cardiac monitoring
- Intravenous or central line access
- Catheterisation for urine output measurement.

Clinical investigations should include:

- *Blood chemistry analysis* – both to monitor renal function and to maintain adequate potassium levels if loop diuretics, such as frusemide, are being administered

- *Cardiac enzymes* – especially for CK, to check for muscular damage
- *Full blood count* – a low haemoglobin would show any evidence of anaemia
- *Arterial blood gases* – monitor frequently to assess respiratory function
- *Chest X-ray* – useful in determining the degree of pulmonary oedema and any evidence of heart enlargement.

Management

The aims of first-line management are:

- to relieve symptoms
- to treat the underlying cause.

Oxygen therapy is vital to counteract the effects of hypoxia. Positioning is also important in LVF, as sitting patients in an upright position reduces venous return. LVF is highly treatable and good nursing and medical care should provide symptomatic relief very quickly for the patient. Symptomatic relief comes in the form of i.v. diuretics, namely frusemide, due to its rapid onset of action. This type of diuretic is a potent 'loop diuretic' causing almost immediate diuresis. In severe cases, inotropic drugs may be required, such as dobutamine, dopamine or adrenaline to increase the contractility of the myocardium and thus to assist the left ventricular function. Other drugs of note include vasodilation agents such as ACE inhibitors (captopril, enalapril), nitrates (isosorbide mononitrate) and calcium channel blockers (diltiazem). These reduce preload and thus enable an increase in the cardiac output.

Cardiogenic shock

Shock is defined as impaired organ perfusion, which if left uncorrected will lead to irreversible cell damage and multiple organ failure and death (Timmis & Nathan 1993). In the case of cardiogenic shock, the degree of heart failure is so severe that the extreme reduction in cardiac output leads to inadequate organ perfusion. The reason behind this is that the heart is failing to pump effectively due to myocardial damage. Cardiogenic shock requires urgent intervention. The most common cause is MI, and 15% of patients admitted to hospital with an acute MI will die from cardiogenic shock (O'Connor 1995). Other causes include:

- cardiomyopathy
- cardiac tamponade
- arrhythmias
- valvular disease.

Assessment

Patients presenting with cardiogenic shock require urgent attention as they are acutely ill. The patient will appear clinically shocked and hence consideration must be given to the following symptoms:

- acute dyspnoea
- profound hypotension
- pale/cyanotic
- cold/clammy
- arrhythmias.

The assessment findings are summarised in Box 26.10.

Box 26.10 – *Assessment findings in cardiogenic shock*

- **Blood pressure.** Severe hypotension, due to a radically reduced cardiac output

- **Pulse.** Tachycardia; the heart rate increases to compensate for the reduced cardiac output, but in profound stages the rate may become weaker and arrhythmias may occur

- **Respirations.** Oxygen therapy is vital if hypoxia is to be restricted. An upright posture will help to reduce venous return. Again, in extreme cases intubation and ventilation may be required. Arterial blood gases must be performed on a regular basis to monitor levels of hypoxaemia and any rise in the carbon dioxide levels.

Priorities for care

Ideally the patients should be cared for in the resuscitation environment with:

- cardiac monitoring
- i.v. access and CVP access
- oxygen therapy
- baseline observations
- catheterisation.

Clinical investigations include:

- *Renal care* – urine measurement is vital to measure the effectiveness of drug therapy and U&Es to monitor potassium levels
- *Blood analysis* – for routine FBC and cardiac enzymes
- *ECG* – may show multifocal ventricular ectopics indicative of an irritable ventricle, or ischaemic changes suggestive of an acute MI
- *Chest X-ray* – evidence of pulmonary oedema and cardiac enlargement may be present.

Management

Close, frequent observations and cardiac monitoring are vital if life-threatening abnormalities are to be detected. Adequate i.v. access is essential if the haemodynamic status of the patient is to be stabilised. Aggressive i.v. diuretic therapy (usually frusemide) should be administered to this end and its effectiveness monitored. Volume replacement is sometimes necessary, but should be titrated to CVP and pump functioning. Vasodilators (i.v. nitrates) and inotropic agents (dobutamine, dopamine or adrenaline) may be used to support the cardiovascular system. On occasions an intra-aortic balloon pump may be required to support the left ventricle. Thought and consideration must be given to the family and/or friends as this is undoubtedly a very stressful experience for them.

Viral/inflammatory Conditions

Pericarditis

Acute pericarditis is defined as an acute inflammation of the pericardium (O'Connor 1995). The presence of a respiratory tract infection may indicate a viral infection. Causes of pericarditis include:

- idiopathic (non-specific)
- bacterial infection
- viral infection
- connective tissue disease, e.g. systemic lupus erythematosus (SLE), arthritis
- following an acute MI
- renal failure
- neoplasm, e.g. breast, lung, etc.
- radiation.

Assessment

The patient with pericarditis presents in A&E with sharp, retrosternal chest pain worsening on deep inspiration, coughing or movement. Other symptoms include (Shabetai 1990):

- dyspnoea
- fever
- production of sputum
- weight loss.

On auscultation of the chest, the sound of a friction rub confirms the diagnosis of pericarditis.

Immediate priorities for care

- Baseline observations

- Cardiac monitor
- Intravenous access
- Oxygen therapy.

Specific investigations should include:

- *ECG* – the classical sign seen on the ECG is the presence of widespread concave ST elevation, often referred to as saddleback
- *Blood analysis* – U&Es due to the possibility of uraemically induced pericarditis as a result of decreased renal function
- *FBC* – a raised white cell count would be indicative of bacterial infections
- *Blood culture* – to investigate for infections
- *Chest X-ray* – this is usually normal, unless the presence of a pericardial effusion shows cardiac enlargement.

Management

The immediate management is pain relief. In the initial stages the use of opiates may be required, e.g. diamorphine, or if the pain is less acute, NSAIDs such as voltarol are given.

To correct the underlying causes of pericarditis, NSAIDs are the drugs of choice. With viral pericarditis no further treatment is required. For bacterial pericarditis, antibiotic therapy should be initiated. If pericarditis is left uncorrected, it can become potentially life-threatening, leading to pericardial effusion and cardiac tamponade.

Endocarditis

Endocarditis is caused by either bacterial or fungal infiltration of the heart valves or endocardium. It is prevalent in a heart already damaged by congenital or acquired heart abnormalities (Snelson *et al.* 1992). The main characteristic of endocarditis is a vegetative growth on the leaflets of the valves, causing dysfunctional or incompetent valvular action.

Assessment

The symptoms of endocarditis include:

- anaemia
- heart murmur
- fever
- chills.
- rigors
- night sweats
- haematuria

Immediate priorities for care

A major complication of endocarditis is heart failure.

Hence, on presentation in the A&E department, the patient, along with the symptoms listed above, may be acutely short of breath, dyspnoeic and pale. Thus, immediate priorities are:

- oxygen therapy where required
- baseline observations – check temperature for recurrent pyrexias
- i.v. access.

Specific investigations include:

- *ECG* – to detect damage or stress to the heart
- *Blood analysis* – FBC for possible raised white cell count in response to an infection
- *U&E* – imbalance may occur if heart failure is present
- *Blood cultures* – these are performed to enable isolation of the causative pathogen, so that the correct antibiotics are used to target the source of the infection.

Management

This is dependent upon the causative factor for endocarditis; there are three approaches:

- Bacterial endocarditis – suggested antibiotics include benzylpenicillin and gentamicin
- Fungal endocarditis – amphotericin is the drug of choice
- Surgical intervention – to replace the diseased valve.
- Antibiotic prophylaxis is required when undertaking any dental work. This is necessary to reduce the risk of reinfection.

Cardiomyopathy

Recent statistics of patients with heart failure show that it often results from cardiomyopathy and not from coronary artery disease as previously thought (Laurent-Bopp 1995). The definition and diagnosis of cardiomyopathy are ambiguous due to the fact that it is a disease of the heart muscle of an unknown cause (Wold 1983).

There are three classifications of cardiomyopathy:

- dilated
- hypertrophic
- restrictive.

Assessment

The majority of patients in the acute phase will be suffering from heart failure due to their cardiomyopathy. Other symptoms include:

- dyspnoea, because of heart failure
- fatigue, because of hypoxia due to inadequate cardiac output
- chest pain related to a decreased cardiac output (mainly with hypertrophic cardiomyopathy)
- syncope
- anxiety
- depression.

Immediate priorities for care

In the presence of heart failure or an acute episode, the priorities should be:

- cardiac monitoring for ventricular arrythmias, suggestive of a stressed heart
- oxygen therapy
- i.v. access
- baseline observations
- ECG
- routine FBC and U&Es
- chest X-ray – this will show cardiac hypertrophy and may show pulmonary oedema.

During non-acute phases, patients with cardiomyopathy are usually asymptomatic.

Management

The only true treatment to offer a cure is heart transplantation. During the interim period, the use of ACE inhibitors such as captopril may be of benefit. Other drugs used in the treatment of cardiomyopathy include:

- diuretics
- amiodarone to control ventricular arrhythmias
- prophylactic anticoagulants, e.g. warfarin – these are indicated as the risk of thrombus formation and subsequent pulmonary embolus is great.

Conclusion

The diversity of cardiac conditions presenting in A&E is vast. It is therefore essential for A&E nurses to understand the principles of a systematic approach to the elements of cardiac care. This chapter has explored one of the most exciting aspects of A&E nursing by identifying distinct aspects of patient care and subsequent management.

References

Advanced Life Support Working Group of the European Resuscitation Council (1998). Guidelines for adult advanced life support. *British Medical Journal* **316**, 1863–1869.

Advanced Life Support Working Party (1997) Guidelines for life support. *Resuscitation* **34**, 16–21.

Alexander MF, Fawcett JN, Runciman PJ. (1994) *Nursing Practice: Hospital and Home – The Adult*. Edinburgh: Churchill Livingstone.

Barrett J (1983) *Accident and Emergency*. Oxford: Blackwell Scientific.

Beeler L (1993) Non-invasive temporary cardiac pacing in the emergency department: a review and update. *Journal of Emergency Nursing* **19**(3), 202–205.

Chamberlain DA (1991) Lignocaine and bretylium as adjuncts to electrical defibrillation. *Resuscitation* **22**, 153–157.

Colquhoun MC, Handley AJ, Evans TR (1995) *ABC of Resuscitation*. London: BMJ.

Cooper MJ, Abinader EG (1979) Atropine-Induced ventricular fibrillation: case report and review of the literature. *American Heart Journal* **99**, 225–228.

Department of Health (1992) *Health of the Nation: a Strategy for Health in England*. London: HMSO.

Erickson BA (1991) Dysrhythmias. In: Kinney MR, Packa DR, Andreoli KE, Zipes DG, eds. *Comprehensive Cardiac Care*, 7th edn. St Louis: Mosby.

Hampton J. (1992) *The ECG Made Easy*, 4th edn. Edinburgh: Churchill Livingstone.

Handley AJ (ed.) (1992) *Advanced Life Support Manual*. London: Resuscitation Council (UK).

Hendrick JA (1994) The challenge of myocardial infarction in accident and emergency nursing. *Accident and Emergency Nursing* **2**, 160–166.

Hillis WS (1998) Acute treatment of myocardial infarction. In: *Current Issues in Cardiology: Management Strategies*. London: BMJ.

Jacobson C. (1995) Arrythmias and conduction defects In: Woods SL, Froelicher ESS, Halpenny JC, Motzer SU (eds) *Cardiac Nursing*, 3rd edn. Philadelphia: J.B. Lippincott.

Jowett NI, Thompson DR (1995) *Comprehensive Coronary Care*, 2nd edn. London: Scutari.

Julian P (1988) *Cardiology*, 2nd edn. London: Baillière Tindall.

Khan MG (1988) *Manual of Cardiac Drug Therapy*, 2nd edn. London: Ballière Tindall.

Lange C (1994) *A Guide to ECG Patterns* (2nd issue) London: Blue Sensor Medicotest.

Laurent-Bopp D. (1995) Cardiomyopathies and myocarditis In:

Woods SL, Froelicher ESS, Halpenny JC, Motzer SU, eds. *Cardiac Nursing*, 3rd edn. Philadelphia: J.B. Lippincott.

Marieb E (1995) *Human Anatomy and Physiology*, 3rd edn. California: Benjamin Cummings.

O'Connor S (1995) *The Cardiac Patient. Nursing Interventions*. London: Mosby.

Office of Health Economics (1990) *Coronary Heart Disease: The Need for Action*. London: HMSO.

Office of Population Census and Surveys (1990) *OPCS Monitor: DH2/90/2*. London: HMSO.

Opie L (1994) *Drugs and the Heart*, 2nd edn. London: WB Saunders.

Peatfield RC, Sillett RW, Taylor D, McNicol MW (1977) Survival after Cardiac Arrest in Hospital. *Lancet* **i**, 1223–1225.

Robertson C, Steen P, Adgey J *et al.* (1998) The 1998 European Resuscitation Council guidelines for adult advanced life support. *Resuscitation* **37**, 81–90.

Quinn T (1996) Myocardial infarction. *Nursing Times* **92**(5), Knowledge for Practice Professional Development Unit (supplement) 25, 1–4.

Quinn T, Thompson DR (1995) Administration of thrombolytic therapy to patients with acute myocardial infarction. *Accident and Emergency Nursing* **3**, 208–214.

Schamroth L (1990) *An Introduction to Electrocardiography*, 7th edn. Oxford: Blackwell Scientific.

Shabetai R (1990) Acute pericarditis. *Clinical Cardiology* **8**, 639.

Skinner D, Vincent V (1997) *Cardiopulmonary Resuscitation*, 2nd edn. Oxford: Oxford University Press.

Smith CE (1988) Assessing chest pain quickly and accurately. *Nursing* **18**(5), 52–60.

Snelson C, Cline BA, Luby C (1992) Infective endocarditis: a challenging diagnosis. *Dimensions in Critical Care Nursing* **12**(1), 4–16.

Timmis AD, Nathan AW (1993) *Essentials of Cardiology*, 2nd edn. Oxford: Blackwell Scientific.

Tortora GJ, Grabowski S (1996) *Principles of Anatomy and Physiology*, 8th edn. New York: Harper Collins.

Wold B (1983) Dilated (congestive) cardiomyopathy: considerations for the coronary care unit nurse. *Heart and Lung* **12**(5), 544–551.

Woods SL, Sivarajan-Froelicher ES, Halpenny CJ, Underhill-Motzer S (eds) (1995) *Cardiac Nursing*, 3rd edn. Philadelphia: JB Lippincott.

Wyatt JP, Illingworth RN, Clancy MJ, Munro P, Robertson CE (1999) *Oxford Handbook of Accident & Emergency Medicine*. Oxford: Oxford University Press.

Chapter 27

Medical Emergencies

Tim Kilner & Rosie Wilkinson

- Introduction
- Respiration
- Asthma
- Pulmonary chronic obstructive disease
- Pulmonary oedema
- Pulmonary embolism
- Anaphylaxis
- Near drowning
- Carbon monoxide poisoning
- Renal disorders
- Urinary tract disease
- Dehydration – fluid volume deficit
- Thermoregulation
- Nervous system
- Glucose regulation
- Haematology
- Conclusion

Introduction

A substantial proportion of the A&E nurse's workload involves dealing with patients who present with medical emergencies. Medical emergencies are many and varied, and it is beyond the scope of this chapter to consider them all. The main conditions are identified and the assessment and management detailed. It is, however, possible to provide initial management of any life-threatening medical emergency by making an assessment of, and interventions to support, the airway, breathing and circulation. Provided these are intact, baseline observations of pulse, respiration and blood pressure should be established. When coupled with effective communication, these 'routine' actions form the beginnings of a therapeutic relationship and ease the distress and suffering of patients and their relatives.

Respiration

Respiration is a process which is fundamental to life itself. In the absence of external respiration, oxygen is not absorbed into the circulation and carbon dioxide is not removed from it. The existence of such factors are clearly incompatible with life and are of an importance few would fail to acknowledge. The process of respiration is considerably more complex than external respiration alone (see Fig. 27.1). Respiration also takes place at a cellular level, known as internal respiration, where oxygen plays a fundamental part in cell energy production, or metabolism, with one of the by-products of this process being carbon dioxide. Internal and external respiration cannot sustain life without the existence of an adequate transport system which enables the oxygen absorbed by external respiration to be delivered to the cells to support internal respiration, and the removal of carbon dioxide produced by internal respiration to the lungs for excretion by means of external respiration.

It is essential that assessment of the respiratory system takes into account *all* of these processes, as

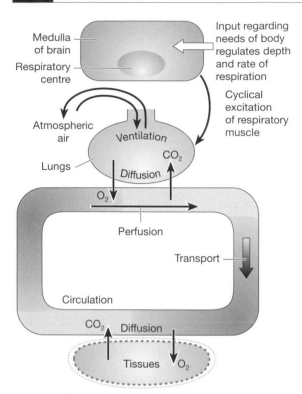

Figure 27.1 – *Process involved in respiration. (After Hinchliff, et al, 1996).*

the presence of one process does not ensure that other processes are functioning. It is equally important that an assessment evaluates the adequacy of these processes and not just their presence or absence.

The mechanics of respiration

Inspiration occurs when intrathoracic pressure falls below atmospheric pressure. This fall in intrathoracic pressure is caused by an increase in the intrathoracic volume, which occurs when muscle contraction causes the rib cage to move upwards and outwards at the same time as the diaphragm is flattening. During normal inspiration it is the movement of the diaphragm that accounts for the greatest change in intrathoracic volume and not the expansion of the rib cage (Ganong 1993). The fall in intrathoracic pressure causes air to be drawn into the lungs.

Expiration occurs when the lungs recoil, at the end of inspiration, bringing the chest wall back to its pre-inspiratory position. The diaphragm domes, returning to its pre-inspiratory state. Air leaves the lungs by this passive process. Movement of gas is proportional to changes in volume. Therefore, small changes in volume will result in small movements of gas, with the risk that inspired air may only be moving in and out of the anatomical dead space, never reaching the site of gas exchange at the alveoli.

Assessment of the mechanics of respiration

For external respiration to be adequate, the chest wall must be intact, the thorax and diaphragm must be able to rise and fall and that movement must be sufficient to create a negative pressure which will draw air beyond the anatomical dead space and to the alveoli. Patient assessment should reflect this and at least include a subjective assessment of the adequacy of respiratory volume. Observation must be made to ascertain whether the chest is moving symmetrically and to note if movement is in any way paradoxical.

Neural control of respiration

The rate, rhythm and volume of respiration are governed by the central nervous system, with the involuntary or automatic component being controlled by the respiratory centre in the medulla of the brain. There is a degree of voluntary control over respiration, for instance when an individual intentionally takes a deep breath, which is controlled by the cortex of the brain.

Chemoreceptors in the carotid and aortic body sense changes in blood pH. As the levels of carbon dioxide rise in the blood, the blood becomes more acid and impulses from the chemoreceptors to the respiratory centre increase. In response to this, the respiratory centre increases the respiratory rate. A similar process occurs in the brain where chemoreceptors in the medulla respond to changes in the pH of cerebrospinal fluid. Chemoreceptors are also responsive to a fall in blood oxygen concentrations, increasing impulses to the respiratory centre as the levels of oxygen fall.

In those individuals with chronic respiratory disease, the respiratory centre becomes unresponsive to the changes in carbon dioxide concentration. In these circumstances the falling oxygen concentrations become the main stimuli for respiration (Despopoulos & Sibernagi 1986). Consequently the administration of high concentrations of inspired oxygen may lead to a fall in respiratory rate or apnoea.

Assessment of respiratory control

Assessment should be made of the rate, rhythm and volume of respiration, as this may give an early indication of the increased carbon dioxide or decreased levels of oxygen in the blood. A further and often more striking indication of these physiological process is the use of the accessory muscles of respiration in the neck, shoulders and abdomen. This is often associated with tracheal tug and recession of the sternum and intercostal muscles.

Bronchial tone

The tone of the bronchi and bronchioles is maintained by the smooth muscle contained within their walls.

Hypoxia

Hypoxia is regarded as being one of the leading causes of preventable death in the trauma patient (Anderson *et al.* 1988), but it is often overlooked as a potential threat to life in the many patients who attend A&E for reasons other than having sustained an injury. Hypoxia, or inadequate tissue oxygenation, falls broadly into four broad groups (see Box 27.1):

- hypoxic hypoxia
- anaemic hypoxia
- stagnant hypoxia
- histotoxic hypoxia.

Assessment of gas exchange

In recent years, there has been an increased reliance upon pulse oximetry in respiratory assessment. In many cases, this technology is helpful in identifying hypoxia. However, pulse oximetry must be used with caution as it has the potential to mislead (Moyle 1994). Pulse oximetry gives an indication of the degree to which the available haemoglobin is saturated with oxygen. A patient with carbon monoxide poisoning may well have an anaemic hypoxia whilst still presenting what appears to be a normal oxygen saturation on the pulse oximeter. Similarly, patients with other forms of hypoxic anaemia may have normal pulse oximetry readings because the pulse oximeter is a reflection of the degree of saturation of each red blood cell and not the total oxygen content of the blood. Again pulse oximetry must be used with caution when there is probe movement or when peripheral perfusion is low, as recorded saturation may be inaccurate (Levine & Fromm 1995).

It must be remembered that pulse oximetry only provides information about the patient's oxygen saturation; it is not able to offer information regarding carbon dioxide in the blood. Consider the patient who is having an acute asthma attack and who has been given oxygen therapy by face mask. She may well have what may be regarded as satisfactory oxygen

---

Box 27.1 – *Types of hypoxia*

- **Hypoxic hypoxia**
  Oxygen is not available to haemoglobin in the red blood cells. This may occur when the patient is in an atmosphere which has a reduced oxygen content, although it is most likely to occur as a result of a decrease in respiratory rate and/or volume. If untreated, conditions such as pulmonary oedema or pneumonia lead to hypoxic hypoxia by preventing the diffusion of oxygen at the alveolar/capillary interface in the lungs.

- **Anaemic hypoxia**
  The oxygen-carrying capacity of the blood is reduced because of a lack of available haemoglobin. In the acute episode, this is likely to be due to hypovolaemia where haemoglobin is lost in proportion to the number of red cells lost. This type of hypoxia may also occur following chronic conditions where the number of red cells is normal but the haemoglobin is either reduced or not readily available, e.g. in iron deficiency anaemia and sickle cell anaemia. Following carbon monoxide poisoning, the carbon monoxide preferentially binds to the haemoglobin, preventing oxygen binding with the haemoglobin and thus resulting in anaemic hypoxia.

- **Stagnant hypoxia**
  This occurs as a result of failure of the circulatory system to transport oxygenated blood to the tissues. Normal diffusion occurs at the alveolar/capillary interface in the lungs, but inadequate circulation prevents the oxygen from being delivered to the tissues. This type of hypoxia is classically associated with physiological shock, be that cardiogenic, neurogenic, anaphylactic etc. This type of hypoxia may also occur at a local level where vascular obstruction causes a reduction in blood flow distal to the obstruction.

- **Histotoxic hypoxia**
  In this case, adequate concentrations of oxygen are transported to the tissues, but the cells are unable to utilise the oxygen. This type of hypoxia usually results from certain types of poisoning, classically cyanide poisoning.

---

saturation, yet have inadequate ventilation with high and increasing levels of blood carbon dioxide. The most accurate way to assess the gaseous content of the circulating volume is by arterial blood gas analysis. Not only does this investigation provide information regarding respiratory gases in the circulation, but it is also a vital tool in the assessment of acid–base balance.

Asthma

Asthma has been described as a localised disease of the airways which results in episodes of increased airflow obstruction. While many of the 10–20% of the population who have asthma are asymptomatic or are well controlled with medication (Edwards *et al.* 1995), there are up to 2000 deaths per year attributed to the disease (Wardlaw 1993). Acute asthma is characterised by an acute attack of bronchospasm in which the airways become swollen, constricted and filled with mucous plugs. The airflow obstruction, which characteristically fluctuates markedly, causes a mismatch of alveolar ventilation and perfusion and increases the work of breathing. Being more marked during expiration it also causes air to be 'trapped' in the lungs. Respiratory arrest may occur within a few minutes of the onset of a severe episode or death may occur from alveolar hypoventilation and severe arterial hypoxaemia in the patient exhausted by a prolonged attack. Severe airflow obstruction is manifested in the symptoms of breathlessness and wheezing (Wardlaw 1993). Acute severe asthma may arise from absence of treatment or from inadequate or unsuccessful treatment and is life-threatening and should be considered a medical emergency.

In the non-asthmatic individual, there is a minimal reaction of the smooth muscle in the bronchial wall to stimulation by inhaled allergens such as the house dust mite, animal hair or pollen. Non-allergenic stimulants such as cold weather, cigarette smoke, anxiety and exercise also have a minimal effect on the reactivity of the smooth muscle. In the individual with asthma, reaction to such stimulation is exaggerated, a response termed bronchial hyperreactivity, which is thought to be associated with an inflammatory process.

Asthma can be broadly divided into two main types: allergic and non-allergic. Allergic asthma, as the name suggests, is triggered by allergens such as the house dust mite and others previously identified. This condition generally appears in childhood and may improve as the child reaches adolescence (Axford 1996). Conversely, non-allergic asthma is triggered by factors such as anxiety or cold weather, first presenting in middle age. The symptoms of non-allergic asthma tend to intensify in both severity and frequency as the individual becomes older (Axford 1996).

Attendance at the A&E department is usually precipitated by one of two events: (1) acute event in the individual who has episodic asthma, i.e. who is symptom-free between distinct acute episodes; or (2) an acute increase in the severity of symptoms in the individual who has chronic asthma, where tightness and wheezing are present most of the time, if not controlled by regular medication.

Initially, the most obvious sign of asthma may be noisy respiration in the form of a wheeze, which is generally expiratory but can also be inspiratory. One must be cautious not to make false assumptions based upon this symptom, for as Axford (1996) notes, 'all that wheezes is not asthma'. Wheezing is a sign of airway obstruction which may or may not be asthmatic in origin. In previously fit asthmatic patients, peak flow recordings of <200 L/min are indicative of severe disease, and values of <100 L/min must be taken as evidence of life-threatening asthma and treated with assisted ventilation if the patient fails to respond.

Assessment

A full and objective assessment is essential and should include:

- *A full history* – it may not be possible to obtain this from the patient, if breathless. In cases of severe and life-threatening asthma, treatment should not be delayed in order to obtain a full history. The history should include:
  — onset of symptoms
  — duration
  — exacerbation.
- *Observation*
  — respiratory effort
  — use of accessory muscles
  — chest movement and symmetry
  — skin colour and appearance, such as sweating
  — respiratory rate, rhythm and depth
  — pulse
  — blood pressure
  — temperature (episode may have been precipitated by a chest infection).
- *Palpation*
  — degree of chest expansion
  — temperature of the skin.
- *Percussion* – resonance of the chest.
- *Auscultation*
  — quality of breath sound
  — degree of air entry
  — silence.
- *Peak expiratory flow rate*
  — measured against predicted and actual normal for that individual
  — should not be done if the patient has signs of severe or life-threatening asthma (i.e. is unable to speak a complete sentence).
- *Pulse oximetry* – use with caution; remember it will not tell you the amount of carbon dioxide the patient is retaining.

Table 27.1 – *Features of severe asthma. (After Greaves et al. 1997)*

Adult	Child
Cannot complete sentences	Cannot talk or feed
Pulse >110 min	Pulse > 140 min
Respiratory rate > 25 min	Respiratory rate > 50 min
Peak flow rate < 50% of predicted	

Table 27.2 – *Features of life-threatening asthma.. (After Greaves et al. 1997)*

Adult	Child
Exhaustion	Reduced conscious level
Cyanosis	Agitation
Bradycardia	Cyanosis
Hypotension	Silent chest
Silent chest	Coma
Peak flow < 33% of predicted	
Coma	

- *Arterial blood gas analysis.*
- *Chest X-ray.*

From the assessment it will be possible to identify those patients with severe and life-threatening asthma who need immediate intervention (see Tables 27.1 and 27.2).

Management

Position the patient to sit upright to maximise ventilation. Administer high-concentration oxygen through a Hudson mask with reservoir bag at a flow rate of 10–15 L/min. The drug regime recommended by the British Thoracic Society guidelines (British Thoracic Society 1997a) includes nebulised salbutamol or terbutaline, and oral or i.v. steroids. In life-threatening asthma, ipratropium should be added to the nebuliser; alternatively, use i.v. aminophylline or salbutamol (not children) or terbutaline (not children). In addition to continued reassessment based upon the initial assessment, monitor the cardiac rhythm. Provide psychological care for patient and family in dealing with their stress and anxiety.

In the less severe episodes, it is important to check out the patient's understanding of the illness and management. It is not uncommon for some individuals with asthma to have a poor understanding of the purpose of their medication, when it should be taken and how to take it correctly. It is important to make use of such opportunities to provide some preventative care. It is also essential that appropriate follow-up is arranged to continue patient education and monitoring in the primary health care setting. Patients with little understanding of their condition and medication regime will continue to attend A&E departments where their symptoms will be treated without resolving the underlying issues.

It is important to differentiate asthma from hyperventilation as the presenting symptoms of both are dramatic and can easily be confused by the inexperienced nurse. A hyperventilating patient will be tachypnoeic but not tachycardic and will usually have oxygen saturation levels of 100%. Hyperventilation is associated with anxiety and responds quickly to rebreathing through a paper bag. Hyperventilating patients generally do not have a history of asthma.

Pulmonary Chronic Obstructive Disease

Chronic obstructive airways (or pulmonary) disease (COAD/COPD) is a collective term for a number of chronic respiratory diseases the most common of which are chronic bronchitis and emphysema (British Thoracic Society 1997c).

Chronic bronchitis

Chronic bronchitis is most frequently seen in adults of middle age and beyond. It is characterised by a productive cough resulting from increased mucous secretion from hypertrophied mucus-secreting glands in the bronchi. The patency of the smaller bronchi is further compromised by inflammation of the mucosa. The cough and associated inflammation last for several months each year and occur on consecutive years.

Assessment

When the individual with chronic bronchitis attends the A&E department, it is usually because of an acute exacerbation of symptoms associated with a superimposed upper respiratory tract infection. Assessment of the individual will include:

- *A full history*, including past history as well as the history of the current episode
  - — onset of symptoms
  - — duration
  - — exacerbation.

- *Observation*
  — signs of chronic respiratory disease, e.g., clubbing of the fingers, barrel chest
  — respiratory effort
  — use of accessory muscles
  — chest movement and symmetry
  — skin colour
  — respiratory rate, rhythm and depth
  — pulse
  — blood pressure
  — temperature.
- *Palpation*
  — degree of chest expansion
  — temperature of the skin.
- *Percussion* – resonance of the chest.
- *Auscultation*
  — quality of breath sound
  — degree of air entry
- *Pulse oximetry* – use with caution; remember it will not tell you the amount of carbon dioxide the patient is retaining.
- *Arterial blood gas analysis* – will be abnormal given the chronic respiratory disease and should be viewed in light of the individual's actual or predicted normal.
- *Sputum sample* – for microbiological examination (microscopy, culture and sensitivity).
- *Chest X-ray.*

Assessment of the patient is likely to reveal the following clinical features:

- purulent productive cough
- dyspnoea
- tachypnoea
- wheezing
- respiratory distress and use of accessory muscles
- poor chest expansion
- cyanosis.

Management

Position the patient sitting upright to maximise ventilation. Oxygen should be given at a low concentration initially, but may need to be increased if improvement does not occur. If the patient needs oxygen, it should be given; however, close monitoring for signs of respiratory depression is required, in the event of which assisted ventilation may be necessary. Antibiotics, bronchodilators and steroids should be given if asthma is an element in the acute episode. In addition to continued reassessment based upon the initial assessment, the cardiac rhythm should be monitored. Psychological care for patient and family should be provided in dealing with their stress and anxiety

Emphysema

Dilation of the alveoli reduces the functional surface area of the lung available for gas exchange. The mechanics of respiration are also compromised by the reduction of elasticity and recoil of the lung. As with other chronic respiratory conditions, emphysema is commonly seen in adults beyond middle age. The individual attends the A&E department with an increase in the severity of the symptoms, often associated with additional respiratory disease or infection.

Assessment should follow the format as for the patient with chronic bronchitis. Such assessment will reveal:

- dyspnoea
- quiet breath sounds
- overinflation of the chest
- forced expiration through pursed lips.

Management of the patient is much the same as that for chronic bronchitis.

Pulmonary Oedema

Although pulmonary oedema for many patients has its origins in the cardiac system, it is a manifest problem in the respiratory system.

Cardiac-related pulmonary oedema

The most common presentation of pulmonary oedema of cardiac origin seen in the A&E department is as a result of left ventricular failure which may or may not be secondary to acute myocardial infarction. Failure of the left ventricle leads to back pressure in the pulmonary circulation. As the pressure builds, fluid is forced from the circulation firstly into the pulmonary interstitial spaces and then, with further increases in pressure, into the alveoli. This fluid within the interstitial spaces and the alveoli reduces the efficacy of gas exchange at the alveolar–capillary interface (British Thoracic Society 1997b).

Other possible causes of pulmonary oedema

It is important to remember that pulmonary oedema is not a disease in itself but is merely a symptom of some other underlying pathology, e.g.:

- opiate overdose
- inhalation of toxic or irritant substances
- allergic reactions
- airway burns/inhalation injury
- circulatory volume overload (overinfusion)
- pulmonary embolism

- hypoalbuminaemia
- near drowning.

Assessment

Onset is usually sudden with the individual attending the A&E department as symptoms worsen and respiratory function deteriorates. Assessment must focus upon the presenting symptoms, but must also aim to consider the possible underlying causes:

- *A full history* (past history as well as the history of the current episode)
  — onset of symptoms
  — duration
  — exacerbation.
- *Observation*
  — airway
  — signs of possible underlying mechanisms, e.g. inhalation injury, substance misuse
  — respiratory effort
  — use of accessory muscles
  — chest movement
  — skin colour
  — respiratory rate, rhythm and depth
  — pulse
  — blood pressure
  — temperature
  — level of consciousness.
- *Palpation*
  — degree of chest expansion
  — temperature of the skin.
- *Percussion* – resonance of the chest.
- *Auscultation*
  — quality of breath sound
  — degree of air entry.
- *Pulse oximetry* – with caution.
- *Arterial blood gas analysis.*
- *Chest X-ray.*

Assessment is likely to reveal:

- dyspnoea
- orthopnoea
- tachypnoea
- exhaustion
- respiratory distress
- noisy respiration
- expectoration of frothy sputum.

Management

Management of the patient is dependent upon the underlying pathology, but will include securing the airway and positioning the patient upright to maximise ventilation. Provide high-concentration oxygen through a Hudson mask with reservoir bag at a flow rate of 10–15 L/min. Diuretics may reduce the fluid load from the circulation. Morphine/diamorphine, if not contraindicated, causes venous pooling, thus reducing venous return on loading on the heart. Opiates will also help in the reduction of anxiety, but one must be vigilant for signs of respiratory depression. Vasodilators, if indicated, again cause venous pooling. Catheterisation should be considered and the patient's fluid output should be carefully monitored. Twelve-lead ECG should be performed to monitor any cardiac changes. In addition to continued reassessment based upon the initial assessment, monitor the cardiac rhythm. Psychological care should be provided for patient and family in dealing with their stress and anxiety.

Pulmonary Embolism

Pulmonary embolism is a common cause of respiratory-related death in the UK, with an estimated 30 000 deaths each year (Edwards *et al.* 1995). It is a commonly associated complication of deep vein thrombosis (DVT) where a fragment detaches from the thrombus to form an embolus (Fig. 27.2). The embolus flows through the circulation until it wedges in narrow branches of the arterial system, classically branches of the pulmonary artery. The pulmonary circulation becomes obstructed, which consequently reduces the efficacy of gas exchange and ventilation perfusion mismatch occurs.

Predisposition to pulmonary embolism, generally speaking, is determined by a predisposition to DVT, i.e.:

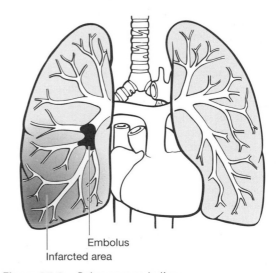

Embolus

Infarcted area

Figure 27.2 – *Pulmonary embolism.*

- sluggish circulation due to:
  — bed rest
  — limb immobilisation
  — heart failure/reduced cardiac output
- venous injury
  — trauma
  — venous cannulation
- increased coagulability
  — drugs, such as oral contraceptives
  — dehydration
  — polycythaemia
- increased age.

Emboli may arise from other mechanisms such as air, fat or amniotic fluid entering the circulation, but these are less common. Symptoms are related to the size of the area of lung affected, the rate of onset and the severity of the symptoms being determined by the size and number of emboli:

Small emboli. These wedge in smaller vessels, close to the alveolar – capillary interface, and affect only a small area of lung.

Medium emboli. These wedge in the larger branches of the pulmonary artery some distance from the alveolar – capillary interface. They affect a larger area of lung than do smaller emboli and result in a greater ventilation – perfusion mismatch.

Large emboli. These wedge in the largest branches of the pulmonary artery, furthest away from the alveolar – capillary interface. They affect very large areas of the lung and result in a massive ventilation – perfusion mismatch.

Assessment

A good assessment is vital as the symptoms of pulmonary embolism are often confused with those of acute myocardial infarction:

- *A full history*, considering predisposition to and evidence of DVT, as well as the history of the current episode:
  — onset of symptoms
  — duration
  — exacerbation.
- *Observation*
  — signs of possible underlying mechanisms, in particular DVT
  — respiratory effort
  — use of accessory muscles
  — chest movement
  — skin colour
  — respiratory rate, rhythm and depth
  — pulse

Table 27.3 – *Features of pulmonary emboli*

Small emboli	Medium emboli	Large emboli
Slow onset	Rapid onset	Sudden onset
Mild – moderate dyspnoea	Pleuritic chest pain	Dyspnoea
Fatigue	Dyspnoea	Chest pain
	Haemoptysis	Haemoptysis
		Tachycardia
		Compromised circulation
		Hypotension
		Cyanosis
		Reduced level of consciousness
		Unconsciousness

  — blood pressure
  — sputum
  — level of consciousness.
- *Palpation*
  — degree of chest expansion
  — temperature of the skin.
- *Percussion* – resonance of the chest.
- *Auscultation*
  — quality of breath sound
  — degree of air entry.
- *Pulse oximetry* – with caution.
- *Arterial blood gas analysis*
- *Chest X-ray.*
- *12-lead ECG.*

Table 27.3 outlines the features of emboli of different sizes. An ECG may reveal an S wave in lead I, a Q wave in lead III and an inverted T wave in lead III. The ECG may also be useful in excluding other diagnoses such as myocardial infarction and pericardial disease.

Management

Position the patient sitting upright to maximise ventilation. Administer high-concentration oxygen using a Hudson mask with reservoir bag at a flow rate of 10–15 L/min. Bloods should be taken for clotting screen. Anticoagulants, such as heparin, are often the only form of treatment given for massive pulmonary embolism. Thrombolytics such as streptokinase and rtPA are indicated primarily in patients who are haemodynamically unstable, particularly in the presence of systemic hypotension (ACCP 1996). The nurse should monitor the patient's cardiac rhythm for changes.

Anaphylaxis

An acute anaphylactic reaction is the result of a severe or overwhelming allergic or hypersensitivity reaction with sometimes fatal consequences. Symptoms will usually occur rapidly within minutes of exposure to the causative allergen, especially if given parenterally. Repeated administration of parental or oral therapeutic agents may also precipitate an anaphylactic reaction.

Contributory factors include:

- antibiotics, e.g. penicillin or other penicillin derivatives
- bee or wasp stings
- insect or snake venom
- foodstuffs, e.g. nuts or shellfish.

Clinical features

The clinical features of anaphylactic shock may occur singly or in combination and may include respiratory distress, cyanosis, bronchospasm, laryngeal obstruction circulatory collapse, hypotension, tachycardia, generalised erythema, urticaria, nausea, vomiting, abdominal pain and diarrhoea. Generally, the faster the onset of symptoms, the more life-threatening the reaction.

Management

The priority is to secure and maintain the airway; intubation may be required especially if laryngeal oedema is present. If the patient is able to maintain an open airway, she should be administered supplemental oxygen by a face mask at a high flow rate of 10–15 L/min. Adrenaline slows the release of cellular chemical mediators and, additionally, causes vasoconstriction. It also has beneficial effects on myocardial contractility, peripheral vascular tone and bronchial smooth muscle. Steroids are no longer thought to be of value.

The A&E nurse should be aware of the dangers of anaphylactic reactions and have knowledge of any relevant patient history. The nurse should avoid giving medication to patients with a known allergic disorder, such as hayfever or asthma, unless absolutely necessary. Ensure that prescribed medication is given by the most appropriate route; anaphylactic reactions are more likely to occur when drugs are given via the parenteral route. Provide education for patients identified as susceptible, and encourage then to carry appropriate first aid measures, such as treatment for insect stings and adrenaline. Patients known to have an allergic history should be encouraged to wear 'medic alert' type identification.

Near Drowning

Near drowning following submersion in water results from one of two main mechanisms: 'dry' drowning and 'wet' drowning. Dry drowning occurs following immersion in cold water, the cold water causing laryngospasm and vagal stimulation which leads to asphyxiation, hypoxia and cardiac arrest. Little or no water enters the lower airways or lungs. More commonly, drowning and near drowning occur as a result of wet drowning. After a period of breath-holding following immersion, the individual is forced to inhale by reflex mechanism. Water is aspirated into the lungs along with the large volumes of water which have been swallowed. The inhaled water obstructs the lower airways and thus prevents adequate gas exchange. Consequently, the individual rapidly becomes hypoxic, which leads to unconsciousness and cardiac arrest (Knopp 1992).

Near drowning is often associated with other factors which complicate the individual's condition. In adults, as much as 25% of cases have been documented as being associated with alcohol use (Mills *et al.* 1995). Hypothermia is common in UK waters. This is inevitable when the water is below 10°C as body heat is lost despite the individual actively exercising (Greaves *et al.* 1997). Near drowning is frequently associated with head and neck injury, when individuals dive into shallow water or water which contains submerged objects.

Significant neurological impairment occurs in up to 25% of near-drowning patients. Neurological injury results from hypoxia and can lead to cerebral oedema and brain stem herniation. Approximately 20% of comatose patients recover completely (Emergency Nurses Association 1994). Hypothermia is an important clinical feature in determining outcome as it decreases the metabolic demands of the body, and severe cerebral hypoxia may be prevented or delayed. Acidosis is a common finding in near-drowning patients. Metabolic acidosis is primarily due to tissue hypoxia, but a respiratory component may be present following aspiration. Hypoxia and acidosis act as myocardial depressants and precipitate circulatory collapse.

Assessment

There are some physiological differences between near drowning in fresh water and that in salt water. These differences are functionally irrelevant in the early management of the individual in the A&E department. Assessment of the individual must ensure that due consideration is given to the mechanism of injury in respect of potential head and neck trauma (Orlowski 1987). This should include:

- *A full history*
  — onset of symptoms
  — duration
  — exacerbation.
- *Observation*
  — airway
  — signs of possible underlying factors; head and neck trauma, alcohol use
  — respiratory effort
  — use of accessory muscles
  — chest movement
  — skin colour
  — respiratory rate, rhythm and depth
  — pulse
  — blood pressure
  — temperature
  — level of consciousness.
- *Palpation*
  — degree of chest expansion
  — temperature of the skin.
- *Percussion* – resonance of the chest.
- *Ausculation*
  — quality of breath sound
  — degree of air entry.
- *Pulse oximetry* – with caution.
- *Arterial blood gas analysis.*
- *Chest X-ray.*

The presentation of the individual following near drowning may be diverse, but is likely to include at least some of the following:

- head and neck trauma
- reduced level of consciousness – unconscious
- apnoea
- tachypnoea
- shallow respiration
- pulmonary oedema
- hypothermia
- arrhythmias
- asystole.

Symptoms may be delayed. Apparently well patients must be observed and reviewed over the subsequent 48 hours.

Management

- Airway management with cervical spine control
- High-concentration oxygen, with intermittent positive pressure ventilation if indicated
- Rewarming if indicated (see hypothermia)
- Management of arrhythmias

- Management of injuries
- Cardiac monitoring
- Continued reassessment based upon the initial assessment
- Psychological care for the patient and family in dealing with their stress and anxiety.

Carbon Monoxide Poisoning

Carbon monoxide poisoning is the commonest cause of poisoning in the UK, and is thought to cause 1000 deaths/year of which approximately one-third result from self-poisoning (Robinson & Stott 1993). Carbon monoxide is a colourless, odourless, tasteless gas produced by incomplete combustion of organic material. Poisoning is usually associated with inhalation of smoke from fires in confined spaces, engine exhausts and faulty heating systems. It is often referred to as the silent killer as victims of accidental exposure often have no idea they are being poisoned, even when they develop severe symptoms. Consequently, victims are likely to remain in a life-threatening environment without realising the dangers. Carbon monoxide combines more readily with haemoglobin than does oxygen; its affinity is more than 200 times that of oxygen. Once combined with carbon monoxide, haemoglobin is unable to bind with oxygen, resulting in a fall in Po_2 and an anaemic hypoxia.

Assessment

Assessment is largely dependent upon a clear history and a high index of suspicion, as symptoms in themselves may not be self-evident:

- *A full history* – has the individual been in a confined space in which carbon monoxide may be present? The history should include:
  — onset of symptoms
  — duration
  — exacerbation.
- *Observation*
  — airway – soot, carbonaceous sputum as evidence of an inhalation injury
  — respiratory effort
  — use of accessory muscles
  — chest movement
  — skin colour – may look pink or flushed (cherry red appearance may not be evident)
  — respiratory rate, rhythm and depth
  — pulse
  — blood pressure
  — temperature
  — level of consciousness.

Table 27.4 – *Presentation of carbon monoxide poisoning*

Carboxyhaemoglobin	Symptoms
<10%	No symptoms
10–20%	Headache Nausea Vomiting Loss of manual dexterity
21–40%	Confusion Lethargy ST depression on ECG Apathy – loss of interest in leaving dangerous environment, and therefore may be fatal
41–60%	Ataxia Convulsions Apnoea Coma
>60%	Usually fatal

- *Auscultation*
  — quality of breath sound
  — degree of air entry.
- *Pulse oximetry* – can be extremely misleading, giving high readings even though the patient is hypoxic.
- *Arterial blood gas analysis*.
- *Bloods for carboxyhaemoglobin*.

Presentation will depend upon the percentage of carboxyhaemoglobin present (see Table 27.4).

Management

The patient should be given high-concentration oxygen, with intermittent positive pressure ventilation if indicated. In the presence of 100% O_2 there is a 50% reduction of carboxyhaemoglobin in the first 20 minutes. Consider hyperbaric oxygen which forces oxygen onto the haemoglobin and reduces the half-life of carbon monoxide as well as decreasing intercranial pressure and cerebral oedema (Driscoll *et al.* 1994). The indications for hyperbaric oxygen (Axford 1996) are:

- conscious patients with levels of carboxyhaemoglobin of >20%
- neurological symptoms other than headache at any time since exposure
- pregnancy
- cardiac arrhythmias.

Renal disorders

The renal system is an important system as it influences a large number of physiological processes, e.g. the control and maintenance of blood pressure, fluid and electrolyte balance, acid–base balance and excretion of by-products of metabolism.

Maintenance of blood pressure

Baroreceptors in the renal arterial system respond to a fall in blood pressure by stimulating the release of renin from the juxta-glomerular apparatus. The renin enters the bloodstream and acts upon angiotensinogen, produced in the liver, to form angiotensin I. Angiotensin I is then converted to angiotensin II by angiotensin-converting enzyme (ACE) found mainly in the lungs and kidney. Angiotensin has a number of effects which raise blood pressure:

- acts directly on arterioles to cause vasoconstriction
- stimulates the circulation centre in the central nervous system resulting in vasoconstriction
- stimulates the thirst mechanism in the hypothalamus
- influences renal blood flow and the glomerular filtration rate by renal vasoconstriction
- stimulates the adrenal cortex to secrete aldosterone, which increases sodium reabsorption by the kidney and so causes water retention.

Fluid and electrolyte balance

A fluid deficit in the circulating blood volume is detected by the osmoreceptors, located in the hypothalamus. This causes the secretion of antidiuretic hormone from the posterior pituitary. This hormone stimulates increased water absorption in the kidney and this is supported by the effects of the renin–angiotensin pathway (described above).

Acid–base balance

In cases where the blood is acidotic the lungs play a major part in the reduction of the acidosis by the excretion of the acid-producing hydrogen ions in the form of carbon dioxide. However, the kidney provides a valuable additional role in the reduction of the hydrogen ion concentration. The kidney provides a back-up in the case of inadequate respiration; it removes acid produced by fat and protein metabolism which cannot be removed by the lungs and it allows bicarbonate to be reabsorbed to supplement that being used in buffering processes. Acid is excreted by the kidney in a buffered form.

Excretion of by-products of metabolism

Carbohydrates and fats are broken down to carbon dioxide and water and are excreted by means of processes as detailed previously. Many substances such as protein and amino acids contain nitrogen, which relies upon the kidney to excrete nitrogenous by-products in the form of urea, uric acid and creatinine.

Assessment of the renal system

The renal system gives an insight into many physiological processes and should not be underestimated when making a patient assessment. Likewise an assessment of the renal system should not be restricted to those patients with renal conditions. The assessment of these processes and of renal function is via the urine output in terms of volume, frequency and content. This may be achieved by accurate fluid balance measurement and recording at intervals appropriate to the patient's condition. Routine urine testing using reagent strips offers a wealth of information, as does visual inspection of the urine which is frequently undervalued in assessment.

Urinary tract infection

Of the many conditions which are of renal or urinary tract in origin, few are seen in the A&E department. Where the patient does attend with an underlying renal or urinary tract pathology, it is generally because of pain rather than any other symptom, the most common conditions being urinary tract infection (UTI) and renal colic.

Urinary tract infection

This is commonly caused by *E. coli* from faeces; other organism groups that cause UTI include *Proteus, Pseudomonas, Streptococcus, Staphylococcus epidermidis* and *Klebsiella* (Edwards *et al.* 1995). Following inoculation, organisms rapidly multiply in the ideal culture material of the urine. The individual will generally present at the A&E department complaining of pain on micturition.

Assessment

- *A full history*
  - onset of symptoms
  - duration
  - exacerbation.
- *Observation*
  - skin colour

- temperature
- urine–colour, opacity, odour.
- *Midstream specimen of urine* – for microscopy, culture and sensitivity.

Symptoms of UTI include:

- dysuria
- frequency of micturition
- haematuria.

In its advanced stages UTI may lead to infection of the kidney or kidneys in the form of pyelonephritis, which may present as:

- signs of UTI
- fever
- loin pain
- nausea
- vomiting.

Management

Management of the condition is based upon:

- antibiotics
- increased oral fluid intake
- patient education.

Renal colic

Renal colic is the most common presentation of renal calculi. Generally affecting men between 30 and 40 years of age, renal calculi are predominantly calcium in origin, although they may be calcium/ammonium phosphate, urate or cystine. The calculi form in the kidney when the urine is saturated with the given solute and the kidney is unable to excrete it. The solute, in its crystalline form, deposits in the kidney causing pain. Pain is at its most intense when the calculi pass through the urinary tract.

Assessment

- *A full history and pain assessment*
  - onset of symptoms
  - duration
  - exacerbation.
- *Observation*
  - skin colour
  - temperature
  - urine – colour, opacity, odour, laboratory stick test. Urine should be filtered through filter paper to identify evidence of grit from the calculi.
- *Midstream specimen of urine* – for microscopy, culture and sensitivity.

Table 27.5 – *Dehydration – fluid deficit. (After Paradiso, 1995)*

	Hypertonic deficit	Isotonic deficit
Mechanism	Occurs when fluid is lost without the loss of electrolytes Extracellular fluid becomes concentrated and fluid moves from the intracellular compartment to the extracellular compartment	Occurs when fluid and electrolytes are in normal physiological proportions Extracellular and intracellular fluid remains unchanged
Possible causes	Severe GI infections, causing fluid loss and sodium concentration Increased insensible loss Low-volume, concentrated feeds (infants or nasogastric) Inability to access water (environmental isolation/entrapment loss of consciousness)	Diarrhoea and vomiting Increased urine output (renal disease, diuretics) Increased sweating Burns Haemorrhage Lack of fluid and electrolyte intake
Symptoms	Decreased skin elasticity Dry mucous membranes Hypotension Tachycardia Increased respiratory rate and volume Increased thirst Pitting oedema	Acute weight loss Dry mucous membranes Hypotension Tachycardia Increased respiratory rate and volume Decreased and concentrated urine output Sunken eyes Pleural effusion Pulmonary oedema Dependent oedema
Management	Water replacement Hypotonic i.v. fluids	i.v. replacement of isotonic fluids Blood and blood products Anti-emetics

The main feature identified by the assessment is likely to be pain; however other features may be present:

- pain – unilateral pain radiates from the loin to left or right lower quadrants. Suprapubic pain may also be present. Pain may be sudden and intermittent in onset
- restlessness
- dysurea
- urgency
- frequency
- haematurea
- proteinurea
- UTI.

Management

- Analgesia – opiates, non-steroidal anti-inflammatory drugs
- Antispasmodics – atropine
- Anti-emetics

- Increase fluid intake – orally or i.v.
- Patient education – advise patient to increase fluid intake especially at night when urine normally concentrates.

Dehydration – Fluid Volume Deficit

The mechanisms leading to dehydration are many and varied. It is likely that the patient will attend the A&E department with a condition resulting in dehydration rather than with dehydration *per se*. It is important to consider the processes involved in the underlying illness to identify the potential for dehydration. There are three main types of dehydration, depending on the type of fluid deficit, i.e. hypertonic, isotonic (Table 27.5).

In an effort to correct dehydration, patients may inadvertently overhydrate, leading to subsequent physiological disturbance. This is covered in Table 27.6.

Table 27.6 – *Overhydration – fluid excess. (After Paradiso, 1995)*

	Hypertonic excess	Isotonic excess
Mechanism	Increased sodium concentrations with fluid volume remaining normal Extracellular fluid becomes concentrated with intracellular fluid moving into the extracellular compartment	Increase in fluid and electrolyte concentrations of normal physiological concentrations No movement of fluid across the compartments
Possible causes	Intake of relatively large volumes of salt water	Excessive intake of isototomic fluids either orally or i.v. Abnormal fluid and electrolyte retention following renal disease Corticosteroid therapy
Symptoms	Circulatory overload Oedema Increased cardiac output Congestive cardiac failure Pulmonary oedema Increased BP Full bounding pulse Decreased level of consciousness Muscle twitching Fitting Coma Hypernatraemia	Circulatory overload Oedema Increased cardiac output Congestive cardiac failure Pulmonary oedema Increased BP Full bounding pulse
Management	Management of underlying disease Removal of sodium with diuretics Replacement of fluid lost by drug-induced diuresis	Diuretics Treatment of underlying disease, e.g. CCF i.v. replacement of hypertonic fluids with caution

Assessment

This should include:

- *A full history*, including past history as well as the history of the current episode:
  — onset of symptoms
  — duration
  — exacerbation.
- *Observation*
  — respiratory effort
  — use of accessory muscles
  — chest movement
  — skin colour
  — respiratory rate, rhythm and depth
  — pulse
  — blood pressure
  — temperature
  — level of consciousness
  — urine – volume, colour and concentration.
- *Palpation*
  — degree of chest expansion

  — skin temperature and elasticity.
- *Auscultation*
  — quality of breath sound
  — degree of air entry.
- *Pulse oximetry* (depending upon respiratory symptoms) – with caution.
- *Arterial blood gas analysis*
- *Chest X-ray.*

Thermoregulation

The control of body temperature takes place in the hypothalamus in response to changes in core temperature, detected by thermoreceptors in the hypothalamus, skin and spinal cord. When the body temperature rises, the hypothalamus responds by increasing sweating, respiration and blood flow to the skin, via the autonomic nervous system.

When the temperature falls, the body aims to raise the body temperature by heat conservation and increased heat production. Heat is conserved by reducing the activity of the sweat glands, erection of the body hair and diverting the blood flow from the periphery to the core. Heat is produced by involuntary muscle activity in the form of shivering and by voluntary muscle activity such as stamping the feet.

Assessment of body temperature

Assessment of the body temperature is reliant upon thermometry, which has traditionally been by means of the clinical thermometer either orally, axillary or rectally. This method often yields inaccuracies in temperature measurement as thermometers are often removed before an accurate temperature has been recorded. With the advent of electronic tympanic thermometers, this has become less of a problem. However, inaccuracies do occur if the ear canal is occluded by either wax or other debris. Again it is important not to discount the value of patient observation as a means of assessment.

Heat illness

Heat illness is inextricably linked to fluid and electrolyte balance. An increase in body temperature is controlled by an increase in sweating as a means of dissipating heat by evaporation. Increased sweating, although a relatively efficient way of reducing temperature, results in the loss of considerable amounts of fluid. Consequently, electrolyte concentrations, especially sodium, become deranged.

A number of factors predispose heat illness. These are rarely of significance individually, but pose a great risk in combination:

■ high ambient temperature
■ high humidity (humidity reduces effective evaporation through sweating)
■ exercise
■ clothing which reduces the skin surface area available for evaporation.

Assessment

Good assessment is important to establish the type of heat illness which has occurred and to guide management:

■ *A full history*, including past history as well as the history of the current episode:
  — onset of symptoms
  — duration
  — exacerbation.
■ *Observation*
  — airway

  — respiratory effort
  — use of accessory muscles
  — chest movement
  — skin colour
  — respiratory rate, rhythm and depth
  — pulse
  — blood pressure
  — temperature
  — level of consciousness.
■ *Palpation*
  — degree of chest expansion
  — temperature and elasticity of the skin.
■ *Blood for urea and electrolytes.*
■ *Pulse oximetry* – with caution.

From the assessment, two conditions may be identified;

Heat exhaustion. The signs and symptoms are:

■ loss of fluid and electrolytes
■ slight increase in core temperature
■ tachycardia
■ headache
■ dizziness
■ sweating.

Heat stroke (life-threatening). Signs and symptoms are:

■ core temperature above 41°C
■ heat increases beyond the body's ability to loose heat (beyond 42°C hypothalamic control of temperature is lost)
■ sweating may be absent
■ hot dry skin
■ nausea and vomiting
■ hypovolaemia
■ hypokalaemia
■ decreased level of consciousness – unconsciousness.

Management

Heat exhaustion

■ Place in a cool environment, with gentle air flow.
■ Remove clothing preventing heat loss.
■ Replace isotonic fluid – orally if conscious and orientated and not vomiting; otherwise by the intravenous route.

Tepid sponging and the use of a fan is not advocated as this causes peripheral vasoconstriction, pooling the blood to the core with a consequential rise in core temperature.

Heat stroke

■ Secure the airway if indicated.

- Administer high-concentration oxygen and assisted ventilation if required.
- Remove clothing.
- Carry out active cooling – consider immersion in cool water, taking into account potential airway and breathing problems. Spraying the skin with cool water in the presence of air flow may be a more practical intervention to reduce body temperature through evaporation.
- Carry out intravenous fluid replacement and correction of electrolyte imbalance.

Nervous System

The brain is highly intolerant to a fall in oxygen and glucose levels and is therefore highly sensitive to changes in its blood flow. This sensitivity is manifest in changes in the level of consciousness and subtle signs such as confusion or disorientation. As the brain is responsible for the control and regulation of many vital functions, such as respiration, cardiac output or movement, by means of the somatic or autonomic nervous system, symptoms may be manifest in these systems or processes.

Neurological assessment

As with all assessment, neurological assessment is about the interpretation of trends in clinical signs and not single observations viewed in isolation. One of the most important and informative signs is the level of consciousness. The accepted tool for this assessment is the Glasgow Coma Scale.

Headaches

Although headaches, when accompanied by other neurological signs, may be an indication of some underlying condition, they are infrequently life-threatening in themselves (Pearce 1996). Headaches with no other neurological signs fall broadly into three main groups: tension, migraine and cluster. In order to differentiate between the three and to identify any serious underlying conditions, a full assessment is essential, with great emphasis being placed upon the history:

- *A full history*; including past history as well as the history of the current episode:
  — location of pain
  — type of pain
  — severity/intensity of pain
  — onset of pain
  — duration of pain
  — frequency of pain
  — context in which pain occurs
  — what exacerbates or relieves pain
  — other associated neurological symptoms
  — health history – has the individual experienced these headaches previously?
  — current medication – especially over-the-counter medications taken for symptom relief, vasodilators or caffeine-containing drugs
  — allergies
  — diet – including intake of caffeine
  — alcohol and substance use
  — smoking.
- *Observation*
  — signs of possible underlying mechanisms, substance misuse for example
  — skin colour
  — respiratory rate, rhythm and depth
  — pulse
  — blood pressure
  — temperature
  — level of consciousness (GCS)
  — photophobia
  — neck stiffness.

Tension headaches

These are associated with stress and can often be associated with identifiable causes, such as increase in workload, financial pressures and bereavement. Pain is usually slow in onset, often increasing in intensity over a number of hours and is described as a dull or nagging ache. Generally the pain is generalised and described as a band around the head, rather than focused in a specific area. Tension headaches are frequently chronic as the underlying stress may be chronic.

Management is based upon managing the stress through relaxation techniques and addressing underlying problems where possible. In the immediate term, pain relief may be achieved with simple over-the-counter analgesics as appropriate in the light of current medication history. Ensure that analgesics do not contain caffeine.

Migraine

Migraine falls into two distinct groups: classic and common. Classic migraine affects 20% of migraine sufferers and common migraine affects the remaining 80% (Pearce 1996). Individuals suffering classic migraine experience an aura, usually in the form of visual or motor disturbance up to half an hour before the onset of the headache. Visual disturbance is often in the form of flashing lights or rods of light in front of the eyes. At the onset the pain is unilateral and is accompanied by nausea, vomiting, numbness of hands, face and tongue, weakness and clumsiness. The pain is described as throbbing or pounding and is often intensified by light. Common migraine has similar clinical features, but without the aura, individuals often being awoken from sleep by the pounding headache.

Individuals often find the symptoms less intense if they are able to lie down in a quiet darkened room. Analgesia, especially containing codeine, may help in symptom relief but should be preceded by an anti-emetic. Analgesia alone is of little benefit as reduced gastric motility prevents its absorption. If vomiting is severe, consideration should be given to administering the anti-emetic per rectum.

The majority of migraine sufferers experience their first episode before the age of 30 and so any individual who presents with a first attack over the age of 40 should be viewed with suspicion and carefully investigated

Cluster headaches

Cluster headaches refer to repeated episodes of headaches occurring several times a day and lasting between 30 minutes and 2 hours, clusters lasting from 1 to 4 months followed by a period of remission. Pain can occur at any time, but often follows a pattern and frequently occurs an hour after falling a sleep. The pain is described as a stabbing, boring pain, which causes the individual to be restless, pacing the floor rather than going to bed. Vomiting is not common. Trigger factors have been linked with alcohol and vasodilators in particular. Treatment is based on analgesia, which is best taken prophylactically prior to expected episodes. Ten minutes of oxygen therapy at 5–10 L/min is also reported as being of benefit.

Headaches with associated neurological symptoms

Serious neurological illness may manifest in the form of headaches, but is likely to be accompanied by other neurological signs. Brain tumours, for example, are often associated with fitting and focal neurological signs. The form of the focal signs is dependent upon the site of the tumour, but may include changes in mood, memory, balance, motor function, gait and coordination. The most serious indication of under-lying pathology is failing vision and or reducing levels of consciousness. Again, a thorough history is important in order to establish trends; single occurr-ences are open to misinterpretation.

Any headache associated with other neurological symptoms must be treated with suspicion and the patient refered immediately.

Subarachnoid haemorrhage

Spontaneous subarachnoid haemorrhage generally results from the rupture of an intercranial aneurysm on a major artery in the circle of Willis. The patient generally presents with sudden onset of an intense headache which may initially be frontal or occipital, but eventually becomes generalised. The blood in the subarachnoid space leads to irritation and neurological signs such as drowsiness, confusion, neck stiffness, photophobia, convulsions and loss of consciousness. Depending upon the location of the bleed, the indi-vidual may have aphasia, hemiparesis or hemiplegia.

Management is focused on supporting the vital functions in terms of airway, breathing and circulation. Particular attention should be given to the monitoring of the blood pressure, as a raised blood pressure may increase the degree of bleeding.

Ischaemic brain injury

The most frequently observed types of brain ischaemia seen in the A&E department are transient ischaemic attacks and ischaemic stroke. In both cases, ischaemia leads to focal loss of cerebral function. As the name suggests, the symptoms of the ischaemia are short-lived, lasting less than 24 hours, the actual ischaemia being shorter in duration than this. When symptoms last more than 24 hours, death occurs from what is thought to be a cerebral vascular event alone (Lott et al. 1999).

The mechanism of ischaemic stroke is thought to be due to infarction in 80% of cases, a primary inter-cerebral bleed in 10% and subarachnoid haemorrhage in the remaining 10% (Warlow 1996).

Assessment

- ■ *A full history*
  — onset of symptoms
  — duration
  — exacerbation.
- ■ *Observation*
  — skin colour, appearance
  — respiratory rate, rhythm and depth
  — pulse
  — blood pressure
  — temperature
  — Glasgow Coma Scale.

The modes of presentation of both transient ischaemia and ischaemic stroke differ little other than in the duration of the symptoms. Symptoms vary depending upon the area of brain affected:

- sudden onset of symptoms, although symptoms may develop more slowly in ischaemic stroke
- hemiparesis
- hemiplegia
- dizziness
- dysarthria
- dysphagia
- dysphasia
- ataxia
- visual disturbances
- confusion
- reduced level of consciousness
- unconsciousness.

Management

As with subarachnoid haemorrhage, management is focused upon supporting the vital functions in terms of airway, breathing and circulation. Particular attention should be given to monitoring of the blood pressure, as a raised blood pressure may increase the degree of bleeding.

Epilepsy

Epilepsy in itself is not a medical emergency, however there are a number of mechanisms which may make it so, the most common being injury sustained during a convulsion and several seizures following on from the previous in quick succession – status epilepticus. Neurones within the brain communicate in a systematic way. During a seizure, discharge from the neurones is chaotic, often manifesting in a tonic-clonic fit, but it may manifest in many other ways. During the tonic phase, the individual loses consciousness, this being accompanied by muscle contraction causing the body to become stiff, jaw to be clenched, air to be forced out of the lungs and possibly incontinence. The tonic phase is followed by the clonic phase which is characterised by rhythmic contractions of the limbs and trunk – convulsions.

Normally when convulsions cease, the individual is drowsy, confused and may have a headache. The main danger for the individual in such circumstances is from injury when falling to the ground or colliding with objects or from having objects forced into the mouth by unwitting 'helpers'. It is important to establish if the fit is related to epilepsy or if it is a symptom of some other condition such as head injury or subarachnoid haemorrhage. Status epilepticus, where as one seizure ends another immediately commences, is a potentially life-threatening condition requiring immediate intervention to break the cycle. Status epilepticus has a significant mortality (2–4%)

and morbidity (10%) with irreversible neurological damage (Appleton 1994). The mainstay of management is intravenous diazepam or phenytoin infusion, remembering to support airway, breathing with high-concentration oxygen and circulation

Glucose Regulation

Two of the hormones secreted by the pancreas, insulin and glucagon, have an important function in the maintenance of blood glucose levels. Insulin is secreted in response to elevated blood glucose levels, its function being to promote the storage of glucose by facilitating its uptake by the cells and by the synthesis of glycogen in the liver, renal cortex and the muscles. Consequently, these actions reduce blood glucose.

Unlike insulin, the stimuli for glucagon release are hunger and a low blood sugar level, the net effect of its release being to raise the blood sugar level. This is achieved by the glycogenolysis, the conversion of stored glycogen into glucose. In addition, glucose is synthesised from lactate, amino acids and glycerol.

Assessment of blood sugar

Patient observation and a nursing history may provide an indication that the patient has an altered blood sugar. The use of single drop of blood laboratory sticks is a rapid and accurate method of providing objective confirmation of your observations. This should always be followed up with a laboratory test of a larger sample of blood drawn by venepuncture. Such assessments should also be considered for those patients who have an altered level of consciousness and where a raised or lowered blood sugar cannot be excluded.

Diabetes mellitus

Diabetes mellitus is a condition whereby the cells are unable to access and utilise glucose taken in through the diet, due to either a lack of insulin or ineffective insulin. A lack of naturally occurring insulin is referred to as type 1 or insulin-dependent diabetes mellitus (IDDM), which generally first appears in childhood. Where naturally occurring insulin is present but is ineffective, the condition is termed type 2 or non-insulin-dependent diabetes mellitus (NIDDM). This usually first appears in later life. As a consequence of the cells' inability to access the glucose, it remains in the circulation, with some being excreted by the kidneys. In the absence of effective glucose metabolism, the body begins to metabolise fats.

Two main conditions occur in diabetes mellitus which may present a threat to life: hypoglycaemia and diabetic ketoacidosis (DKA), resulting from the incomplete metabolism of fats. Because the brain is highly sensitive to altered levels of glucose, especially low levels, the main presentation of this condition is an alteration in the level of consciousness.

Assessment

Assessment of the neurologically impaired patient is important regardless of the suspected mechanism:

- *A full history*
  — onset of symptoms
  — duration
  — exacerbation
- *Observation*
  — skin colour, appearance
  — respiratory rate, rhythm and depth
  — pulse
  — blood pressure
  — temperature
  — odour on the breath
- *Reagent strip blood test for glucose*
- *Formal blood sample for laboratory blood glucose measurement*
- *Assessment for dehydration.*

Hypoglycaemia

Symptoms and signs

- Blood glucose of less than 3.0 mmol/L
- Rapid in onset in IDDM, where synthetic insulin intake oversupplies glucose intake or where there is an increased glucose demand
- Slower in onset in NIDDM
- Early signs
  — weakness
  — sweating
  — tachycardia
  — palpitations
  — tremor
  — irritability
  — confusion
  — amnesia
  — visual disturbance
- Later signs
  — unconsciousness
  — fitting.

All individuals with a reduced level of consciousness, especially if associated with alcohol, should routinely have blood glucose measured by use of a reagent labstick.

Management

The conscious individual

- Fast-acting sugar in the form of a drink, e.g. sugar in tea or coffee, soft drink – *not* diet/low calorie
- Longer-acting sugar, e.g. a sandwich or biscuits.

The unconscious individual

- Maintain the airway
- Support breathing
- Glucogon by injection – converted into glucose by the body; benefits are temporary and so it must be followed up with oral long-acting sugar when consciousness returns and the individual is able to protect his own airway
- 50% glucose i.v. – must be into a large vein as hypertonic fluids are highly irritant.

Diabetic ketoacidosis

Symptoms and signs

- Blood glucose persistently above 15 mmol/L
- Usually IDDM, but can be NIDDM
- Osmotic diuresis – water following glucose excreted by the kidney
- Thirst
- Polyuria
- Oliguria
- Fatigue
- Warm dry skin
- Nausea
- Vomiting
- Electrolyte imbalance
- Loss of consciousness.

Management

- Airway management as required
- Support of breathing
- Rehydration with i.v. isotonic fluids
- Insulin – guided by measured blood glucose
- Correction of electrolyte imbalance.

Haematology

The blood has a number of important functions, many of which impinge on other systems and processes. It plays a vital role in the transportation of respiratory gases, maintenance of body temperature, acid–base balance, fluid and electrolyte balance and immunity. Blood, by volume, is predominantly plasma, in which are suspended red blood cells, white blood cells and platelets. Red blood cells are predominantly involved in the transportation of oxygen by means of the haemoglobin. The red cells are produced in the bone marrow and remain in the circulation for about 120 days. Changes in blood concentration, infection and some drugs are known to easily damage the relatively fragile red blood cells.

White cells are produced in the bone marrow and are considerably less numerous than the red blood cells. The white cells are of three main types: granulocytes (neutrophils, eosinophils and basophils), lymphocytes and monocytes. Collectively these cells form the basis of the body's defence system. Platelet formation also takes place in the bone marrow; 60–75% of platelets stay in the circulation and the bulk of the remainder are found in the spleen (Hinchcliff et al. 1996). Platelets are predominantly involved in clotting processes.

The plasma, as well as being a transport medium for the red cells, white cells and platelets, contains a number of salts and proteins. The proteins have a wide range of functions, including maintaining the osmotic pressure of the blood, clotting and immunity.

Haematological assessment

Much of the assessment may be based upon patient observation and the nursing history. However, much information may be gained from the appropriate haematological and biochemical tests and the interpretation of the results.

Sickle Cell Disease

Although commonly viewed as affecting only black people, sickle cell disease is in fact also seen in Mediterranean, Middle Eastern and Indian communities (Franklin 1990). Sickle cell disease is thought to have evolved over a considerable time in malaria endemic areas, as a defence against malaria. The evolutionary changes have resulted in a change in the structure of the haemoglobin, which in sickle cell disease can lead to a change in the shape of the red blood cell to form the classically sickle-shaped blood cell. The evolutionary nature of the disease has resulted in changes in the genetic material, accounting for the hereditary element of sickle cell disease (Davies & Oni 1997).

The most commonly occurring crisis experienced by sufferers of sickle cell disease is painful crisis and this accounts for over 90% of hospital admissions for patients with sickle cell disease (Brozovic et al. 1987). Sickled cells can cluster together causing occlusion of small blood vessels. Such obstruction reduces the blood flow to the distal tissues and causes the acute pain. It is the acute pain which precipitates the attendance at the A&E department, but it is essential that an adequate assessment is made to identify factors which may have triggered the episode, such as:

- reduced oxygenation – often following exercise
- cold or excessive heat
- dehydration
- fever
- infections
- stress.

Assessment

The identification of such factors are important in guiding patient management.

Assessment

Assessment will include:

- *A full history*, including past history as well as the history of the current episode:
  — onset of symptoms
  — duration
  — exacerbation.
- *Observation*
  — respiratory effort
  — use of accessory muscles
  — chest movement and symmetry
  — skin colour
  — respiratory rate, rhythm and depth (respiration may be compromised if sickling occurs in the pulmonary circulation)
  — pulse
  — blood pressure
  — temperature
  — Glasgow Coma Scale as sickling in cerebral vessels can lead to ischaemic stroke.
- *Palpation*
  — degree of chest expansion
  — temperature of the skin.
- *Auscultation*
  — quality of breath sound
  — degree of air entry.
- *Pulse oximetry* – with caution.
- *Chest X-ray*.

Clinical features

These include severe pain which commonly starts in the limbs, but may occur in the back and chest. Other clinical features may be associated with the precipitating factors, such as dehydration.

Management

This includes rapid and adequate analgesia, usually requiring opiate analgesics. These should not be delayed by undertaking a detailed examination (Department of Health 1993). Seek specialist advice from the haematologist. Ensure the patient is adequately hydrated, warm and able to rest. Oxygen therapy should be given if indicated, however oxygen will be of little or no benefit to most individuals in sickle cell crisis as the problem is associated with obstructed blood flow and not oxygenation of that blood. It is highly recommended that each department has a policy for managing individuals with sickle cell disease and information on where to access specialist advice and support locally.

Conclusion

In the modern A&E department, a 'medical emergency' can range from a full cardiac arrest to a GP referral patient with an exacerbation of a chronic condition. This chapter has considered the more common medical conditions which may result in A&E attendances. The A&E nurse plays an important role in identifying and alleviating symptoms and conditions which can be debilitating for the patient. While many medical conditions are chronic, the exacerbation of these conditions may require the patient to attend A&E for subsequent admission. The provision of supportive care can alleviate the suffering and disruption caused by these medical emergencies.

References

ACCP (1996) Consensus Committee on Pulmonary Embolism: opinions regarding the diagnosis and management of venous thromboembolic disease. *Chest*, **109**, 233–237.

Anderson ID, Woodford M, de Dombal T, Irving M (1988) A retrospective study of 1000 death from injury in England and Wales. *British Medical Journal*, **296**, 1305–130.

Appleton R (1994) *The Nursing Times Guide to Epilepsy*. Basingstoke: Macmillan.

Axford J (1996) *Medicine*. Oxford: Blackwell Science.

British Thoracic Society (1997a) The British guidelines on asthma management 1995 review and position statement. *Thorax*, **52**(Suppl. 1).

British Thoracic Society (1997b) Suspected acute pulmonary embolism: a practical approach. *Thorax*, **52**(Suppl. 4), S1–24.

British Thoracic Society (1997c) BTS Guidelines for the management of chronic obstructive pulmonary disease. *Thorax*, **52**(Suppl. 5), S1–28.

Brozovic M, Davies SC, Brownell AI (1987) Acute admissions of patients with sickle cell disease who live in Britain. *British Medical Journal*, **294**, 1206–1208.

Davies SC, Oni L (1997) Management of patients with sickle cell disease. *British Medical Journal*, **315**, 656–660.

Department of Health (1993) *Report of a Working Party of the Standing Medical Advisory Committee on Sickle Cell, Thalassaemia and other Haemoglobinopathies*. London: HMSO.

Despopoulos A, Sibernagi I (1986) *Color Atlas of Physiology*. New York: Thieme.

Driscoll P, Gwinnutt P, LeDuc Jimmerson C, Goodall. (1994) *Trauma Resuscitation: the Team Approach*. Basingstoke: Macmillan.

Edwards CRW, Bouchier IAD, Haslet C, Chilvers ER (1995) *Davidson's Principles and Practice of Medicine*, 17th edn. Edinburgh: Churchill Livingstone.

Emergency Nurses Association (1994) *Emergency Nursing Core Curriculum*, 4th edn. Philadelphia: WB Saunders.

Franklin I (1990) *Sickle cell disease: a guide for patients, carers and health workers*. London: Faber & Faber.

Ganong WF (1993) *Review of Medical Physiology*, 16th edn. Connecticut: Appleton & Lange.

Greaves I, Hodgetts T, Porter K (1997) *Emergency Care: A Textbook for Paramedics*. London: WB Saunders.

Hinchliff S, Montague S, Watson R (1996) *Physiology for Nursing Practice*, 2nd edn. London: Baillière Tindall.

Knopp RK (1992) Near drowning. In: Rosen P, Barkin RM, Braen G, *et al.*, eds. *Emergency Medicine: Concepts and Clinical Practice*. St Louis: Mosby Year Book.

Levine RL, Fromm RE (1995) *Critical Care Monitoring: from Pre-hospital to the ICU*. St Louis: Mosby.

Lott C, Hennes HJ, Dick W (1999) A medical emergency. *Journal of Accidental Emergency Medicine*, **16**(1), 2–7.

Mills K, Morton R, Page G (1995) *Colour Atlas and Text of Emergencies*, 2nd edn. London: Mosby-Wolfe.

Moyle J (1994) *Pulse Oximetry*. London: BMJ.

Orlowski JP (1987) Drowning, near-drowning and ice water submersion. *Pediatric Clinics of North America*, **34**, 75–92.

Paradiso C (1995) *Fluids and Electrolytes*. Philadelphia, JB Lippincott.

Pearce (1996) Headaches. In: Weatherall DJ, Ledingham JGG, Warrell DA, eds. *Oxford Textbook of Medicine*, 3rd edn. Oxford: Oxford University Press.

Robinson R, Stott R (1993) *Medical Emergencies: Diagnosis and Treatment*, 6th edn. Oxford: Butterworth Heinemann.

Wardlaw AJ (1993) *Asthma*. Oxford: Bios Scientific.

Warlow (1996) Cerebrovascular disease. In: Weatherall DJ, Ledingham JGG, Warrell DA, eds. *Oxford Textbook of Medicine*, 3rd edn. Oxford: Oxford University Press.

Chapter 28

Surgical Emergencies

*Peter Dowds**

■ Introduction
■ Anatomy and physiology of the abdomen
■ Nursing assessment of the acute abdomen
■ Acute abdominal emergencies
■ Vascular disorders
■ Genitourinary disorders
■ Preoperative preparation
■ Conclusion

INTRODUCTION

The management of patients presenting with surgical emergencies relies upon rapid assessment, diagnosis and appropriate management to reduce morbidity and mortality. The emergency nurse may be the first person to assess the patient, and therefore finely tuned assessment skills are vital. Some of the physical examination skills described in this chapter will require both instruction in the technique and repeated practice. However, for patient assessment to be safe and thorough, the skills of inspection, palpation, auscultation and percussion should be utilised appropriately during patient consultations. This chapter will describe non-traumatic surgical emergencies of the abdominal and pelvic regions, according to the following classification: acute abdomen, vascular and genitourinary emergencies.

Anatomy and Physiology of the Abdomen

The abdomen can divided into sections by imaginary lines, a process which assists in identifying areas for examination. A vertical line can be drawn from the xiphoid process of the sternum to the symphysis pubis, and a horizontal line can be drawn across the abdomen through the umbilicus. This divides the abdomen into four segments or quadrants: right upper quadrant, right lower quadrant, left upper quadrant and left lower quadrant (Fig. 28.1).

Oesophagus

This muscular tube extends from the pharynx to the stomach. It is about 25 cm long and lies in front of the vertebral column and behind the trachea within the mediastinum. The oesophagus transports food

*The editors would like to thank Ruth Gower-Smith for her contribution to earlier drafts of this chapter.

Right upper quadrant

Right iobe of liver
Gallbladder
Pylorus
Duodenum
Head of pancreas
Upper right kidney

Left upper quadrant

Left lobe of liver
Spleen
Stomach
Left kidney
Body of pancreas
Splenic flexure of colon

Right lower quadrant

Lower right kidney
Cecum
Appendix
Ascending colon
Right fallopian tube (female)
Right ovary (female)
Right ureter
Bladder (distended)

Left lower quadrant

Descending colon
Sigmoid colon
Left fallopian tube (female)
Left ovary (female)
Left ureter
Bladder (distended)

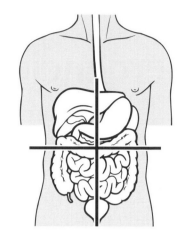

Figure 28.1 – *Abdominal contents.*

from the pharynx, and upper and lower oesophageal sphincters regulate the movement of food into and out of the oesophagus. Lubrication of the food is provided by mucous glands coating the inner surface of the oesophagus.

Stomach

The stomach is a 'J'-shaped organ lying under the diaphragm in the epigastric, umbilical and left hypochondrial regions of the abdomen. The most superior part of the stomach is called the fundus. The largest part is the body, which has a convex area laterally called the greater curvature and a concave area medially called the lesser curvature. The final part of the stomach is the pylorus which provides the opening into the first part of the small intestine.

The muscular coats of the stomach consist of three layers: a longitudinal outer layer, a middle circular layer and an inner oblique layer of muscle fibres. The lining mucosa of the stomach is arranged into folds called rugae. These folds allow the stomach to stretch, and they disappear as the stomach is filled. The cells in the stomach produce mucus, hydrochloric acid, intrinsic factor, regulatory hormones and pepsinogen, which is involved in protein digestion.

The small intestine

The small intestine is about 6 m in length and is composed of three parts: the duodenum, the jejunum and the ileum. The duodenum is about 25 cm long, the jejenum is 2.5 m long and the ileum is 3.5 m long. The

duodenum nearly completes a 180° arc which contains the head of the pancreas. The common bile duct from the liver and the pancreatic duct both empty into the duodenum. The surface area of the duodenum is greatly increased by tiny projections called villi, which are covered by columnar epithelium. The villi are about 1 mm high, and with around 10–40 mm^2, the surface area is greatly increased for absorption of nutrients. About 9 L of water enter the small intestine each day, most of which is reabsorbed, with only about 1 L reaching the large intestine. The jejunum and the ileum are similar in structure to the duodenum. The junction between the ileum and the large intestine is the ileocaecal sphincter which has a one-way valve.

The large intestine

The large intestine is responsible for the elimination of food residue and the maintenance of water and electrolyte balance. It consists of the caecum, colon, rectum and anal canal. The caecum is the first part of the large intestine and has a 9 cm long blind tube called the appendix attached. The colon is about 1.8 m long, consisting of ascending, transverse, descending and sigmoid colons. The lining of the large intestine contains many mucus-producing goblet cells and columnar cells which reabsorb water. About 1 L of water enters the large intestine each day, but only about 100 ml is lost in the faeces – the rest is reabsorbed. The circular muscle layer is complete, with an incomplete longitudinal layer of muscle. Contraction of this longitudinal layer gives the colon a pouched appearance called haustra. The rectum is a straight muscular tube running from the sigmoid colon to the anal canal. This canal is about 3 cm long and is the final part of the digestive tract.

Peritoneum

The abdominal cavity is lined by a serous membrane called the parietal peritoneum, with the organs being covered by the visceral layer of the peritoneum. There is a potential space between these two layers called the peritoneal cavity which contains serous fluid. A small amount of fluid in the peritoneal cavity allows the abdominal organs to move freely. The intestines are supported in the abdominal cavity by a fan-like structure of connective tissue called the mesentery. The mesentery connecting the lesser curvature of the stomach to the liver and diaphragm is called the lesser omentum. The greater omentum connects the greater curvature of the stomach to the transverse colon and the posterior abdominal wall. The greater omentum also covers the front of the abdominal organs. It contains a lot of adipose tissue and looks like a fatty apron hanging over the organs. If infection occurs in the peritoneum, the greater omentum tries to wall off the infection by surrounding it, to prevent its spread. The mesenteries contain blood and lymphatic vessels and nerves that supply the abdominal organs.

Abdominal organs which lie against the posterior abdominal wall have their anterior surface covered by peritoneum and are described as retroperitoneal organs. These are the duodenum, pancreas, ascending colon, rectum, kidneys, adrenal glands and the bladder.

Abdominal wall

The abdominal wall is composed of skin, fascia and four pairs of flat, sheet-like muscles called rectus abdominis, external and internal oblique and transverse abdominis. The linea alba is a tough, fibrous band of tissue which stretches from the sternum to the symphysis pubis and is made up of the aponeurosis of the abdominal muscles. Part of the external oblique muscle forms the inguinal ligament, which runs from the anterior superior iliac pubic tubercule. Just superior to the medial end of this ligament is the superficial inguinal ring which is the outer opening of the inguinal canal. This canal contains the spermatic cord and the ilio-inguinal nerve in males and the round ligament of the uterus and the ilio-inguinal nerve in females. The posterior abdominal wall is composed of the bones of the lumbar spine and the hip bones, along with the psoas, quadratus lumborum and iliacus muscles.

Nursing Assessment of the Acute Abdomen

The nurse should ensure before beginning this assessment that the airway, breathing and circulation have been assessed and appropriate interventions performed.

History

- What is the patient's main complaint?
- How does the patient describe associated symptoms?
- What is the duration?
- Previous medical history – has the patient suffered from diabetes, ischaemic heart disease, epilepsy, stroke, rheumatic fever, asthma or tuberculosis?
- Social history – occupation, family history, activity level
- Drug history – current medications, alcohol, tobacco, allergies, recent foreign travel.

To establish a full clinical picture, the nurse should also ask the patient about the following:

Appetite. This will be depressed in severe illness, and recent alterations in dietary habits should be noted. Does the patient avoid certain foods for any reason? Has there been any change in the patient's weight? Do the patient's clothes still fit? Is there any ascites?

Tongue. The state of the tongue gives some indication of the state of hydration of the body. If the patient has been ill for some time with a gastro-intestinal problem, frequently he will have a fluid and electrolyte deficit. A dry brown tongue may be found in any severe illness, uraemia or acute intestinal obstruction.

Skin. Is there any change in skin colour, bruising or itching? These may be signs of liver disease.

Bowel habits. Is there any constipation, diarrhoea, blood or mucus in the stool?

Energy. Are there any feelings of lethargy or changes in mental status?

Assessment of pain

Abdominal pain is due to:

- contraction of muscle tissue
- irritation of the mucosa
- stretching of an organ
- inflammation of the peritoneum
- irritation of nerves in the area.

The body is programmed to appreciate pain from areas under voluntary control and the skin. We are

---

Box 28.1 – *Assessing abdominal pain using mnemonic TROCARS*

T	Timing – duration of the pain
R	Radiation – does the pain go anywhere else?
O	Occurrence – when does the pain start?
C	Characteristics – colicky, sharp, dull
A	Aggravating factors – food, exercise
R	Relieving factors – rest, medicines
S	Site and Severity – location and pain score

Table 28.1 – *Hand examination*

Clinical finding	Cause
Pallor	Anaemia
Clubbing	Cirrhosis Crohn's disease Ulcerative colitis
Palmar erythema	Liver disease
Spoon-shaped nails	Iron deficiency

therefore not able to appreciate the precise location of the source of visceral pain. In pain originating in the heart, for example, impulses pass along the dermatomes of T_1–T_4, so the patient experiences pain across the chest and down the arms. Pain may therefore be referred to a site far from its origin; for instance, pain from the spleen may be referred to the left shoulder due to irritation of the phrenic nerve. There are several aspects to consider when assessing a patient's pain, which can be usefully remembered by the mnemonic TROCARS (see Box 28.1).

Examination

Begin the assessment of the gastrointestinal tract by examining the patient's hands to discover signs of disease (see Table 28.1). Next examine the patient's eyes for pale conjunctiva as this is indicative of anaemia. Enlarged lymph nodes may be found in the supraclavicular fossa, suggestive of secondaries from a gastric carcinoma.

The abdomen has to be relaxed during the examination and this will be facilitated if the patient has privacy, is given a full explanation of the procedure and is kept comfortable. The patient should be placed in a supine position with the head resting on a small pillow and the arms resting by the sides. In some cases the patient may be more comfortable with a small pillow under the knees, to help relax the abdominal muscles. Although it is necessary to expose the area from the sternum to the pelvis, the patient should be kept as warm as possible during the procedure, which should be performed quickly and efficiently. The patient should be examined from his right side, in a gentle manner, with warm hands. It is important when examining the abdomen that the patient's face is observed for any sign of discomfort (McGrath 1998).

Inspection

Look for any visible peristalsis and bruising, and note any visible pulsations. Pulsation of the abdominal aorta may be observed in thin patients or in those with an aortic aneurysm. The nurse should look for any scars, which may be recent (pink) or old (white). The location of operation scars may give clues as to the type of surgery previously performed. The abdomen is normally symmetrical, and may be asymmetrical due to bowel obstruction, hernia or spinal deformity. It is useful to try to visualise the underlying organs during the examination. For example, asymmetry of the lower abdomen may be due to a distended bladder, masses of the ovary, uterus or colon. Distended veins around the umbilicus signify portal hypertension. Generalised distension of the abdomen may be due to one of the five Fs:

- fat
- fluid
- faeces
- flatus
- fetus.

Gastric distension is also a complication seen in young children following head injury (Yates & Redmond 1985). The abdomen should move freely with respiration, but this will be diminished or absent in generalised peritonitis. Children are naturally abdominal breathers and therefore abdominal pain may alter their breathing pattern.

Auscultation

Following inspection, the abdomen should be auscultated for abdominal sounds. Experience can be gained by listening to many normal abdomens to establish a baseline. Initially, it is best to listen using the diaphragm of the stethoscope to the right of the umbilicus. Bowel sounds should be checked for at least 1 minute in all four quadrants, before declaring that they are absent. Absent bowel sounds are a feature of paralytic ileus, late obstruction and generalised peritonitis.

In an obstructed patient, the absence of bowel

sounds suggests strangulation or ischaemia. In small bowel obstruction the bowel sounds are exaggerated initially, with frequent low-pitched gurgles, rising to become high-pitched tinkling sounds as peristalsis increases above the obstruction. The presence of these sounds coincides with the peristalsis and the colicky abdominal pain suffered by the patient. In between these painful episodes, the bowel is quiet. The bowel is also hyperactive in gastroenteritis and severe diarrhoea.

Normally, blood flow along arteries cannot be heard using a stethoscope. However, when the vessel becomes diseased the resultant turbulence, as the blood flows over atheromatous plaques, produces soft high-pitched sounds called bruits. These bruits may be heard using the bell of the stethoscope over a diseased aorta and renal, hepatic, splenic or femoral vessels. Check the aorta by listening in the mid-epigastric region above the umbilicus. Renal bruits may be heard in this area, and additionally in the flanks or posteriorly over the kidneys. Femoral bruits may be heard in the groin. Bruits are heard even if the patient changes position.

Percussion

Light percussion is performed to determine the presence of masses, enlargement of an organ or abdominal distension. The middle finger of the left hand is placed on the area to be percussed, and the back of its middle phalanx is struck with the tip of the middle finger of the right hand. The percussing finger should be bent, so that when the blow is delivered, its terminal phalanx is at right angles to the metacarpal bone it is striking. Tympany is the normal percussion note and is a hollow resonant sound heard over the abdomen, apart from over the solid organs. Dull percussion notes will be heard over dense organs such as the liver and spleen, tumours or over a fluid-filled bladder.

Palpation

If the patient is not relaxed, the abdominal muscles will tense, making examination impossible. Start far away from the area where the pain is being experienced. Using a warm hand flat on the abdominal wall, gently palpate all four quadrants. Palpation of specific organs requires practice, and further description is beyond the scope of this chapter. When pain is found, test for rebound tenderness by pressing the examining hand gently and slowly into the abdomen; sudden release of the pressure produces pain. Ask the patient where the pain was felt, as it may be far removed from where the pressure was applied. Rebound tenderness is a feature of an inflamed appendix and peritonitis. Check for the presence and equality of the femoral pulses, and assess the femoral and inguinal lymph nodes for tenderness or enlargement.

Vomit

The strongest stimuli for vomiting are irritation and distension of the stomach. Nerve impulses are transmitted to the medulla, and returning impulses to the upper gastrointestinal organs, diaphragm and abdominal muscles. The stomach is then squeezed between the diaphragm and the abdominal muscles. Prolonged vomiting will lead to loss of gastric juice and fluid. This can lead to disturbance in fluid and acid–base balance. If bleeding is severe, the vomit may look like pure blood or it may be dark with clots. Bleeding may be altered to a dark brown or black colour by gastric juice. The dark colour is due to the conversion of haemoglobin into haematin. The altered blood is sometimes compared to 'coffee grounds'. Blood in vomit may have been swallowed from mouth injuries or epistaxis. Vomit may have a faecal odour in advanced intestinal obstruction.

Faeces

Black stools may be due to the presence of blood or iron. Bleeding high in the intestinal tract produces offensive 'tarry' stools. If bleeding is from the large intestine, the blood may be less mixed with the faeces and may be seen as streaks. Stools may be pale in obstructive jaundice, diarrhoea or malabsorption.

Shock

Shock is a condition which results from inadequate blood supply to the tissues, leading to a decreased supply of oxygen and other nutrients, which are essential to maintain the metabolic needs of the body. Without oxygen, the cells shift from aerobic to anaerobic metabolism. Anaerobic metabolism is a less efficient method of extracting energy, and the cells begin to use up their stores of adenosine triphosphate (ATP) faster than they can be replaced. This disturbs the cell electrolyte balance, causing sodium to be retained and potassium lost. Excessive sodium in the cell means that it becomes waterlogged. This immediately affects the cells of the nervous system and myocardium leading to depression of their function. The water that leaks into the cells is coming from the interstitial space and will be replaced from the intravascular space, causing further hypovolaemia. Anaerobic metabolism produces large quantities of acid. This increase is detected by the brain, which increases the respiratory rate to reduce the carbon dioxide level and correct the imbalance.

As the supply of oxygen and nutrients fails to meet the demand, the body responds by activating compensatory mechanisms to improve perfusion to the vital organs. As the blood volume decreases, the peripheral blood vessels constrict due to sympathetic stimulation, which increases peripheral resistance and raises the blood pressure. As a result the patient looks pale and has cold clammy skin. As perfusion of the vital centres in the brain is reduced, the patient becomes anxious and restless.

The increase in peripheral resistance may be detected clinically by a *rise* in the diastolic blood pressure. Eventually as the body loses the battle, the systolic pressure will begin to fall. Reduced blood flow to the kidney, because it is not a vital organ as far as the body is concerned, causes the release of certain chemicals which increase sodium retention, increase water retention and increase vasoconstriction. The release of adrenaline causes glycogen to be broken down to supply the additional glucose needed; increased blood sugar levels may be noticed in these patients.

The management of the patient who has lost blood or body fluids is the most important aspect of dealing with surgical emergencies. It is vital that the condition is recognised and treated promptly to reduce both morbidity and mortality. The management of the patient with haemorrhage may be surgical, or in certain cases conservative. In assessing these patients, trends are noted in their vital signs such as pulse, respiratory rate and blood pressure. It is appropriate to measure these regularly, perhaps every 15 minutes initially and decreasing later as the patient's condition becomes more stable. Accurate measurement of intake as well as losses of body fluids such as vomit, are important in the management of the patient's fluid balance. One of the best indicators of perfusion is to measure urinary output hourly – approximately 1 ml/kg per hour is indicative of effective circulating volume.

Management principles

It is important to provide emotional support for the patient, since fear and anxiety can aggravate the condition.

- Administer oxygen via a non-rebreather mask at 12–15 L/min.
- Initiate intravenous fluid replacement. Two large-bore cannulae, 14 or 16 gauge, should be placed in the antecubital fossa and well secured to provide an adequate flow rate. Either crystalloid (normal saline 0.9% or Hartmann's solution) or colloid (Haemaccel or Gelofusine) may be ordered. An initial bolus of 1–2 L may be given to an adult patient as rapidly as possible. It is important to assess the patient's response to this bolus by rechecking vital signs. The rate of flow is usually slowed as the blood pressure increases: too rapid an increase in blood pressure can cause further bleeding. When the intravenous cannulae are inserted, blood should be taken for typing and cross-match. Patients who do not adequately respond to the fluid bolus are likely to require blood transfusion. In extreme emergencies it may be necessary to give the patient O-negative blood (universal donor), while awaiting type-specific blood. Fluids may be given rapidly using a pressure device, but should be warmed to prevent inducing hypothermia. Hypothermia results in decreased tissue extraction of oxygen from haemoglobin and impaired cardiac contract. Hypothermia also causes problems with blood clotting due to disruption of cellular enzymes and platelets, and increased fibrinolysis.
- Provide prescribed analgesia.
- Prepare the patient for surgery.
- The patient may be positioned with the legs slightly elevated to increase venous return to the heart and so increase blood pressure.
- Gastric distension can lead to vomiting; inserting a gastric tube will allow decompression of the stomach and provide a sample for testing.
- Inserting a urinary catheter will allow accurate fluid balance and provide evidence of successful fluid volume replacement.
- Monitor the temperature to determine hypothermia, or pyrexia due to infection.

Acute Abdominal Emergencies

Bowel obstruction

Obstruction to the passage of contents may occur in the small or large bowel and is a serious life-threatening condition. Obstruction of the small bowel is more common because the ileum is the narrowest segment, and therefore more easily obstructed. Obstruction of the large bowel tends to develop more slowly. The most common cause of small bowel obstruction is postoperative adhesions, with hernias being the second most common cause. Adhesions are bands of scar tissue following inflammation which can constrict the intestine. Other causes of bowel obstruction are:

- *volvulus* – twisting of bowel more common in the elderly
- *intussusception* – segment of intestine prolapsed into an adjacent part, usually in infants
- *mesenteric embolus* – interferes with blood supply, foreign bodies (drug smugglers swallowing packages), faecal impaction, tumours
- *paralytic ileus* – peristalsis may be interrupted by disturbance of the nerve supply following peritonitis, pancreatitis, shock, spinal cord lesions, or after abdominal surgery.

Pathophysiology

Obstruction of the bowel causes fluid, gas and air to collect near the obstruction site. The bowel tries to force its contents past the obstruction by increasing peristalsis. This causes damage to the intestinal mucosa, which results in further swelling at the site. This increased pressure exceeds venous and capillary pressure, causing reduced blood supply to the bowel. As the bowel wall swells, instead of performing its normal function in this area, it starts to secrete water, sodium and potassium, leading to dehydration. Gas-forming bacteria collect in the area and aggravate distension by fermentation, which produces more gas. If untreated, the interruption of the blood supply to the bowel will lead to gangrene, perforation of the bowel and peritonitis. patients who develop septicaemia in these cases have a 70% mortality rate (Emmans 1993).

Assessment

Obstruction of the small bowel is commonly associated with sudden onset of colicky abdominal pain radiating over the whole abdomen. Appendicitis is characterised by a dull pain in the right lower quadrant, accompanied by an elevated temperature. The pain of pancreatitis is constant, not colicky, and the pain of diverticulitis usually occurs in the left lower quadrant and may be accompanied by blood in the faeces (Clemings *et al.* 1990). In large bowel obstruction, the pain has a more gradual onset.

In small bowel obstruction there is vomiting of gastric juice, mucus and bile in high obstructions. If the obstruction is in the ileum or large bowel, the patient may vomit faecal contents. This loss of fluid by vomiting and increased intestinal secretion leads to severe dehydration and electrolyte imbalance. The extravasation of plasma from the capillaries adds to the accumulation of fluid in the intestines, which compresses the veins, reducing venous return and contributing to the shock.

The patient will display the classic features of shock as previously described: rapid weak pulse, restlessness, low blood pressure and cold, clammy skin. There is constipation and no flatus is passed. The patient suffers abdominal distension due to the accumulation of gas and fluids, with active tinkling bowel sounds initially, progressing to absent bowel sounds as peristalsis diminishes. The stretched weakened intestinal wall becomes permeable to organisms and perforation of the bowel may lead to peritonitis. Obstruction of the large bowel is less acute with complete constipation (obstipation) and slowly developing distension. The pain is described as colicky, with vomiting and dehydration occurring later.

Investigations

Blood should be sent for full blood count, electrolytes, amylase, glucose and cross-match. Radiographs may reveal bowel distortion and distension, with air or fluid levels. In small bowel obstruction, a central gas shadow may be seen, with no air in the large bowel. In large bowel obstruction, gas can be seen proximal to the blockage but not distal to it.

Management

The most life-threatening problem for this patient is fluid volume deficit and therefore the initial priorities are to treat the shock due to the hypovolaemia and to prevent further complications. Give the patient 100% oxygen via a non-rebreather mask at 12–15 L/min. Initiate large-bore intravenous infusions, using crystalloids such as normal saline. Do not give anything orally, and insert a gastric tube to decompress the stomach as fluid shifts can be more severe as the bowel becomes decompressed. Accurate recording of fluid balance and vital signs is essential. Assist the patient into a comfortable position, and give prescribed analgesia and antibiotics, which reduce the risk of sepsis if the bowel perforates.

In less urgent cases of large bowel obstruction, the patient may be given an enema to attempt to clear the obstruction. Intestinal obstruction other than paralytic ileus is treated surgically. In some cases, it may be possible to delay surgery to improve the patient's general condition, but if there is evidence of compromised blood supply to the intestines, emergency surgery is indicated. If the bowel is strangulated or if there is gross distension, surgery should take place within 1 hour to avoid perforation.

The extent of the surgery required will depend upon the cause of the obstruction. Simple adhesions may be divided, but if the blood supply to the bowel has been interrupted, the bowel is checked for viability and, if gangrenous, will require resection with anastomosis or a stoma. Stomas may be temporary or permanent. Paralytic ileus is commonly seen post-operatively and is treated conservatively with a gastric tube to drain secretions and reduce distension. Intravenous fluids will correct electrolyte deficiencies, and the condition usually resolves gradually.

Peritonitis

This is a life-threatening condition due to inflammation of the visceral and parietal peritoneum. This follows perforation of an abdominal organ, causing leakage into the normally sterile peritoneal cavity. This chemical and bacterial invasion causes an inflammatory response, with depressed intestinal motility and distension of the bowel with gas and fluid.

Pathophysiology

The peritoneal cavity is a closed sac, which normally contains a little fluid to allow the abdominal organs to move freely. The great omentum is a sheet of peritoneum which is reflected off the stomach and hangs down in front of the intestines like a curtain. If peritonitis occurs, the great omentum tries to wall off the infection by surrounding it, to prevent spread of infection. Peritonitis may follow ruptured appendix, ruptured diverticuli or penetrating abdominal trauma.

Assessment

The patient usually lies very still and looks unwell. There is a sudden onset of severe abdominal pain which may initially be localised, but as time passes and more of the peritoneum becomes involved, the pain becomes more generalised. The abdomen is distended, rigid like a board and there is rebound tenderness, with absent bowel sounds. Signs of shock may be present (tachycardia, pallor, sweating, low blood pressure), along with pyrexia, nausea and vomiting. Respirations may be shallow due to interference by extreme abdominal distension. The peritoneal membrane becomes oedematous, with loss of protein and electrolyte fluid into the peritoneal cavity aggravating the shock.

Investigations

Radiographs may show distension of both small and large bowels, or air under the diaphragm. As little as 20 ml of air will produce a gas shadow between the liver and the diaphragm (Wilson & Flowers 1985). Blood should be sent for full blood count, glucose, electrolytes, amylase (to exclude pancreatitis), gases and cross-match.

Management

Give the patient 100% oxygen via a non-rebreather mask, at 12–15 L/min. Insert two large-bore intravenous cannulae and give intravenous fluids to treat the hypovolaemia. Do not give anything orally, and insert a gastric tube to decompress the stomach. Blood transfusion may be given to treat shock and replace the protein lost in the inflammatory response in the peritoneum. Provide prescribed analgesia and treat the infection with i.v. antibiotics. The patient may require surgery to seal off the source of the leak or to resect the affected area. The patient's history may require the perforation to be treated conservatively, using gastric suction, antibiotics, analgesics and i.v. fluids.

Appendicitis

This is a common cause of acute abdominal pain and is the commonest surgical emergency. It is more common in children, adolescents and young adults. Early diagnosis prevents complications. Several factors are claimed to predispose the patient to appendicitis, including:

- faecoliths – hard pellets of faeces
- food residues
- enlargement of lymphoid tissue in response to a viral infection in children.

All of these causes will lead to blockage of the appendix, allowing secretions to collect.

Pathophysiology

The appendix is a narrow blind tube which is attached to the inferior part of the caecum. It has no special function, and if diseased it can be removed. Inflammation begins in the mucosa after a breach in the epithelium, allowing the entry of bowel bacteria. The appendix is a blind tube, and if secretions cannot pass the obstruction they will accumulate, causing enlargement and pain. The resulting infection leads to ulceration of the mucosa, which eventually spreads causing peritonitis. Inflammation can cause the greater omentum to become adherent to the appendix in an attempt to wall off the infection. If the area has time to be walled off and the appendix then ruptures, an abscess will form. However, the build-up of pressure within the wall can lead to the distal part of the appendix becoming gangrenous and perforating, causing generalised peritonitis, before it has time to be walled off.

Assessment

The patient complains of dull abdominal pain, which may initially be centred around the umbilicus or mid-epigastric region The pain is described as steady, persistent or constant by the patient. As the inflammation spreads through the walls of the appendix, involving the parietal peritoneum, it becomes confined to the right lower quadrant. The pain is not usually described as stabbing or colicky in nature (Bourg *et al.* 1986). This classic presentation is found in 70% of patients (Norton & Abernathy 1993). Pain is aggravated by coughing, and on rectal examination there is increased pain on the right side. There may be rebound tenderness in the right lower quadrant, although rebound tenderness in other areas suggests that the appendix has perforated and caused peritonitis. There is also nausea, anorexia, vomiting and a low-grade pyrexia of 38–39°C. The patient will try to avoid sudden movements, which increase the pain, and may keep the right thigh flexed to provide pain relief.

The pain of appendicitis may be demonstrated by the following signs:

■ McBurney's point – tenderness on palpation in an area about 2 inches from the anterior superior iliac spine on a line with the umbilicus
■ Aaron's sign – pain or distress in the area of the heart or stomach when McBurney's point is palpated
■ Rovsing's sign – pain in the right lower quadrant, when the left lower quadrant is palpated
■ Psoas sign – increased pain in the abdomen when the right thigh is flexed up towards it.

Investigations

Blood should be sent for full blood count which may reveal a leucocytosis. Leucocyte count is raised above 10 000 in 90% of cases. Other blood tests may include glucose, amylase (to exclude pancreatitis) and electrolytes. Females with lower abdominal pain should always have their beta human chorionic gonadotrophin (B-HCG) checked, to help exclude ectopic pregnancy. A urine specimen may help to exclude urinary tract infection or urinary calculi as a cause of the pain. Abdominal radiographs are rarely necessary, but may help to exclude bowel obstruction or perforation.

Differential diagnosis

Adults

■ Right-sided lobar pneumonia or pleurisy
■ Perforated ulcer
■ Acute cholecystitis
■ Intestinal obstruction
■ Gastroenteritis
■ Acute salpingitis.

Children

■ Mesenteric adenitis
■ Gastroenteritis
■ Intussusception
■ Meckel's diverticulum.

Management

Initiate intravenous fluids to rehydrate the patient, but do not give anything orally. Provide prescribed analgesia. Preoperative antibiotics can decrease the rate of wound infections in patients with a gangrenous appendix from 30% to 8%. They also decrease the rate of wound infections in acute appendicitis from 7% to 2% (Norton & Abernathy 1993). If the condition is still located within the appendix, and it has not perforated, an appendectomy is performed. If it has progressed to peritonitis, the patient may be managed conservatively with antibiotics and intravenous fluids. Surgery can be arranged at a later stage to remove the appendix.

The appendix may be removed by open appendectomy or laproscopic appendectomy. The laproscope is particularly useful in young women to allow widespread visualisation of the abdomen and pelvis. This allows differentiation of appendicitis from gynaecological disease with minimally invasive surgery. The laproscope also reduces hospital stay by decreasing postoperative ileus because the tissues are handled less. There are fewer adhesions and there is less scarring from smaller incisions.

Vascular Disorders

Oesophageal varices

These refer to the localised dilation of veins in the lower oesophagus, due to the impairment of portal blood flow through the liver.

Pathophysiology

In patients suffering from cirrhosis of the liver, the blood flow from the portal vein meets resistance in the damaged organ. This increased resistance causes

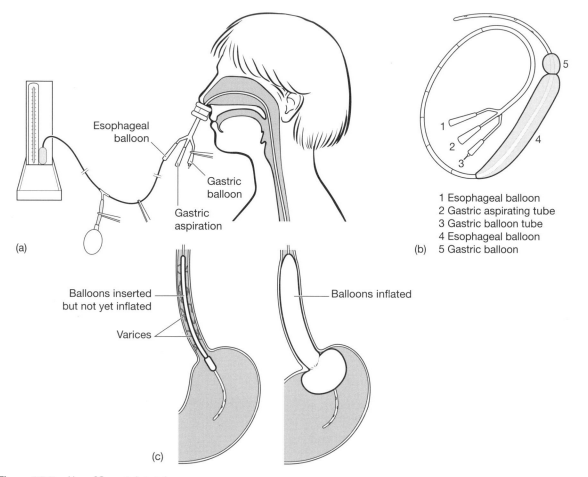

Figure 28.2 – *Use of Sengstaken tube.*

back pressure into the veins that normally empty into the portal system. The veins most affected are those at the lower end of the oesophagus. The veins become weak and varicosed, lifting the mucosa so that they protrude into the oesophagus, where they can be damaged by passing food, coughing, vomiting or straining. Patients with liver disease may also have abnormal blood clotting, which exacerbates the problem. Bleeding from these veins can be both dramatic and fatal; because of the high pressure within the vascular bed, hypovolaemia occurs quickly

Assessment

The patient may have a history of alcohol abuse and ascites, without abdominal pain. Painless haematemesis is suggestive of varices. Haematemesis following peptic ulceration may cause significant vomiting of bright red blood, but is usually accompanied by abdominal pain. In bleeding there

may be a dramatic haematemesis, occasionally preceded by feelings of dizziness, as the bleeding into the stomach causes the blood pressure to fall. There may be a history of previous episodes. Features of portal hypertension are splenomegaly and ascites. Some of the blood will pass through the intestinal tract and will appear later as melaena. Patients with portal hypertension may be asymptomatic until they suddenly suffer catastrophic haemorrhage.

Investigations

Full blood count, electrolytes, glucose, gases, clotting factors and liver function tests should be requested.

Management

This is a life-threatening condition with the patient requiring prompt emergency treatment. These patients often require aggressive resuscitation. There is a 40–70% mortality rate with the first bleed. Ensure that there are adequate receivers and working suction to hand, as bleeding can be sudden and profuse. In massive haemorrhage, the patient may lose consciousness and therefore airway clearance will be a priority. Provide 100% oxygen via a non-rebreather mask at 12–15 L/min. Establish at least two large-bore intravenous lines and be prepared to give large quantities of warmed fluid. A cannula may be inserted into a central vein to monitor the central venous pressure as a guide to fluid replacement. Immediately cross-match at least six units of blood (O-negative can be used initially). The patient and relatives will require a lot of emotional support.

Insert a urinary catheter and maintain accurate fluid balance records. A Sengstaken triple-lumen tube may be inserted orally to apply pressure to the bleeding veins and to allow aspiration from the stomach and upper oesophagus (see Fig. 28.2). Digestion of blood in the intestine produces nitrogenous wastes which, when absorbed, predispose the patient to hepatic coma. If time permits, the tube may be chilled prior to insertion. This makes the tube more rigid and aids insertion. Insertion of the tube is a fairly unpleasant procedure for the patient, and it may remain in position for up to 12 hours. Leaving the tube in for longer than this can cause oedema, ulceration and perforation. Inflation of the oesophageal balloon will make swallowing difficult for the patient, and suction may be required. Suction should be available before, during and after removal of the tube.

The nurse should maintain a vigilant assessment of the patient's respiratory status after the tube has been inserted. If signs of respiratory distress or obstruction develop, the nurse should immediately cut away the valves from the end of the tube and remove it (Cooper 1988). Care should be taken to ensure that the correct balloons are inflated and deflated. Inadequate inflation will be ineffective at controlling bleeding, while excessive pressures will cause tissue damage. The doctor may order deflation of the balloon at regular intervals to reduce the risk of tissue ischaemia. Regularly monitor the patient's vital signs and fluid balance. Gastric aspirate should gradually decrease, and the doctor may order lavage of the stomach with ice water to induce vasoconstriction.

Vasopressin

This may be given to produce arterial vasoconstriction, which will reduce the amount of blood entering the portal system. Twenty units of vasopressin in 200 ml of 5% dextrose may be given over 15 minutes via the central line to induce vasoconstriction. This is successful in 80% of patients (Kumar & Clark 1994).

Vasopressin may also be injected directly into the superior mesenteric artery with the assistance of angiography.

Endoscopic sclerotherapy

In this technique a coagulating substance is injected into the varices which seals the bleeding veins by coagulation and is the primary method of treatment. The patient will require repeated treatments at regular intervals for a few years.

Percutaneous transhepatic portal vein embolisation

This may be done under X-ray control to insert embolic material directly into the blood vessels. Emergency surgery carries considerable risk and it is preferable to stabilise the patient's condition and undertake surgery when bleeding is controlled. Various options are available:

- a portacaval shunt – this makes an anastomosis between the portal vein and the inferior vena cava
- a splenorenal shunt
- a mesocaval shunt between the superior mesenteric vein and the inferior vena cava
- a transoesophageal ligation of the bleeding vessels.

Surgery will reduce the risk of further ruptured varices, but will not resolve the underlying liver disease. Other procedures involve oesophageal transection and anastomosis, or ligation of bleeding veins. In patients with oesophageal varices, there is a 60–80% recurrence over 2 years, with 20% mortality during each further episode of bleeding.

Aortic aneurysm

An aneurysm is a localised dilation of a blood vessel which has been weakened by atheroma. The commonest site for aneurysms is the aorta, although they can occur elsewhere.

Pathophysiology

The largest diameter arteries, such as the aorta, have a greater proportion of elastic tissue and a smaller proportion of smooth muscle compared with other arteries. Elastic arteries are stretched when the ventricles of the heart pump blood into them. The elastic recoil prevents blood pressure from falling rapidly and maintains blood flow while the ventricles are relaxed. As the arteries become smaller, they undergo a gradual transition from having walls containing more elastic tissue than smooth muscle to having walls with more smooth muscle than elastic tissue. This allows these arteries (radial, brachial etc.) to have a greater degree of vasoconstriction and vaso-dilation, allowing them to alter blood flow according to local demands.

Arteries are composed of three layers. From the inside to the outer wall the layers are:

■ *tunica intima* – an endothelium composed of simple squamous cells and a small amount of connective tissue
■ *tunica media* – the middle layer consists of smooth muscle arranged circularly around the blood vessel
■ *tunica adventitia* – composed of connective tissue.

The walls of the arteries undergo changes as they age, mainly in the large elastic arteries such as the aorta, coronary arteries serving the heart and carotid arteries serving the brain. Atherosclerosis refers to the deposition of material in the walls of arteries to form plaques. This fatty material contains cholesterol and may be replaced by connective tissue and calcium deposits. Atherosclerosis increases resistance to blood flow, as the deposits reduce the internal diameter of the arteries. The rough plaques attract passing plate-lets, which adhere to them increasing the chances of thrombus formation. As the tunica media becomes weakened, the wall of the aorta begins to bulge.

The aneurysm may form a sac or it may separate through the layers of the vessel, called a dissecting aneurysm, without a visible dilation (see Fig. 28.3). Dissecting aneurysms can spread for some distance along the aorta and affect other organs, such as the kidneys. Aneurysms can also send off emboli to distant sites. If the aneurysm ruptures, the sudden loss of blood will almost always prove fatal.

Assessment

Abdominal aortic aneurysms tend to affect middle-aged to elderly people. There may be a history of atherosclerosis and the patient may have suffered a previous myocardial infarction or stroke or may have peripheral vascular disease. If the aneurysm is pressing on other structures, there may be abdominal pain radiating to the back or groin. There may be few initial indications that the patient has an aneurysm, until it is large and causes pressure on other struc-tures, or it starts to leak. The immediate problem is of sudden abdominal pain and collapse. Patients with a dissecting aneurysm may complain of a sudden tearing or ripping pain. There is no history of hae-matemesis, which tends to exclude oesophageal varices or perforated ulcer.

The patient has signs of hypovolaemic shock, pale, cold, clammy skin and rapid respirations. The blood pressure may be low with an accompanying tachy-cardia. Physical examination may reveal a pulsatile mass in the centre of the abdomen, and in extreme cases pulsation may be visible. A pulsatile mass can be found in 80–90% of patients (Drake 1993). The patient's femoral pulses may be weak or absent. Impaired blood supply to a limb can be assessed by its lower skin temperature. The skin of the foot may be cold, pale or cyanosed and capillary refill after blanching with light finger pressure may be delayed.

Differential diagnosis

■ Pancreatitis
■ Renal colic
■ Biliary disease
■ Musculoskeletal back pain.

Investigations

Blood should be cross-matched urgently – initially at least 10 units in anticipation of surgery. Also request full blood count, amylase, glucose, gases and clotting studies. Further investigations should be tailored to the clinical condition of the patient. Chest and abdominal X-rays waste time in unstable patients who need to go to theatre. Ultrasound can be performed in the emergency department, allowing continual monitoring of the patient in a controlled environment. CT scan is time-consuming and involves moving the patient to the X-ray department. Angiography provides very detailed information and is best reserved for stable patients.

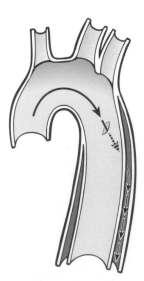

Figure 28.3 – *Dissecting aortic aneurysm.*

Management

A senior surgeon should be involved early in the care of these patients, and in unstable patients limited investigations should be undertaken prior to surgery. Provide 100% oxygen via a non-rebreather mask at 12–15 L/min. Initiating large-bore intravenous access with 14 gauge cannulae and controlled fluid resuscitation is critical for a patient with an aneurysm.

The patient's blood pressure should be maintained at 100–120 mmHg to decrease the pressure of ventricular systole against the fragile aorta. Attempting to increase blood pressure beyond this range may rupture the aneurysm, with fatal consequences for the patient (Kitt 1990, Page 1988). Fluids should be warmed to prevent hypothermia and coagulopathy. Regularly monitor the patient's fluid balance and vital signs, including cardiac monitoring and pulse oximetry. Analgesia can be given intravenously and titrated according to the patient's response, without adversely affecting blood pressure. Antibiotics may be prescribed to reduce postoperative infection. Surgery may involve a trouser graft being inserted to replace the diseased aorta. There is a 21–70% mortality among treated patients, and 100% mortality in untreated patients.

Arterial embolism

Occlusion of an artery may follow external compression, thrombosis or embolism. This deprives the tissues of vital blood supply. An embolus is a mass of material which can lodge in a blood vessel, occluding the lumen and obstructing the blood flow. This may have been introduced from outside the body or it may have arisen from within. Most often it is a thrombus which has become dislodged from the wall of a blood vessel.

Pathophysiology

Emboli travel along blood vessels until they reach a point where the vessel diameter stops them from going any further. The effect on the tissue supplied by that vessel depends upon the presence of collateral circulation to that area. The most common emboli are derived from thrombi in the circulatory system. Thrombi can develop in peripheral blood vessels due to atheroma, aortic aneurysms or trauma. Thrombi in the arterial system can form within the heart on areas of dead myocardium, where the circulating platelets are exposed to the rough collagen, thus encouraging clot formation. Atrial fibrillation causes blood to stagnate in the heart, allowing thrombi to form.

Emboli from the right side of the heart or the veins cause pulmonary embolism, while emboli from the left side can travel to the brain, viscera or limbs.

If the occlusion has been gradual, collateral circulation will have developed, so that blood is able to flow around the occlusion. However, if the occlusion is sudden, there will be no collateral vessels, and blood flow will stop at the occlusion. The resulting ischaemia may cause necrosis, gangrene and loss of the limb if circulation is not restored quickly. In the case of the abdominal organs, death of a small part of the kidney will leave a scar, whereas death of a small area of the bowel will lead to perforation and peritonitis. Thromboses tend to occur in association with atheroma at areas of turbulent blood flow, such as at the bifurcation of arteries.

Assessment

The limb may feel cold to the touch compared with the other limb, and the skin may appear pale or cyanosed. Peripheral pulses below the obstruction disappear. In the lower limb, the following peripheral pulse sites may be assessed: femoral popliteal, posterior tibial and dorsalis pedis.

The likely findings can be remembered as the six Ps:

- *pain* – this may be sudden and severe in embolic episodes, or occur over several hours in the case of thrombosis; it is aggravated by flexion and extension of the limb
- *pulseless* – with decreased or absent capillary refill, this is a very late sign
- *pallor* – the limb will look pale
- *paraesthesia* – the patient may complain of tingling sensations in the limb
- *perishing cold* – the limb feels cold to the touch
- *paralysis* – there is loss of function due to the decreased blood supply to the nerves and muscles.

Investigations

Blood should be sent for full blood count, electrolytes, glucose and clotting studies (as a baseline prior to treatment). Assess blood flow in the limb using Doppler or angiography. ECG and chest X-ray are also required.

Management

Provide 100% oxygen via a non-rebreather mask at 12–15 L/min. Establish intravenous access in the unaffected limb. Keep the limb warm and in a dependent position to encourage vasodilation. Carry out regular monitoring of vital signs and distal pulses in the affected limb, as well as cardiac monitoring and pulse oximetry in the normal limb. Provide prescribed analgesia; anticoagulants may also be prescribed, such as heparin 15 000 units every 12 hours.

Surgery should be undertaken as soon as possible, and is most effective within 6–12 hours of occlusion. Embolectomy can be done using local or general anaesthesia. In some cases, more advanced surgery requiring patch grafting of the blood vessels may be required. In the case of arterial reconstruction, the percentages of limbs saved in survivors are 80% in femoropopliteal bypass grafts and 60% in femorotibial bypass grafts (Hope 1993).

Genitourinary Disorders

Retention of urine

Pathophysiology

The urethra exists the bladder inferiorly and anteriorly near the entrance of the two ureters. The ureters and bladder are lined with transitional epithelium which is specialised to stretch as the volume of urine increases. The walls of the ureter and bladder have smooth muscle, and waves of muscle contraction propel the urine along from the kidneys to the bladder. Contraction of muscle in the bladder will force urine to flow along the urethra to exit the body.

At the junction of the urethra and bladder, the smooth muscle of the bladder forms the internal sphincter. The external sphincter is skeletal muscle surrounding the urethra as it extends through the pelvic floor. These sphincters regulate the flow of urine through the urethra. Enlargement of the gland causes stretching and distortion of the urethra, which obstructs the bladder outflow. The bladder muscle enlarges in an attempt to overcome the obstruction, causing high pressures to be generated. Eventually the bladder becomes dilated and the muscle hypotonic.

Assessment

Urinary retention may be acute or chronic. Urinary retention may develop in males with previous symptoms of prostatic obstruction (hesitancy, poor stream, dribbling). Benign prostatic enlargement occurs most often in men over the age of 60 years. Retention may be precipitated by constipation, 'holding on too long', infection, neurological disease or postoperatively. Chronic retention is relatively painless, and although the bladder is distended it is not tender because the distension is more gradual. There

may be a history of frequency, with overflow incontinence usually at night. The patient may present with severe lower abdominal pain or discomfort, a palpable distended bladder, and feeling the need to pass urine but unable to do so. The nurse should consider the last time of voiding, intake and output and relevant history. In addition, vital signs to establish a baseline should be checked.

Investigations

Urine, when available, should be taken for culture and routine analysis. Blood should be sent for full blood count, electrolytes and acid phosphatase (a marker of disease activity). Further investigations will be arranged at a later time (ultrasound, urine flow rates etc.).

Management

Patients with retention of urine can be quite distressed and will need reassurance. It may be possible to overcome the retention by ensuring privacy for the patient and altering his position if possible. Warm baths and letting the patient listen to running water may help; however, in a number of cases the patient will require catheterisation, by either the transurethral or suprapubic method.

If retention has been acute, not more than 1000 ml of urine should be drained initially, and then 300 ml each hour until the bladder is empty (Royle & Walsh 1992). Sudden decompression of the bladder can result in an inflow of blood to the area and some capillary bleeding. The sudden emptying of an overdistended bladder can result in an atonic bladder wall. The suprapubic route may be chosen when there is trauma to the urethra or when it has proved impossible to pass a urethral catheter. It is a surgical procedure and, in common with urethral catherisation, requires aseptic technique. It may be performed under local or general anaesthesia. The catheter is sutured in place and taped to the abdomen to reduce traction on the tube.

Urinary catheters

Although urinary catheterisation is seen as a last resort for urinary retention, it remains a common procedure for short-, medium- and long-term management. The urethra may become inflamed in response to the materials used in the manufacture of the catheter. This risk increases as the catheter is left in over several weeks. Latex catheters are particularly irritant, plastic catheters cause less reaction, and silicone virtually no reaction. Silicone permits gas diffusion and these catheters tend to have problems with balloon deflation over time, but they are inert causing less irritation and seldom encrusting.

Blockage of the catheter by debris within the urine is particularly common in those with a urinary tract infection who are catheterised (Srinvasan & Clark 1972). Encrustation of the catheter will reduce the rate of urine flow through it and may eventually obstruct it completely (Bruce *et al.* 1974). Most catheters will become encrusted to some extent, although some materials may lessen the incidence.

Bypassing of urine around the catheter can be an alarming and distressing experience for the patient. Patients with larger catheters tend to experience more bypassing problems than those with smaller catheters (Britton & Wright 1992). Catheters with smaller balloons allow the catheter tip to sit lower in the bladder, leaving less residual urine. The use of large catheters with large balloons apart from irritating the bladder, may cause pressure on the bladder neck and lead to necrosis, particularly if they are not secured to relieve traction (McGill 1982). The main rule, therefore, is to choose the smallest catheter that will drain adequately, i.e. 12, 14 or 16 Ch, and if there is heavy haematuria, perhaps a size 18 Ch may be required. It may be concluded that where bypassing is a problem, inserting larger catheters or adding water to the balloon is not the solution; in fact it is likely to irritate the bladder further. It is not necessary to try to occlude the urethra by using a large catheter. The urethral folds will normally close upon themselves. There should be enough space around the catheter for the paraurethral glands to drain freely. Large catheters will obstruct these glands, leading to abscess and stricture formation (Blandy & Moors 1981).

Discharge advice

Adequate provision for the discharge of patients from emergency departments is recognised as a priority for all those concerned with the quality of care offered to patients. There is evidence of a distinct lack of communication between members of the multidisciplinary team and patients regarding discharge arrangements. More recent evidence suggests that discharge planning is still not a high priority (Ferguson 1997, 1998).

Although patients with retention of urine may have previous experience of catheter insertion, it is vital that the nurse ensures adequate after-care arrangements. It is sometimes assumed that patients do not ask questions because they know all the answers! Do not assume that the patient has received adequate education in the management of his condition. The nurse should ensure that the patient, and in certain cases the carers, understands the importance of adequate fluid intake to sustain the urine output and hydration, as well as the routine care of the catheter. Patients should have some point of contact in the community if they experience problems.

Torsion of the testis

Torsion of the spermatic cord involves twisting of the testis and epididymis on their axis. It is important to recognise the condition early and to treat it as a surgical emergency to save the testis.

Pathophysiology

The scrotum is divided into two by a connective tissue septum which separates the testes. Beneath the skin of the scrotum there is a layer of loose connective tissue and a layer of smooth muscle called the dartos muscle. In cold temperatures the dartos muscle contracts, causing the skin of the scrotum to become firm and wrinkled and thus reducing its overall size. At the same time, extensions of the abdominal muscles, called cremaster muscles, which extend into the scrotum, contract. The testes are then pulled nearer to the body and their temperature is raised. During warm weather the process is reversed and the testicles descend away from the body, which lowers their temperature. If the testes become too cold or too warm, the normal sperm production does not occur.

The outer part is a white connective tissue capsule. Part of the capsule extends to the interior of the testis, dividing it into about 250 lobules with tubules in which sperm cells develop. Interstitial cells secrete the hormone testosterone. Sperm cells move from these tubules to the epididymis, where they mature in a few days and develop their capacity to function as sex cells. The vas deferens passes from the epididymis via the inguinal canal through the abdominal wall to the prostate gland. The urethra is a passage for both urine and male reproductive fluids. While semen is passing through the urethra, a reflex causes the urinary sphincter muscles to contract, stopping urine from passing from the bladder to the urethra.

Torsion of the testis is due to an anatomic abnormality in which the testicle is not attached to the scrotum (see Fig. 28.4) Torsion produces an initial occlusion of the venous return from the testis, although the arterial supply continues for some time. There follows congestion of the testis, with haemorrhagic infarction as the arterial system becomes impaired. The infarction produces a shrunken, fibrotic testis.

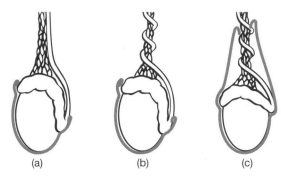

Figure 28.4 – *Testicular torsion.*

Assessment

Torsion is often precipitated by exertion which causes contraction of the cremaster muscle producing the torsion. The patient is usually 15–30 years old, with sudden onset of pain in one testis. Pain may radiate up to the abdomen, the original site of the testicles in the embryo. Nausea and vomiting are common, and on examination the patient is found to have a hot swollen testis.

Differential diagnosis

- Epididymitis
- Testicular tumour
- Trauma
- Hydrocele.

Investigations

Use of a Doppler on the spermatic cord is an attempt to measure arterial blood flow to the involved testis. While absence of blood flow obviously supports the diagnosis, the presence of blood flow does not exclude torsion. Ultrasound may be helpful, although most would agree that if there is a doubt it is best to perform surgical exploration.

Management

The patient may be in considerable pain and will require both emotional support and prescribed analgesia. Surgery should be performed as soon as possible, and certainly within 4–6 hours. Testicular loss can occur within 2 hours of the onset of symptoms (Glichrist & Lobe 1992). Informed consent will include an explanation by the surgeon that the testis may have to be removed if it is found to be non-viable at operation, as well as an explanation that both testes

will be fixed by suturing. Torsion is a bilateral phenomenon, so the uninvolved testis should also be fixed to the scrotum during the operation to prevent subsequent torsion. If the testis is viable at operation, it is sutured to the scrotal wall, and if it is deemed unsalvageable it is removed.

Preoperative Preparation

The length of time available for the preparation of the patient will depend upon the patient's clinical condition. The chief objective is to ensure that the patient goes to surgery in the best physical and psychological condition. There will be some overlap between the medical and nursing input in the preparation of the patient. It is important that the nurse is present during the surgeon's explanation to the patient to allow for continuity. If other relatives arrive when the patient has already gone to surgery, the nurse will then be able to provide the necessary information.

Psychological

While surgical procedures and their preparation may be relatively routine for staff in A&E, for patients and their relatives, the need for surgery may come as quite a shock with little time for psychological preparation. Adequate explanation of the operative procedure and postoperative events is essential. Allow the patient some time to consider the information, and be available to answer the patient's questions. Jaworski & Wirtz (1995) noted that during an acute crisis the patient may seem to understand, but information and instructions may have to be repeated. It has been shown that providing patients with information preoperatively leads to more favourable postoperative outcomes (Owens & Hutelmyer 1982). It has also been demonstrated that informing patients about anticipated pain and giving them some control over the pain experience decreased apprehension, increased pain tolerance and resulted in earlier discharges (Vorshall 1980). Even where the patients's condition is grave and surgery is being undertaken as a desperate last measure, it remains important to be truthful to both patients and their relatives without unduly frightening them.

Consent

Informed consent suggests that the patient has been given information by the doctor about the exact nature of the procedure and possible complications, and that the patient understands this information and has agreed to the operation. Informed consent protects the patient against unauthorised procedures, and protects the hospital and its staff from litigation.

When signing the consent form, the patient should be rational and not under the influence of drugs or alcohol that may impair comprehension. As far as the law is concerned there is no specific requirement that consent should be given in a particular way; however, consent in writing is by far the best method for all procedures involving risk. In an emergency, where the patient's life is in danger and the patient is not able to consent, the doctor may proceed and do what is required without formal consent. This is rarely necessary, and even in the unconscious patient, consent should be sought where possible from the next of kin.

Skin preparation

Specific preparation by shaving or depilation prior to surgery is no longer recommended. Research suggests that avoiding these procedures reduces infection (Alexander *et al.* 1983, Cruse & Foord 1980).

Preoperative checklist

In emergencies, preparation is limited to the essentials:

- Informed consent
- Psychological preparation
- Gastric tube to empty the stomach
- Establishment of intravenous access, bloods for cross-matching, electrolytes, full blood count, clotting studies, glucose
- Urine specimen to test for abnormalities (diabetes/ impaired renal function); catheterise if necessary
- Patient identity bracelet; mark operation site
- Remove prosthetics, cosmetics and jewellery
- Assemble records including vital signs, fluid balance, drug history, allergies, property
- Notification of relatives.

In more controlled circumstances additionally:

- Chest x-ray
- ECG
- Special investigations specific to the patient's condition.

Conclusion

The management of surgical emergencies in this chapter covers the full spectrum of patients, from those suffering the discomfort of urinary retention to these with a life-threatening aortic aneurysm. Rapid assessment, diagnosis and intervention remain the key to ensuring the best outcome for the patient.

References

Alexander JW, Fischer JE, Boyajian M, Palmquist J, Morris MJ, (1983) The influence of hair removal methods on wound infection. *Archives of Surgery*, **118**, 347–352.

Blandy JP, Moors J (1981) *Urology for Nurses*. Oxford: Blackwell Scientific.

Bourg P, Sherer C, Rosen P (1986) *Standardised Care Plans for Emergency Departments*. St Louis: CV Mosby.

Britton PM, Wright ES (1992) Nursing care of catheterised patients. In: Horne EM, Cowan T, eds. *Staff Nurses Survival Guide* 2nd edn. London: Wolfe.

Bruce AW, Sira SS, Clark AF, Awad SA (1974) The problems of catheter encrustation. *Canadian Medical Association Journal* **111**, 238–241.

Clemings L, Duda J, Duda J (1990) Gastrointestinal emergencies. In: Kitt S, Kaiser J, eds. *Emergency Nursing: a Physiological and Clinical Perspective*. Philadelphia: WB Saunders.

Cooper K (1988) Gastrointestinal emergencies In: Mowad L, Ruhle DC, eds. *Handbook of Emergency Nursing: the Nursing Process Approach*. Norwalk, CT: Appleton & Lange.

Cruse PJE, Foord R (1980) The epidemiology of wound infection. *Surgical Clinics of North America* **60**(1), 27–40.

Drake T (1993) Aortic aneurysm and aortic dissection In: Markovchick VJ, Pons PT, Wolfe RE, eds. *Emergency Medicine* 3rd edn. Philadelphia: Hanley & Belfus.

Emmans LS (1993) Bowel disorders. In: Markovchick VJ, Pons PT, Wolfe RE, edn. *Emergency Medicine Secrets*. Philadelphia: Hanley & Belfus.

Ferguson A (1997) Discharge planning in A&E: part 1 *Accident & Emergency Nursing* **5**(4), 210–214.

Ferguson A (1998) Discharge planning in A&E: part 2. *Accident & Emergency Nursing* **6**(2), 53–57.

Gilchrist BF, Lobe TE (1992) The acute groin in paediatrics. *Clinical Paediatrics* **31**, 488–496.

Hope RA (1993) *Oxford Handbook of Clinical Medicine* 3rd edn. New York: Oxford University Press.

Jaworski MA, Wirtz KM (1995) Spinal trauma. In: Kitt S, Selfridge-Thomas J, Proehl J, Kaiser J, eds. *Emergency Nursing: a Physiological and Clinical Perspective*. Philadelphia: WB Saunders.

Kitt S (1990) Abdominal trauma. In: Kitt S, Selfridge-Thomas J, Proehl J, Kaiser J, eds. *Emergency Nursing: a Physiological and Clinical Perspective*. Philadelphia: WB Saunders.

Kumar P, Clark M (1994) *Clinical Medicine*. London: Baillière Tindall.

McGill S (1982) Catheter management. It's the size that's important. *Nursing Mirror* **154**, 148–149.

McGrath A (1998) Abdominal examination and assessment in A&E. *Emergency Nurse* **6**(4), 15–18.

Norton D, Abernathy C (1993) Appendicitis. In: Markovchick VJ, Pons PT, Wolfe RE, eds. *Emergency Medical Secrets*. Philadelphia: Hanley and Belfus.

Owens JF, Hutelmyer CM (1982) The effect of post operative delirium in cardiac surgical patients. *Nursing Research* **31**(1), 61–62.

Page BW (1988) Cardiovascular emergencies. In: Mowad L, Ruhle DC, eds. *Handbook of Emergency Nursing: the Nursing Process Approach*. Norwalk, CT: Appleton & Lange.

Royle JA, Walsh M (1992) *Watson's Medical and Surgical Nursing* 4th edn. London: Baillière Tindall.

Srinvasan V, Clark SS (1972) Encrustation of catheter materials in vitro. *Journal of Urology* **108**, 473.

Vorshall B (1980) The effects of pre-operative teaching on post operative pain. *Topics in Clinical Nursing* **2**(1), 39–43.

Wilson DH, Flowers MW (1985) *Accident and Emergency Handbook*. Oxford: Butterworths.

Yates DW, Redmond AD (1985) *Lecture Notes on Accident and Emergency* Oxford: Blackwell Scientific.

Chapter 29

Gynaecological and Obstetric Emergencies

Lynda Holt & Orla Devereux

- Introduction
- Anatomy and physiology
- Emergency care of the non-pregnant woman
- Sexual assault
- Emergency care of the pregnant woman
- Conclusion

Introduction

This chapter considers women's health in both pregnant and non-pregnant patients. Although many of the principles of management are similar, significant anatomical differences exist, and many of the signs and symptoms have different implications. Conditions relating to female reproduction form a relatively small part of A&E work, however many women actively choose A&E for both emergency care and preventative intervention. As well as its physical implications, for many patients an obstetric or gynaecological condition can be distressing and value-laden. This chapter seeks to equip the A&E nurse to rapidly assess the patient's condition and intervene appropriately. It will provide an outline of relevant anatomy and physiology before identifying conditions commonly treated in A&E.

Anatomy and Physiology

The female reproductive organs consist of:

- uterus
- ovaries
- fallopian tubes
- vagina
- external genitalia.

They are situated outside of the peritoneal cavity (see Fig. 29.1).

The uterus is located in the anterior pelvis above the bladder. It is a pearshaped organ with thick walls, made up of three layers: an outer serous membrane, a middle layer of smooth muscle, and the mucosal inner layer of endometrium, which is extremely vascular. The top of the uterus is called the fundus; it is the height of this which is measured to determine the gestation of pregnancy (see Fig. 29.2).

The neck of the uterus is called the cervix. This opens into the vagina, the opening of which is called the os. The status of the os is an important consideration in assessing bleeding in early pregnancy. The

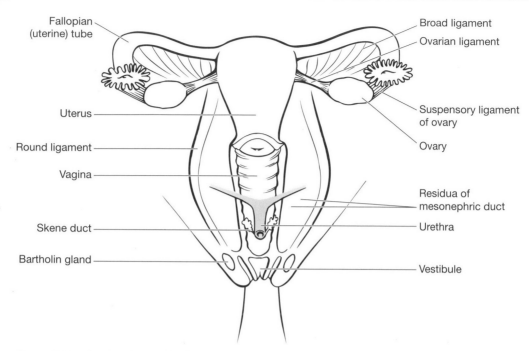

Figure 29.1 – *The female reproduction system.*

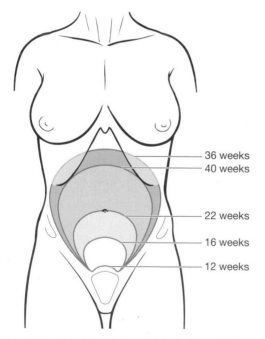

Figure 29.2 – *Change in fundal height during gestation.*

ovaries sit bilaterally to the uterus, on the lateral pelvic wall, and are connected to the uterus by fallopian tubes. The fallopian tubes have a funnel-like opening below the ovaries, which collects the ova and trans-

ports them by peristalsis to the uterus. The tubes are made up of smooth muscle and mucous membrane. The vagina is an elastic tube leading to the external genitalia. There are two small glands either side of the vaginal opening called Bartholin's glands which can be prone to cyst formation in some women.

During child-bearing years, the female reproductive cycle varies in length between 21 and 35 days, but for most, the average cycle is 28 days. The cycle consists of ovulation and menstruation, and is governed by changes in hormone levels. The first 5–7 days of the cycle represent menstruation. This is followed by a 7–8 day follicular phase preparing the endometrium for a implantation of a fertilised egg. At around days 14–15 of the cycle, ovulation occurs. Once the ovum is released from the follicle, the luteal phase then commences: the collapsed follicle becomes an endocrine gland called the corpus luteum. It secretes oestrogen and progesterone to support the egg if fertilised. If the egg is not fertilised the luteal phase is responsible for the degeneration of the corpus luteum, after which the thickened lining of the endometrium sheds and the cycle begins again. If the egg is fertilised, the corpus luteum continues to secrete hormones until about 3 months into the pregnancy when the placenta takes over.

Fertilisation of the ovum takes place in the fallopian tube, and during the first few days it passes slowly towards the uterus while a series of cell divisions take place forming a mass of embryotic cells. The embryo reaches the uterus between 3 and 5 days after fertilisation. It then begins to implant into the uterine wall by about days 6–7 after fertilisation. The placenta forms around where the embryo is embedded and, after a few weeks, begins to provide oxygen and nutrients to support fetal growth for the rest of the pregnancy. By 5 weeks after implantation the fetal heart is pumping well, and nutrients pass from the maternal blood supply across the placental membrane to nourish the fetus. The pregnancy is divided into trimesters of growth: in the first the internal organs develop; in the second the fetus grows in length and systems begin to mature; and in the last trimester the fetus fattens out and builds up reserves for birth. Physiological changes in pregnancy are plentiful, and an overview of key changes is given in Box 29.1; however, a detailed description is beyond the scope of this text and only those changes related to emergency care in A&E will be discussed.

Emergency Care of the Non-pregnant Woman

History

Obtaining an accurate history is vital to establish the severity of a patient's condition. Because of the personal nature of gynaecological complaints, the nurse should ensure that assessment is carried out in private and in a sensitive and non-judgmental manner. Box 29.2 highlights the information that should be obtained.

Assessment

General assessment of the woman with a gynaecological condition should include baseline observations of pulse, respiration, blood pressure and temperature to detect signs of shock or infection. The level of pain should be determined, together with the exact location. Gentle abdominal examination will assist in this. If clinically indicated, a vaginal examination should be carried out once, either by the nurse, or more commonly, by the doctor. Assessment should include urinalysis to detect a urinary tract infection as a primary cause of pain. Initially this can be diagnosed by the presence of leucocytes, protein and blood in urine, but culture and sensitivity should follow to ensure appropriate antibiotic therapy. A pregnancy test should also be carried out routinely to exclude unknown pregnancy. Abdominal pain is often the primary reason women with gynaecological complaints attend A&E (Gondeck 1998). Conditions causing acute abdominal pain are shown in Box 29.3.

Menstrual pain

Mid–cycle pain

This is known as Mittelschmerz disease and is a benign condition associated with ovulation. Pain is usually unilateral and lasts 24–48 hours. Some women experience this every month as part of their usual cycle; for others it is an unexpected pain sometimes

---

Box 29.1 – *Physiological changes in pregnancy*

Cardiovascular
- Blood vascular increases by 30%
- Red cell mass rises by 20%
- Plasma increases by up to 50%
- Peripheral resistance decreases, reducing diastolic BP in the first and second trimesters
- Heart rate increases by up to 20 beats/min
- CVP falls by 65% by term
- Cardiac output increases by up to 30%

Respiratory
- Oxygen consumption increases by 20%
- Respiratory rate increases
- Pulmonary function alters, residual capacity decreases, minute volume increases by 40–50% and tidal volume increases

Renal
- Renal plasma flow and glomerular filtration rate increase steadily throughout pregnancy to a 50% greater capacity by term
- Speed of urine formation increases
- Water and sodium reabsorption rates are increased

Gastrointestinal
- Smooth muscle relaxes, and therefore gastric emptying is faster
- Intestines are relocated into the upper abdomen
- Acid regurgitation is common

Endocrine
- Base metabolic rate increases by up to 25%
- Anterior pituitary hypertrophy occurs
- Thyroid hypertrophy occurs

Other
- Anaemia develops because of rapid increase in iron requirements
- Cell-mediated immunity is depressed
- Autoimmunity disease eases during pregnancy

Box 29.2 – *History related to gynaecological assessment*

- Duration of symptoms
- Type and location of any pain
- Is there any redness of itching?
- Date of last menstrual period, and duration
- Was menstrual period normal?
- Is there any possibility of pregnancy?
- Is the patient sexually active? What (if any) contraception is being used?
- Is there any abnormal vaginal discharge or bleeding? If so, what is the discharge like?
- How heavy is bleeding, i.e. how often are pads or tampons being changed?
- Past history of pregnancy
- Coexisting medical problems/drug therapy
- Is there a history of assaults?

Box 29.3 – *Causes of acute abdominal pain in gynaecology*

- Menstrual cycle
  - mid-cycle pain
  - menstruation
- Ovarian cyst
- Pelvic inflammatory disease (PID)

---

associated with per vaginal (PV) bleeding which causes enough discomfort and anxiety for the patient to seek emergency health care. Mittelschmerz pain is thought to be caused by a combination of local irritation due to blood, follicular fluid and prostaglandins released after ovulation, and increased peristalsis in the fallopian tubes (Hinchliff *et al.* 1996). At this time, most women experience microscopic PV bleeding, a few regularly have overt bleeding and most women will have an occasional mid-cycle PV bleed. This is due to a temporary fall in hormone levels between the follicular and luteal phases of the menstrual cycle. Bleeding usually lasts only a few hours.

Mittelschmerz disease is diagnosed by relating the type of pain to the stage of the woman's menstrual cycle. It should only be diagnosed once other causes, such as ovarian cyst and pelvic inflammatory disease, have been ruled out (Reedy & Brucker 1995). The

condition is self-limiting, and therefore treatment involves symptom control and education. Non-steroidal anti-inflammatory drugs (NSAIDs), such as ibruprofen, are usually the most effective analgesia. The patient should be made aware of the cyclical nature of the condition, and the possibility of recurrence.

Dysmenorrhoea

In most cases, dysmenorrhoea (period pain) is self-diagnosed and treated at home; however, when symptoms are unusually severe, some women seek emergency care. Two types of dysmenorrhoea exist: primary and secondary dysmenorrhoea. In the former, uterine spasm involves A nerve fibres, responsible for acute pain, and C nerve fibres responsible for chronic and referred pain (Golub 1992); (see also Ch. 24). Primary dysmenorrhoea is most common in adolescents and young women who have not had children.

Secondary dysmenorrhoea is more common in women over 30 with gynaecological problems like endometriosis. In both types of dysmenorrhoea, the patient will have crampy, low abdominal pain either at onset of menses or 24 hours prior to onset. The woman may have referred pain in the back and legs. Associated symptoms include breast tenderness, nausea/vomiting, diarrhoea and headache, all due to rapid hormonal changes.

Diagnosis should be made only after other causes of pain and bleeding have been excluded. Management revolves around symptom control, and the condition is self-limiting. NSAIDs are the analgesia of choice because they inhibit intrauterine synthesis of prostaglandin (Weissmann 1991) as well as decreasing pain. Small quantities of alcohol are effective in the treatment of dysmenorrhoea because it reduces oxytocin and vasopressor activity, therefore reducing uterine spasm. Ethically, however, this method of pain control should only be advocated for women who understand the potential dangers of alcohol ingestion and are legally old enough to use it (Reedy & Brucker 1995). Discharge information should include the commonality of dysmenorrhoea and, in the case of secondary dysmenorrhoea, information and advice about the predisposing condition.

Ovarian cyst

These usually result from a dysfunction in the menstrual cycle, when a collection of fluid forms around the corpus luteum. Cyst formation is more common in endometriosis and most are benign and self-limiting. In some instances, the cyst increases in size and becomes symptomatic at about 5 cm diameter (Lichtman & Papera 1990). Eventually, if growth persists, bleeding, rupture or torsion can occur. Ovarian cysts are uncommon in women using oral contraception (Selfridge-Thomas 1997).

Assessment

The patient will have abdominal pain, worse on the affected side, with possible guarding on examination. Onset of pain is usually during the latter half of the menstrual cycle or the week prior to menses where the cycle is regular. The patient will experience prolonged menstruation. If a small cyst ruptures, the fluid collected in it is reabsorbed without any clinical evidence. Rupture of a large cyst can cause potentially life-threatening hypovolaemia.

Assessment of vital signs should be ongoing as a mild tachycardia can quickly deteriorate into severe hypotension and shock in ovarian cyst rupture. Prior to rupture, a large cyst can twist around the vascular pedicle causing ovarian torsion. This is identified by a sudden onset of intermittent but sharp pain. Nausea or vomiting is an early sign of ovarian torsion.

Management

Cysts not causing haemodynamic compromise tend to be managed conservatively with follow-up investigation from a GP or gynaecological clinic. If adequate pain control cannot be achieved, hospital admission should be considered. If the patient has mild to moderate signs of hypovolaemia, intravenous fluid support should be established, and laproscopic surgical decompression of the cyst should be considered. In cases of severe hypotension or torsion, fluid resuscitation and urgent surgical intervention are necessary. These women will need both information and psychological support during a time which potentially threatens their fertility.

Pelvic inflammatory disease

Pelvic inflammatory disease (PID) is an increasing gynaecological problem, with approximately 20% of female infertility attributed to it (Reedy & Brucker 1995). It is also linked to an increase in ectopic pregnancy. PID is a generic term used to describe infection of the pelvic peritoneum, connective tissue and reproductive organs – most commonly the fallopian tubes (also termed salpingitis). PID results from:

■ sexually transmitted diseases (STDs), particularly gonorrhoea and *Chlamydia*

■ termination of pregnancy
■ childbirth with assisted delivery
■ the use of intrauterine devices for contraception
■ gynaecological surgery.

Sexually transmitted diseases are the most common cause of PID. The infection occurs in the genital area and spreads along mucosal surfaces causing transient bouts of inflammation. Infection tends to settle in fallopian tubes, causing scar tissue and adhesions. This makes ovum passage more difficult and increases the likelihood of ectopic pregnancy because the fertilised egg is unable to pass to the uterus and implants in the tube. PID is most common in young women with multiple sexual partners, and within that group has a higher incidence in women from lower socioeconomic groups (Wolner Hanbseen 1991). The most common age group is 15–19 years of age (Selfridge-Thomas 1997), which has considerable implications for future health care and fertility therapy.

A patient with PID will present with moderate to severe abdominal pain, worse with walking, urination, bowel action and intercourse. She may be tachycardic and will have a pyrexia. If STD is the cause, the patient will have a thick, vaginal discharge. If pelvic abscess or peritonitis is developing, the patient will also have nausea or vomiting. Lichtman & Parera (1990) highlighted three grades of PID (see Box 29.4).

> **Box 29.4** – *Grades of pelvic inflammatory disease*
>
> **Grade I** Infection confined to tube(s) or ovary(s)
> **Grade II** Infection complicated by abscess or tissue mass
> **Grade III** Infection spread beyond pelvis due to a ruptured abscess. Peritonitis is commonly present

Management

Pain relief is a priority for management of all types of PID. The strength of analgesia needed will vary depending on the severity of infection and the patient's individual perceptions of her condition. Grade I infection can be treated with broad-spectrum antibiotics, usually cefotaxime or tetracycline, and the patient can be discharged and followed up in the STD clinic. Grade II conditions warrant hospital admission for i.v. antibiotics. Grade III PID is uncommon, but necessitates hospitalisation and surgical intervention as well as antibiotic therapy.

If the woman is pregnant or has not responded to, or complied with, oral antibiotics, hospital admission should be considered. If the patient is discharged from

A&E, it is essential that she has appropriate health education to enable her to recognise a recurrence and get treatment. This is important in reducing potential long-term health problems, such as infertility. If the PID originates from an STD, the patient's partner should be encouraged to attend an STD clinic and advice should be given about the use of barrier methods of contraception during intercourse.

Bartholin's cyst

The Bartholin's glands lie on either side of the vagina and secrete fluid onto the surface of the labia. In normal health these cannot be seen or palpated. If the duct becomes blocked, a small cyst forms; these are usually benign and self-limiting. They can, however, become infected with *E. coli* or STDs such as gonorrhoea. If infection occurs, the labium becomes inflamed and oedematous to the extent that the patient may have difficulty walking. This is a painful and distressing condition, which is resolved by early excision and drainage of the cyst. This is usually performed as an inpatient. Antibiotic therapy is also indicated (Walters 1992).

Sexually transmitted disease

Patients may present to A&E because of its relative anonymity compared with GP attendance. Many people are still unaware of the existence and accessibility of STD clinics. Broadly common symptoms of STD are genital irritation or pain, infection, discharge and sometimes bleeding. Specific symptoms and management are shown in Table 29.1.

The role of the A&E nurse in caring for patients with STDs is twofold: firstly, to provide immediate therapy to resolve the acute episode with appropriate STD clinic follow-up; and secondly, to provide non-judgmental health education aimed at preventing the spread of STDs. All direct sexual contacts of the patient should be advised to have a health check. It is not possible for the A&E nurse to personally follow up patient contacts, but the nurse can support the patient in informing a current partner, and information can then be cascaded to anyone else who may be involved. Patients should refrain from sexual activity until the infection is clear. Advice about barrier contraception should also be given (Howe 1996).

Emergency contraception

Postcoital contraception is available in the form of oral oestrogen-based pills taken within 72 hours of intercourse or an intra-uterine contraceptive device (IUCD) which needs to be inserted within 5 days of intercourse.

Oestrogen–based pills

Oestrogen-based pills work by a combination of pituitary influence and action on the ovary and endometrium. The luteal phase of the menstrual cycle is shortened. The endometrial biochemistry is also altered to make it hostile to implantation. The way the pill works is important in differentiating between contraception which prevents pregnancy and drugs which induce abortion, which the oestrogen pill does not.

Many patients need this differentiation spelt out for

Table 29.1 – *Sexually transmitted disease*

Organism	Incubation	Symptoms	Discharge	Treatment
Neisseria gonorrhoea	3–5 days	Dysuria	Yellow	Cefotaxime
Chlamydia trachomatis	5–10 days	Urethral itching	Mucopurulent vaginal discharge	Tetracycline
Trichomonas vaginalis	1 week	Vaginal itching	Thin, frothy, greenish, foul-smelling	Metronidazole
Gardinerella vaginalis	5–10 days	Itching	Thin, white, fishy odour	Metronidazole
Candida albicans	Variable	Inflammatory itching	Thick white discharge	Clotrimazole
Herpes simplex II	2–12 days	Painful, genital lesions	–	Acyclovir
Genital warts	1–6 months	Wart – type lesions on genitals spreading up genital tract	–	Paint with 5% acetic acid

long-term peace of mind. Before the postcoital pill is prescribed, it is important that the patient is aware of the risks associated with its use. The patient must be warned that a small teratogenic risk exists if the fetus survives, similar to continued use of daily oral contraception pills. As yet, however, oestrogen teratogenesis has only been proved where repeated high doses are used in early pregnancy (Stevens & Kenney 1994). It is advisable to document that this information was given to the patient.

Administration of the drug is in two doses, which should be taken within 72 hours of unprotected intercourse. Nausea and vomiting are significant side-effects of oral postcoital contraception and some doctors prefer to prescribe prophylactic antiemetics with the pill. Follow-up care should be sought around 3 weeks after postcoital contraception. It is because these facilities are not available in A&E that some consultants choose not to offer emergency postcoital contraception. Most women will commence menses within 21 days of the postcoital pill. If this does not happen, a pregnancy test should be performed; however, the failure rate of the postcoital pill is less than 5% (Stevens & Kenney 1994). The patient should be advised about contraception in the short term while still in A&E. The patient must also be advised to use barrier methods of contraception for the rest of this cycle as the postcoital pill alters the timing of ovulation. Longer-term contraception will be discussed in the follow-up check. It should also be noted that, because the postcoital contraceptive pill prevents uterine implantation, it does not preclude ectopic pregnancy. The patient should be advised of the symptoms of ectopic pregnancy and advised to seek medical care should these be experienced.

Intrauterine contraceptive device

The IUCD may be used up to 5 days after ovulation, or after unprotected intercourse if the date of ovulation is not known. It also works by preventing implantation, and failure is rare. There are disadvantages to its use in nulligravida women because of pain associated with insertion. It is not ideal for women with existing pelvic infection as it could exacerbate this. Irregular vaginal bleeding is also common after IUCD insertion. The advantage of this method is that it provides longer-term contraception.

Sexual assault

Rape and sexual assault are violent crimes. Police forces are increasingly caring for physically injured survivors of rape in dedicated rape suites equipped for the privacy and comfort of women who have been

---

> **Box 29.5** – *Reporting/non-reporting sexual assault care paths. (After Holloway 1994)*
>
> **Incident reported to police**
> - Police officer allocated to support patient
> - Examination carried out by forensic medical examiner (FME)
> - Entrance to victim support scheme
> - Police statements obtained
> - Police officer support throughout court case
>
> **Incident not reported**
> - Medical examination by senior A&E doctor
> - Support agency contacted
> - Follow-up at STD clinic
> - Nurse support throughout
> - Retain option of police involvement

---

assaulted. A&E departments should have a rape protocol that has been discussed with the local police force and rape support groups. This should ensure that the patient's best interests are served in terms of both immediate health care and her subsequent ability to produce evidence to prosecute the assailant. A&E nurses should attempt to reinstate the patient's perception of control over what happens to her. Unless associated injuries prevent it, the patient should be encouraged to give explicit consent, either written or verbal, for any investigations or examination she undergoes.

The decision to report sexual assault is entirely that of the patient and A&E staff must support that decision and plan care around it. Box 29.5 shows care paths for reporting and non-reporting of sexual assault. If the patient does not have significant physical injury, it may be appropriate to obtain a full history with the police if the patient wishes to report the attack. This is simply to prevent the patient having to describe the incident several times, which can be unnecessarily distressing. The decision to take a joint history should be the patient's. Box 29.6 highlights the essential information needed.

It is important that any potential forensic evidence is preserved. This is equally important in a patient who is unconscious or who has significant physical injury. A paper sheet should be placed under the patient to collect debris if possible; otherwise linen used should be saved. A mobile patient should be asked to stand on a paper sheet while undressing so that debris can be saved. Physical examination should be carried out at once by a forensic medical examiner (FME) (Holloway 1994). In some areas, the FME will take on this role whether or not the patient intends to

Box 29.6 – *Obtaining a history from a survivor of sexual assault*

■ Establish the date, time and location of the attack

■ Circumstances of assault:
  - where injured, i.e. in mouth, skin, breast, anus, vagina
  - was condom used?
  - removal or damage to clothing by assailant
  - number of assailants
  - drugs/alcohol used
  - any associated physical injuries

■ Action taken after assault:
  - cleaned teeth, mouthwash gargled
  - wash/shower/bath
  - changed clothes
  - urinated/bowels opened
  - changed tampon/pad
  - subsequent sexual intercourse

■ Alcohol/drugs (prescribed or recreational) taken prior to the attack or since

■ Previous sexual intercourse, if within 2 weeks

■ Menstrual stage, date of last period and usual method of birth control if of child-bearing age

■ Medical and obstetric history

prosecute. The first priority must lie in protecting the patient from further humiliation and distress, and on those grounds alone, one examination is good practice. For evidence to be submissible, the examination, evidence collection and documentation should follow local police policy. The primary role of the A&E nurse is in supporting the patient and assuring her privacy and safety until examination can take place. Box 29.7 shows what evidence should be collected and how it should be preserved.

Once the medical examination has been carried out, the patient needs to be advised about pregnancy risk and offered emergency contraception if appropriate. The patient should also be offered follow-up STD screening and it is imperative she has either actual contact with a rape survivors' support counsellor or contact telephone numbers for later use should she wish to do so. Rape trauma syndrome (RTS) is experienced by most sexual assault survivors in some form (Burgess & Holmstrom 1974). Good, sensitive, non-judgmental care immediately following the attack can help to reduce the impact of RTS. It is important that A&E nurses understand the progression of this syndrome, both for immediate care of attack survivors and to help recognise and rationalise associated symptoms of patients some time after the assault. Box 29.8 outlines the stages of RTS.

Box 29.7 – *Forensic evidence from survivors of sexual assault. (After Stevens & Kenney 1994)*

■ Observe and document the condition of clothing, i.e. damaged, stained, debris attachment to it. Clothing should be placed in a paper bag for dry storage

■ Full medical examination, documenting injuries in detail; provide photographs if possible

■ Obtain following samples:

Sample	Collect in	Store in
Blood group/DNA profile	EDTA bottles	Fridge
Blood alcohol	Fluoride oxadate bottle	Fridge
Saliva/sperm group	Universal container	Fridge
Urine/drugs/alcohol screen	Sodium fluoride	Fridge
Skin swabs	Plastic tube	Freeze
Vaginal/cervical swabs	Plastic tube	Freeze
Anal swabs	Plastic tube	Freeze
Loose hairs/debris	Plastic bag	Dry storage
Fingernail clippings	Plastic bag	Dry storage
Tampon/sanitary towel	Plastic bag	Freeze

Box 29.8 – *Rape trauma syndrome. (After Holloway 1994)*

Acute phase (during the attack and the period afterwards)
■ Shock
■ Disbelief and terror
■ Anxiety·
■ Vulnerability
■ Guilt
■ Physical pain
■ Suppressed/controlled emotions

Adjustment phase (during weeks and months following)
■ Sleep disturbance
■ Flashbacks
■ Phobias
■ Eating disorders
■ Voluntary isolation and rejection of close friends/relatives
■ Denial of incident
■ Insecurity

Long-term implications
Most women carry emotional scars for the rest of their lives. Some common problems include:
■ Depression
■ Inability to trust others
■ Inability to maintain intimate relationships
■ Constant reminders triggered by smells, sounds etc.
■ Some women have persistent flashbacks

Box 29.9 – *Obtaining an obstetric history*

■ Number of previous pregnancies
  – terminations
  – miscarriages
  – live births – combinations in pregnancy, delivery, postnatal care

■ This pregnancy
  – gestation
  – antenatal care
  – PV bleeding to date
  – other complications
  – ultrasound scans
  – fetal abnormality tests

Most patients receiving antenatal care in the UK have patient held notes which contain a detailed account of their obstetric history.

Emergency Care of the Pregnant Woman

History

As with other aspects of health care, an accurate history of events leading to A&E attendance is imperative. In the case of a pregnant patient, a full obstetric history should be obtained as well as the history of the presenting complaint. Box 29.9 highlights the information needed for an obstetric history.

Assessment

General assessment should include baseline observations of pulse, blood pressure, respirations and temperature to detect signs of shock, infection or pre-eclampsia. Routine urinalysis should also be carried out for glucose and protein. The progress of the pregnancy should be assessed in terms of the height of the fundus compared with estimated gestation, and after about 14–16 weeks, fetal heartbeat should be assessed. Any vaginal discharge or bleeding should only be assessed in terms of type, quality and odour. Vaginal examination should only be carried out if it is necessary to determine the state of the cervical os or to identify causes of fresh vaginal bleeding. During assessment and care, maternal health should be paramount whatever the gestation of the fetus.

Miscarriage

Miscarriage is also termed 'spontaneous abortion' and describes the delivery of a non-viable fetus before 24 weeks' gestation. There are six types of miscarriage and these are listed in Table 29.2.

Miscarriage is extremely common and up to 20% of confirmed pregnancies spontaneously abort (Miscarriage Association 1996). Where a cause is investigated, pathological abnormalities with the fetus or placenta are commonly found (Creasy & Resnick 1993). Immunological incompatibility with the father, maternal infection, substance misuse and malnutrition have also been linked with spontaneous abortion (Reedy & Brucker 1995).

Despite the relative commonality of miscarriage, it is devastating for the woman and her partner. Apart from the physical pain associated with miscarriage, the woman and her family are grieving for the loss of a baby, the dreams and plans they will have had for that baby, and their identity as a family (Duncan 1995). It is essential that A&E nurses recognise the enormity of this loss and do not attempt to trivialise it with

Table 29.2 – *Categorisation of miscarriage*

Type	Bleeding	Passed tissue	Cervical os	Pain	Size of uterus
Threatened	Slight	No	Closed	Mild	Normal for gestation
Inevitable	Moderate–heavy	No	Open	Moderate–severe	Normal for gestation
Incomplete	Heavy	Yes	Open with tissue present	Severe	Smaller than expected for gestation
Complete	Slight	Yes	Closed	Mild	Smaller than expected for gestation
Missed	None	No	Closed	Nil	Smaller than expected for gestation
Septic	Varies, foul odour often accompanies loss	Sometimes	Open	Moderate – severe High temperature	Normal or small for dates

comments like 'you can have another', or by functional care avoiding conversation about the miscarriage. Parents want their loss acknowledged and it is much better for the nurse to express condolences for the loss of their baby (Standing 1997).

Assessment

This should revolve around maintaining maternal health, as little can be done to alter fetal prognosis (Regan 1992). The patient's heamodynamic stability should be assessed, in terms of heart rate, respirations and blood pressure, as well as blood loss. When enquiring about blood loss, the nurse should seek to establish quantity in terms of the number of pads used per hour. The type of loss should also be noted, whether it is fresh or dark blood, and whether clots or tissue have been passed. This will help to determine the category of miscarriage occurring.

The amount and location of pain should be established, and appropriate analgesia given. A urine sample should be obtained to confirm pregnancy and to rule out urine infection as a cause of bleeding. Blood should also be taken to confirm rhesus status in case the patient is rhesus negative and anti-D serum is required. A vaginal examination will confirm the status of the cervical os, rule out a vaginal source for bleeding and identify and products of conception in the cervix or vagina. An ultrasound scan should be organised to confirm clinical findings, i.e. to identify a potentially viable pregnancy or retained products of

conception. For humanitarian reasons, this should be done as soon as possible as most patients and their partners need confirmation of a visible heartbeat to believe that everything is all right or, more commonly, they need the reinforcement that their baby is dead, or has been miscarried, in order to come to terms with their loss.

Management

In most cases of miscarriage, A&E care revolves around symptomatic management and psychological support. If the patient shows signs of hypovolaemia, intravenous fluid replacement should be commenced. Adequate analgesia should be given, particularly if the pregnancy is not viable. If the miscarriage has been an incomplete or missed abortion, the patient should be prepared physically and emotionally for an evacuation of retained products of conception (ERPC) in theatre. Psychological support for both the woman and her partner is important throughout their stay in A&E as the initial handling of their loss will impact on the grieving process they must work through (see also Ch. 13).

The use of the term 'spontaneous abortion' should be avoided at this time, as many people associate abortion with voluntary termination of pregnancy. Miscarriage, on the other hand, is seen as involuntary (Reedy & Brucker 1995). Using the term abortion can therefore cause unnecessary distress.

The length of the gestation may alter physical

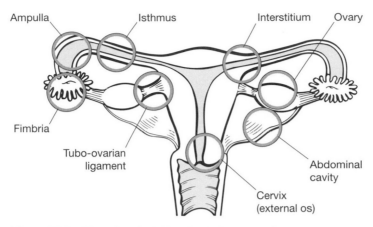

Figure 29.3 – *Sites of implantation of ectopic pregnancies.*

symptoms, but it does not alter emotional ones. All patients should be offered contact numbers for support groups or specialist counsellors. It is also useful to reinforce their need to grieve, and identify times which may be hard, like the period around the baby's estimated delivery date. This helps the patient and her partner to legitimise their feelings. Some hospitals offer bereavement counselling and a book of remembrance for babies; others also offer the services of the hospital chaplain.

Ectopic pregnancy

This occurs when a fertilised ovum implants somewhere other than the endometrium. The most common site is the fallopian tube (Blackburn & Loper 1992), but implantation can also occur in the ovaries and abdominal cavities (see Fig. 29.3).

The incidence of ectopic pregnancy is about 0.5–1% of pregnancies (Stevens & Kenney 1994). This ratio has risen over the last decade and indications are that it will continue to rise with the increase in PID and IUCD use (Stovall & Ling 1992). The use of oral postcoital contraceptives and some fertility treatments also appear to increase the risk of ectopic pregnancy. Ectopic implantation appears to occur because of delay in passage of the fertilised egg. This passage is induced by muscular contraction and ciliary activity. If the fallopian tubes are damaged due to adhesions following infection, the ciliary activity is reduced and the egg cannot pass into the uterus, so it implants in the tube. Hormonal changes of the corpeus luteum continue as, physiologically, the pregnancy is still viable at this stage. As a result, the uterus grows and softens as it would with a normal uterine pregnancy. The products of conception continue to expand causing pain and vaginal bleeding in a 'spotting' form.

It is usually at this stage that the woman seeks health intervention. If left unchecked, the products of conception will continue to grow until rupture of the tube occurs and devastating haemorrhage follows.

Assessment

Most patients will give a history of abdominal pain, sometimes unilateral or generalised lower abdomen and pelvic pain. The patient usually has intermittent vaginal bleeding or spotting and, as a result, may or may not be aware that she is pregnant. Most embryos die within 6–12 weeks of gestation due to lack of placental development. For this reason, most women with ectopic pregnancy suffer a lot less nausea than those with a uterine pregnancy with a healthy developing placenta. Once the embryo dies, endometrium is shed and a large PV bleed ensues. This is different to the potentially life-threatening haemorrhage which occurs with a ruptured fallopian tube. The degree of haemodynamic compromise determines the urgency of intervention, and therefore accurate assessment of basic haemostasis is vital. Slight tachycardia would be expected because of the emotion and anxiety attached to ectopic pregnancy, but bradycardia together with an increase in respirations and postural and persistent hypotension should be treated seriously. As part of the assessment, a urine sample should be taken to confirm pregnancy, and an ultrasound scan will show the location of pregnancy after about 6 weeks' gestation. Table 29.3 highlights the clinical differences between a threatened miscarriage and an ectopic pregnancy.

Management

Early management revolves around symptom control and psychological support. Pain relief and routine

Table 29.3 – *Differential diagnosis of ectopic pregnancy vs. threatened miscarriage. (After Stevens & Kenney 1994)*

Symptom	Ectopic		Threatened miscarriage	
	Nature	Percentage of patients affected	Nature	Percentage of patients affected
Abdominal pain	General or affected side	90	Midline, crampy	10
Shoulder tip pain		26		None
General abdominal	General	45	Usually non-tender	
tenderness	Lower	25		
	Unilateral	30		
Vaginal bleeding	Light/spotting	64	Light	100
Amenorrhoea		75		90
Uterus size	Normal	80	Right for dates	100
Shock		17		None
Dysuria		11		None
Rectal pain		9		None

intravenous access should be established. If the woman demonstrates signs of shock, fluid replacement should commence. Once the diagnosis has been made, early surgical intervention is necessary to prevent tubal rupture. In many cases the fallopian tube can be saved in ectopics diagnosed in early gestation. This is achieved by a laproscopic salpingostomy. This carries an increased risk of future ectopic pregnancies because of scar tissue. If salpingostomy is not possible, the fallopian tube is removed, with obvious implications for future fertility.

If ectopic rupture is suspected, the patient should be considered to have a life-threatening condition. Ruptured ectopic pregnancy is the highest single cause of maternal death (Rita 1998). Death usually occurs as a result of uncontrolled haemorrhage. This is because occult bleeding into the abdominal cavity can occur as well as PV loss; therefore, blood loss can be underestimated. The patient compensates initially, then becomes rapidly shocked. It is important to commence vigorous fluid resuscitation. Urgent surgical intervention is necessary to preserve maternal life. The woman and her partner's psychological needs should not be overlooked. As well as the physical distress, they are also coming to terms with the loss of their baby and the threat to future fertility that surgery brings. The nurse needs to acknowledge, not minimise, these feelings. A full description of psychological care and appropriate follow-up is given in the section on miscarriage (p. 420).

Pre-eclampsia/eclampsia

Pre-eclampsia, or pregnancy-induced hypertension, occurs in about 7% cent of pregnancies (Stevens & Kenney 1994). Its causes have not been proven, but several theories exist, the most common being that susceptibility to eclampsia is a hereditary trait linked to a recessive gene (Chesley 1985). Other theories link eclampsia to a possible immunological cause where an antigenic reaction to the fetus causes maternal symptoms. Historic linkage of eclampsia to socioeconomic status has no foundation in research (Reedy & Brucker 1995). Women most susceptible to pre-eclampsia/eclampsia are those at either end of the child-bearing age range, i.e. younger than 16 or older than 35 years of age. It is most common in first pregnancies and in those women expecting twins or more, and there appears to be a familial link. Women with pre-existing health problems, such as diabetes and chronic hypertension, are more susceptible to pre-eclampsia.

The disease usually has a gradual onset, the pre eclampsia phase. Because of good antenatal screening, most patients are identified and treated early. Therefore, the use of A&E for care in the pre-eclampsic phase is uncommon, but it is important to understand the disease process in order to treat life-threatening eclampsia in A&E. Pre-eclampsia has a multisystem impact (see Box 29.10).

Pre-eclampsia

A triad of symptoms exists:

- hypertension – 30 mmHg or more above the woman's usual systolic BP or 15 mmHg above her usual diastolic BP
- proteinuria

Box 29.10 – *Multisystem impact of pre-eclampsia/eclampsia*

Cardiovascular
- Hypertension – increased peripheral resistance
- Damage to blood vessels – vasopression traumatises vessels and induces coagulopathy
- Haemorrhage – due to reduced platelets

Haematological
- Thrombocytopenia – results from coagulopathy and reduces platelets and fibrinogen activity
- Abnormal clotting
- Disseminating intravascular coagulopathy

Renal
- Impaired glomerular function – glomerular filtration rate (GFR) and renal blood flow are increased in pregnancy; with pre-eclampsia a decrease occurs
- Proteinuria – due to renal impairment
- Sodium/potassium retention – contributes to oedema
- Acute renal failure

Neurological
- Headache – due to cerebral oedema. In severe cases cerebral infarct/haemorrhage may occur
- Hyperreflexia – nerve-end irritation due to vasospasm
- Visual disturbance – due to retinal oedema; can lead to retinal detachment
- Convulsions – late sign of eclampsia

Respiratory
- Pulmonary oedema – due to cardiovascular and renal complications
- Haemorrhage – due to thrombocytopenia

Hepatic
- Abnormal liver enzymes
- Periportal haemorrhage – secondary to other system changes
- Infarction
- Rupture

Placental/fetal
- Placental infarction
- Abruptio placentae
- Fetal intrauterine growth retardation
- Fetal death

- oedema – where this is present in the face or upper limbs it is of greater concern. Lower limb oedema, particularly of the feet or ankles, is usually mechanical in nature.

If any two of these symptoms are present, the woman is considered to have pre-eclampsia. Persistent hypertension should be treated, and initially close maternal and fetal monitoring will necessitate admission.

Eclampsia

This is usually defined as the onset of fitting after 20 weeks' gestation, with or without preceding pre-eclampsic symptoms (Stevens & Kenney 1994). Prior to fitting, most patients complain of headache, visual disturbance, shortness of breath or right hypochondriacal pain. They may also have oliguria and appear confused. These symptoms are all derived from the physiological processes described in Box 29.10. While some women present in A&E at this stage, more appear as emergency admissions once fitting has commenced. Eclampsic fitting is life-threatening to both the mother and fetus. It must be brought under control rapidly using small doses of diazepam, 10 mg i.v. repeated up to five times. It is administered in this manner to prevent fetal depression. Intravenous infusion of chlormethiazole or phenytoin should also be considered. Occasionally, short-term ventilation and paralysis may be necessary. Other presentations of impending eclampsia include severe right hypochondriacal pain and shock as a result of hepatic rupture.

Urgent laparotomy is indicated to control haemorrhage and preserve maternal life. In these circumstances, however, it has a mortality of about 70%. Symptoms of disseminating intravascular coagulopathy (DIC) accompany about 7% of eclampsic conditions (Stevens & Kenney 1994). Once pre-eclampsia reaches this stage, or fitting has occurred, urgent preparation to deliver the fetus should be made. Delivery usually resolves maternal symptoms, although in some cases they may persist for up to 10 days (Reedy & Brucker 1995). The baby has a greater chance of survival even if delivered premature.

Abrupto placentae

This is more commonly treated in obstetric units than in A&E departments. It occurs as a result of premature separation of the placenta from the uterine wall. Haemorrhage and blood usually track between the uterus and placental membranes, causing PV bleeding and pain. Bleeding can be occult in about 10% of cases, and therefore diagnosis should not be made simply by the presence of PV bleeding. A pelvic ultrasound should be used to confirm diagnosis. Predisposing factors include substance misuse, pre-eclampsia, a maternal age of 35 or more, multiple gestation and as a result of trauma.

Emergency childbirth

The majority of births are normal deliveries requiring little assistance and the duration of labour is usually long enough for the woman to seek maternity care. Occasionally, however, it is necessary to deliver a baby in A&E, if there is insufficient time to reach the delivery unit. The most common causes of emergency childbirth include multiparous women with precipitous (rapid) deliveries and adolescents girls who successfully conceal their pregnancy until they present with abdominal pains or do not recognise the signs of active labour. Some women in pre-term labour may also have precipitous deliveries.

Labour can be described as a process by which the fetus, placenta and membranes are expelled through the birth canal. Normal labour begins spontaneously at approximately 40 weeks' gestation, referred to as 'term', with the fetus presenting by the head or 'vertex' (Bennet & Brown 1990). Box 29.11 outlines the stages of labour.

> **Box 29.11 –** *The three stages of labour*
>
> **■ First stage**
> This is the longest phase during which the body prepares for delivery. The cervix effaces then dilates. There is usually a pink, mucous 'show' as this begins, and the amniotic membranes rupture as the cervix dilates. If this has not already occurred, contractions gradually increase in frequency and intensity. Transition to second stage occurs once the cervix is fully dilated to 10 cm. This phase usually lasts several hours, however the time reduces with the number of pregnancies.
>
> **■ Second stage**
> This is from full dilation until after delivery of the baby. During this phase, the baby's head travels down the birth canal. When it reaches the outlet, it flexes to present occiput first. This is a complicated but natural process. The visible occiput is termed 'crowning' and highlights the imminence of delivery. The head is followed by the shoulders, then the trunk and legs. This usually lasts up to 1 hour.
>
> **■ Third stage**
> This is from the delivery of the baby until complete delivery of the placenta and membranes and control of haemorrhage.

First stage labour management

The nurse's role in the care of a woman facing imminent childbirth is to provide physical and emotional support in a calm, relaxed manner. The nurse should obtain enough information to assess the woman's immediate circumstances:

- What parity is the woman?
- At what gestation is the pregnancy?
- What signs of onset of labour has she experienced?
- Has she a history of precipitous labour?
- What are the frequency and duration of the contractions?

The assistance of a midwife, obstetric and neonatal team should be obtained immediately, and provision for the imminent birth should be made. Signs of imminent childbirth include:

- the mother experiences tension, anxiety and intense contractions
- blood 'show' as a result of rapid dilation of the cervix
- bulging or gaping of the anus as a result of descent of the fetal presenting part
- bulging or fullness of the perineum
- 'crowning' of the fetal head at the introitus, which occurs when the fetal skull escapes under the pubic arch and no longer recedes (Fig. 29.4)
- the mother saying 'the baby is coming'.

In multiparous women, the last sign is symptomatic of imminent birth; however, in primaparous women, birth may take up to 30 minutes. Birth is near when the head stays visible between contractions. The mother should be made to feel in control, protecting her dignity, and should be kept informed of all that is happening. Her partner should be included as a source of constant support and encouragement to the mother at this time. The mother should be encouraged to adopt a position which is most comfortable for her, which is usually sitting on the trolley with her back well supported with pillows or a foam wedge.

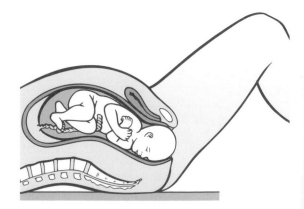

Figure 29.4 – *Cross-sectional view of crowning.*

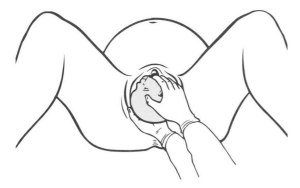

Figure 29.5 – *Hold infant's head gently in both hands.*

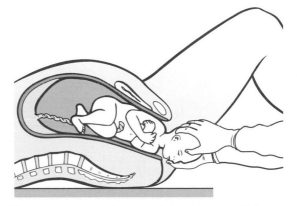

Figure 29.6 – *Carefully support infant's head as it is born.*

Nitrous oxide is the preferred method of pain relief when birth is imminent and the mother should be encouraged to inhale the gas while she is feeling the contractions. As well as providing pain relief, it is also an effective means of providing extra oxygen to both the mother and the fetus.

Baseline recordings of maternal temperature, pulse, respirations and blood pressure should be obtained. The fetal heartbeat is also recorded and may be auscultated using a fetal stethoscope or fetal Doppler when the head is presenting. The fetal heart sounds are more commonly located close to the midline below the umbilicus. The normal fetal heart rate is between 120 and 160 beats/min. A further assessment of fetal condition includes observation of the amniotic fluid or 'waters'; these are normally straw-coloured, but they may become green as a result of meconium.

Second stage labour management

The attending nurse/midwife should open a sterile delivery set and wash the woman's vulva with sterile swabs and warmed antiseptic solution. With the next contraction, the woman should be encouraged to inhale deeply and bear down to facilitate the delivery. The nurse should place his fingers over the advancing head to prevent expulsive 'crowning', which may result in perineal tearing and a heightened risk of intraventricular haemorrhage to the newborn infant (Fig. 29.5). As the fetal head advances and gradually distends the perineal tissue, the mother should be encouraged to pant to facilitate a controlled delivery and reduce maternal trauma. Once the baby's head emerges, the nurse should slip a finger over the occiput to feel if the cord is round the baby's neck. If this has happened, the cord should be released either by slipping it over the head or, if this is unsuccessful, by applying two artery forceps 2–5 cm apart and cutting the cord between them.

The nurse should continue to support the head, taking care not to put any traction on it (Fig. 29.6). Mucus should be removed with a sterile swab, but the eyes should not be cleansed due to the risk of infection. At the next contraction, the anterior shoulder should be delivered by gentle downward traction of the head. Then the baby should be raised and the posterior shoulder will deliver rapidly, followed by the trunk and legs. The baby should be dried and placed in a warm towel as a cold baby has an increased oxygen consumption and cold babies more easily become hypoglycaemic and acidotic; they also have an increased mortality (Advanced Life Support Group 1997). The newborn baby should be allowed to lie on the bed or be placed on the mother's abdomen, allowing her to see and touch the baby. The umbilical cord should be clamped and cut if this has not already been done and Syntometrine given intramuscularly to the mother. This contains oxytocin and ergometrine. The oxytocin provides marked uterine contraction after approximately 3 minutes but is short-lived, and as its effects begin to wear off, the ergometrine begins to act and provide longer-lasting uterine contractions, reducing the risk of postpartum haemorrhage (Greaves *et al.* 1997).

The time of the delivery and those involved in it should be recorded accurately. The Apgar score should also be recorded. This is a numerical scoring system used to assess the newborn baby's condition at 1 minute after birth and reassessed again after 5 minutes. While Kelnar *et al.* (1995) stress that assessment at 1 minute is important, it has been shown that an assessment at 5 minutes is much more reliable as a predictor of death during the first 28 days of life and of the child's neurological state and risk of major handicap at the age of 1 year (Nelson & Ellenberg 1981, Rehnke *et al.* 1987). The factors assessed are

Table 29.4 – *Apgar scores*

	Score		
Factor	0	1	2
A = appearance (colour)	Blue	Blue limbs, pink body	Pink
P = pulse (heart rate)	Absent	<100 beats/min	>100 beats/min
G = grimace (muscle tone)	Limp	Some flexion	Good flexion
A = activity (reflexes irritable)	Absent	Some motion	Good motion
R = respiratory effort	Absent	Weak cry	Strong cry

heart rate, respiratory rate, muscle tone, reflex response to stimulus, and colour. A score of 0–2 is given to each sign in accordance with the guideline in Table 29.4. A normal infant in good condition at birth will achieve an Apgar score of between 7 and 10. A score below 7 indicates some degree of asphyxia which requires some form of resuscitation (Michie 1990).

Third stage labour management

The third stage of labour is from delivery of the baby to delivery of the placenta and usually takes about 5–20 minutes. A sterile receiver should be placed between the woman's thighs to collect any blood lost, and the umbilical cord is placed in the receiver. Once the signs of placental separation are observed, i.e. lengthening of the umbilical cord, a fresh gush of blood and contraction of the uterus causing the fundus to rise to the level of the umbilicus, the mother should be asked to bear down as for delivery to expel the placenta and membranes. Once delivered, the placenta should be examined for completeness. The fundus of the uterus may be massaged to promote contractions, expel blood clots and control haemorrhage. The woman's vagina and perineum should be examined for tearing which may require suturing. The mother's temperature, pulse and blood pressure should be recorded and her lochia, i.e. PV loss, observed. The baby should also be examined, weighed and have a rectal temperature taken. Two identity bands should also be placed on the baby. Both mother and baby should then be transferred to the nearest maternity unit for post-natal care.

Postpartum haemorrhage

Postpartum haemorrhage occurs in 3–5% of pregnancies and accounts for almost 10% of maternal deaths (Beischer & Mackay 1986). It can be described as any bleeding from the genital tract which adversely affects the mother's condition following the birth of a baby, up to 6 weeks post-delivery. A blood loss of 500 ml or more at delivery is regarded as post-partum haemorrhage, irrespective of maternal condition.

There are two types of postpartum haemorrhage:

- *Primary postpartum haemorrhage*, which occurs within the first 24 hours post-delivery.
- *Secondary postpartum haemorrhage*, which occurs at any time after the first 24 hours, up to 6 weeks post-delivery, but most commonly occurs between 7 and 14 days postpartum. It can be described as bleeding in excess of the normal lochial loss and may be associated with retained placental tissue or uterine infection.

Assessment

History should include the following information:

- duration of symptoms
- quantity of bleeding in terms of number of pads used per hour
- type of blood loss, i.e. red, brown clots
- type of pain
- location of pain
- date of delivery and any subsequent period/PV bleeding
- any infection
- any trauma
- other related medical history.

The woman will have a enlarged 'boggy', uterus. On palpation the uterus will feel soft, distended and lacking in tone. The fundal height will rise above the umbilicus as a result of retained blood in the uterus preventing uterine contraction. A low-grade pyrexia, rising pulse and falling blood pressure characterise postpartum haemorrhage together with lower back and abdominal pain, and general restlessness.

Sanitary pads should be checked to evaluate the amount of bleeding and note the presence or absence of clots or odour.

Management

The aim of A&E management is to control haemorrhage and maintain blood volume. Blood should be taken for group and cross-match, and large-bore i.v. lines for warmed crystalloids and blood should be established. Oxygen should also be administered. An i.v. injection of ergometrine or Syntometrine may be given in order to cause uterine contraction, which assists in haemorrhage control. If the uterus is palpable, it may be massaged to enable it to contract and expel any clots. The presence of retained products of conception should be excluded on pelvic ultrasound. If debris is found or haemorrhage is not controlled, urgent evacuation of retained products of conception (ERPC) should be performed in theatre.

Conclusion

This chapter has considered the common gynaecological and obstetric reasons for presentation to A&E. Many of these conditions have a life-long impact on the patient and her family, in terms of either physical or, more commonly, psychological well-being. It is imperative that A&E staff are sensitive to the needs of the woman and her partner, and can offer privacy and compassionate, non-judgmental care. Inappropriate assessment or intervention can have catastrophic consequences. The information provided in this chapter should enable the nurse to make an informed assessment and plan therapeutic care for this emotionally and physically vulnerable group.

References

Advanced Life Support Group (1997) *Advanced Paediatric Life Support. a Practical Approach.* London: BMJ.

Beischer NA, Mackay EV (1986) Ante natal care: education of the patient. In: Beischer NA, ed. *Obstetrics and the Newborn* 2nd edn. London: Baillière Tindall.

Bennett RV, Brown LK (1990) The first stage of labour: physiology and early care. In: Bennett RV, Brown LK, eds. *Myles Textbook for Midwives.* Edinburgh: Churchill Livingstone.

Blackburn S, Loper D (1992) *Maternal, Fetal and Neonatal Physiology.* Philadelphia: WB Saunders.

Burgess A, Holmstrom L (1974) *Rape: Victims of Crisis.* Maryland: RJ Brady.

Chesley L (1985) Hypertensive disorders in pregnancy. *Journal of Nurse-Midwifery* 30(2), 99–104.

Creasy R, Resnick R (1993) *Maternal Fetal Medicine.* Philadelphia: WB Saunders.

Duncan D (1995) Fathers have feelings too. *Modern Midwife* 5(1), 30–31.

Golub S (1992) *Periods.* Newberry Park: Sage.

Gondeck J (1998) Gynecologic emergencies. In: Newberry L, ed. *Sheehy's Emergency Nursing: Principles and Practice* 4th edn. St Louis: Mosby.

Greaves I, Hodgetts T, Porter K (1997) Childbirth. In: Greaves I, Hodgetts T, Porter K, eds. *Emergency Care: a Textbook for Paramedics.* London: Baillière Tindall.

Hinchliff S, Montague S, Watson R (1996) *Physiology for Nursing Practice* 2nd edn. London: Baillière Tindall.

Holloway M (1994) Care of the sexually assaulted woman. *Emergency Nurse* 2(3), 18–20.

Howe J (1996) Aetiology, treatment and control of gonorrhoea. *Nursing Standard* 11(9), 46–48.

Kelnar CJH, Harvey D, Simpson C (1995) *The Sick Newborn Baby* 3rd edn. London: Baillière Tindall.

Lichtman R, Papera S (1990) *Gynecology: Well Woman Care.* Norwalk, CT: Appleton & Lange.

Michie MM (1990) The baby at birth. In: Bennett RV, Brown LK, eds. *Myles Textbook for Midwives.* Edinburgh: Churchill Livingstone.

Miscarriage Association (1996) *Why Did it Happen to Us? – a summary of Causes, Tests and Treatment* Wakefield: Miscarriage Association.

Nelson KB, Ellenberg JH (1981) Apgar scores as predictors of chronic neurologic disability. *Pediatrics* 68, 36–44.

Reedy N, Brucker M (1995) Emergencies in gynecology and obstetrics. In: Kitt S, Selfridge-Thomas J, Prochl JA, Kaiser J, eds. *Emergency Nursing: a Physiologic and Clinical Perspective* 2nd edn. Philadelphia: WB Saunders.

Regan L (1992) Managing miscarriage. *The Practitioner* 236, 1513, 374–378.

Rehnke M, Carter RL, Hardt NS *et al.* (1987) The relationship of Apgar scores, gestational age and birthweight to survival of low birthweight infants. *American Journal of Perinatology* 4, 121–124.

Rita S (1998) Obstetric emergencies. In: Newberry L, ed. *Sheehy's Emergency Nursing: Principles and Practice.* St Louis: Mosby.

Selfridge-Thomas J (1997) *Emergency Nursing: an Essential Guide for Patient Care.* Philadelphia: WB Saunders.

Standing J (1997) Miscarriage in A&E: a review of the literature. *Emergency Nurse* 5(5), 25–29.

Stevens L, Kenney A (1994) *Emergencies in Obstetrics and Gynaecology.* Oxford: Oxford University Press.

Stoval R, Ling F (1992) Some new approaches to ectopic pregnancy. *Contemporary Obstetrics and Gynaecology* 35(5), 35–70.

Walters BA (1992) Caring for the patient with a disorder of the reproductive system. In: Royle JA, Walsh M, eds. *Watson's Medical-Surgical Nursing and Related Physiology* 4th edn. London: Baillière Tindall.

Weissmann G (1991) The actions of NSAIDs. *Hospital Practice* 26, 60–76.

Wolner Hanbseen P (1991) Incidence and diagnosis of acute salpingitis. *Contemporary Obstetrics and Gynaecology* 36(2), 67–72.

Chapter 30

Ophthalmic Emergencies

Janet Marsden

- Introduction
- Anatomy and physiology of the eye
- Assessing ophthalmic conditions
- Ocular burns
- Penetrating trauma
- Major closed trauma
- Minor trauma
- Eyepads
- Eyedrops
- Red eye
- Health promotion
- Conclusion

Introduction

A significant proportion of the workload of the A&E department is made up of patients with ophthalmic problems, ranging from 6% (Edwards 1987) to 8%. Tan *et al.* (1997) found a lack of basic ophthalmic training for A&E SHOs leading to a lack of confidence on their part in the management of eye emergencies. This lack of confidence on the part of junior doctors is reflected in the nursing teams of many A&E departments and, combined with the apparent health of many ophthalmic patients, can lead to inappropriate management in the A&E department.

Being able to see and make a visual assessment of surroundings is taken for granted by most people and the sudden decline in or loss of sight is an extremely frightening experience. In A&E, patients attend with acute and chronic ophthalmic conditions of varying degrees of severity. For some, immediate intervention can be sight-saving. This chapter will equip A&E nurses to assess, identify and initiate care for patients with common ophthalmic conditions. Anatomy and physiology of the eye and surrounding structures will aid nurses in using mechanism of injury, signs and symptoms to assess the patient's condition. The chapter will address ophthalmic conditions in terms of assessment findings, which can be broadly categorised into two groups:

- trauma
- non-traumatic red eye.

Anatomy and Physiology of the Eye

Orbit

The orbit is a large bony socket which contains the eyeball or globe with its associated muscles, nerves, blood vessels, fat and most of the lacrimal apparatus (see Fig. 30.1). Each of the two orbits is roughly pyramidal in shape with the apex lying posteriorly. The

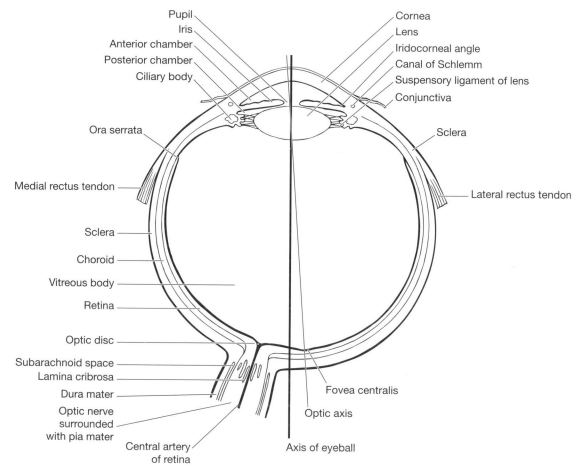

Figure 30.1 – *Basic structure of the eye.*

orbit is made up of seven individual bones: the maxilla, palatine, zygoma, sphenoid, frontal ethmoid and lacrimal bones.

Eyelids

The lids are layered structures covered on their outer surfaces by skin and on their inner surfaces by conjunctiva (see Fig. 30.2). In between is subcutaneous tissue, the orbital septum of which thickens within the lids to form fibrous tarsal plates which give structure to the lid. The upper lid contains the levator muscle and the lower contains the inferior tarsal muscle, which retracts it. The lids are maintained in position by the medial and lateral canthal tendons which attach to the periosteum. The lids are closed by the orbicularis muscle.

Within the lid structure are a number of glands. Tarsal or Meibomian glands are arranged perpendicular to the lid margin on the conjunctival surface of the tarsal plate; when blocked and infected, these are known as chalazia. The eyelashes are more numerous on the upper lid than on the lower. Sebaceous and modified sweat glands open into each lash follicle – infection produces a hordeolum or stye.

Behind the lashes is the join between the conjunctiva and the skin of the lids. This is known as the grey line because of its relative avascularity. The lids protect the eye by preventing contact with foreign bodies and by preventing drying of the cornea and conjunctiva. Lid closure and blinking help to spread the tear film over the front of the eye and move it into the lacrimal drainage apparatus.

Lacrimal system

The tear film is composed mainly of watery fluid from the lacrimal gland which is situated in the orbit. The other important components of the tear film are mucin from the conjunctival goblet cells and oil from the

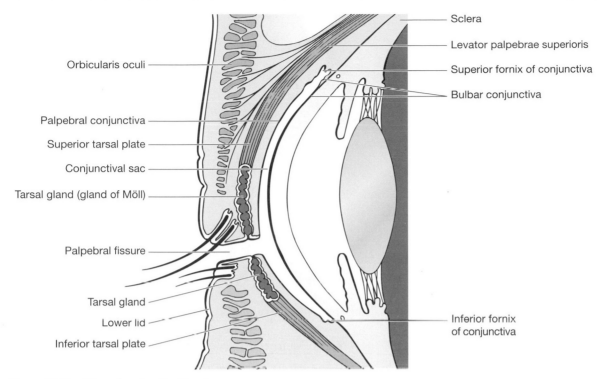

Orbicularis oculi

Palpebral conjunctiva

Superior tarsal plate

Conjunctival sac

Tarsal gland (gland of Möll)

Palpebral fissure

Tarsal gland

Lower lid

Inferior tarsal plate

Sclera

Levator palpebrae superioris

Superior fornix of conjunctiva

Bulbar conjunctiva

Inferior fornix
of conjunctiva

Figure 30.2 – *Lids and conjunctival formices.*

Meibomian (tarsal) glands and the glands of Möll and Zeiss. The tear film is distributed over the surface of the eye by gravity, capillary action of the puncta and canaliculi and the eyelids. The tears leave the eye by evaporation and by way of the puncta, the upper of which takes 25% of the tears and the lower 27%. From the puncta, the tears flow into the canaliculi, into the common canaliculus and then into the lacrimal sac and through the nasolacrimal duct (see Fig. 30.3).

Conjunctiva

The conjunctiva is a thin, transparent mucous membrane lining the inner surface of the eyelid (palpebral conjunctiva), reflecting back on itself at the upper and lower fornices and covering the sclera as far as the corneoscleral junction (bulbar conjunctiva). The conjunctiva is adherent to the lid and rather less so to the Tenon's capsule overlying the sclera. It is most adherent at the corneoscleral junction (limbus). The conjunctiva is quite mobile in the fornices and over the globe and can absorb a large volume of fluid and become oedematous. The epithelium of the conjunctiva is continuous with the corneal epithelium. It contains goblet cells which secrete mucus. The main body of the conjunctiva is connective tissue housing blood vessels, nerves and other glands.

Cornea

The transparent cornea forms the anterior one-sixth of the globe. Its curvature is higher than that of the rest of the globe and it is the main structure responsible for the refraction of light entering the eye. It is an avascular structure which is nourished by the aqueous humour, the capillaries at its edge and from the tear film. Microscopically, it consists of five layers:

- *The epithelium* – consists of five layers of cells centrally, 10 or more at the limbus. Running between the cells are the nerve endings of sensory nerve fibres, which are sensitive mainly to pain. The epithelium regenerates by the movement of cells from the periphery towards the middle.
- *Bowman's layer* – is acellular and consists of collagen fibres.
- *Substantia propria or stroma* – comprises 90% of the thickness of the cornea. It is transparent and fibrous, and is made up of lamellae of collagen fibres arranged parallel to the surface. This arrangement ensures corneal clarity.

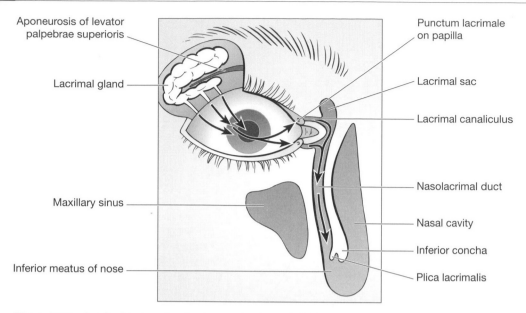

Figure 30.3 – *Lacrimal system showing tear production and drainage.*

■ *Descemet's membrane* – a strong membrane which is the basement membrane of the endothelium.
■ *Endothelium* – a single layer of flattened cells which plays a major role in controlling the hydration of the cornea by a barrier and active transport method. Loss of endothelial cells leads to corneal oedema and lack of clarity.

Sclera

Sclera forms the posterior five-sixths of the eye. It is 1 mm thick posteriorly and thinnest (0.3 mm) immediately posterior to the insertion of the recti muscles. The sclera forms the 'white' of the eye; its outer surface is smooth, except for where the six orbital muscles are attached. It is perforated posteriorly by the optic nerve at an area known as the lamina cribrosa. In this area, the sclera forms a meshwork rather than a solid structure to allow nerve fibres and the central retinal artery and vein to pass through it. The sclera is weakened at this point. Raised intraocular pressure can make the lamina cribrosa bulge outwards, producing a cupped disc.

The sclera is composed of two main layers: the episclera, a loose connective tissue which provides most of the nutritional support of the sclera via a vascular plexus; and the main body of the sclera, which is a dense fibrous tissue that is relatively avascular. The function of the sclera is to protect the intraocular contents and preserve the shape of the globe, maintaining the placement of the optical system. It provides the insertion for the muscles.

The uveal tract

The uveal tract is composed of the iris, the ciliary body and the choroid. The iris is a thin pigmented diaphragm with a central aperture or pupil. It is located between the cornea and the lens. The pupil varies in size from 1 to 8 mm and differs in size on the two sides in 25% of 'normal' people. The iris divides the anterior segment into anterior and posterior chambers. Its periphery is attached to the ciliary body. The colour of the iris is produced by pigment in melanocytes within its structure. The main body of the iris consists of highly vascular connective tissue; it also contains nerve fibres, the muscle of the sphincter pupillae and the dilator pupillae. The sphincter forms a ring of smooth muscle around the pupil. When it contracts in bright light and during accommodation, the pupil constricts. The dilator is a thin layer of muscle extending from the iris root to the sphincter pupillae. When the dilator pupillae contracts in low-intensity light and during sympathetic activity such as fear, the pupil enlarges.

The ciliary body is continuous with the choroid and the margin of the iris. It contains the ciliary muscle used to change the shape of the lens during accommodation. Its outer, pigmented layer is continuous with the retinal pigment epithelium. Its inner, non-pigmented layer produces aqueous humour. The lens attaches to the ciliary body by a suspensory ligament whose fibres are known as zonules.

The choroid is a thin, soft, brown coat covering the inner surface of the sclera. It extends from the optic nerve to the ciliary body at the ora serrata. The inner surface of the choroid is firmly attached to the pigment layer of the retina. The main body of the choroid is a vascular layer, the choriocapillaris, which supplies nutrition to the external half of the retina and the macula. Its outer layer consists of larger vessels and collecting veins.

The angle and aqueous

The anterior segment of the globe is divided into two chambers. The anterior chamber lies between the cornea and the root of the iris. At the periphery of the anterior chamber is a junction between the cornea, sclera, ciliary body and iris, known as the angle. Within this angle is the trabecular meshwork. The posterior chamber is a slit-like cavity between the back of the iris and the ciliary processes and lens.

Aqueous humour is a clear fluid which fills both of these chambers. It is formed by the ciliary processes of the ciliary body. From the ciliary processes, the aqueous flows through the pupil into the anterior chamber and from there through the trabecular meshwork into a sinus, the canal of Schlemm. From this structure, it drains into the aqueous veins and into the general circulation. There is a continuous dynamic production and drainage of aqueous which supplies the metabolic needs of the lens and cornea. Pathologically high pressure, such as glaucoma, is usually due to reduced outflow of aqueous and causes damage to the retina.

The lens

The lens is a transparent, biconvex structure situated behind the iris and in front of the vitreous. It is flexible and kept in position by suspensory ligaments attached to the ciliary body. The convexity of its anterior surface is less than that of its posterior surface and it contributes to the refractive power of the eye. The lens consists of a capsule, an epithelial layer on its anterior surface and the lens fibres. The capsule is elastic and encloses the whole lens. The lens fibres constitute the main part of the lens. Epithelial cells change to become lens fibres throughout life. No cells are lost and therefore the centre of the lens becomes denser and less pliable over time. With age, the nucleus becomes dense and yellow; if it becomes opaque, it is known as a cataract.

Contraction of the ciliary muscle moves the ciliary body forwards. This relieves pressure on the fibres of the zonule and allows the lens to relax and become more spherical. At the same time, the sphincter pupillae contracts allowing light to enter through the thickest part of the lens. Light is therefore enabled to focus on the retina. The power to accommodate reduces as the lens becomes less flexible with age.

Retina

The retina is the nervous coat of the eye and the internal layer of the globe. It is a thin, transparent membrane, continuous with the optic nerve and extending to the ora serrata behind the choroid. The retina consists of a pigmented layer next to the choroid which absorbs light and releases vitamin A, which is necessary for the functioning of the photoreceptors. The neural retina consists of photoreceptors and then a number of layers of nerve cells which serve to amplify and transmit the impulses from the photoreceptors to the optic nerve and from there to the brain.

Two types of photoreceptors are present within the retina: 'rods', which allow vision in dim light and in black and white; and 'cones', which are adapted to bright light and can resolve fine detail and colour. Rods are absent at the fovea and rise rapidly in numbers towards the periphery of the retina. Cones are most dense at the fovea and reduce in number towards the periphery. Light impinges on the photoreceptors, producing a chemical reaction which results in an electrical impulse. This is amplified by the various nerve cells and synapses in the neural retina and transmitted through the nerve fibre layer to the optic nerve.

Vitreous

The vitreous body fills the posterior segment of the eye. It is a clear, jelly-like substance consisting of a collagen framework with hyaluronic acid. Collagen fibrils attach the vitreous to the retina at the ora serrata and the optic disc. Its function is to transmit light and to contribute slightly to the resolving power of the eye. It supports the posterior surface of the lens and assists in holding the neural part of the retina in place against its pigment layer.

Assessing Ophthalmic Conditions

History

Establishing the exact history of a patient's condition is fundamental to making an accurate diagnosis. The history of the presenting problem should include:

- How long the patient has had symptoms for and whether they are getting worse

Box 30.1 – *Determining mechanism of injury*

■ Chemical involvement – identify type of chemical substance.

■ Force of injury and size of projectile

■ Possibility of penetration – may be small and high speed

■ What first aid has taken place?

■ Rapidity and mode of onset
■ Was heat/light a factor? (see Box 30.1)
■ Degree, type and location of pain
■ Is vision reduced and to what degree?
■ Has the patient had this, or a similar problem before?
■ Are there any concurrent systemic problems?
■ Is the patient photophobic?
■ Is there any discharge or watering?
■ Does the patient wear glasses/contact lenses?

Discussion of systemic problems and medication is important as it can point to possible ophthalmic problems. For example, there is a link between ankylosing spondylitis and uveitis, and a link between rheumatoid arthritis and dry eyes, and there are many ophthalmic side-effects of systemic drugs. The assessing nurse needs to investigate any pre-existing ophthalmic or other medical conditions. Of particular importance are conditions such as glaucoma, iritis and blepharitis; systemic conditions such as diabetes and rheumatoid arthritis; and any drug therapy, as all of these may affect the health of the eye.

Visual acuity

Assessment of visual acuity should be undertaken at triage for any ophthalmic patient, before any other investigations or treatment, except irrigation or instillation of local anaesthetic. The patient's affected or poorer seeing eye should be tested first, and the other occluded with a card or the patient's hand. Any distance glasses should be worn. He should be asked to read down from the top of the Snellen chart, making an attempt at all possible letters. Visual acuity should be recorded as:

Distance at which the eye is being tested (usually 6 m)
―――――――――――――――――――――――――――――――
Last line read by the patient

The number for this line is indicated on the Snellen chart, just above or just below the letters. If part of a line only is read, this may be recorded as the line

above plus the extra letters, or the line below minus the missed letters. For example, if the patient reads the '12' line except for one letter, at 6 m, it should be recorded as 6/12 – 1.

If the patient's vision appears poor (less than 6/9), a pinhole (a small hole in a card or a commercial pinhole) can be held in front of the eye to negate the effects of any refractive error. The visual acuity should be recorded with and without pinholes and a note should be taken of whether distance glasses or contact lenses are worn. If the patient is unable to read the top letter, the distance should be reduced until the patient can see the top letter on the chart, i.e. 5/60, 4/60, etc. to 1/60. If the patient cannot see the top letter at 1 m, it should be ascertained whether he can count fingers (CF), see hand movements (HM) or just perceive light (PL) at 1 m. Lack of light perception is recorded as NPL. Normal visual acuity is 6/6, but normal visual acuity *for the patient* may be less for a variety of reasons.

Problems in accurate visual acuity assessment may occur if the patient does not speak English or is not able to read. Strategies to overcome this may include:

■ using a recognition chart so that the patient may match letters or shapes
■ obtaining the services of an interpreter or family member to translate for the patient
■ with children, using picture tests such as the Kay picture test and making the procedure into a game – this will usually encourage greater cooperation.

Patients who are in pain should have a drop of local anaesthetic instilled so that any corneal pain is alleviated and the patient can cooperate more fully with the procedure, thus achieving an accurate visual acuity. Patients sometimes feel that this is a test that they have to pass and 'cheat' by looking through their fingers etc. It should be explained that the nurse is attempting to obtain an *accurate* assessment of their vision and that it is important that they are not tempted to make it seem better than it really is.

Examining the eye

Eye examination must be systematic. It is very easy to assume a diagnosis from the history and, in that way, miss less obvious problems. The eye should be examined from the 'outside' – the eye position and surrounding structures – working 'in' to consider the globe itself. Considerations for a thorough eye examination are given in Box 30.2.

Remember to compare the findings with the normal eye. What appears to be an abnormality may be bilateral and normal for the patient.

Equipment to aid assessment

An adequate eye assessment can be performed with minimal equipment. A bright light source, such as a pen torch or adjustable light, is essential for examination of the eye. Ophthalmoscopes are useful for retinal examination, but not for general examination as they only produce a small spot of light. Magnification is a useful aid, particularly in the hunt for foreign bodies. A hand-held magnifier, head loupe or ring light can be used. Cotton buds are used to evert the eyelids, remove foreign bodies and during irrigation.

Fluorescein drops or strips which stain damaged epithelial tissue are useful in examining abrasions. The stain is inserted and then the eye is viewed through a cobalt blue filter, as a penlight attachment, slit lamp or ophthalmoscope filter. While slit lamps (a binocular microscope for eye examination) offer the optimum provision for examination, they are expensive and not vital to initial assessment. Local anaesthetic, such as amethocaine 1% or benoxinate 0.4%, should be available in single-dose applications for pain relief and to facilitate examination.

Contact lenses

If the patient is wearing contact lenses, the lens should be removed from the injured eye, or from both eyes if inflammation or swelling is present. If possible, the patient should remove his own lens; each contact lens wearer develops his own way of doing it.

Removal of lenses

To remove hard lenses, the nurse should stretch the skin of the eyelid by pulling gently in a lateral direction from the outside corner of the patient's eye. Once the skin is stretched, the nurse should push the upper and lower lids together using a finger from each hand. This movement catches the edges of the lens and breaks its suction to the cornea. Once this happens, the lens will fall out (see Fig. 30.4). Alternatively, the

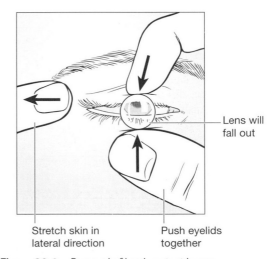

Lens will fall out

Stretch skin in lateral direction

Push eyelids together

Figure 30.4 – *Removal of hard contact lenses.*

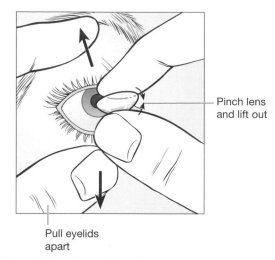

Pinch lens
and lift out

Pull eyelids
apart

Figure 30.5 – *Removal of soft contact lenses.*

nurse could put a (washed) index finger on the lens and gently move away from the cornea. The lids can then be used to lever the edge of the lens away from the cornea, and as the adhesion to the cornea breaks, the lens can be gently removed (Stollery 1997).

Hard lenses can also be removed using a specifically designed suction cup. The cup should be soaked in saline and then gently pressed against the contact lens. This forms a stronger suction than that of the lens to the cornea. The lens can then be lifted away from the eye. Other suction extractors must be squeezed before applying to the lens. The lens should be put into a labelled container with normal saline. If any significant corneal infection is present, such as an ulcer or abscess, the lens must be kept for microbiological culture.

Removal of soft lenses is demonstrated in Figure 30.5.

Triage decisions

Similar to other illness and injury, ophthalmic conditions vary considerably in severity and urgency. Using the Manchester Triage Group guidelines (Mackway-Jones 1996), eye complaints can be prioritised as follows:

- *Priority one (red)* – chemical injury; failure to act to dilute or neutralise chemical agents results in increased tissue damage and can lead to vascular damage and ischaemia and is therefore sight-threatening.
- *Priority two (orange)* – severe pain, penetrating trauma or recent, sudden total loss of vision. These presentations have the potential to be sight-

threatening or result in further damage if not treated promptly.
- *Priority three (yellow)* – moderate pain, reduced visual acuity or unclear/inappropriate history.
- *Priority four (green)* – pain, red eye, recent problem/injury.
- *Priority five (blue)* – chronic complaint without acute exacerbation.

Ocular Burns

Ocular burns may be divided most commonly into chemical, thermal and radiation (UV) burns.

Chemical burns

These are the most urgent category of ocular burns and are usually caused by alkalis, acids or solvents. Alkali burns are usually caused by sodium or potassium hydroxide, used as cleaning agents; calcium hydroxide, found in plaster and mortar; and ammonia, which is found in fertiliser and used in liquid form. Alkalis penetrate rapidly through corneal tissue, combining with cell membrane lipids, and result in cell disruption and tissue softening. A rapid rise in the pH in the anterior chamber may cause damage to the iris, ciliary body and lens. Damage to vascular channels leads to ischaemia. Alkali burns can be divided into acute and later stages.

Acids are less penetrating, and most damage is done during and soon after initial exposure (Tannen & Marsden 1991). Acid substances precipitate tissue proteins, forming barriers against deeper penetration and localising damage to the point of contact, although they can still be devastating. Acid burns are often due to car battery (sulphuric) acid or more complex organic and inorganic compounds. Hydrofluoric acid is exceptional in that it causes progressive damage similar to an alkaline substance. Solvent burns, although very painful, usually cause only transient irritation and damage. Thermal and/or contusion injuries due to the temperature or pressure of the chemical may be superimposed on the chemical injury (Marsden 1999a).

Primary management

A prompt and effective response to a chemical injury is vital to minimise tissue damage. One of the main determinants of ultimate outcome is duration of contact (Waggoner 1997), and as Glenn (1995) suggested, the initial treatment given by the nurse in the case of chemical eye injury may have more impact on the final vision than any subsequent care by the ophthalmologist.

Irrigation

The initial treatment involves copious irrigation to dilute the chemical and remove particulate matter. Irrigation should commence immediately, using whatever source is available. Herr *et al.* (1991) found no difference in the efficacy of irrigation fluids and therefore, in the A&E department, the irrigating fluid of choice is normal saline (0.9%) administered via a giving set to provide a directable and controllable jet. Sterile water is also used. The eyelids should be held open and contact lenses removed. A drop of local anaesthetic should be instilled prior to irrigation to assist in patient compliance and minimise pain. All aspects of the cornea and conjunctiva (exposed by everting the upper lid) should be thoroughly irrigated. All particulate matter should be removed, by wiping with a cotton-tipped applicator if necessary.

Any delay caused by attempting to identify the chemical or an appropriate neutralising solution adds to the contact time and increases the risk of more severe injury. It is best to assume that any previous irrigation is inadequate and carry out adequate irrigation in the department. It is impossible to specify an exact time for irrigation or a volume of fluid which should be used, as this depends on the nature of the chemical and its physical state as well as the patient's condition. Waggoner (1997) suggested that it is impossible to over-irrigate a chemically injured eye and recommended irrigation for 15–30 minutes.

The use of pH paper to check for adequate irrigation may be debated. In alkaline injury in particular, the chemical will leach out of the eye for a number of hours after injury, thus altering the pH. Delay in therapy of a number of hours until the pH is back to normal will delay healing. Waggoner (1997) suggested that the pH of the tear film should be recorded after 5 minutes without irrigation in order to be sure that the tear film is tested rather than the irrigating fluid. However, if the pH then proves to be abnormal, the eye has had a long period without irrigation in which further damage may take place; therefore this practice is not recommended. Ultimately, indicator paper is no substitute for prompt, adequate and thorough irrigation. Following irrigation, the patient's visual acuity should be checked to provide a baseline measurement.

Ophthalmic management

All but the most trivial chemical injuries should be referred to an ophthalmologist. The eye may look deceptively normal due to tissue blanching and ischaemia, which needs urgent assessment and treatment.

Ophthalmic management usually includes:

- mydriatics, which are used to dilate the pupil, reduce pain due to ciliary spasm and prevent adhesions between the iris and the lens (posterior synechiae)
- topical antibiotics – prophylactic use prevents secondary infection
- topical steroids to reduce and control inflammation
- potassium ascorbate drops or systemic ascorbic acid – these are often used in the treatment of alkali burns to restore levels of potassium ascorbate in the anterior chamber and thus aid healing
- admission to hospital may be required.

Solvent injury

This may be seen after staining with fluorescein as punctate stains on the cornea. They may be treated with a mydriatic drop to dilate the pupil and chloramphenicol ointment to prevent secondary bacterial infection and aid comfort. They usually resolve very quickly.

Thermal burns

These usually involve damage to the lids and are often associated with facial burns. Treatment is similar to that of thermal burns elsewhere on the body. Thermal burns range from very mild, such as those caused by tobacco ash which may be treated as an abrasion, with dilation of the pupil and chloramphenicol ointment, to the very severe caused by molten metal and glass which may require reconstruction of the globe and surrounding structures. Thermal burns involving the lids should be referred due to the possibility of aberrant healing, leading to lid closure and mobility problems (see also Ch. 10).

Radiation burns

These are likely to be caused by ultraviolet light in the form of sun lamps or from welding equipment. The symptoms are similar, ranging from mild discomfort to severe pain, photophobia and lacrimation. The condition is usually bilateral and symptoms are delayed by 6–10 hours. Local anaesthetic drops may be used to facilitate examination but should not be given to the patient to use at home. Treatment may include dilation of the pupil and topical chloramphenicol ointment. The most affected eye may be double padded. The condition resolves spontaneously within 24–36 hours.

Patients who have been using a MIG welder may need a fundal check if there is any residual loss of visual acuity after epithelial healing. The intensity of the light produced by this type of equipment may cause retinal burns (Marsden 1999b).

Infrared radiation burns are more severe than ultraviolet radiation burns; however, they are becoming rare since the development of protective eyewear. Infrared radiation burns can cause permanent loss of vision secondary to absorption of infrared rays by the iris and increased lens temperature, which leads to cataract formation (Egging 1998).

Penetrating trauma

Penetrating injuries and intraocular foreign bodies may cause eye damage by:

- disruption of the ocular tissues at the time of injury
- introduction of infection
- scar tissue formation (corneal, disrupting vision, retinal detachment caused by contracting scars inside the eye)
- reaction of the eye to foreign bodies – from organic material introducing infection or inflammation and from the deposition of pigments caused by degrading metal foreign bodies.

Large penetrating eye injuries are very obvious, but small perforations may be easily missed. The eye may look intact if the perforation is small and the wound may be sealed by iris tissue. It is very important, therefore, that a *systematic* eye examination is carried out and the particular circumstances of the incident are ascertained (Marsden 1996). Corneal perforations always leave a full-thickness scar, even if it is very small. Scleral perforations may be masked by overlying subconjunctival haemorrhage.

The use of Seidel's test may help to identify a full-thickness laceration. This involves instilling a drop of fluorescein into the eye and watching for dilution of it from escaping aqueous. The cobalt blue filter on the slit lamp or pen torch will identify a bright fluorescence from escaping aqueous.

Patients with penetrating trauma should be referred urgently to an ophthalmologist. Wounds with retained foreign bodies should be protected with a rigid shield such as a cartella shield or a gallipot. Retained foreign objects should not be removed from the eye. In the case of other penetrating injuries, the eye should be covered with a single pad, so no pressure is applied to the eye, and a cartella shield if possible. The patient should be transported lying flat in order to reduce the possibility of further injury or loss of ocular contents.

Major Closed Trauma

A direct blow to the eye from a blunt missile such as a clenched fist, squash ball or champagne cork may produce one or a combination of the following:

- ecchymosis (or black eye)
- hyphaema
- dislocation of the lens
- blow-out fracture of the orbital floor or nasal wall
- iridodialysis
- traumatic mydriasis or miosis
- traumatic uveitis
- traumatic angle recession
- posterior segment problems such as retinal oedema (commotio retinae), choroidal rupture and retinal detachment.

Patients with reduced vision following blunt trauma should be referred to an ophthalmologist.

Ecchymosis

Ecchymosis is more commonly known as a 'black eye'. It results from a blow to the orbit which leads to bruising and oedema of the eyelids. In itself, it is a relatively minor injury, treated with ice packs to relieve swelling. The force needed to cause this sort of injury may cause contusion or concussion injuries to any or all of the structures within the eye, as well as orbital rim or floor fractures. It is important, therefore, that the eye and surrounding structures are assessed carefully. The patient may be able to assist in opening the lids enough for the clinician to be able to assess the eye.

Hyphaema

Traumatic hyphaema may only be detectable with a slit lamp, when red blood cells may be seen floating in the anterior chamber, or alternatively it may be visible with the naked eye, when blood may fill the whole of the anterior chamber. The signs and symptoms of hyphaema are:

- history of trauma
- reduced visual acuity
- reddish haze present diffusely through the anterior chamber, a settled layer of blood inferiorly or complete filling of the anterior chamber
- pain – due to raised intraocular pressure and other eye injury
- pupil irregular or poorly reactive
- drowsiness – particularly in children.

Admission may be necessary in the treatment of hyphaema in children, and in the treatment of large hyphaema with raised intraocular pressure in adults. Patients with minimal bleeding may be advised to rest at home. Daily intraocular pressure monitoring by an ophthalmologist is usual, and treatment with agents such as Diamox, glycerol or mannitol may be indicated if the intraocular pressure is raised.

The ophthalmologist will examine the retina after the hyphaema has settled. The pupil is not usually dilated while a hyphaema is present, as the view of the fundus will not be ideal and there is a risk of retraumatising the iris vessel and causing further bleeding. Patients who need to be transported to an ophthalmic unit should be transported sitting upright to allow the blood cells to settle and the visual axis to clear.

Luxation or subluxation of the lens

A patient with a total dislocation of the lens or a partial dislocation (subluxation) can also present to A&E. It may be the result of trauma, hereditary, or associated with certain syndromes, such as Marfan's syndrome (Stollery 1997). Vision will be disturbed, but the degree of visual disturbance will depend on the degree of dislocation; if 25% or more of the zonules of the lens are ruptured, the lens is no longer held securely behind the iris. The signs and symptoms of luxation or subluxation of the lens are:

- deepening of the anterior chamber due to tilting of the lens posteriorly – the anterior chamber may be shallow if the lens moves anteriorly
- pupil block – this may occur if the lens occludes the pupil
- a tremulous iris (iridodonesis).

The patient should be referred to an ophthalmologist. In general, if no complications occur, dislocated lenses are best left untreated. If complications do occur, such as acute glaucoma, these should be treated before cataract extraction is attempted, as surgery in these instances is difficult.

Orbital fractures

The orbits are each composed of seven bones, the thinnest of which are the *lamina papyracea* over the ethmoid sinuses, along the medial wall, and the maxillary bone on the orbital floor.

Medial orbital fractures

The lacrimal secretory system, especially the nasolacrimal duct, may be damaged and the medial rectus muscle may be trapped within fractures of the *lamina papyracea*.

Orbital floor fractures

These are often referred to as 'blow-out fractures' because they are produced by transmission of forces through the bones and soft tissues of the orbit by a non-penetrating object such as a fist or a ball. These fractures may be complicated by the entrapment of muscles and orbital fat which limit ocular motility. They are often found by plain X-rays, but CT scans are used to investigate them further. Symptoms resolve without surgery in almost 85% of patients, as oedematous tissues usually settle, freeing muscles and allowing correct motility (Egging 1998). Signs and symptoms of orbital floor fracture include:

- diplopia
- enophthalmos
- surgical emphysema
- infraorbital anaesthesia.

Orbital fractures are not considered an ocular emergency unless visual involvement or globe injury is present. Discharge instructions should include cautions about Valsalva's manoeuvres, such as straining at stool and nose blowing. Antibiotics may be prescribed to prevent orbital cellulitis.

Iridodialysis

This is the disinsertion of the iris base from the ciliary body and it is often associated with hyphaema. No immediate treatment is undertaken. Whether or not surgical intervention is undertaken depends on the effect of iridodialysis on visual acuity after a suitable recovery period.

Traumatic mydriasis or miosis

This may be present after blunt trauma. Additionally, the pupil may react only minimally to light, or not at all, and may have an irregular shape. This deformity is indicative of complete or partial rupture of the iris sphincter. It may be permanent or transient.

Traumatic uveitis

A mild inflammatory reaction of the iris and/or ciliary body is frequently seen after blunt trauma. The patient complains of aching in the eye and cells, and flare may be seen in the anterior chamber. Treatment is as for any uveitis, i.e. dilation and topical steroids by an ophthalmologist.

Angle recession

Angle recession refers to a separation or posterior displacement of the tissues at the anterior chamber angle at the site of the trabecular meshwork. At least

20% of patients with a hyphaema have some degree of angle recession and are followed up, as secondary glaucoma may eventually follow damage to the trabecular meshwork.

Cataract

A cataract is an opacity of the lens of the eye. It prevents light entering the lens properly and causes dimness of vision. When the structure of the lens is altered, e.g. as a result of a blunt (contusion) injury from a squash ball, aqueous enters the lens substance, causing it to swell and become cloudy. Contusion cataracts may occur as an immediate or long-term consequence of blunt trauma.

Posterior segment problems

A number of posterior segment problems may result from blunt trauma. Their common feature from the patient's perspective is a reduction in visual acuity which may be relatively temporary, usually a matter of weeks, or permanent. It is not possible to give the patient an accurate prognosis for vision initially as this may take some time and early referral to the ophthalmologist is important.

Minor Trauma

The vast majority of eye injuries are relatively minor and involve the anterior segment only. It is important, however, to bear in mind the possibility of more major trauma and not to rule it out without a comprehensive examination. If it is assumed that the eye injury is likely to be trivial, sight-threatening injuries may easily be missed. The degree of pain following eye trauma is not a good indication of the severity of the injury. Corneal abrasions can be extremely painful, whereas a sight-threatening perforating injury may be virtually painless.

Traumatic subconjunctival haemorrhage

This is common after a variety of injuries and is, in itself, relatively minor. Fluorescein should be used to rule out a conjunctival laceration. The condition is self-limiting and does not require treatment. A traumatic subconjunctival haemorrhage which extends backwards so that the posterior border is not visible may be an indication of significant orbital trauma and may warrant further investigation if the history and other signs and symptoms are indicative of this. The patient should be reassured that the haemorrhage will resolve, usually over a period of weeks.

Corneal abrasion

Corneal abrasions are very common as the corneal epithelium is easily damaged. The damage to the cornea exposes superficial corneal nerves, causing tearing, eyelid spasms and pain. The degree of pain may be considerable and visual acuity is likely to be reduced. Providing the deeper layers of the cornea are not involved, there should be no visual impairment after the abrasion has healed. Topical anaesthetic may be needed in order to examine the eye effectively. The eye should be stained with fluorescein, and the extent of the abrasion documented.

Eye pain is difficult to control. The pain associated with a breach in the corneal epithelium has a component of ciliary muscle spasm which can be relieved, along with a degree of the patient's pain, by the use of a dilating drop such as cyclopentolate 1%. Any breach in the corneal epithelium places the eye at risk of infection. A prophylactic antibiotic is necessary and chloramphenicol is usually the antibiotic of choice. In the treatment of corneal abrasions, this is often prescribed in ointment form, as this provides a lubricant layer over the eye, which enables the lid to slide over the damaged epithelium, and is therefore much more comfortable for the patient.

If the eye is painful, eyepads may be applied after instillation of ointment and the patient instructed not to disturb them for 24 hours. After this time, chloramphenicol ointment should be instilled four times daily for 5–7 days. Corneal abrasions generally heal within 48–72 hours. Abrasions which appear slow to heal or involve loose epithelium should be referred to an ophthalmologist.

In some instances, the cornea is at particular risk of infection, slow healing or recurrent abrasion. This is particularly the case in human, animal or vegetable material scratches. It is important, therefore, that the patient uses the antibiotic ointment at night for a period of 3–4 weeks to prevent this occurring. Follow-up visits are not usually necessary unless the abrasion is particularly large, involves the deeper layers of the cornea or the patient is a child.

Conjunctival abrasion and foreign body

Foreign bodies do not often penetrate the conjunctiva and are therefore easily wiped off using a moistened cotton bud after instillation of local anaesthetic. The resulting (and any concurrent) abrasion may be treated with antibiotic ointment. A pad is not usually necessary and the degree of pain experienced is much less than with corneal trauma

Subtarsal foreign body

In this case, the patient often presents with a foreign body sensation and a history of something falling or blowing into the eye. Management involves everting the upper lid using a moistened cotton-tipped swab. Any foreign material trapped underneath the lid may be wiped off with the swab. The eye should then be stained with fluorescein to rule out any corneal abrasion. If corneal abrasions are present, they are often linear, superficial and quite characteristic of this type of injury. If the corneal injury is minimal, a stat dose instillation of antibiotic ointment is usually sufficient. If larger abrasions are present, they should be treated as corneal abrasions.

Corneal foreign body

These commonly occur from grinding wheels and other industrial machines, from DIY and even wind-borne materials. The patient may present with a foreign body sensation, especially when opening or closing the eye. Superficial foreign bodies are often easily removed with a moistened cotton bud after instillation of local anaesthetic. Dry cotton buds should not be used as they can stick to the corneal epithelium, which is moist, and this may result in a large abrasion, complicating the injury.

Impacted corneal foreign bodies need to be removed using the edge of a 21 gauge needle held tangentially to the cornea with the hand resting on the patient's cheek or nose. The needle may be mounted on a cotton-tipped applicator or syringe for easier manipulation. After the initial removal of the foreign body, a rust ring often remains. This must be removed completely, but this is easier after 24–48 hours of treatment with antibiotic ointment.

Removal of corneal foreign body with a needle is a procedure which must be carried out with extreme care. Although the cornea is tough, it is quite possible to penetrate it with a needle and, if the foreign body is 'dug' out too enthusiastically and the deeper layers of the cornea are damaged, a corneal scar will result. This might cause major visual problems if it involves the visual axis. It is therefore important that if the A&E department possesses a slit lamp, it is utilised for the removal of corneal foreign bodies so that both a high degree of magnification and support for the patient's head are possible. A&E staff may feel most comfortable removing only peripheral foreign bodies and referring on central ones. If in any doubt, the patient should be referred to an ophthalmic unit.

After removal of the foreign body, treatment is as for a corneal abrasion, although often the patient is happier without a pad as little corneal epithelium is lost and therefore pain is minimal. Many patients have repeat visits for removal of corneal foreign bodies and treat them as an occupational hazard. Opportunities should be taken for providing health education regarding eye protection. X-ray examination is only indicated if there is a definite history of a high-speed foreign body hitting the eye, such as a hammer and chisel, and no foreign body can be found. It is most unlikely that one foreign body would penetrate the eye while another stayed on the cornea.

Eyepads

Although there is no evidence that prolonged padding of the eye is therapeutic, experience suggests that patients are, on the whole, much more comfortable with the eye padded for 24 hours after injury. If the eye is padded and uncomfortable, it should be suggested that the patient remove the pad. If no pad is used, the patient does not have a choice of treatment. A single pad will not keep the eye closed and further damage to the cornea may be caused by the surface of the pad. If padding is required, the following method should be used;

Fold one pad in half and place over the closed eyelids after instilling the necessary medication. Place the second pad, flat, over the first and secure with two or three pieces of tape. It is unnecessary to pad an eye merely because local anaesthetic has been used. Anaesthetic drops last for only around 20–30 minutes and the risk of the patient sustaining any further injury because of the local anaesthetic drop is minimal (Cheng et al. 1997) (see Fig. 30.6).

The A&E nurse should not pad the eye of a patient who is driving home. If the patient leaves the eyepad on and drives anyway, he is breaking the law, invalidating his insurance and driving extremely dangerously. If the patient takes it off to drive, time, materials and effort have been wasted. The patient is much more likely to comply with advice if allowed to drive home and advised how to apply the eye pad there. A drop of local anaesthetic will facilitate driving home safely. Patients should never have both eyes padded at once, as this is extremely disorientating and disabling. If both eyes are affected, the worst should be padded and pads given for the other eye for use at home, if necessary.

Eyedrops

Local anaesthetic drops are a very valuable tool for examination purposes. They 'magically' remove all the

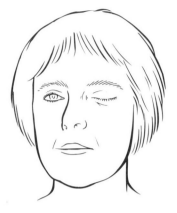 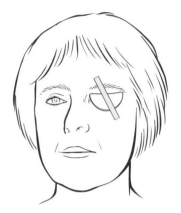 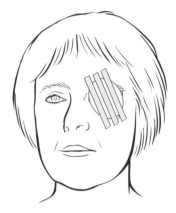

Eye closed after instillation of antibiotic ointment

Single folded pad over the closed lid and taped down – ensures the patient cannot open his eye under the pad

Second pad – open (unfolded) over the first and taped firmly to the face

Figure 30.6 – Use of eye pads.

patient's pain and he may be very keen to have some to take home so that this pain-free state may continue. Unfortunately, local anaesthetic drops also inhibit epithelial healing. The patient will be pain-free, but the epithelial defect will not heal.

Mydriatic and cycloplegic drops, such as cyclopentolate, dilate the pupil and paralyse accommodation. The patient's near vision is therefore blurred for a period of time. This does not mean that the patient should not drive. If he feels safe to do so, there is nothing to stop him driving as, in practice, only distance vision is used for driving. However, he should be warned that, if it is a bright day, he may be quite dazzled by sunlight and should wear sunglasses and take extreme care. Steroid drops should not be prescribed in the A&E department as the effects of steroids on the eye in a misdiagnosed condition can be catastrophic.

Red Eye

Ophthalmic trauma is fairly easy to recognise with the aid of a history and a brief eye examination. However, ophthalmic medical problems are, on the whole, less easily diagnosed and therefore may be dealt with less well than other problems. The differential diagnosis of the red eye (Marsden 1997) is shown in Table 30.1.

Subconjunctival haemorrhage

Patients may present with a spontaneous subconjunctival haemorrhage. Often, the patient has not noticed any irritation but has been prompted to attend by others noticing the haemorrhage. This presents as a deep red patch of blood under the conjunctiva which may be quite small and circumscribed or may be severe enough for the conjunctiva to appear like a 'bag of blood'. Providing there is no history of trauma, no treatment is needed. Subconjunctival haemorrhage may occasionally be associated with hypertension so it might be useful to check the patient's blood pressure.

Patients with clotting disorders or those on anticoagulants may be prone to repeat episodes. Because the patient's eye appears much worse than it is, a lot of reassurance may be needed. Subconjunctival haemorrhages will take up to 3 weeks to resolve and, because the conjunctiva is an elastic membrane, the blood may spread under it and actually appear worse before it begins to resolve.

Blepharitis

This chronic eyelid condition is very common. The patient is likely to present with gritty, sore eyes and red-rimmed eyelids with crusting, which may be mild to very severe, along the lid margin – the lash line. Treatment involves regular lid cleaning, using a cotton bud dipped in a solution of baby shampoo and water to 'scrub' the lid margin along the lash line to remove all the crusts. When the condition is acute, antibiotic ointment should be rubbed into the lid margin after lid hygiene two to four times a day. As this is a chronic condition, lid cleaning should continue even after the symptoms have resolved, or the condition will recur. Occasionally, punctate staining may occur at the corneoscleral junction. This is marginal keratitis, an

Table 30.1 – *Differential diagnosis of the red eye*

	Blepharitis	Conjunctivitis	Uveitis	Glaucoma	Corneal ulcers
Lids	Red margins ?Trichiasis	? Swollen follicles	✓	✓	May be swollen
Conjunctiva	May be injected	Injected	Injected	Injected	Injected
Cornea	?Marginal keratitis	?Punctate staining	✓	Very hazy	Opacity/stains with fluorescein
Anterior chamber	Deep	Deep	Deep	Shallow or flat	Deep
Iris	3	✓	May look 'muddy'	May be difficult to see	✓
Pupil	3	✓	Slight miosis (compared with fellow), sluggish	Fixed, oval, semi-dilated	Usually normal, may be slightly sluggish
Pain	Gritty	Gritty	Deep pain in eye	Severe pain in and around eye and head	Gritty
Discharge	Crusting and discharge on lids	Pus/watery/sticky in morning	May water	No	May water
Photophobia	Unlikely	If severe	Yes	No	Not usually
Systemically	Well	?Flu-like symptoms (URTI)	Well	Nausea, vomiting, severe abdominal pain, dehydration	Well

inflammatory change. The patient should be referred to an ophthalmologist.

Conjunctivitis

Inflammation of the conjunctiva is by far the most common cause of red eyes. Bacterial conjunctivitis in adults is much less common than is often thought (Tullo & Donnelly 1995) and most conjunctivitis in adults is caused by a virus, often a type of adenovirus. Conjunctivitis in children is more likely to be bacterial.

Bacterial conjunctivitis

The patient is likely to present with a red, irritable eye, describing the sensation as 'gritty' rather than painful. Discharge is likely to be purulent and profuse, and the lashes may be coated with it. There will be no corneal staining with fluorescein. Treatment is usually with a broad-spectrum antibiotic such as chloramphenicol or fucidic acid, applied topically in the form of drops. Drops are often prescribed quite frequently during the first 48 hours; for example, in the case of chloramphenicol drops, 2 hourly application would not be unreasonable.

Health education information, particularly on how to control the spread of infection, should be given and the nurse must ensure that the patient understands how to use his medication before leaving the department. Information on how to keep the lids clean and free from discharge may be needed, e.g. using cooled, boiled water and cotton wool or tissues, especially by parents of small children who may also need extra help instilling the prescribed medication effectively. Patient education should also, where appropriate, incorporate discussion of cross-contamination through eye make-up, pillows and towels. (Egging 1998).

Viral conjunctivitis

Viruses, often types of adenovirus, are by far the most common cause of conjunctivitis in adults. Once again, the patient is likely to complain of a gritty sensation, but the discharge is much less likely to be purulent than profuse watering, with stickiness often only in the morning when the watery discharge has dried and the lids are stuck together. If the lid is everted, the conjunctiva covering it will appear very bumpy rather than smooth. These 'bumps' are follicles and are inflamed lymphoid tissue. This roughness of the conjunctiva is what makes the eye feel so gritty and irritable. The patient with viral conjunctivitis often complains of dryness, along with a watery eye. The tears, although profuse, are inadequate in quality and dry up very quickly; the eye responds to the irritation and dryness by producing more. There may be punctate erosions on the cornea when stained with fluorescein.

Some types of adenovirus, of which there are about 30, cause upper respiratory tract infection and this, when combined with an eye infection, is known as pharyngoconjunctival fever. The patient may feel generally unwell with flu-like symptoms and the preauricular lymph node may be enlarged. Treatment of viral conjunctivitis is based on controlling the symptoms. Unless the eye is particularly sticky, antibiotics are not indicated. Artificial tears may help to control the feeling of dryness and irritation and these may be used very frequently, e.g. every 30 minutes. A bland ointment such as simple eye ointment may also be helpful. Cold compresses on the lids may ease the irritation of this very distressing condition The patient should be aware that viral conjunctivitis may persist for 3–6 weeks and the symptoms of dryness may last much longer.

Adenoviral conjunctivitis is a condition with symptoms out of all proportion to its relative clinical importance. Once the symptoms have peaked, however, the patient may be said to be no longer an infection risk. Adenovirus is highly infectious and infection control is of paramount importance, both for the patient and for the department. Handwashing is the first line of defence in infection control and is vital to stop the spread of viral conjunctivitis.

Allergic conjunctivitis

This is very common and presents acutely in two distinct ways. Firstly, the patient may have red eyes with itching and watering and an appearance of large bumps (papillae) on the subtarsal conjunctiva. This presentation is particularly common during the 'hay fever' season and may therefore be associated with a runny nose, sneezing etc. Treatment is with systemic antihistamines and/or topical treatment such as Alomide.

The second presentation is an acute and frightening atopic reaction which involves massive chemosis or swelling of the conjunctiva which the patient often describes as 'jelly' on the eye. This is usually due to the patient rubbing the eye with an allergen present on the hand or finger. Common allergens include some plant juices and cat hairs. This condition is completely self-limiting and requires no treatment unless the chemosis is severe and protruding from the closed lids. In this case, lubricant drops may be necessary. Reassurance about the condition is likely to be necessary and, if the reaction is severe, the patient may need to be monitored for systemic effects of the allergen.

Anterior uveitis (also known as uveitis, iridocyclitis, iritis)

Uveitis is an inflammatory condition which may be associated with systemic disease such as ankylosing spondylitis but which is often idiopathic. It may also occur secondary to trauma. The most common presenting symptoms are photophobia, pain due to iris and ciliary spasm, conjunctival redness (infection), which may be more marked around the corneoscleral junction (limbus), and decreased visual acuity. The reduction in vision is due to protein and white blood cells which are part of the inflammatory reaction in the anterior chamber. The pupil, because of spasm and inflammation, is likely to be small (miosed) compared with the unaffected eye and may react sluggishly. There will be a clear reflection of light when the cornea is illuminated, demonstrating the lack of corneal involvement, and there will be no staining with fluorescein. Treatment is with topical corticosteroids, and mydriatics to dilate the pupil to reduce inflammation and prevent adhesions of the iris and lens. Prompt referral to an ophthalmologist is required.

Acute glaucoma

In acute glaucoma, the outflow of aqueous in the eye is obstructed by the peripheral iris covering the trabecular meshwork. As aqueous continues to be produced, the pressure inside the eye increases rapidly. This results in the sudden onset of severe pain, due to the increased intraocular pressure, and blurred vision due to corneal oedema. Haloes may be seen around lights. The pain is not likely to be localised in the eye, but may involve the whole head and may be accompanied by nausea, vomiting and abdominal pain due to vagal stimulation. Patients are usually elderly and are likely to be hypermetropic (long-sighted). On examination, the patient's eye will be red and the reflection of light from the cornea will be very diffuse, showing that the cornea is oedematous. The pupil will be semi-dilated, oval and fixed.

Acute glaucoma is an ophthalmic emergency and the patient should be referred to an ophthalmologist urgently, including emergency ambulance transportation if necessary. Prolonged raised ocular pressure at this level will cause permanent loss of vision which may be severe and will occur relatively quickly. Treatment will involve the use of carbonic anhydrase inhibitors, such as acetazolamide intravenously, constriction of the pupil once the pressure has reduced and, eventually, laser treatment when the pressure is back to normal. In the A&E department, analgesia and antiemetics may be required. Occasionally, patients present having coped with these symptoms for some time and may be dehydrated due to prolonged vomiting. Rehydration may therefore be necessary, started in the A&E department or the ophthalmic unit. A great deal of explanation, reassurance and care are needed by these ill and often terrified patients.

Corneal ulcers

There are three main types of corneal ulcer which are likely to be seen in the A&E department. All should be referred to an ophthalmic unit because differentiation between the different types of corneal ulcer is sometimes difficult and the treatment is completely different.

Bacterial ulcers occur as 'fluffy' white demarcated areas on the cornea which stain with fluorescein. They are cause by a number of organisms, some of which, e.g. *Pseudomonas*, are very difficult to treat. All need a number of investigations to be carried out, such as Gram stain and culture which will be done in the ophthalmic unit without delay. Patients may be treated with frequent antibiotic drops on either an outpatient or, if the infection is severe, an in-patient basis. Delay in treatment of infected corneal ulcers can result in devastating intraocular infection.

Marginal ulcers appear as ulcerated areas which stain with fluorescein and are usually close to the limbus. They are part of a hypersensitivity response by the eye to staphylococcal exotoxins and are usually treated with steroid eye drops by an ophthalmologist.

Viral ulcers caused by herpes simplex virus are known as 'dendritic' ulcers because of their branching, tree-like shape when stained with fluorescein. They are treated with acyclovir eye ointment, again only by an ophthalmologist.

Health Promotion

Many patients with ophthalmic conditions are only seen for a short period of time in A&E, before either discharge or referral, and there is therefore limited time to advise patients. It is important, however, that patients leave the department with a basic knowledge of their condition, in order to understand the importance of drug treatment and follow-up requirements and instruction on correct eyedrop instillation and side-effects of any drug therapy. Patients with newly diagnosed conditions should also be aware of recurring symptoms which should prompt them to seek early treatment.

Many activities in the home and workplace cause eye injuries, due to equipment, materials, chemicals and radiation. Patients with such injuries should be encouraged to wear eye protection or to check that any equipment already in use is of a suitable standard. All eye protection should conform to British Standard BS 2092 requirements. Children, in particular, are vulnerable to eye injuries. Parents need sympathetic health education to minimise the risks of sight-damaging injury (Kutsche 1994).

Conclusion

While ocular emergencies do not present a threat to the patient's life, sight is precious and the A&E nurse can have a critical impact on a patient's vision. Once lost, vision cannot be replaced, and therefore knowledge of the management of the most common ophthalmic conditions will assist the nurse in protecting sight and promoting health.

Further reading

Eagling EM, Roper-Hall MJ (1986) *Eye Injuries: an Illustrated Guide*. Sevenoaks: Butterworth.

Hinchliff S, Montague S, Watson R (1996) *Physiology for Nursing Practice*, 2nd edn. London: Baillière Tindall.

Kanski JJ (1990) *Synopsis of Ophthalmology*. London: Wright.

Okhravi O (1997) *Manual of Primary Eye Care*. Oxford: Butterworth Heinemann.

Perry JP, Tullo AB (eds) (1995) *Care of the Ophthalmic Patient*, 2nd edn. London: Chapman and Hall.

Snell RS, Lemp MA (1989) *Clinical Anatomy of the Eye*. Oxford: Blackwell Scientific.

References

Cheng H, Burdon MA, Buckley SA, Moorman C (1997) *Emergency Ophthalmology*. London: BMJ.

Edwards RS (1987) Ophthalmic emergencies in a district general hospital casualty department. *British Journal of Ophthalmology* **71**, 938–942.

Egging D (1998) Ocular emergencies. In: Newberry L, ed. *Sheehy's Emergency Nursing: Principles and Practice* 4th edn. St Louis: Mosby.

Glenn S (1995) Care of patients with chemical eye injury. *Emergency Nurse* **3**(3), 7–9.

Herr RD, White GL, Bernhisel K *et al.* (1991) Clinical comparisons of ocular irrigation fluids following chemical injury. *American Journal of Emergency Medicine* **9**, 228–231.

Jones NP, Hayward JM, Khaw PT, Claove CM, Elkington AR (1986) Function of an ophthalmic 'accident & emergency' department: results of a six month study. *British Medical Journal*, **292**, 188–190.

Kutsche PJ (1994) Ocular trauma in children. *Journal of Ophthalmic Nursing and Technology*, **13**(3), 117–120.

Mackway-Jones K (ed.) (1996) *Emergency Triage: Manchester Triage Group*. London: BMJ.

Marsden J (1996) Ophthalmic trauma in accident and emergency. *Accident and Emergency Nursing*, **4**(1), 54–58.

Marsden J (1997) Identifying and managing non-traumatic red eye in A&E. *Emergency Nurse*, **5**(9), 34–40.

Marsden J (1999a) Ocular burns. *Emergency Nurse*, **6**(10), 20–24.

Marsden J (1999b) Painless loss of vision. *Emergency Nurse*, **6**(9), 13–18.

Stollery R (1997) *Ophthalmic Nursing*, 2nd edn. Oxford: Blackwell Science.

Tan MMS, Driscoll PA, Marsden JE (1997) Management of eye emergencies in the accident and emergency department by senior house officers: a national survey. *Journal of Accident and Emergency Medicine*, **14**, 157–158.

Tannen M, Marsden J (1991) Chemical burns of the eye. *Nursing Standard*, **30**(6), 24–26.

Tullo AB, Donnelly D (1995) Conjunctiva. In: Perry JP, Tullo AB, eds. *Care of the Ophthalmic Patient*, 2nd edn. London: Chapman and Hall.

Waggoner MD (1997) Chemical injuries of the eye: current concepts in pathophysiology and therapy. *Survey of Ophthalmology*, **41**(4), 275–313.

Chapter 31

Ear, Nose and Throat Emergencies

Tim Kilner, Philip Docking & Elaine Hayward

- Introduction
- The ear
- Infections of the ear
- Mechanical obstruction
- Foreign bodies
- Perforation of the tympanic membrane
- The nose
- Foreign body
- Epistaxis
- Nasal fracture
- Rhinorrhoea
- Allergic rhinitis
- Sinusitis
- The throat
- Oral cavity
- Pharynx
- Conclusion

Introduction

Ear, nose or throat (ENT) conditions presenting at the A&E department are often trivialised, even though some can subsequently become life-threatening. For those patients who attend the A&E department with an ENT disorder, the onset of symptoms is likely to be acute, but the nurse should be alert to the fact that the current episode may also be a feature of a chronic condition. The A&E nurse should also be conscious of the danger of viewing the patient only in terms of the presenting symptoms.

It is often the case that such conditions are accompanied by systemic illness precipitated by local infection. Equally important is the fact that the individual may have psychological, social and emotional needs as well as the presenting pathophysiological needs. This may be obvious in the case of an individual who has hearing loss as a direct result of being in close proximity to the seat of an explosion, but may be less apparent in the individual whose hearing loss results from wax impaction, but who is concerned that she may be becoming permanently deaf.

This chapter broadly examines ENT conditions in terms of infection, trauma and foreign bodies. The nursing care of patients is discussed in relation to presenting conditions.

The Ear

The attendance at the A&E department of a patient with an ear-related problem is usually precipitated by one or more of the following symptoms:

- pain
- discharge from the ear
- hearing loss
- foreign bodies in the ear canal
- direct trauma to the external structure of the ear.

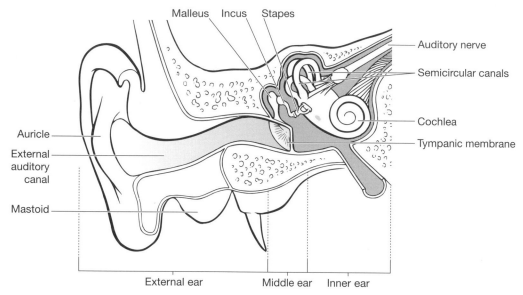

Figure 31.1 – *Anatomy of the ear.*

Anatomy of the ear

The ear is divided into three sections: external, middle and inner ear (see Fig. 31.1). The outer ear funnels sound into the middle ear which serves to transmit the sound to the auditory apparatus of the inner ear. The external ear consists of the aurical (or pinna), ear canal and tympanic membrane. The S-shaped ear canal is approximately 2.5–3.0 cm long and terminates at the tympanic membrane. The canal is lined with glands that secrete cerumen, a yellow waxy material that lubricates and protects the ear. Ear wax sloughed off skin cells and dust may impair sound transmission through the outer ear, especially if a plug of wax attaches to the eardrum.

The tympanic membrane (or eardrum) is a thin, translucent, pearly grey oval disc separating the external ear from the middle ear. It can easily be observed with an otoscope. The tympanic membrane vibrates and moves in and out in response to sound. The middle ear is an air-filled cavity containing three tiny bones, the ossicles, which are individual called the malleus (hammer), the incus (anvil) and the stapes (stirrup), so named because of their appearance. The malleus is attached to the tympanic membrane by a set of ligaments. The incus is attached to the malleus and they move as one. The stapes attaches to the oval window, the membrane separating the middle and inner ear. When the tympanic membrane vibrates in response to sound, the malleus and incus are displaced, and the stapes vibrates against the oval window continuing the transmission of sound. The pharyngo-tympanic tube, formerly known as the Eustachian tube, which connects the middle ear with the naso-pharynx, allows the passage of air to equalise pressure on either side of the tympanic membrane. The inner ear is composed of several fluid-filled chambers encased in a bony labyrinth in the temporal bone. The semicircular canals are also important for balance.

Presentation to A&E may be prompted by a single symptom, such as hearing loss resulting from wax impaction. The patient may alternatively have multiple symptoms, resulting from, for example, an ear infection where pain, discharge and hearing loss may be present in combination with systemic illness.

Infections of the Ear

Acute otitis externa

The external auditory meatus is a canal-shaped structure which extends from the external opening of the ear to the tympanic membrane. The integrity of the canal is protected from pathogens by its lining. The lateral one-third is composed of skin which is a continuation from the concha, which is the depression in the centre of the shell-shaped external structure of the ear – the pinna. The lining continues as an epithelial layer, protecting not only the medial two-thirds of the external auditory meatus but also the tympanic membrane.

The protective lining of the external auditory meatus may be easily breached by direct trauma, although pre-existing dermatological conditions, typically eczema and psoriasis, as well as external mediators such as maceration by water, may influence the resilience of the lining (Ludman 1997). Dermatological conditions may be precipitated by a range of chemicals which make contact with the external auditory meatus, such as shampoos and cosmetics (O'Donoghue *et al.* 1992).

Clinical evidence and management

Acute otitis externa is essentially a localised or diffuse infection of the lining of the external auditory meatus. Acute otitis external frequently occurs following bathing or swimming when the external auditory meatus is cleaned out using the corner of a dirty towel. For this reason it is often referred to as 'swimmer's ear'. Infection may be diffuse within the external auditory meatus or it may be focal in the form of a local swelling known as a furuncle which may be extremely painful. Taking swabs for microbiological studies may not be well tolerated by the patient. It is essential that careful preparation of the patient takes place before any attempt is made to take a swab, especially if the individual is a child. Attempts to take a swab from an uncooperative child should be avoided as there is a risk that the tympanic membrane may be perforated by the swab if the child moves her head.

As the external auditory meatus contains no mucus-secreting cells, discharge from the ear is minimal, however any discharge which does occur is usually thick and foul-smelling infected wax. The canal may also contain cell debris, which is unlikely to cause hearing loss, but may contribute to the intense irritation the individual may experience.

Treatment is based upon cleaning and drying the external auditory meatus. This should only be done following medical examination to determine that the tympanic membrane is intact. Following cleansing of the external auditory meatus, topical medication may be instilled. The type of medication is dependent upon the infecting organism, i.e. fungal or bacterial infection.

Acute otitis externa largely results from identifiable causes and therefore lends itself to prevention strategies. The focus of much of the nursing care may revolve around prevention of future exposure by identifying high-risk behaviour and educating those individuals in ways of reducing the risks. O'Donoghue *et al.* (1992) suggested that certain occupational groups may be exposed to the risk of acute otitis externa. Typically these are individuals who work in occupations where they are required to wear inserts in their ears, such as telephonists and workers using internal ear defenders, as well as doctors and nurses sharing a communal stethoscope.

Although these individuals are at risk, the likelihood of subsequent infection may be reduced through careful history-taking and appropriate health education regarding aural hygiene and cleansing of equipment. Single operator use should also be advocated, thus reducing the risks of the individual infecting others and reinfecting themselves. Patients should be provided with the advice and support necessary for them to instil any prescribed medication.

Acute otitis media

An acute infection of the middle ear, i.e. medial to the tympanic membrane, may cause pain, a feeling of pressure in the ear and hearing loss, the symptoms being caused by infective material splinting the tympanic membrane. Discharge from the external ear may be present, but in order for this to occur, the tympanic membrane must have been damaged, usually as a result of the increased pressure causing perforation.

Clinical evidence and management

Acute otitis media is often associated with systemic illness and pyrexia (Ludman 1997), which may be attributed to the otitis media alone or occur in conjunction with coincidental upper respiratory tract infection. Acute otitis media is characterised by rapid onset of ear pain, headache, tinnitus, hearing loss, and nausea or vomiting. Infants and young children may present with irritability, crying, rubbing or pulling the ear, restless sleep and lethargy (Olson 1998). Children are often prone to acute otitis, as the infection frequently results from upper respiratory tract infection of bacterial or viral origin. (Strome *et al.* 1992).

Uncomplicated otitis media is treated with systemic antibiotics, supported by analgesia with antipyretic properties. If otitis media is not treated aggressively, serious complications can develop, including meningitis, mastoiditis, intracranial abscess, permanent hearing loss and neck abscess (Emergency Nurses Association 1994).

Patient education may focus upon the medication regime to ensure the efficacy of the antibiotics, analgesia and antipyretics. Antibiotic treatment regimes have a failure rate of 5–10% and recurrent episodes of otitis media are common (Criddle 1995). Female patients of child-bearing age who are prescribed antibiotics should be warned that they may reduce the efficacy of oral contraceptives. It should also be noted that bottle-fed infants are at higher risk of otitis media (Benson 1991).

If the tympanic membrane has perforated, the individual should be advised to keep the ear dry and prevent water entering the ear. However, the ear should not be packed, and the patient should be advised not to do this at home, as it may prevent the discharge draining from the ear. In some cases, where the tympanic membrane is intact, the infective material may cause the membrane to bulge, resulting in considerable pain with associated loss of hearing. In such cases, admission to hospital is required in order that the tympanic membrane may be surgically perforated under general anaesthetic and grommets inserted to allow the discharge to drain out freely.

Mechanical Obstruction

Impacted wax

The lateral one-third of the external auditory meatus contains cells which secrete a waxy substance called cerumen, the purpose of which is to act as a defence against dust and other foreign material entering the external auditory meatus.

Clinical evidence and management

Cerumen may build up in the external auditory meatus causing mechanical obstruction, which may be exacerbated by cleaning the ear with cotton-tipped buds. Such activities often cause cerumen to be pushed deep into the canal, causing impaction against the tympanic membrane. Obstruction in either case may cause a reduction in hearing, but rarely causes complete deafness. Impacted cerumen is often hard and resistant to removal by syringing alone; thus, in the A&E department, the most appropriate management is to initiate a regime to soften the cerumen using commercially available ear drops.

Patient education involves self-administration with advice to contact their GP in 2–3 weeks to arrange for ear syringing. Ear syringing is rarely indicated in the A&E department. Poor technique and failure to take adequate precautions may cause the patient serious harm; it is therefore imperative that ear syringing is carried out by a nurse who is suitably trained in the technique.

Foreign Bodies

Clinical evidence

Older children and adults may present with a history of having a foreign body in the ear. Young children have a tendency to put foreign bodies in their ears, but as they often do not disclose this information, the nurse should be suspicious of children who present with earache, hearing loss and discharge from the ear.

Small insects may also crawl into the ear canal and become trapped, causing a great deal of discomfort if still alive and buzzing.

Management

Some foreign bodies may be removed with alligator forceps, under direct vision, by individuals skilled in such techniques. Care should be taken to ensure that this process does not impact the foreign body further in the ear, causing trauma to the external auditory meatus and the tympanic membrane. If the object is not retrieved at the first attempt, the patient should be referred to the ENT department.

If the tympanic membrane is intact and the foreign body is not vegetable in nature, then syringing the external auditory meatus with warm water may flush the foreign body out. However, this should only be carried out by those skilled in the technique. If the foreign body is vegetable matter, this technique should be avoided as it is likely to cause the foreign body to swell and impact in the external auditory meatus.

Where insects have entered the external auditory meatus causing the patient severe distress, Barkin & Rosen (1994) suggest that the insects should be killed in situ by the instillation of alcohol into the external auditory meatus, prior to removal. For patients whose personal convictions dictate that no harm befalls the insect, the use of penlight may attract a live insect out of the ear canal. Analgesic and/or antibiotic treatments should be prescribed as necessary. Safe removal of a foreign body from the external auditory meatus requires a skilled operator and a cooperative patient, which is not always possible to achieve in the A&E department. If in any doubt, the patient should be referred to the ENT department.

Perforation of the Tympanic Membrane

Perforation of the tympanic membrane may be caused by two main mechanisms – either direct or indirect trauma. In both cases the symptoms are much the same, i.e. hearing loss, pain and possibly bleeding from the external auditory meatus.

Direct trauma

This is commonly caused by the insertion of objects either to clean the ear or to relieve itching, although any object inserted into the external auditory meatus has the potential to cause tympanic perforation. Objects frequently used are cotton-tipped buds and hair grips. In most cases, the ruptured tympanic membrane will heal spontaneously in 1–3 months (Strome *et al.* 1992), however ENT opinion should be sought. Pain relief and prophylactic antibiotics may be required, especially if the mechanism of injury includes contamination by water or a foreign body.

This provides the A&E nurse with a health education opportunity in terms of prevention of subsequent episodes particularly in relation to aural hygiene. The importance of keeping the ear dry at all times must be stressed. A protective cotton plug coated with petroleum jelly will enable the patient to shower safely; however, swimming and generally getting the ears wet should be avoided.

Indirect trauma

Perforation of the tympanic membrane may be caused by high pressure transmitted along the external auditory meatus to the tympanic membrane. This barotrauma to the tympanic membrane results from significant changes in atmospheric pressure causing air trapped in the external ear canal or behind the tympanic membrane to expand or contract enough to rupture the eardrum. This pressure may be generated by such forces as a slap to the ear, flying, diving or exposure to an explosion. Pressures of 7 pounds per square inch (psi) on the tympanic membrane are likely to cause it to rupture (Owen-Smith 1983), although in the explosion scenario some individuals will be protected from these pressures because of the orientation of the external auditory meatus to the blast wave (Maynard *et al.* 1989). As it is unlikely that data will be available regarding blast wave pressure, all individuals who have been in close proximity to an explosion should be carefully assessed and referred to the ENT department if appropriate.

Although tympanic membrane rupture may be seen in isolation from other injuries following an explosion, the nurse should be aware of other injuries which may have occurred, such as lung and gastrointestinal injury, which may be covert in nature. The nurse should also be aware of the emotional and psychological crisis the patient will be experiencing, not only from the incident itself, be it explosion or assault, but also from anxieties about the permanency of hearing loss and the problems associated with communication. As perforation of the tympanic membrane may be caused by a slap to the ear, such injuries in children may be resultant of a non-accidental injury.

External trauma

Wounds to the external ear or pinna in most cases may be closed by conventional wound closure methods. However, if the cartilage of the pinna is involved, scrupulous wound cleansing is required as any subsequent infection is likely to lead to permanent deformity of the pinna (Wardrope & Smith 1992). Blunt trauma to the pinna, commonly occurring in contact sports, may result in haematoma formation. The haematoma, if untreated, may lead to the necrosis of the underlying cartilaginous skeleton of the pinna. O'Donoghue *et al.* (1992) advocate early incision and drainage as the most appropriate course of action in order to reduce morbidity. This is likely to require a general anaesthetic, and therefore referral to the ENT department is pertinent.

The Nose

Anatomy and physiology

The nose is a structure with a bony and cartilaginous skeleton which is attached to the skull via the frontal bone and the maxilla. It is a vascular structure whose prime functions are to interface with the respiratory system, to warm, filter and moisten inhaled air and to act as a sense organ involved in the enjoyment of food and the detection of danger in the case of smoke and gas (O'Donoghue *et al.* 1992). The upper third of the nose, where the frontal and maxillary bones form the bridge, is bony (see Fig. 31.2).

Foreign Body

A foreign body in the nose usually occurs in children and they often will be accompanied by parents who are distressed and anxious about their child's well-being.

Clinical evidence and management

Usually the child will have told the parents that she has put something up her nose, or the parents will have noticed that the child has a purulent discharge from one nostril. Unilateral discharge is highly suggestive of a foreign body in the nose, however children are not averse to placing foreign bodies in each nostril, resulting in a bilateral discharge.

The child should be seated in a dental chair or on a parent's lap in a semi-recumbent position. Initial assessment and history should ascertain the type of foreign body present, how long it has been in the nostril and whether there has been any bleeding or discharge. Careful explanation and instruction regarding the procedure for removal are required and psychological support for both parents and child is essential both for humanitarian reasons and to gain

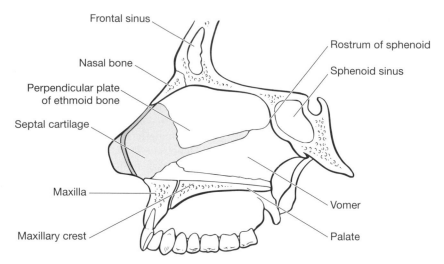

Figure 31.2 – *Anatomy of the nose.*

their cooperation during the procedure. Removal can be attempted using some topical anaesthetic spray, a ring curette or alligator forceps (Budassi Sheehy 1990). Care should be taken to prevent damage to the highly vascular nasal septum and mucosa during removal of a nasal foreign body. If the child is too distressed, the foreign body is too far into the nostril or there is any evidence of trauma to the nostril already, then the child should be referred to the ENT surgeon.

Epistaxis

Epistaxis is often seen as a relatively minor problem in the A&E department. However, something as simple as a nose bleed can quickly turn into a life-threatening condition if it is not treated swiftly and correctly (Moulds 1992). Most nose bleeds come from ruptured blood vessels on the nasal septum. Epistaxis can commonly occur in (Budassi Sheehy 1990):

- children
- adults, usually aged 50–80 years, with hypertension
- patients with blood dyscrasias
- patients on anticoagulant/aspirin treatment
- patients with alcoholism
- patients with allergies
- patients with recent nasal trauma – often following an assault.

Clinical evidence and management

The patient will present with active bleeding from the nose, or a recent history of bleeding which may have stopped. The leading cause of epistaxis is nose picking, otherwise known as digital manipulation or 'epistaxis digitorum' (Joyce 1991). The main aim of treatment is to stop the epistaxis. If the bleeding is from the anterior end of the septum – Littles' area – bleeding can usually be alleviated by seating the patient upright and advising her to hold the front soft part of the nose very firmly (Solomon 1989). The patient's head should be tilted forward over a bowl.

This compression must be applied for at least 30–40 minutes without interruption (Walsh 1996). The use of ice can be helpful for its vasconstricting action, however, toleration may be a problem for children and the elderly. The patient should be encouraged to expectorate blood rather than swallow it, as this can lead to vomiting which makes measurement of blood loss difficult. Haematemesis is also very anxiety provoking for the patient.

If the bleeding is from the posterior part of the nose, indicated by continuous bleeding after compression or as seen on examination, the patient may need to have the nose packed or the area cauterised. In this case, the patient is usually referred to the ENT surgeon. If it is to be done in the A&E department, a spray of cocaine solution (2.5–10%), a good head light and mirror, silver nitrate sticks and nasal packing are needed.

If the patient is hypertensive on presentation an antihypertensive, such as nifedipine, may need to be administered.

Occasionally, the patient with an epistaxis may need resuscitative care due to blood loss. The siting of a large-bore intravenous line and commencement of replacement fluid, monitoring of vital signs, and taking of blood for a full blood count and cross-match are necessary in this case (Bird 1999). All patients with epistaxis have the potential to become shocked if bleeding is not stopped. Initial assessment involves an estimate of the amount of bleeding, the length of time active bleeding has been taking place and any previous relevant medical history. Physical assessment of the patient should always include monitoring of vital signs.

Nasal Fracture

This is the most common facial fracture, usually caused by blunt trauma and commonly seen in the A&E patient who has been assaulted (Walsh 1996). Clinically, the injury can usually be recognised immediately afterwards by the distortion from normal shape, although this soon becomes obscured by soft tissue swelling (Ludman 1997).

Clinical evidence and management

There will be a history of trauma to the nose, swelling deformity and occasionally epistaxis. It is important to examine the nose for any evidence of cerebrospinal fluid (CSF) rhinorrhoea and any indication of fractures to the cribiform plate (Criddle 1995). Normal CSF is clear and slightly yellow, but CSF nasal drainage is frequently mixed with blood. Little can be done for patients following a fracture of the nose until 5–10 days after the initial injury, due to soft tissue swelling. The patient should therefore be referred to the ENT outpatients department. Since the nasal bones will become firmly set within 3 weeks of the injury, the need for treatment should be assessed after a week, and, if necessary, reduction under general anaesthetic will be planned for the following week. X-rays are often requested for medicolegal reasons, but are not strictly necessary (see also Ch. 9).

Rhinorrhoea

Otherwise known as a 'runny nose', this is caused by excess mucus being produced by an inflamed nasal mucosa.

Clinical evidence and management

The patient presents with a runny nose or the sensation of something dripping down the back of the throat. The discharge may be clear or purulent (O'Donaghue et al. 1992). The causes are:

- allergy
- infection
- foreign body
- underlying tumour.

The patient may need a foreign body removed. If an allergy is suspected, antihistamines may be prescribed, and advice should be given on avoidance of common allergens, i.e. grass/tree pollen, dust and cat or dog fur. The patient may also need to be referred to an allergy clinic. Infective rhinosinusitus may need treatment with antibiotics. If a tumour is suspected, urgent referral to ENT will be necessary.

Advice, explanation and health education regarding the taking of antihistamines (whose main side-effect is drowsiness) and antibiotics should be given to the patient. If the rhinitis is viral in origin, antibiotics will have little or no effect, and they should therefore not be seen as a panacea for this, or any other, condition.

Allergic Rhinitis

This can be seasonal or perennial. The symptoms are those of sneezing, nasal obstruction and rhinorrhoea. There is often itching of the nose, eyes and palate. This condition may form part of a broader clinical picture, which may include other conditions such as asthma (Solomon 1989). Patients should be advised to avoid common allergens as much as possible, such as grass/tree pollen, cat or dog fur and house dust. They should be given antihistamines and advised to see their GP for further prescription of any topical decongestants and for referral to a local allergy clinic (Bryoch 1993).

Sinusitis

Sinusitis is an inflammatory, and usually infective, condition of the paranasal sinus, which usually occurs after a viral infection of the upper respiratory tract. Complications of untreated or inadequately treated acute sinusitis include chronic sinusitis, orbital abscess, meningitis, brain abscess, cavernous sinus thrombosis and osteomyelitis of the maxillary or frontal bones (Selfridge-Thomas 1995).

Clinical evidence and management

The main symptoms a patient can present with in the A&E department are headache and facial pain which are worse when bending forward, and a recent history of upper respiratory tract infection. The patient may be very worried about her sinusitis headache. A set of baseline observations of pulse, blood pressure, temperature and respirations will aid diagnosis. This, along with a clinical history, may help to rule out other diagnoses such as hypertension or subarachnoid haemorrhage.

Treatment usually involves prescription of a broad-spectrum antibiotic. Advice can be given to take analgesia and to use a decongestant spray. The patient should be advised to see her GP if symptoms persist, as referral to the ENT department may be necessary.

The Throat

Anatomy and physiology

The throat, or pharynx, consists of the nasopharynx, oropharynx and laryngopharynx. It is a funnel-shaped tube that starts at the internal nares (nasal passages) and extends to the level of the cricoid cartilage. Its wall is composed of skeletal muscles and lined with mucous membrane. The central portion (oropharynx) provides a common passage for air, drink and food (Hinchliff *et al.* 1996). Pharyngeal constrictor muscles propel food or liquid into the oesophagus. These muscles are also responsible for the gag reflex, which is controlled by the cranial nerves. The larynx helps to prevent aspiration, assists in coughing and serves as the organ for speech.

Airway obstruction

Many patients who attend the A&E department with either an apparently trivial throat condition or more severe conditions are potentially at risk of airway obstruction. Thus the potential for a life-threatening condition to be overlooked is ever-present, unless there is a high index of suspicion and a rigorous assessment of these patients takes place (see also Ch. 2).

Airway obstruction can be partial or complete and is dynamic in nature. In the case of oedema, where the airway may initially be partially obstructed, it can progress rapidly to complete obstruction as the oedema progresses. Relatively large foreign bodies inhaled into the airway may well rapidly obstruct it, while oedema of the airway in response to an allergic reaction may obstruct it in a more progressive manner.

Should the airway become compromised, by whatever means, patency must be achieved as a matter of urgency, in order for ventilation to occur. Airway management should initially be in the form of basic techniques, such as positioning the patient and the Heimlich manoeuvre where the obstruction is caused by a foreign body. The Heimlich manoeuvre must not be performed on infants under 1 year (Advanced Life Support Group 1997).

Circumstances such as complete obstruction by an impacted foreign body or rapidly progressing oedema may dictate the early use of advanced techniques, such as endotracheal intubation, cricothyrotomy and surgical airway. Oxygen should be administered to all patients with actual and potential airway obstruction. Admission must be considered for observation of patients whose airway has been compromised and where deterioration is a possibility.

A number of events can compromise the airway. If these are dealt with effectively, complete obstruction can be prevented. These events will be discussed under the headings traumatic, infective and reactive.

Oral Cavity

Traumatic

Trauma to the oral cavity can cause a great deal of tissue swelling. Extensive bleeding can occur because of the vascular nature of the region, which is why lacerations to the tongue can bleed dramatically. Teeth can be dislodged or broken and inhalation can occur. Fracture of the mandible may also cause problems and these are dealt with in Chapter 9. Injuries to the oral cavity are common in young children (Rowe & Williams 1986).

A visual assessment is vital in determining the extent of any injury. Suction may be required to enable visual assessment to take place. Blind suction should be avoided as this can exacerbate trauma and increase the likelihood of additional problems, such as vomiting. X-rays can be of benefit in suspected fractures or in locating lost teeth when inhalation is suspected. Where an assault has occurred, photographs may be of use for medicolegal purposes. Bleeding from tooth sockets can usually be arrested with haemostatic agents and slight pressure. Antibiotics may be prescribed prophylactically.

It is essential that anxiety is reduced by reassuring the patient at the time of initial assessment. In the case of children, injuries frequently appear worse than they really are, especially when bleeding is profuse, and parents require as much reassurance as the children. Not all lacerations in the mouth will require sutures. Small lacerations, particularly to the inside of the lip, will usually heal well without intervention, other than advice on oral hygiene and the use of medicated mouth washes. Similarly, lacerations of the tongue bleed profusely, but they too usually heal well. Sutures inside the oral cavity should be soluble so that removal is not required. Those patients with extensive lacerations in the oral cavity will require appropriate referral. External cold compresses may be helpful in reducing swelling.

Infective

Infections of the oral cavity most commonly involve the teeth and gums and referral to a dentist may be the most appropriate action.

Clinical evidence and management

Abscesses of the teeth may need drainage and/or antibiotic therapy, which is most appropriately carried out by a dental practitioner. Frequently the most appropriate course of action is to refer the patient to her GP, but in the interim the patient may be prescribed antibiotics and analgesia. Patient education may focus upon the safe and efficacious use of prescribed medication.

Reactive

Reactions occur as a result of exposure to foreign substances to which the body has developed an allergy, resulting in a local or systemic allergic reaction which in severe cases may manifest as anaphylactic shock.

Aetiology of anaphylactic shock

Anaphylaxis is an acute allergic reaction following exposure to a foreign protein to which the patient has been previously sensitised. The individual becomes sensitised to the allergen by the production of antibodies in response to this exposure. These bind to basophils in the blood and sensitise the cells. Common sensitising substances are antibiotic medication, especially penicillin and penicillin derivatives, bee stings, foodstuffs such as peanuts and non-steroidal anti-inflammatory medications. When the allergen re-enters the body, this stimulates the release of mediators of anaphylaxis, e.g., histamine, serotonin, slow-release substances of anaphylaxis (SRS-A) and platelet-activating factors (PAF), which result in cellular damage.

Clinical evidence of anaphylactic shock

Physiological changes include:

- increased blood capillary permeability – causing localised oedema
- smooth muscle contraction (bronchioles)
- increased gastric secretion
- increased mucus secretion
- inhibited coagulation.

These changes may result in some or all of the following symptoms:

- wheezing
- urticaria
- pruritis
- stridor
- respiratory difficulty
- tachypnoea
- hypotension
- collapse.

The severity of the reaction can vary, ranging from a mild episode to severe shock and collapse. Generally, the faster the onset of symptoms, the greater the reaction. Patients may present at the A&E department with mild symptoms of an allergic reaction following the ingestion of an allergen. Local swelling of the face, lips and tongue (angio-oedema) is not uncommon, but should heighten awareness of potential airway obstruction. Similarly, patients may attend A&E with mildly noisy breathing due to laryngeal oedema. A careful history is important to establish the cause of the noisy breathing, as it is easy to assume that the patient suffers from asthma and that the noisy breathing is due to long-standing respiratory pathology. People with asthma are not immune to anaphylaxis.

Management of anaphylactic shock

The treatment is dependent upon the severity of the reaction. Mild episodes, such as skin rashes, may require oral antihistamines. More severe occurrences may require adrenaline by intramuscular injection, to reverse the effects of altered physiology, supported with high-flow oxygen to combat potential hypoxia. Where adrenaline is administered, the patient should be admitted for a period of observation. If possible, the allergen should be identified to enable the patient to avoid this in the future.

Those patients with mild reactions and who are discharged home require advice on the safe and efficacious use of any prescribed medications, most likely antihistamine tablets. Specifically they should be warned of the sedative effects of this type of medication and thus the implications for driving and operating machinery while taking the medication. Subsequent exposure to an unidentified allergen may cause a more severe reaction which could be potentially fatal. It is crucial that these patients are offered advice on identifying the allergen which caused the reaction. This is perhaps best achieved by referral to their own GP who may arrange appropriate tests and support.

Pharynx

Swelling in this region is more likely to compromise the airway than in the oral cavity because of the smaller diameter of the lumen of the airway. This is highly significant in children, where as little as 1 mm of oedema may cause 75% occlusion of the airway.

Traumatic

Clinical evidence

External as well as internal trauma may cause oedema in this region. People who have attempted suicide by hanging or strangulation and those involved in accidents involving strictures around the neck account for a proportion of this group of patients. In cases of strangulation and hanging where the patient is unable to self-advocate, for whatever reason, consideration should be given to any medicolegal implications, and where appropriate the police may need to be informed. Victims of road traffic accidents may also suffer trauma to this region of the body which can be easily overlooked in the presence of more obvious injuries, highlighting the importance of thorough primary and secondary surveys. Where neck injuries are apparent, the possibility of trauma to the internal structures should be considered.

Inhalation injury due to hot gases and flames may be present in burn-injured patients. Signs of inhalation injury from hot substances are not always evident, but a useful sign to look for is singed nostril hairs. If the gas was hot enough to damage these hairs then airway damage should be expected. Similarly, the ingestion of corrosive substances may also cause burns and swelling to the pharynx area. Inhalation of small foreign bodies, such as fish bones, rarely causes airway obstruction, but they can be troublesome, causing irritation, increased salivation and coughing because they are lodged in the pharynx. Patients should be advised that fish bones can often scratch the side of the throat on the way down, leaving them with the feeling that the foreign body is still there.

Management

The airway is the number one priority. Careful and accurate assessment of the patient and the extent of injuries must be carried out early. If the patient is conscious, a history of the event and mechanism of injury will give an indication of the stresses involved. Signs of airway obstruction such as noisy breathing should be noted and monitored for deterioration. Admission is essential where there is a degree of swelling which is likely to increase, leading to the airway becoming compromised.

For patients with small foreign bodies in their pharynx, X-ray examination may be helpful and could reveal radio-opaque objects. A plain lateral soft-tissue X-ray of the neck can provide valuable information about tissue swelling.

Infective

Clinical evidence

There will be a number of patients attending the A&E department with simple sore throats. They often only need reassurance and simple advice, possibly with referral to their GP if symptoms persist. There will be some adults among them with a peritonsillar abscess that will require further intervention. Children are less likely to complain of a sore throat but often go off their food and generally feel unwell and are pyrexial. These children may present with dysphagia, a wheeze or stridor and will need careful assessment. The possible cause of these symptoms is epiglottitis, which is a potentially fatal inflammation of the epiglottis and pharynx as a result of infection. Presentation is usually in late infancy and childhood, with a peak incidence of 2–3 years (Eaton 1993).

Management

Peritonsillar abscesses in need of drainage will require the attention of the ENT team. The patient should be referred as soon as the diagnosis has been made. As a general anaesthetic may be required, the patient should be kept nil by mouth, and unnecessary examination of the throat should be avoided as this is likely to be very uncomfortable.

Children with epiglottitis will require urgent assessment and admission by the paediatric team. It is essential that the child is kept calm and is not distressed, that examination in A&E is kept to a minimum, and that insertion of instruments, such as thermometers or tongue depressors, should not take place as this may cause the epiglottis to be pushed onto the larynx, thus occluding the airway completely. Endotracheal intubation should only be carried out by those who are extremely experienced in these techniques. If the airway becomes occluded then patency should be ensured by means of cricothyrotomy.

Conclusion

This chapter has examined the care of the individual who attends the A&E department with a condition relating to the ear, nose or throat. For practical purposes, care has been artificially described in terms of specific conditions, when in reality many of the identified conditions form only a part of a broader clinical picture. Care should encompass the psychological, emotional and social needs of patients and their families. What may be regarded as a minor condition to the A&E nurse is often a terrifying experience for the affected individuals.

The key element in care with these individuals, as with all aspects of A&E care, is communication. Patients who attend the A&E department with an acute ENT condition are often regarded as having a trivial condition, yet many of these conditions have the potential to become life-threatening. Patients who have traumatic injuries are rightly given high priority and are treated aggressively, yet the preventable causes of death in both groups of patients are the same, i.e. hypoxia and hypovolaemia – hypoxia resulting from a foreign body impacted in the airway, and hypovolaemia resulting from epistaxis. People die from acute ENT conditions and, in many instances, these deaths are preventable. The A&E nurse has a critical role to play in reducing the number of these preventable deaths.

Further reading

Bryoch M. (1993) Understanding is the means to Control: Management and Treatment of Seasonal Rhinitis. Professional Nurse. 8, 10, 662–6.

Bull PD (1991) Lecture Notes on Diseases of the Ear, Nose and Throat Oxford, Blackwell Scientific.

Butler K Malem F. (1993) Nurse aid management of Ear and Nose Emergencies. British Journal of Nursing 2, 17, 875–8.

Colman B (1992) Diseases of the nose, throat and ear, and head and neck Edinburgh, Churchill Livingstone.

References

Advanced Life Support Group (1997) *Advanced Paediatric Life Support* London: BMJ.

Barkin RM, Rosen P (1994) *Emergency Paediatrics: a Guide to Ambulatory Care*, 4th edn. St Louis: Mosby.

Benson N (1991) Earache. In: Hamilton GC, Saunders AB, Strange GR, Trott, eds. *Emergency Medicine: an Approach to Clinical Problem Solving*. Philadelphia: WB Saunders.

Bird D (1999) Managing epistaxis in A&E. *Emergency Nurse*, **7**(3), 10–13.

Bryoch M (1993) Understanding is the means to control: management and treatment of seasonal rhinitis. *Professional Nurse*, **8**(10), 662–666.

Budassi Sheehy S (1990) *Mosby's Manual of Emergency Care*. St Louis: CV Mosby.

Criddle LM (1995) Maxillofacial trauma and ear, nose and throat emergencies In: Kitt S, Selfridge-Thomas J, Proehl JA, Kaiser J, eds. *Emergency Nursing: a Physiologic and Clinical Perspective*, 2nd edn. Philadelphia: WB Saunders.

Eaton CJ (1993) *Essentials of Immediate Medical Care*. Edinburgh: Churchill Livingstone.

Emergency Nurses Association (1994) *Emergency Nursing Core Curriculum*, 4th edn. Philadelphia: WB Saunders.

Hinchliff S, Montague S, Watson R (1996) *Physiology for Nursing Practice*. London: Baillière Tindall.

Joyce SM (1991) Epistaxis. In: Hamilton GC, Sanders AB, Strange GR, Trott AT, eds. *Emergency Medicine: an approach to Clinical Problem Solving*. Philadelphia: WB Saunders.

Ludman H (1997) *ABC of Otolaryngology*, 4th edn. London: BMJ.

Maynard RL, Cooper GJ, Scott R (1989) Mechanisms of Injury in Bomb Blasts and Explosions. In: Westaby S, ed. *Trauma Pathogenesis and Treatment*. Oxford: Heinemann Medical Books.

Moulds A (1992) Managing a nosebleed. *Practice Nurse*, **4**(18), 467–473.

O'Donoghue GM, Bates GJ, Narula AA (1992) *Clinical ENT: an Illustrated Textbook*. Oxford: Oxford University Press.

Olson CM (1998) Dental, ear, nose and throat emergencies. In: Newberry L, ed. *Sheehy's Emergency Nursing: Principles and Practice*, 4th edn. St Louis: Mosby.

Owen-Smith M (1983) Bullet wounds: explosive blast injuries. In: Hughes S (ed.) *The Basis and Practice of Traumatology*. Rockville, MD: Aspen.

Rowe N, Williams N (eds) (1986) *Maxillofacial Injuries*. Edinburgh: Churchill Livingstone.

Selfridge-Thomas J (1995) *Manual of Emergency Nursing*. Philadelphia: WB Saunders.

Solomon NB (1989) *Practical Introduction to ENT Disease*. New York: Springer-Verlag.

Strome M, Kelly JH, Fried MP (1992) *Manual of Otolaryngology Diagnosis and Therapy*, 2nd edn. Boston: Little, Brown.

Wardrope J, Smith JAR (1992) *The Management of Wounds and Burns*. Oxford: Oxford University Press.

Walsh M (1996) *Accident & Emergency Nursing – A New Approach*, 3rd edn. Oxford: Heinemann Nursing.

Part 7

Practice issues in A&E

32. Primary Care: the A&E Dimension   **461**

33. Health Promotion   **469**

34. Nurse Triage   **475**

35. Nurse Practitioners   **485**

Chapter 32

Primary Care: the A&E Dimension

Robert Crouch

- Introduction
- Legitimacy of attendance
- A&E: the primary care role
- Providing for primary care in A&E
- Developing the primary care role of A&E nurses
- Bridging the gap between A&E and primary care
- Changing the culture
- Nurse practitioners
- Telephone consultation: extending the primary care role
- Future implications: out-of-hours care delivery
- Conclusion

Introduction

The A&E department is at the interface between primary and secondary care. This chapter explores issues of providing primary care in the A&E environment, identifying the need to challenge and change long established cultures. The traditionally held beliefs about legitimacy of attendance will be considered in the context of triage and the broader aspects of A&E nursing, focusing on developing a primary care orientation for A&E nurses and identifying the primary care role of the A&E department. The chapter will consider background research into attitudes towards patients at triage and an innovative educational exchange scheme designed to help break down barriers between primary and secondary care. With the changing emphasis on out-of-hours care and the need to explore alternative methods of patient consultation, the implications of these initiatives will be explored.

As an interface between primary and secondary care, the A&E department should provide an open access facility for delivering health care. A review of the literature infers that this philosophy is not universally accepted. The literature on the use and abuse of A&E implies that certain types of patients are seen as undesirable, resulting in suggestions for control over who uses the service (Jeffery 1979, Calnan 1982). This view is incongruent with the philosophy of open access. The prejudicial labelling of patients as 'inappropriate attenders' has been widely debated (Dolan 1999). The issues surrounding primary care provision in A&E are complex; to understand them fully, several key issues need to be explored, including the legitimacy of attendance, the A&E primary care role and the departmental culture.

Legitimacy of Attendance

The first element is legitimacy of attendance and the disparity between the professional and public view of the A&E service. Roth (1972) suggested that despite limited information available about patients in the

A&E setting, judgments are made about the patients' moral fitness, social worth and the appropriateness of their visit to the department. He believes that patient assessment in A&E is influenced by the evaluation of a person's social worth in the context of the wider society, and the staff's concept of their own work role. Roth (1972) also suggested that the perceived social worth of the patient is directly related to treatment by staff. Some staff take a morally superior stance to patients in lower social classes and also to patients seen as responsible for their illness. Jeffery (1979) also identified this concept of 'good' patients and 'normal rubbish', asserting that some patients were viewed negatively when it was thought that they were in some way responsible for their predicament. These views are further reinforced by the findings of Sbaih (1997), in her work describing the work of A&E nurses. Her account highlights nurses describing why patients attend A&E in the context of 'recognising the deserving patient'.

Roth (1972) suggested that 'the negative evaluation of patients is strongest when they combine an undeserving character with illegitimate demands'. Thus, a patient presenting with a minor medical complaint at an inconvenient hour is more vigorously condemned if he is a 'welfare case' than if he is a 'respectable citizen'. On the other hand a 'real emergency' can overcome moral repugnance.

Calnan (1982) suggested that ascribing patients' attendance as illegitimate may have more to do with professional autonomy. Other specialties in hospital medicine have a screening process for referral, allowing the doctor to select those patients to be treated. This enables them to build their speciality, and enhances their perceived professional autonomy. The lack of screening for admission to A&E results in staff attempting to exert control over patients by other means, such as defining an 'appropriate' attendance.

One group of patients commonly regarded as illegitimate are those attending A&E with primary care needs. Restricting access to health care in the A&E department to those who are 'genuine' accident or emergency cases could be supported by a perceived need to curb the number of annual attendances. 'Inappropriate attenders' are blamed for stretching scarce resources (Edmonds 1997, Rock & Pledge 1991) and jeopardising the care of those who really need it, namely the critically ill or injured. However, no evidence is provided to support this premise.

There is a move by some emergency departments to turn people away who are considered not to need formal assessment in A&E (Derlet & Nishio 1990). In this situation, triage is used as a screening process for eligibility to attend, and patients not thought appro-

priate to the A&E department could be referred to other clinics for continuation of their care. Driscoll et al. (1987) and Crouch (1992) suggested that refusing care may be unwise because of the difficulty in excluding the risk of harm to a proportion of patients. The policy of refusing care at an emergency facility raises questions about the patient's legitimate right to choose where to receive health care. It also leaves the nurse faced with the ethical dilemmas of performing a gate-keeping role.

A&E: The Primary Care Role

It is important to explore the reasons why people use A&E for primary care. The reasons for patients attending A&E are varied and complex but include such factors as the patient's perception of the urgency of his problem, the perceived need for X-ray or other investigation, advice from friends, not wishing to bother the GP and the presumed availability of a doctor (Cliff & Wood 1986, Dale et al. 1991, Singh 1988). A&E staff are constantly exposed to patients with primary care needs and often view their attendance at A&E as a failure of either the GP or the primary health care facility.

There have been many attempts to dissuade the public from using the A&E department for primary care, such as changing the name from 'casualty' to 'accident and emergency' (Standing Medical Advisory Committee 1962), positioning notices close to the entrance outlining the function of the department, challenging patients as to why they haven't seen their GP and redirection following triage (Derlet & Nishio 1990). All of these have had limited success (Cliff & Wood 1986, National Audit Office 1992, Worth & Hurst 1989).

It is not immediately apparent why such initiatives to dissuade the public from using A&E for primary care have failed. Educating the public to the appropriate use of the A&E department has been heralded as the key to decreasing the prevalence of primary care attenders. Nurses' views on 'inappropriate attenders' revealed agreement that patient education is important in the appropriate use of A&E but disagreement about the 'appropriateness' of individual patients' attendance (Green & Dale 1990). Any guidelines for the public regarding the 'appropriateness' of A&E attendance could, therefore, only be written in the broadest of terms and would be unlikely to have a significant impact on attendance rates. Education about the use of A&E is targeted at the patient on arrival at A&E, however studies examining who advised the patient to come to A&E (Dale et al. 1991) have found that the decision to attend A&E was complex and often involved advice from family and friends. Targeting education at patients may therefore have a limited effect as their decision is influenced by others.

One of the essential elements of providing for primary care in A&E is to address the culture of the department. Predominantly negative attitudes towards primary care attenders in A&E have been highlighted (Crouch & Dale 1994, Roth 1972). Nurses may be viewed as the main determinants of the A&E culture because of their length of service in an A&E department compared with junior doctors. Hughes (1988) suggested that nursing staff alert medical staff to the social character and abuse of the department. Disparate views of professionals and consumers may be seen regarding the function of the A&E department. These disparate perceptions have led to challenge and confrontation. The provision of primary care services in A&E may begin to address this issue.

Providing for Primary Care in A&E

A project to assess demand for an A&E-based primary care service was initiated in 1988 at King's College Hospital, London. Consultation activities and styles of A&E SHOs, registrars and GPs were compared. The study compared the process and outcome of care for primary care attenders. A system for prospective identification of patients at triage was developed (Dale et al. 1995a). A&E SHOs, registrars and GPs were allocated sessions to see patients triaged as 'primary care'. Dale et al. (1995b) found striking differences between these practitioners in the utilisation of resources such as X-ray, blood tests and referral to outpatient departments, as well as usage of consultation time. Primary care consultations made by A&E medical staff resulted in greater use of investigations (such as X-ray or haematological tests), outpatient and specialist services than those made by GPs (Dale et al. 1995b). Primary care patients seen by SHOs and registrars were twice as likely to have an X-ray than those seen by GPs. However, there were a similar identification rates of clinically significant findings on the X-rays between all three groups; in many cases the X-rays ordered by A&E SHOs showed no abnormalities. This seemed to indicate that GPs were able to be more specific when ordering radiological tests without losing sensitivity.

The style of consultation was explored by videoing consultations. Analysis of this data suggested that GPs had a more patient-centred approach to consultation, which was demonstrated by their use of consultation time. The comparison of patients who attended general practice with those who attended A&E with primary care needs revealed that patients attending A&E perceived they needed an investigation, such as an X-ray or blood test. The findings of Dale et al. (1995b) suggest that patients attending A&E with primary care needs who are seen and treated by A&E doctors are more likely to receive an investigation than if seen by a GP. Receiving these investigations may reinforce their decision to attend A&E, which may be reflected in future use of the A&E department.

Dale et al. (1996) noted that more patients who were seen by the GP said that they would either self-treat of visit their own GP in the future. It appears that the style of consultation may empower the patient to make a more informed choice about care-seeking behaviour in the future. This form of education by primary care practitioners, through the consultation, may be a more effective means of ensuring that patients receive the most appropriate form of health care in the future (Dale et al. 1996, Freeman et al. 1999, Ward et al. 1996).

The researchers found that there were only a small group of A&E attenders who were using the A&E department as their primary care facility regularly. Dale & Green (1991) stated that 'for the majority of patients, their decision to attend [A&E] was an understandable and convenient response to perceived health care needs given their circumstances, experience and beliefs'. The findings of Dale et al. (1995 a,b) of differences in resource utilisation by GPs as compared with A&E medical staff have been confirmed in subsequent studies in other departments (Murphy et al. 1996, Ward et al. 1996).

Developing the Primary Care Role of A&E Nurses

As noted above, nurses are probably the strongest influence on the A&E culture. Crouch & Dale (1994) described the development of a self-monitoring tool to highlight the beliefs, attitudes and feelings of triage nurses towards primary care attenders. The study identified marked differences in the feelings of nurses towards patients triaged as primary care attenders compared with those triaged as A&E attenders. The feelings towards primary care attenders involved less sympathy, more irritation and less motivation to help. The primary care attenders were perceived to have less urgent needs than those of 'A&E-type' patients. The information gained is an important measure of departmental culture and can be used to highlight the need for change as well as monitoring resultant cultural shifts.

For the effective provision of primary care in A&E, there needs to be a method of prospective identification of primary care patients. This would usually occur at triage. One approach, adopted as part of ongoing research and development into A&E primary care, has been to develop a decision framework to identify patients with primary care needs and those whose needs required the intervention of A&E doctors. This framework allows not only for the identification of primary care patients, but also for their prioritisation in terms of both their clinical and psychosocial needs (Crouch *et al.* 1993).

The triage framework for prospective identification of primary care patients utilises four key questions (see Box 32.1). The patient is allocated a priority based on clinical need or psychological state. Recognising that triage is a dynamic process, the priority rating can be adjusted at any time according to changing condition or need. The triage model developed enables the nurse to assign a priority of care to patients whether they are classified as primary care or A&E. This acknowledges that patients with primary care needs are not necessarily 'non-urgent'. This decision tree is used to identify the patients to be seen by the relevant practitioner and can be used in conjunction with the National Triage Scale (Crouch & Marrow 1996).

Through the research and development, the need to develop greater links between A&E and local general practice became apparent. An educational exchange scheme between A&E and practice nurses was developed.

Box 32.1 – *Patient assessment*

■ Is the patient likely to require follow-up by A&E or referral to a specialist team?

■ Is the patient likely to require admission to hospital?

■ Has the patient been referred to the A&E department or to an on-call team by a general practitioner?

■ Does the patient have a wound that will require suturing or a wound that will require surgical debridement?

■ If the answer to any of these questions is 'yes' the patient should be triaged as 'A&E'; if 'No', then the patient should be triaged as 'primary care'.

Bridging the Gap Between A&E and Primary Care

The work of Dale & Green (1991) identified that a negative view of general practice is held by A&E nurses. To facilitate a greater understanding of general practice and the A&E departments' role in providing for primary care, an educational exchange scheme has been piloted to foster more defined links between traditionally perceived primary and secondary care providers (Crouch *et al.* 1996a). The principal objectives of this exchange scheme are outlined in Box 32.2.

Box 32.2 – *Principal objectives of the Educational Exchange Scheme*

■ To facilitate an appreciation of the working environments of the A&E department and general practice and to identify the similarities and differences

■ To allow the exchange of ideas relating to nursing practice and research with relevance to A&E and general practice work

■ To enhance the understanding of each other's roles in caring for patients with primary care needs

---

Specific objectives for the A&E nurses and practice nurses were also set as part of the scheme. For the A&E nurse, these included gaining insight into the role of the practice nurse in health education, health and lifestyle screening and caseload management. The A&E nurses were also asked to observe the practice nurses' consultation style and content and to compare it with those used in A&E. For the practice nurses, the objectives included gaining insight into the varying needs of patients attending the A&E department, observing the assessment and management of patients in the different areas of the department, and comparing the management of patients attending the A&E department with primary care needs to that in the general practice setting.

During the evaluation of the scheme, nurses from both the A&E department and the primary care settings identified surprising similarities between their workloads (Crouch *et al.* 1996a). The educational exchange scheme is an effective means of providing insights into care in general practice. The adoption of such schemes has been beneficial in fostering closer liaisons between A&E and local general practice.

Changing the Culture

Over the past few years, increasing numbers of A&E departments in the UK have started providing a designated primary care service. For these initiatives to be successfully implemented, there is a need to challenge the traditional A&E culture and to establish new systems of training and practice. This process requires organisational change in terms of shared ownership of goals and service development (Dolan *et al.* 1997). To help meet these needs a workshop series was organised aimed at developing the primary care orientation of a number of A&E departments in England and Scotland. This included providing a framework of skills for the management of change to enable individual A&E departments to develop primary care services appropriate to their local circumstances.

The workshop series sought to influence clinical practice by sharing the experience of researchers and practitioners in a supportive environment. The use of this approach offered an effective means of bridging research and practice development and the theory–practice gap. The 'true' effectiveness of this method of disseminating research and effecting change cannot be readily assessed. It is suggested that this is a method to be explored for effective practice development and change management (Crouch *et al.* 1997).

Nurse Practitioners

There has been a significant increase in the numbers of nurse practitioners in A&E departments in recent years. Most of the nurse practitioner schemes developed in A&E use protocols and standing orders to see and treat a predetermined group of patients.

Many patients attending the A&E with primary care problems could have their needs addressed by a nurse practitioner with the necessary skills. The key to dealing effectively with primary care patients is the clinical background and educational preparation of the practitioner. Dale *et al.* (1991) identified marked differences in the management and outcomes of patients seen by the SHO and those seen by a GP. Would the same differences be seen if a similar comparison were made between an emergency nurse practitioner and a GP? The nurse practitioner working in the A&E department should have a background understanding and knowledge of primary care skills. The following question should be asked: Is a nurse with an A&E background suited to providing a nurse practitioner service to primary care patients? To ensure that A&E nurses are able to provide a service to primary care attenders, there is a need to develop education and training in primary care skills, which may well include time spent in general practice. These should focus on the consultation style and content and the utilisation of resources such as X-ray and haematological studies. This should be an integral part of their educational preparation.

A study of nurse practitioners across a number of A&E departments in west London found considerable variation in the scope of services provided. This included wide interpretations and understanding of the role and activity of the practitioner (Dolan *et al.* 1997). There is still a considerable amount of work to be undertaken before consensus as to the role and scope of the nurse practitioner in A&E is reached.

Telephone Consultation: Extending the Primary Care Role

Patients contact A&E not only for the treatment of urgent and emergency problems, but also to seek reassurance and advice about medical conditions (Crouch & Dale 1998a,b). Patients in the latter group often telephone for advice before they attend A&E. There are, at present, few hospitals in the UK with standardised responses to telephone enquiries; one survey of 18 major and 16 minor A&E departments in Wales identified that no department had guidelines, protocols or offered staff training in telephone consultation (Evans *et al.* 1993). Where such schemes exist, the system has been developed essentially as a means of managing the A&E workload and often forms part of the triage nurse's role (Buckles & Carew-McColl 1991). The guidelines produced for telephone consultation have been limited. However, the British Association for Emergency Medicine (1992), identify the need to document calls. This can be achieved either by using a telephone consultation record and recording the patient's name, age, telephone number, presenting complaint and advice given (Crouch *et al.* 1996b), or by using an automatic tape recorder (Egleston *et al.* 1994).

The role of telephone advice services in general is becoming increasingly important. Within the context of cost-conscious, consumer-oriented health care, telephone consultation clearly has an important part to play (Dale & Crouch 1997). A review of developing emergency services in the community recommended that consideration be given to setting centralised helplines as a means of providing immediate assessment and advice and, where necessary, referral to an appropriate service provider (NHS Executive 1996a,b). This proposal has been translated into the concept of NHS Direct, a nurse-led 24-hour telephone advice and information service to cover the nation by the year 2000 (Department of Health 1997).

The need for formal protocols and the provision of better, more specific training for telephone advice has been identified (Aitken *et al.* 1995, Crouch 1992, Peters 1994). There are, however, many unanswered questions about the service and the extent to which it will create, rather than manage, demand, and augment or duplicate the activities of current service providers (Crouch 1998). It may provide the opportunity to centralise resources, and formalise and integrate telephone advice services by redirecting advice calls to the service provider who is most appropriate for the patient's needs (Dale 1998). This model may be more cost-effective in terms of acheiving reliability and consistency in telephone advice than the development of this role in all A&E departments and MIUs.

Two studies report the use of computer-based decision support for telephone triage (Crouch *et al.* 1996c, Srinivas *et al.* 1996). These systems vary significantly in the level of decision support offered, with the system described by Srinivas *et al.* (1996) offering advice with prompts on an information screen. The system described by Crouch *et al.* (1996c) offers interactive assessment questions that will open different assessment pathways, levels of acuity dependent upon the complaint and standardised advice. The latter system has been evaluated in both A&E and primary care settings and found to be acceptable to both patients and staff. Telephone advice now plays an important part in the provision of out-of-hours primary care and this service is being increasingly offered by nurses.

Future Implications: Out-of-Hours Care Delivery

There is increasing demand on GPs for the provision of out-of-hours care, but there is no evidence to suggest that individuals are suffering more health problems needing urgent attention (Hallam et al. 1996). Over the last few years, there have been marked changes in the provision of out-of-hours care, with the formation of many GP cooperatives (Jessop *et al.* 1997), a number of which have bases that are sited alongside A&E departments. In one case, the cooperative has recognised the possibility for income generation and has negotiated a contract to provide a primary care service for the local A&E department (Dale 1996). The provision of care has shifted significantly from home visiting to telephone advice and to patient consultation at bases (Jessop *et al.* 1997). A&E nurses are having an impact in providing care in these services, playing a key role in telephone advice services to patients (Dale & Crouch 1997, Dinsdale 1996). Working in partnership with GP cooperatives will further establish A&E as part of the community.

Conclusion

There is a persistent and consistent demand for primary care in A&E. To make the A&E service more responsive to patients with primary care needs, a new way of thinking is required. To challenge the long established culture requires re-education of those who have been 'brought up' with the traditional beliefs and socialised into the established and accepted culture. Greater emphasis should be placed on 'appropriate' skill mix when recruiting staff to work in A&E. In recent years there has been a growing recognition that victims of trauma require intervention by specially trained personnel; the same is true of patients with primary care needs, and while their problems may not be so obvious, they still require specialist intervention. There is a need to challenge the traditional view of A&E as simply a department within the hospital and to replace it with one that identifies A&E within a broader community context. This requires leadership, organisational change, new systems of training, audit and professional development.

References

Aitken ME, Carey MJ, Kool B. (1995) Telephone advice about an infant given by after-hours clinics and emergency departments. *New Zealand Medical Journal,* **108**, 315–317.

British Association for Accident and Emergency Medicine Clinical Services Committee (1992) *Guidelines on the handling of telephone enquires in Accident and Emergency Departments.* London: The Royal College of Surgeons.

Buckles E, Carew-McColl M (1991) Triage by telephone. *Nursing Times,* **86**(6), 26–28.

Calnan M (1982) The hospital accident and emergency department: what is its role? *Journal of Social Policy,* **11**(4), 483–503.

Cliff KS, Wood TCA (1986) Accident and emergency services. *The Ambulant Patient Hospital and Health Services Review,* **82**(2), 74–77.

Crouch R (1992) 'Inappropriate attender' in A&E. *Nursing Standard (Emergency Nurse* Supplement), **6**(27), 7–9.

Crouch R (1998) Demanding Times. *Nursing Standard,* **12**(16), 14–15.

Crouch R, Dale J (1994) Identifying feelings engendered during triage assessment in A&E: the use of visual analogue scales. *Journal of Clinical Nursing,* **3**, 289–297.

Crouch R, Dale J (1998a) Literature review: telephone triage –

identifying the demand. *Nursing Standard*, **12**(34), 33–38.

Crouch R, Dale J (1998b) Telephone triage – how good are the decisions? (part 2). *Nursing Standard*, **12**(34), 33–38.

Crouch R, Dale J, Haverty S. (1993) *New Challenges in Accident and Emergency: Developing the Primary Care Role of A&E Nurses*. London: Department of General Practice and Primary Care, King's College School of Medicine and Dentistry.

Crouch R, Dale J, Haverty S, Winsor S (1996a) Piloting an A&E and practice nurse educational exchange. *British Journal of Nursing*, **5**(22), 1387–1390.

Crouch R, Dale J, Patel A, Williams S, Woodley H (1996c) *Ringing the Changes: Developing, Piloting and Evaluation of a Telephone Advice System in Accident and Emergency and General Practice Settings*. London: Departments of A&E Medicine and General Practice and Primary Care, King's College School of Medicine and Dentistry.

Crouch R, Haverty S, Westcott J, Dale J (1997) Primary care in the A&E department: meeting the challenge – a workshop series for A&E nurses. *Nurse Education Today*, **17**(6), 481–486.

Crouch R, Marrow J (1996) Towards a UK triage scale. *Emergency Nurse*, **4**(3), 4–5.

Crouch R, Patel A, Williams S, Dale J (1996b) An analysis of telephone calls to an inner-city accident and emergency department. *Journal of the Royal Society of Medicine*, **89**, 324–328.

Dale J (1996) Where to site an emergency centre. *Management in General Practice*, **19**, 16–19.

Dale J (1998) Wired for sound. *Health Services Journal*, **108** (5589), 24–27.

Dale J, Crouch R (1997) It's good to talk. *Health Service Journal*, **107** (5536): 24–26.

Dale J, Green J (1991) How do nurses working in hospital accident and emergency departments perceive local general practitioners? A study in six English hospitals. *Archives of Emergency Medicine*, **8**, 210–216.

Dale J, Green J, Glucksman E, Higgs R (1991) *Providing For Primary Care: Progress in A&E*. London: Department of General Practice and Primary Care, King's College School of Medicine and Dentistry.

Dale J, Green J, Reid F, Glucksman E (1995a) Primary care in the accident and emergency department: I. Prospective identification of patients. *British Medical Journal*, **311**, 423–426.

Dale J, Green J, Reid F, Glucksman E, Higgs R (1995b) Primary care in the accident and emergency department: II. comparison of general practitioners and hospital doctors. *British Medical Journal*, **311**, 427–430.

Dale J, Lang H, Roberts J, Green J, Glucksman E (1996) Cost effectiveness of treating primary care patients in accident and emergency: a comparison between general practitioners, senior house officers and registrars. *British Medical Journal*, **312**, 1340–1344.

Department of Health (1997) *The New NHS: Modern and Dependable*. London: HMSO.

Derlet R, Nishio D (1990) Refusing care to patients who present to an emergency department. *Annals of Emergency Medicine*, **19**(3), 262–267.

Dinsdale P (1996) Can nurses take over night duty? *Management in General Practice*, **19**, 20–21.

Dolan B (1999) Whose need does A&E serve? *Emergency Nurse*, **6**(9), 1.

Dolan B, Dale J, Morley V (1997) Nurse practitioners: the role in A&E and primary care. *Nursing Standard*, **11**(17), 33–38.

Driscoll PA, Vincent CA, Wilkinson M (1987) The use of the accident and emergency department. *Archives of Emergency Medicine*, **4**, 77–82.

Edmonds E (1997) Telephone triage: 5 years' experience. *Accident and Emergency Nursing*, **5**, 8–13.

Egleston CV, Kelly HC, Cope AR (1994) Use of a telephone advice line in an accident and emergency department. *British Medical Journal*, **308**, 31.

Evans RJ, McCabe M, Allen H, Rainer T, Richmond PW (1993) Telephone advice in the accident and emergency department: a survey of current practice. *Archives of Emergency Medicine*, **10**, 216–219.

Freeman GK, Meakin RP, Lawrenson RA, Leydon GM, Craig G (1999) Primary care units in A&E departments in North Thomes in the 1990s: initial experience and future implications. *British Journal of General Practice*, **49**, 107–110.

Green J, Dale J (1990) Health education and the inappropriate use of accident and emergency departments: the views of accident and emergency nurses. *Health Education Journal*, **49**, (4), 157–161.

Hallam L, Wilkin D, Roland M (1996) 24 Hour Responsive Health Care. *Primary Care Briefing Paper*. Manchester: NPCRDC, University of Manchester.

Hughes D (1988) When nurse knows best: some aspects of nurse/doctor interaction in a casualty department. *Sociology of Health and Illness*, **10**(1), 1–22.

Jeffery R (1979) Normal rubbish: deviant patients in casualty departments. *Sociology of Health and Illness*, **1**(1), 90–108.

Jessop L, Beck I, Hollins L, Shipman C, Reynolds M, Dale J (1997) Changing the pattern of out of hours care: a survey of general practitioner cooperatives. *British Medical Journal*, **314**(7075), 199–200.

McGovern M (1993) Uninvited guests. *Nursing Times*, **89**(12), 38–40.

Murphy A, Bury G, Plunkett P, Gibney D, Smith M, Mullan E, Johnson Z (1996) Randomised controlled trial of general practitioner versus usual medical care in an urban accident and emergency department: process, outcome, and comparative cost. *British Medical Journal*, **312**, 1135–1142.

National Audit Office (1992) *The Report of the Comptroller and Audit General: the NHS Accident and Emergency Departments in England*. London: HMSO.

NHS Executive (1996a) *Developing Emergency Services in the Community: Volume 1 – Emerging Conclusions*. London: Department of Health.

NHS Executive (1996b) *Developing Emergency Services in the Community: Volume 2 – The Evidence Base*. London: Department of Health

Peters RM (1994) After-hours telephone calls to general and subspecialty internists: an observational study. *Journal of General Internal Medicine*, **9**, 554–557.

Rock D, Pledge M (1991) Priorities of care for the walking wounded: triage in accident and emergency. *Professional Nurse*, **6**(8), 463–466.

Roth C (1972) Some contingencies of the moral evaluation and control of clientele: the case of the hospital emergency service. *American Journal of Sociology*, **77**(5), 839–856.

Sbaih L (1997) The work of accident and emergency nurses: part 1. An introduction to the rules. *Accident and Emergency Nursing*, **5**(1), 28–33.

Singh S (1988) Self referral to accident and emergency department: patients' perceptions. *British Medical Journal*, **297**, 1179–1180.

Srinivas S, Poole F, Redpath J, Underhill TJ (1996) Review of a computer based telephone helpline in an A&E department. *Journal of Accident and Emergency Medicine*, **13**, 330–333.

Standing Medical Advisory Committee (1962) *Accident and Emergency Services (Platt Report)*. London: HMSO.

Ward P, Huddy J, Hargreaves S, Touquet R, Hurley J, Fothergill J (1996) Primary care in London: an evaluation of general practitioners working in an inner city accident and emergency department. *Journal of Accident and Emergency Medicine*, **13**(1), 11–15.

Worth C, Hurst K (1989) Accident and emergency: false alarm? *Nursing Times*, **85**(15), 24–27.

Chapter 33

Health Promotion

Stewart Piper

- Introduction
- Health persuasion techniques
- Legislative action for health
- Community development
- Personal counselling for health
- Conclusion

Introduction

It is interesting to consider Beattie's (1991) observation that each major health care profession is increasingly claiming that health promotion forms the basis of their work. Interesting because while copious references and articles exploring health promotion in nursing are easily accessible in any nursing library, the emphasis tends to be on practice and 'doing' rather than on asking fundamental questions such as what is its purpose, or on theoretical scrutiny of the different approaches that can be adopted and their pertinence for nursing. The need for such debate has now been given fresh impetus for nursing in general by the *Health of the Nation* (HON) (Department of Health 1992), the government strategy for health in England, which has placed health promotion explicitly on the nursing agenda, and for A&E nurses in particular, as accidents form one of the five key areas of the strategy. Indeed, the HON (Department of Health 1993) highlights that 'Tertiary prevention by Accident and Emergency departments ... will contribute to the overall objective of reducing ill health, disability and death from accidents'.

A critique of the relationship between nursing and HON in general can be found in Brown & Piper (1997). Given this current emphasis on health promotion, the intention of this chapter is to clarify the distinctions and relationships between the various models of health promotion, to outline their mode and focus of intervention, and specifically to move the debate beyond any narrow or traditional view of health promotion as simply a form of information or advice giving. There will also be an emphasis on the aims, methods, impact and outcomes of two key approaches that can be operationalised and applied and which seem most relevant to A&E nursing practice. To facilitate this process and to aid conceptual understanding, Beattie's (1991) framework is utilised to map out and contextualise the discrete approaches to health promotion and is outlined in Figure 33.1. In addition, to avoid the debate surrounding the distinction between health

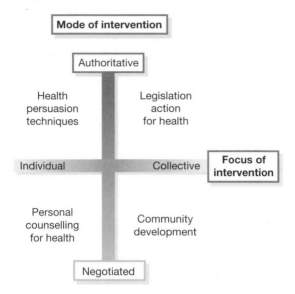

Figure 33.1 – *Models of health promotion. (After Beattie 1991.)*

education and health promotion, for the purpose of this chapter, the definition of health promotion by Tones (1990), who stated that it 'incorporates all measures deliberately designed to promote health and handle diseases', will be adopted.

Health Persuasion Techniques

'Health persuasion techniques' reflects a 'medical model' approach to health promotion. Health is seen as optimum biological functioning and equates with the absence of disease, illness and injury. Although some, such as Kiger (1995), may disagree slightly with the following exposition and others roughly concur (Tones & Tilford 1994), herein primary, secondary and tertiary health promotion are posited as inherent aspects of the health persuasion element of Beattie's grid. Primary health promotion refers to intervention to prevent disease or injury. Secondary aims to prevent presenting pathology becoming chronic or irreversible, and to restore patients to their former health status. Tertiary health promotion aims to optimise a patient's health experience within the constraints imposed by a chronic disease, such as diabetes, asthma, HIV, injury or concomitant disability, and to prevent restrictions or further complications.

At a primary level, an assumption is made that individuals make rational, conscious decisions about their health-related behaviour in response to 'factual' information selectively derived from objective medically based research. Health promotion interventions take the form of edicts from health care professionals and the ever present mass media awareness raising campaigns such as the 'clunk click' television campaigns of yesteryear, encouraging the use of cycle helmets, 'no smoking day' and drug awareness week etc.

It is suggested to the public that if they follow (or don't follow) a prescribed course of action, their 'health' will be at risk. The aim is to act as a trigger to bring about 'do it yourself' attitudes and then behaviour/lifestyle changes consistent with the recommended advice given. 'Health persuasion techniques' as a primary health promotion intervention would engage A&E nurses in an information-based approach. This could include themed displays in the waiting room on a variety of topics such as accident prevention, first aid, the dangers of alcohol misuse, HIV and sexual health, and healthy eating. These must be visually appealing, regularly changed and could tie in with national initiatives such as Drinkwise Day or World Aids Day. They should be supported by a wide range of leaflets in display racks, posters strategically placed around the A&E department, and health promotion videos showing in the waiting room if it is suitably equipped. This process can be assisted by contacting local health promotion specialists who are an important source of information, resources and expertise.

It is important to acknowledge that, while effective at raising awareness about particular health risks, when operating as a sole strategy for attitude and behaviour change the outcomes are likely to be at best uncertain (Brown 1996, McEwan & Bhopal 1991). In emphasising the personal controlling of risks and the correcting of individual inadequacies, it is also assumed that free choice exists and that lifestyle is the primary cause of ill health. In isolation, such an approach denies that health is a social product, and ignores and implicitly condones inequalities and minimal state intervention. For an excellent, albeit old and general, critique of such a stance, the reader is referred to Mitchell (1982).

The purpose of secondary health promotion intervention, primarily aimed at those discharged home from the A&E department, is patient compliance with treatment regimes, with the goal of optimum management of injury and disease by patients to maximise chances of full recovery and to minimise the risk of complications or relapse. The A&E nurse determines the specific behaviour(s) required and supplies the appropriate information, discharge advice and reassurance to achieve this. Obvious examples of daily practice include advice and information on how to care for a fractured limb in a plaster cast, a sprained ligament or minor head injury, and an outline of what potential problems to be alert to, what rehabilitative

Table 33.1 – *Health persuasion techniques*

Aims	Methodology	Impact	Outcome
Health-related behaviour to prevent disease and injury	Mass media campaigns	Change in health-related behaviour	Reduction in accidents:
	Professional advice giving		■ Mortality
Compliance with treatment regimes	Patient teaching	Conforming to advice	■ Morbidity
	Discharge advice		■ Complications
	Patient information		■ Relapse

and preventive actions the patient can take, and so on. This is reinforced by an information sheet that patients and their significant others can take away for reference, and the A&E department's contact telephone number should a problem arise.

Tertiary health promotion essentially adopts the same methods as secondary but it is applied to patients presenting to the A&E department with exacerbations of chronic problems. The author concedes, however, that the severity of the presenting condition may warrant emergency admission and thus health promotion may be problematic, ineffective and inappropriate. The aims, methods, impact and outcomes for health persuasion interventions are summarised in Table 33.1.

These latter two approaches (secondary and tertiary) can be likened to an electrical system model (Hills 1979). This undermines the complexity of the nurse – patient interpersonal interaction by reducing it to a mechanistic relationship, but may serve a purpose for illustration as follows:

Input > Coding > Channel > Decoding > Output

The nurse provides the input and the coding and the patient is the decoder. The method is concerned with the sender (A&E nurse/expert) validating facts and transmitting knowledge to the receiver (patient), with the latter feeding back information on how the sender's messages have been received. Ewles & Shipster (1984) took this one step further and refer to it as a three-stage process:

■ giving information or advice to a patient about her injury/disease
■ ensuring that the patient understands and remembers that information or advice
■ ensuring that the patient is able to act on the information or advice.

They stressed the need to define the objectives and desired outcome for the intervention, to give the infor-

mation in a structured way, emphasising and repeating the important aspects, and to use short words and short sentences to avoid any misunderstanding. This is now moving into the realms of patient teaching and an excellent source for more substantial reading is Kiger (1995). If there are any dangers with this crucial facet of A&E nursing, it is that the process becomes a 'telling rather than listening' top-down one-way 'didactic model of nurse patient relationships' (Macleod-Clark *et al.* 1991) reinforcing the status of the nurse, and engendering patient deference and dependence. The emphasis on professionally determined needs may potentially fail to consider patients' needs, experiences and social, economic or environmental context and to achieve their participation in care.

Legislative Action for Health

For 'legislative action for health', social factors and social conditions are the major determinants of health status. Social class is considered to be beyond the control of individuals but the instrumental influence in shaping their way of life and thus health status. The poor health experiences and higher accident rates of the lower occupational groups are attributed to these class differentials and concomitant socioeconomic inequalities, including the unequal distribution of income, wealth and capital (Blackburn 1991, Townsend & Davidson 1990, Whitehead 1990).

Contributions to collective health gain can be achieved by legislative and environmental interventions governing issues such as welfare provision, taxation, the distribution of resources and pollution. The action of industry and persuasive advertising can be monitored and controlled and laws can be enacted. With regard to the latter, and with a particular resonance for A&E nurses, Tones & Tilford (1994) report that education (health persuasion techniques) to encourage the wearing of front seat belts was successful to a degree, but that legislation has been

Table 33.2 – *Legislative action for health*

Aims	Methodology	Impact	Outcome
Structural change (national/local) Health-promoting accident department	Lobbying re: ■ Inequalities in health ■ Social chapter ■ Health & Safety issues ■ Car design ■ Traffic calming Policy development and change Interagency work Education and training Collaborative care planning Clinical audit	Reduction in inequalities Increase in safety Organisational change: ■ Staff rostering ■ Timing of clinics ■ Skill mix (ALS/ATLS) ■ Use of protocols ■ Trauma scoring ■ Trauma teams ■ Risk registers Liaison Change in health-related behaviour Conforming to advice	Reduction in accidents: ■ Mortality ■ Injury ■ Disability ■ Complications

much more successful in enforcing their use and has changed the pattern of injury following a road traffic accident, helping to reduce mortality and morbidity.

Although not a feature of patient interaction, a 'legislative action for health' approach could engage A&E nurses in collecting data to construct a profile of the pattern of local accidents, and use this data to campaign for traffic calming measures in residential areas or improved street lighting. This would involve nurses lobbying local policy makers by submitting written and verbal evidence to appropriate forums, within the boundaries of confidentiality and UKCC guidelines, and taking every opportunity to sit on multi-agency working groups. Nationally, A&E nurses can lobby power holders through their professional organisations and specialist forums. These can align themselves with other pressure groups to address such issues as poverty and welfare provision, car design, drinking and driving, health and safety laws governing the workplace and advertising bans, such as tobacco or the emphasis placed on the high performance of cars.

More closely related to patients, this frame of reference can be applied from an organisational perspective to an A&E department and focus on policy development, education and training issues and collaborative care planning, all of which are concerned with promoting collective health gain. Policy development

drawing on evidence-based research could enhance standards of care delivery or specify minimum standards to be expected within the department and could embrace issues of skill mix, such as the numbers of nurses on a shift having undergone recognised post-registration training courses, trauma scoring, use of nationally recognised protocols such as those for advanced life support, asthma etc., and the establishment of trauma teams. These are just some examples of how legislative action for health might be adapted and applied by A&E nurses and they are summarised in Table 33.2.

Community Development

Community development (CD) occupies a smaller, though potentially important, role in the health promotion repertoire of A&E nurses. CD also sees the social environment, as opposed to individual characteristics, as the key determinant of health. Rather than addressing power structures and institutions at a national level, CD seeks to improve health by an analysis of community perceptions of social and economic determinants. Like-minded allies share and articulate their social discontents and, through community action, mobilise local resources to force 'bottom up' change.

Although not strictly community development, A&E

nurses can employ a similar approach by having a knowledge of the existence of self-help and support groups in their area and nationally, and direct appropriate patients towards these. This would necessitate A&E departments holding directories of local activities and key contacts. Such groups enable patients and/or their relatives and loved ones to use their collective resources to determine their common needs, shape their agenda for 'health' and build support networks. The group members can share experiences, offer coping strategies and draw strength from each other (Cudmore 1998). They can also challenge the medical and nursing professions and lobby for change in both service provision and societal attitudes.

Personal Counselling for Health

Of the three previous strategies for health promotion explored, legislative action for health is indirect in its involvement in patient care; health persuasion techniques involves direct patient interaction but is professionally directed; and community development is keen to establish and enable the collective health agenda of like-minded patients. None so far has set out with the purpose of achieving individual patient-centred health promotion in a non-hierarchical, non-coercive way, aiming at active patient participation and empowerment. 'Personal counselling for health' seeks to achieve this by enabling and supporting patients to set their own health promotion agendas and to develop scope for personal choice and change following individual patient reflection and clarification of existing health-related behaviours and their relative desirability.

Providing information about the cause and effect of disease may be an important facet of such health promotion, but fundamentally A&E nurses would 'listen rather than just tell'. They would strive towards patient empowerment through ensuring that patients were aware of the options open to them, and enable and acknowledge their right to actively participate in decisions on clinical matters. A&E nurses would support patients during this process, act as advocates when required and assist them to acknowledge and draw on their personal resources and strengths to maximise their autonomy. As such, existing power relations between the nurse and the patient are challenged and equalised, and the distance between the two parties is minimised.

A model currently in vogue and seen as compatible with the personal counselling for health approach is the 'stages of change' model (Prochaska & Diclemente 1982), and the reader is referred to the author's original work for a clear exposition of this process as a detailed outline is beyond the scope of this chapter. Briefly, however, the cycle has stages through which people who change successfully move whatever the variety of behaviour. 'Contemplation', the point at which people enter the cycle, represents a form of cognitive dissonance where people become aware of themselves, the nature of their behaviour and its negative consequences, and think about the positive consequences of change. At this stage they continue the behaviour, such as smoking. 'Action' is when a person has decided to effect change, 'maintenance' is the point at which there is a belief in the ability to maintain change, and 'relapse', an integral part of the cycle, is where the behaviour and contemplation or pre-contemplation stage are reverted to.

It is unrealistic to think that A&E nurses would accompany a patient through the entire cycle of change, but the process is flagged up for further reading as it is desirable to have an understanding greater than that alluded to here to enable appropriate intervention dependent upon the stage the patient has reached.

Conclusion

This chapter has endeavoured to combine a brief theoretical discussion on the nature of health promotion with a translation of how the complementary and contradictory approaches, each with different aims, methods and evaluatory criteria, relate to A&E nursing.

It is the author's contention that health promotion is an intrinsic part of holistic A&E nursing and that the four models outlined enable legitimate A&E health promotion activity, but to varying degrees. Hence, the limited contribution of community development to A&E is acknowledged, and personal counselling for health, although important in terms of the absolute right of patients to have control over their own health and health-related decision-making where possible, is otherwise in reality likely to be subordinate to health persuasion and legislative action interventions due to the very nature of A&E nursing. Clearly, health persuasion health promotion has considerable and obvious application for individual patients, but equally importantly the collective patient agenda can be addressed by legislative action for health, which also delivers valuable indirect health gain. Finally, the author is aware that this chapter may relabel as health promotion, rather than reshape, elements of existing practice.

References

Beattie A (1991) Knowledge and control in health promotion: a test case for social policy and social theory. In: Gabe J, Calnan M, Bury M eds. *The Sociology of the Health Service*. London: Routledge.

Blackburn C (1991) *Poverty and Health*. Buckingham: Open University Press.

Brown PA (1996) A review of mass media campaigns as a form of health education. *Journal of the Institute of Health Education*, **34**(2), 1–6.

Brown PA, Piper SM (1997) Nursing and the health of the nation: schism or symbiosis? *Journal of Advanced Nursing*, **25**, 297–310.

Cudmore J (1998) Critical incident stress: management strategies. *Emergency Nurse*, **6**(3), 22–27.

Department of Health (1992) *The Health of the Nation: a Strategy for Health in England*. London: HMSO.

Department of Health (1993) *The Health of the Nation: Key area handbook: Accidents*. London: HMSO.

Ewles L, Shipster P (1984) *One to One Health Education*. London: South East Thames Regional Health Authority.

Hills P (1979) *Teaching and Learning as a Communication Process*. London: Croom Helm.

Kiger A (1995) *Teaching for Health*, 2nd edn. Edinburgh: Churchill Livingstone.

McEwan R, Bhopal R (1991) HIV/AIDS health promotion for young people: a review of theory, principles and practice. *HIV/AIDS and Sexual Health Programme Paper 12*. London: Health Education Authority.

Macleod-Clark J, Wilson Barnett J, Latter S (1991) *Health Education in Nursing Project: Results of a National Survey on Senior Nurses' Perceptions of Health Education Practice in Acute Ward Settings*. London: Kings College, University of London, Department of Nursing Studies.

Mitchell J (1982) Looking after ourselves: an individual responsibility? *Royal Society of Health Journal*, **4**, 169–173.

Prochaska JO, Diclemente CC (1982) Transtheoretical therapy: toward's a more integrated model of change. *Psychotherapy: Theory, Research and Practice*, **19**(3), 276–288.

Tones K (1990) Why theorise?: ideology in health education. *Health Education Journal*, **49**(1), 2–6.

Tones K, Tilford S (1994) *Health Education: Effectiveness Efficiency and Equity*. London: Chapman and Hall.

Townsend P, Davidson N (1990) *Inequalities in Health: The Black Report*. London: Penguin.

Whitehead M (1990) *Inequalities in Health. The Health Divide*. London: Penguin.

Chapter 34

Nurse Triage

Cherine Woolwich

- Introduction
- The concept of nurse triage
- Direct nurse triage
- Providing a nurse triage system
- Patient assessment
- The triage decision
- Documentation
- Training
- Audit
- A national triage scale
- Conclusion

Introduction

Nursing staff in most A&E departments carry out some form of face-to-face triage in order to assess each patient's complaint/injury. The differences in practice lie in the degree of assessment and the subsequent medical and nursing pathways that follow from that initial assessment. Currently, nurse triage is seen as an integral part of the A&E nurse's role. It has followed its own path of development and bears little resemblance to medical triage used in military and disaster settings. It has been developed within the A&E department as a means of assessing patients, prioritising their care and treating them within the department at a level appropriate to their individual needs.

The introduction of the *Patient's Charter* (Department of Health 1991) requires all patients attending A&E departments to be immediately assessed by a registered nurse. This has prompted nurses and managers to both acknowledge and formalise their triage systems. There are two types of nurse triage:

- *Direct triage* is a face-to-face assessment of patients arriving in the A&E department. This is the type of triage that most A&E nurses refer to when discussing nurse triage
- *Indirect triage* is a more recent development, whereby patients are triaged via the telephone. This a relatively new development in the UK and its use is controversial (Coleman 1997, Glasper & McGrath 1993). While the purpose of telephone triage remains the same, to assess the clinical needs of the patient, the skills required of the nurse and the tools used are very different (Wheeler & Siebelt 1997).

This chapter will focus on direct nurse triage and address some of the issues that surround the formalising and development of this crucial A&E role.

The Concept of Nurse Triage

(From the French *trier*, 'to sort). The origins of triage are well documented (Rund & Rausch 1981). It was originally used as a means of grading the quality of goods such as coffee beans and wool, and was first adopted for use in a medical context during the Napoleonic wars. For the first time, casualties were treated on the basis of medical need rather than rank or social status. It has been used in every war since, as a means of managing mass casualties. While the term triage is used in both military/disaster triage and A&E departments, it must be recognised that the two processes fulfil very different functions.

Rund & Rausch (1981) suggested that while military triage involves little more than identifying 'salvageable' cases for evacuation, nurse triage prioritises emergency patients into a system of care as part of an integral process. Peacetime nursing triage emerged in the United States in the early 1960s, during the war in Vietnam. Highly trained paramedics moved across into civilian hospitals, taking their triage skills with them and adapting the process for use within A&E. It was not until the 1980s that the concept of nurse triage became popular in the UK (Edwards 1999). A&E departments began introducing schemes around this time, based largely on the experiences of American nursing colleagues.

Accident and emergency attenders

The unpredictability of workloads within A&E departments and the steadily increasing numbers of attenders are well recognised and documented (Mallet & Woolwich 1990, Nutall 1986, Selvig 1985). During a 24-hour period a wide spectrum of accidents and emergencies may be seen, sometimes stretching the resources of the department and staff to their limit. In addition, the number of acute hospital closures has had negative impact on waiting times for patients in A&E departments (Allen & Hughes 1993).

Prior to nurse triage, the waiting room was an unknown quantity for the A&E staff. It could be full of patients with a diverse range of illnesses and injuries, of varying degrees of severity. The danger of a patient's condition deteriorating while waiting to be seen was very real. It was also widely recognised, however, that a significant number of attenders, while requiring medical treatment, did not need to receive that treatment in an A&E department. It is inevitable that with the ever-increasing demands on a finite service, longer waiting times will develop for the most vulnerable group of patients: those who are seriously ill and in need of immediate emergency care and treatment. Recognition of all these factors highlights the need for all patients to be assessed on arrival in the A&E department by a person skilled in triage.

The purpose of nurse triage

The purpose of nurse triage is not to reduce the overall waiting time for all patients. Selvig (1985) acknowledged that waiting times for patients are not significantly reduced by triage and Mallet & Woolwich (1990) have shown, in line with other studies, that while the waiting times for the more seriously ill have been reduced, overall departmental waiting times have steadily increased. The purpose of triage is to 'make the best possible use of the available medical and nursing personnel and facilities' and it is there to assist in determining 'which patients need immediate care ... and which patients can wait' (Potter 1985).

For some patients, their only access to the health care system may be through attending an A&E department and nurse triage should not be seen as a means of restricting this entry. It should be seen as an opportunity, rather than an obstacle, for all attenders to receive access to health care.

The role and aims of nurse triage

Budassi & Barber (1981) defined the role of triage as 'the process of deciding the priorities for the therapeutic interventions of a given individual or individuals and the place where these interventions should occur'. Therefore, the primary aim of the triage nurse must be the early assessment of patients, in order to determine the priority of care according to the individual's clinical need. There are other aspects of care, however, that nurse triage can meet (Handyside 1996). There is the more efficient use of the department facilities and resources as patients are allocated to the most appropriate clinical areas within the department and are seen and treated within an appropriate time. Regular reassessment of patients ensures that the appropriateness of the care implemented can be modified as necessary.

The early and appropriate requesting of medical records or relevant previous X-rays will aid the clinical assessment and diagnosis. Essential first aid measures can be taken without delay.

Control of infection may be initiated as soon as the patient has been assessed, promoting a safer environment for patient care. The waiting area is now a known quantity and patient flow can be controlled and organised (Ramler & Mohammed 1995). Patients and their relatives have an easily identifiable and reliable source of information for any enquiries. This helps to relieve anxiety and reduce aggression and can increase patient satisfaction with the service (Dolan 1998).

Appropriate first aid measures can be taken without delay. This initial meeting can also be valuable in terms of health promotion and education. The triage nurse can offer verbal and written information about the availability of primary health care and community services, including self-help and support groups, or social services.

Direct Nurse Triage

Five types of direct nurse triage used in the United States have been identified by Estrada (1979) and used by Bland (1988), of which three are currently in use in the UK.

Non-professional triage. Patients arrive in the A&E department, register with the receptionist and then sit in the waiting area, without any form of assessment, until they are called to be seen by the doctor. The receptionist will only call a nurse if there appears to be some reason for concern.

In the UK, non-professional triage can still be found functioning in some departments and is more frequently used at certain times, e.g. at night when staff and resources are limited. Mallet & Woolwich (1990) identified this as an area of great concern in their study of nurse triage in an inner city A&E department and recommended the provision of a nurse triage service during the night shift. Their concerns are echoed in the findings of a large study of the use of health care assistants (HCAs) in English A&E departments, which found that HCAs assessed patients on arrival in 28.7% of the 282 departments that responded to the survey (Boyes 1995).

Basic triage. The patient is assessed by a registered nurse, a priority rating is determined and the patient is allocated to a treatment area. Although there is some documentation initiated, it does not become part of the patient's medical records. Basic triage can be recognised in the UK as 'informal triage' and often functions on the basis of 'when time and staffing levels allow'. Within such systems there may not be an identified triage role or designated triage nurse. A written policy, protocols and training of staff for the role may not be available. Documentation of assessments is often poor and unstructured. For many departments, it was this level of triage that developed into more formal systems when the *Patient's Charter* was introduced (Department of Health 1991).

Advanced triage. This is the most comprehensive system carried out by a registered nurse. It includes an initial assessment of the patient, the initiation of appropriate diagnostic procedures, such as X-rays or phlebotomy, limited physical examination, documentation and referral to an appropriate resource, often to outside agencies away from the emergency department. Nurses functioning at this level are highly experienced emergency nurses who have undergone specific training for the role. This is, at present, still beyond the remit of many A&E departments in the UK, although as A&E nurses expand their skills and expertise, it may become more commonplace.

In addition to these three types of triage, Estrada (1979) also referred to *physician triage* and *team triage*, but, as mentioned above, neither of these is currently used in the UK.

Over the last 10 years many UK A&E departments have developed more formal direct nurse triage systems. These improvements have resulted in the development of an 'intermediate triage', which lies between basic and advanced triage.

Intermediate triage

In addition to the assessment and prioritising of care, nursing interventions such as vital signs, ECG, test strip urinalysis and pregnancy testing, and the administration of Entonox therapy may be commenced for a patient's identified complaint. Protocols may allow the early administration of analgesia for some patients. In a growing number of departments, the triage nurse is able to request X-rays for patients with certain injuries. They may also have limited referral options, e.g. to specific outpatient clinics, GPs and practitioners, or to family planning clinics.

Where A&E nurses undertake intermediate triage, there is a need to establish standards and policies which must be adhered to by both medical and nursing staff. Training is essential and needs to be given before the role is undertaken. Regular auditing of triage decisions must take place. These criteria legitimise the job of the triage nurse, recognising the role and making the nurse accountable for both her actions and decisions as well any omissions (UKCC 1992a).

The *Patient's Charter* (Department of Health 1991) opened the door for the widespread development of nurse triage when it required that patients should be assessed on arrival in the A&E department. This provided the opportunity for nurses to ensure that nurse triage gained recognition as a skilled and vital part of their role. Patients arriving in the department are no longer being seen on a 'first come, first serve' basis, nor are patients arriving by ambulance automatically seen before those arriving by other means.

Nurse triage has become an essential part of the A&E service and, once established, it cannot be easily withdrawn. It can no longer be offered on an 'ad hoc' basis and, as such, the triage nurse becomes of paramount importance, with the triage function becoming pivotal for the effective management of the department (Budassi & Barber 1981). The relationship between the medical and nursing staff has altered, because it is the triage nurse who determines patient flow through the department. In some departments this has been seen as a radical change in departmental work practice and philosophy.

Providing a Nurse Triage System

Staffing levels may need to be adjusted to allow for a designated triage nurse. The provision of a 24-hour professional nurse triage system is costly and may represent up to 15% of the nursing budget of a medium-sized A&E department (Audit Commission 1996). In order to secure adequate funding, specific targets around the delivery of quality care in A&E need to be highlighted. Specific goals for the service vary in relation to the size of the department, the number of attendances, staffing levels and legal or administrative constraints. They need to be realistic and achievable, and should relate to early assessment, identification of the chief complaint, priority setting and documentation. A comprehensive role description for the triage nurse needs to be developed, setting out the duties and responsibilities of the role holder. This will legitimise the role for nurses undertaking triage, for the medical staff accepting the service and for the hospital management team or Trust board, who will be asked to accept vicarious liability for nurses carrying out triage functions.

Rapid patient assessment is of paramount importance, and therefore the triage nurse should not become involved with aspects of clinical practice that impede the effectiveness of the triage service. Baseline observations, for example, should not automatically be included in the remit of triage (Rund & Rausch 1981). First aid measures should also be limited to the basics. If the situation is deemed life-threatening, then life-saving measures such as cardiopulmonary resuscitation and controlling severe haemorrhage should be initiated and assistance summoned to allow the triage nurse to resume her triage function as quickly as possible (Bland 1988).

In some departments, the triage nurse has other clinical responsibilities in addition to the triage role. This is not considered ideal, unless the workload of the department is so small and sporadic that it would be impractical for one nurse to be allocated in this way (Buschiazzo 1984). In all but the most minor departments, there is the danger that, by one nurse taking on two distinct roles within the department, patient care may become compromised if the workload of either role becomes of secondary importance.

The role of the triage nurse is one of the most stressful in A&E. The workload is variable and patients often arrive in pain and frightened, the nature of their complaint or injury as yet undetermined. The role demands quick and safe decisions to be made based on a brief assessment of each patient. Colleagues managing and working in the clinical areas rely on the judgement and the decisions of the triage nurse. If vital information is not picked up at the initial assessment, the result could be disastrous for the patient. While the safety net of 'over-triage' can be used to make a difficult decision safe, the overuse of this practice can increase the pressure on colleagues, delay treatment of other patients unnecessarily and undermine the effectiveness of the whole triage service.

Patient Assessment

Nurse triage should be a rapid, superficial assessment taking no longer than a few minutes. Its purpose is to elicit information from the patient in order to determine the chief complaint. While in some cases this may be a quite straightforward process, e.g. a patient presenting with a clear history of simple uncomplicated trauma to an extremity, a significant proportion of attenders to the A&E department present with a more complex history involving various contributing factors which pre-empted their current illness or injury. It is the latter presentation that calls on the skills of the triage nurse.

Various assessment tools have been developed which will aid the nurse in decision-making and encourage standardisation of patients' assessments and subsequent collation of information. SOAP is an assessment tool devised by an American, Dr Lawrence Weed, in 1969 (Lee & Fraser 1981). It is perhaps the most well known of the assessment tools used by triage nurses, and in the US is referred to and used extensively in the relevant literature (see Box 34.1). [An 'I' for 'implementation' has been added after SOAP and an 'E' to emphasise the need for continual evaluation (Blythin 1988a, b).]

One of the potential problems with using this tool for the less experienced nurse is that by working systematically through the acronym, the nurse

Box 34.1 – *The SOAP model of triage*
S **Subjective assessment** – the patient's evaluation of his illness or injury
O **Objective assessment** – an evaluation based on observable and measurable data
A **Assessment** – the clinical impression
P **Plan of care**

becomes caught up with the S – subjective assessment – and fails to reach the A, the actual assessment. Although S is the first letter, A and O are crucial elements of the tool. It is the objective assessment (O) which is often the best indicator of a patient's urgency for need of care. There is a rapid absorption of data which combines with a mental comparison with previous cases as the general appearance of the patient is assimilated by the triage nurse from the moment he comes into view. Along with a triage first impression (A), the objective assessment is often the critical factor when making a triage decision. It needs to be understood that the documentation of a triage decision using any of the assessment tools devised, is secondary to the process of making that decision (see also Ch. 37).

The mnemonic PQRST is another assessment tool commonly used by triage nurses (Budassi & Barber 1981) (see Box 34.2). Yet another tool suggested by Budassi & Barber (1981) involves the use of the five senses – looking, listening, smelling, touching and thinking – to evaluate a patient's chief complaint (see Box 34.3).

Box 34.2 – *PQRST model of triage assessment*

P **Provokes**   What makes the pain better or worse?

Q **Quality** – What does it feel like? Suggestions may be offered to encourage a description, such as 'burning', 'stabbing', 'crushing'

R **Radiates** – Where is the pain? Where does it go? Is it in one spot? Show me where it is.

S **Severity** – Give the pain a score out of 10

T **Time** – How long have you had it? When did it start? When did it end?

Box 34.3 – *Systematic assessment model of triage*

Eyes List all the thing that you can see

Ears What is the patient saying and *not* saying? Listen for breath sounds, audible wheeze

Nose Smell for ketones, alcohol, incontinence, infection

Hands Take the pulse, feel the skin temperature, assess capillary perfusion. Touch 'where it hurts'

Brain Use an assessment tool to aid your triage decision, e.g. SOAP or PQRST

The Triage Decision

Having assessed the patient, the triage nurse must make a triage decision. Symptom clustering is a method used to assist in determining the clinical need of the patient. Using existing knowledge and experience, the nurse groups together symptoms and aims to identify the severity of the patient's condition. In this manner, 'chest pain' can be more easily associated with a cardiac condition if the symptom cluster includes nausea, shortness of breath on exertion, grey or clammy pallor, radiation of pain to the jaw or left arm, 'crushing' type pain or a 'tight band' across the chest. Conversely, a symptom cluster which includes increased pain on coughing and deep inspiration, shortness of breath on talking, and a productive cough would be more indicative of a respiratory or pulmonary condition (Rund & Rausch 1981).

'Clinical portraits' present another invaluable aid for the triage nurse when seeking the elusive triage decision. There are some illness and injuries that are so easily recognisable and that present so often in the A&E department that a very clear 'clinical portrait' can be recognised. A symptom cluster narrows the options to a recognised injury or disease process in a particular system; this is followed up with some discriminating questions. The knowledge of a typical clinical portrait allows the nurse to compare the current presentation with previously learned patterns (Rund & Rausch 1981).

The effective and appropriate use of these assessment and decision-making tools is clearly dependent on the expertise of the triage nurse. This expertise cannot be defined solely by the nurse's years of service. It must encompass the ability to understand and make use of decision-making processes. Benner's (1984) model of skill acquisition looks at the way in which expertise in an area develops through an individual nurse's experience. It is the expert nurse's use of experience and intuition when making decisions that differentiates her from the novice nurse; the professional judgement of the triage nurse, her clinical expertise and her use of intuition are crucial components of the triage process and her decision making (see also Table 37.1, p. 510, which compares the characteristics of expert and novice nurses). In addition, the triage nurse must ensure that her decisions are ethically sound (Handyside 1996, Jones 1993).

It has been suggested that if the triage groups are clear and unequivocal, the role of the triage nurse can be carried out by any nurse, novice or expert, after the minimum training (Burgess 1992). The presence of a series of signs or symptoms will inherently warrant a particularly priority, usually through the adherence to a written protocol in the form of flow charts, algorithms or simply lists of conditions in pre-designated priority categories.

While they will certainly standardise the response of the triage nurse and facilitate audit and evaluation of triage decisions, their use is limited. They can be useful for reference purposes and as teaching aids for less experienced staff (Rice & Abel 1993), but they are conservative and usually too inflexible for experienced A&E staff, not allowing them to use either their judgement or intuition (Rund & Rausch 1981). No assessment of the patient is required beyond establishing a symptom and allocating a predetermined priority.

A patient suffering from a myocardial infarction, however, does not always give a clear history of crushing, left-sided chest pain, with radiation to the jaw or left shoulder. The main complaint of the patient may be some tingling of the fingers with no loss of function, It may require some skilful probing to elicit any other pertinent history, if indeed there is any. The skill of the triage nurse lies in her intuition and the ability to ask discriminating questions which lead quickly to a triage decision. While this may be seen as a learned skill, it must also be recognised that the ability to ask the 'minimum of questions with the maximum of value' (Rund & Rausch 1981) comes with experience in the clinical area.

Priority setting

A reliable system of establishing priorities of care is the linchpin which determines the effectiveness of nurse triage. There may be circumstances whereby there is little data on which to determine a priority. Poor communication due to language difficulties is not uncommon, and the age or the condition of the patient may also hinder the triage nurse in making an initial assessment. If in doubt, a higher priority rating should be given. There are numerous different systems for setting priorities. When compared with each other, it is clear that the level and timing of interventions required are similar regardless of the system used. It is important, therefore, to adopt a system that will best suit the needs of a particular department.

There is usually a range of between two and five categories. The advantage of the four or five category systems is that they lessen the risk of ambiguity and allow for more precise priority setting to take place. Categories may be identified by a number, word or colour. The degree of urgency dictated by the category may include criteria relating to the length of wait considered to be appropriate for safe practice, identification of the chief complaint and potential risks or severity,

and the amount of nursing intervention over an average time required by the patient.

Documentation

The accurate documentation of nurse triage findings cannot be overemphasised. Estrada (1981) argued that it is a 'professional judgement made by a professional nurse' deserving of careful documentation. It is a means of communication and becomes an integral part of the patient's permanent medical record. As such, it also becomes a legal document for which the triage nurse becomes accountable and responsible. Indeed, the principle of personal accountability is fundamental to current nurse practice under both the *Code of Professional Conduct* (UKCC 1992a) and the *Scope of Professional Practice* (1992b). Documentation should be generated for all patients presenting to the A&E department. If the patient leaves the department without waiting to see the doctor, it may be the only record of his attendance (Southard 1989).

When documenting the triage findings, a diagnosis should not be made. The purpose of nurse triage, as previously discussed, is not to establish a diagnosis. The initial assessment made by the triage nurse is no substitute for a full clinical examination, as diagnostic investigations may need to be carried out prior to any definitive diagnosis being made. In quieter departments, if the size of the caseload allows, other clinical information may be added: past medical history, allergies, medication etc. This data may be used to initiate patient care plans and structured around the nursing model being used in the department. Duplications of information should be avoided, however, as the patient will be asked similar questions by the doctor or nurse practitioner (Jenkins 1996) (see Box 34.4).

It is essential that the system allows for some degree of flexibility. If the triage area is busy, patients must be sorted rapidly in order for the overall effectiveness of nurse triage to be maintained. Patients who appear to have an urgent problem must be seen immediately even if the triage nurse has to leave a patient that is already being triaged. As a result, inevitably, there will be times when initial assessment may be relatively incomplete. The higher the workload of the triage nurse, the less documentation there will be (Rund & Rausch 1981) (see also Ch. 39).

Training

In the UK at present, there is no nationally recognised training for nurses undertaking nurse triage. In-service training does take place in some departments,

Box 34.4 – *Summary of the principles underpinning records and record keeping (UKCC 1993)*

The following principles must apply:

■ The record is directed primarily to serving the interests of the patient or client to whom it relates and enabling the provision of care, the prevention of disease and the promotion of health

■ The record demonstrates the accurate chronology of events and all significant consultations, assessments, observations, decisions, interventions and outcomes

■ The record and activity of record-keeping form an integral and essential part of care and not a distraction from its provision

■ The record is clear and unambiguous

■ The record contains entries recording facts and observations written at the time of, or soon after, the events described

■ The record provides a safe and effective means of communication between members of the health care team and supports continuity of care

■ The record demonstrates that the practitioners' duty of care has been fulfilled

■ The systems for record-keeping exclude unauthorised access and breaches of confidentiality

■ The record is constructed and completed in such a manner as facilitates the monitoring of standards, audit, quality assurance and the investigation of complaints

---

but the criteria for selecting staff and minimum requirements for undertaking the role vary considerably. In the United States, training is seen as an essential component of nurse triage schemes. It is usually part-time and combines lectures, discussion, role-play, audiovisual material and clinical practice. A wide range of skills is a requirement for the role, including assessment and decision-making skills, problem-solving, good communication skills and intuition, a good working knowledge of departmental, hospital and district policies and protocols, and the ability to avoid conflict and manage aggression (Bland 1988).

Participants observe experienced triage nurses at work and are supervised by triage nurses when undertaking the role. At the end of the period of formal training, assessment takes place to ensure an agreed level of competence has been reached and documentation of approval is commonplace. Nurses

are expected to be experienced in all areas of A&E work prior to participating in the course. A minimum of 2 years' critical care experience and at least 6 months in A&E are the requirements advocated for nurses wishing to become triage nurses. While some of the skills of nurse triage can be described as intuitive (Benner 1984), many are learned and require experience that can only be gained by working in the clinical area coupled with specific training (Budassi & Barber 1981).

Audit

Regular audit of both the triage system and the staff is necessary to ensure quality standards. It is essential that all the staff are appraised in order to verify that they are both confident and competent at performing in the triage role. The completion of an initial training programme and the implications of the *Code of Professional Conduct* (UKCC 1992a) and *Scope of Professional Practice* (UKCC 1992b) documents are not enough to ensure that staff are meeting the required standards of practice. The most confident are not necessarily the most competent.

Decisions need to made about who will be responsible for carrying out the audit. In some departments, the A&E consultant audits nurses performing in a triage capacity, while in others it is felt it should be done by the nurses themselves. The format of the audit needs to be agreed. Areas that need to be examined include:

■ how triage decisions were made
■ why a particular decision was made
■ the accuracy of triage decisions
■ the appropriateness of priority ratings
■ the quality of documentation
■ the lessons that can be learned from errors of judgement that have been identified.

There are various tools that can be used. One method is multidisciplinary case review. As the name suggests, a multidisciplinary group meets and discusses, in an open forum, a selection of case notes. The various audit outcomes are addressed and any other issues or problems that have arisen are discussed together. An alternative tool is that of individual case review in one-to-one sessions, where an individual nurse's performance can be discussed confidentially. In this setting, problem areas can be discussed in a less confrontational manner. Audit of the triage system ensures that levels of staff and patient satisfaction with the service can be ascertained and measures taken to act upon shortcomings as they are identified. After a predetermined length of time, in-depth, formal evaluation of the scheme should be carried out. The original goals that were identified may need modification if the process of triage is not meeting the department's expectations or requirements.

A National Triage Scale

While the *Patient's Charter* has focused attention on patient assessment, the issue of uniformity and triage practice has been the subject of considerable discussion and debate. Following similar initiatives in Australia and Canada, a joint working party with members from both the Royal College of Nursing (RCN) A&E Association and the British Association for A&E Medicine (BAEM) led to the development of a standard five-point triage scale (Crouch & Marrow 1996). The scale is defined in terms of the time the patient should wait before recovery treatment (see Box 34.5 and p. 480).

The RCN and BAEM believe the next step for nurse triage in the UK is the development of a reliable and reproducible method of allocating emergency treatment according to patient priority. They believe that such a method will ensure that comparisons between staff and their departments will be more meaningful. A recently developed approach uses a series of presentational flowcharts that identify 'discriminators' which lead the triage nurse to a clinical priority (Mackway-Jones 1996). The method has been developed by a group of A&E physicians and nurses known as the Manchester Triage Group. The interest in formalising triage is such that their method is being adopted in A&E departments before it has been in use long enough for any evaluation or audit of its effectiveness, reliability or reproducibility to have been carried out. This method utilises flowcharts and predesignated lists of conditions, and as a result has all the limitations outlined previously when discussing their use. The patient's presenting complaint must be fitted into one of only 52 options, two of which relate to major accidents. While seven of the charts are specifically written for children, patients presenting with indigestion, for instance, do not have a flowchart and would probably be channelled into those designated 'chest pain' or 'abdominal pain'. While this aids audit, it should be asked whether it is appropriate for the patient. An interesting feature of the model is the use of a pain assessment tool. The early management of pain in A&E is an area that has been undoubtedly neglected in the past. The emphasis that has been placed on this element of a triage assessment, however, is such that, if applied as described, a common self-limiting illness such as sore

---

Box 34.5 – *The standard triage scale with colour codes and target times*

The times are intervals between arrival and first attention by a practitioner able to institute treatment – this may be a doctor or a nurse.

1 **Immediate resuscitation (red)**
   ■ Patients in need of immediate treatment for the preservation of life
   ■ All patients to be seen on arrival
   ■ These patients would usually be met by a team 'standing by' after prior notification by the ambulance service

2 **Very urgent (orange)**
   ■ Seriously ill or injured patients whose lives are not in immediate danger
   ■ All these patients should be seen within 10 minutes of arrival

3 **Urgent (yellow)**
   ■ Patients with serious problems, but apparently in a stable condition
   ■ All these patients should be seen within 60 minutes of arrival

4 **Standard (green)**
   ■ Standard A&E cases without immediate danger or distress
   ■ The aim should be for these patients to be seen within 120 minutes
   ■ The percentage which can be seen within this time depends on resources available. Few Departments in the UK can achieve rates above 80%

5 **Non–urgent (blue)**
   ■ Patients whose conditions are not true accidents or emergencies
   ■ If these patients are to be treated in the A&E department, the standard should be that they will not have to wait more than 240 minutes to be seen. The percentage seen with 240 minutes will depend on resources available. Patients in this category may be redirected to more appropriate facilities

---

throat could be elevated alongside cardiac-type chest pain. (see also Ch. 24).

When using this model, the response of the triage nurse can certainly be standardised, facilitating audit, but it may have limited use. Novice triage nurses will certainly find it useful, but for the experienced, expert practitioner described by Benner (1984), it may be too restrictive. Although Benner's skills acquisition is acknowledged in the Introduction to this model (Mackway-Jones 1996), it is not clear how intuition or judgement fit into the method described. There are other flaws with this model, both in its presentation and application. The authors refer to the importance of validity and reproducibility, but do not produce any evidence that either has been applied to their model. Mackway-Jones (1996) does not include any evidence to support the statements or assumptions made within the text.

In developing a national model of triage to be implemented across the UK, several issues need to be addressed. It may be desirable within the context of carrying out audit, but is it the most effective way of implementing and developing triage? There may be too many variables for this to be practical. These might include:

- geographical location
- size of department
- numbers of nursing and medical staff on duty at any one time
- the level of experience and expertise of staff
- senior medical and nursing support
- throughput of patients
- numbers of attenders
- the diversity of conditions/complaints.

In addition, the infrastructure supporting the A&E department needs to be taken into account, in terms of accessibility of on-site specialist care, beds for emergency or acute admissions, and so on.

The most effective system for a particular department is the one that best meets the needs of that department. While that undoubtedly will include standards relating to the triage process and of audit, it should not be assumed that any one model can be applied to all departments. Nurse triage is an assessment tool, not an audit tool. A uniform triage model that staff are obliged to follow, but which does not meet the requirements of the service that they are trying to provide, will quickly become obsolete, with

staff overriding the protocols set down within it. For most A&E departments implementing triage, it has been an evolutionary process, beginning with basic triage and gradually formulating more sophisticated systems as staff have adapted to the role and as their skills and expertise have developed. Adjustments and revisions take place over time to meet the particular needs of a department, with the insight of the staff into particular problems or difficulties that they encounter being incorporated. In this way, the process of learning facilitates understanding and a sense of ownership and commitment to the triage model being used. A national triage model, with all its inherent restrictions on an individual's practice, rather than encouraging development and innovation, may inadvertently stifle the natural process of nurse triage.

Conclusion

As well as putting nurse triage into its historical context and outlining the why and how of direct nurse triage, this chapter has looked at some of the clinical and professional issues surrounding both its implementation and development. Direct nurse triage can provide a safe and effective response to the increasing expectations of the patient and also to government requirements in respect of A&E services. It is becoming accepted as a key position in the A&E department, pivotal to safe patient throughput and effective management of nursing and medical resources.

Although the concept of nurse triage is not new in the UK, A&E nurses have been slow to develop schemes to their full potential. The impetus behind its widespread implementation during the 1990s was, to a large extent, due to external forces, a by-product of the *Patient's Charter*. This has created, however, an opportunity for A&E nurses to use nurse triage as a means of enhancing the quality of the A&E service. Those involved in implementing, developing and undertaking nurse triage should be seeking to exploit the concept to gain the greatest benefit for patients and to encourage staff development.

References

Alexander M (1996) Two important lessons: caution with telephone triage and believing the caregiver. *Journal of Emergency Nursing*, **22**(2), 149–150.

Allen D, Hughes D (1993) Going for growth. *Health Services Journal*, **103**, 33–34.

Audit Commission (1996) *By Accident or Design?: Improving A&E Services in England*. London: HMSO.

Benner P (1984) *From Novice to Expert: Excellence and Power in Clinical Nursing Practice*. Menlow Park, CA: Addison-Wesley.

Bland E (1988) Triage. In: Mowad L, Ruhle D, eds. *Handbook of Emergency Nursing: the Nursing Process Approach*. Connecticut: Appleton and Lange.

Blythin P (1988a) Triage – a nursing care system. In: Wright B, ed. *Managing and Practice in Emergency Nursing*. London: Chapman and Hall.

Blythin P (1988b) Triage in the UK. *Nursing*, **3**(31), 16–20.

Boyes A (1995) Health care assistants: delegation of tasks. *Emergency Nurse*, **3**(2), 6–9.

Budassi S, Barber JM (1981) *Emergency Nursing Principles and Practice*. St Louis: CV Mosby.

Burgess K (1992) A dynamic role that improves the service – combining triage and nurse practitioner roles in A&E. *Professional Nurse*, **7**(5), 301–303.

Buschiazzo L (1984) Patient classification in the A&E department. *Journal of Emergency Nursing*, **10**(4), 183.

Coleman A (1997) Where do I stand?: legal implications of telephone triage. *Journal of Clinical Nursing*, **6**, 227–231.

Crouch R, Marrow J (1996) Towards a UK triage scale. *Emergency Nurse*, **4**(3), 4–5.

Department of Health (1991) *The Patient's Charter*. London: HMSO.

Dolan B (1998) A dynamic process (Editorial). *Emergency Nurse*, **6**(4), 1.

Edwards B (1999) What's wrong with triage? *Emergency Nurse*, **7**(4), 19–23

Estrada EG (1979) Advanced triage by an RN. *Journal of Emergency Nursing*, **5**(6), 15–18.

Estrada EG (1981) Triage systems. *Nursing Clinics of North America*, **16**(1), 13–24.

Glasper A, McGrath K (1993) Telephone triage: extending practice. *Nursing Standard*, **7**(16), 34–36.

Handyside G (1996) *Triage in Emergency Practice*. St Louis: Mosby.

Jenkins A (1996) Nurse's notes. In: Guly HR, ed. *History Taking, Examination and Record Keeping in Emergency Medicine*. Oxford: Oxford University Press.

Jones C (1993) Triage decisions: how are they made? *Emergency Nurse*, **1**(1), 13–14.

Lee G, Fraser S (1981) ED nursing SOAP notes. *Journal of Emergency Nursing*, **7**(5), 216–218.

Mackway-Jones K (ed.) (1996) *Emergency Triage: Manchester Triage Group*. London: BMJ.

Mallet J, Woolwich C (1990) Triage in accident and emergency departments. *Journal of Advanced Nursing*, **15**, 1443–1451.

Nutall M (1986) The chaos controller. *Nursing Times*, **82**(20), 66–68.

Potter D Ov (ed.) (1985) *Emergencies Nurses Reference Library*. Pennsylvania: Springhouse Corporation.

Ramler CL, Mohammed N (1995) Triage. In: Kitt S, Selfridge-Thomas J, Proehl JA, Kaiser J, eds. *Emergency Nursing: A Physiological and Clinical Perspective*, (2nd edn.) Philadelphia: WB Saunders.

Rice M, Abel C (1993) Triage. In: Budassi-Sheehy S, ed. *Emergency Nursing: Principles and Practice*, 3rd edn. St Louis: Mosby.

Rund DA, Rausch TS (1981) *Triage*. St Louis: CV Mosby.

Selvig MR (1985) Triage in the emergency department. *Nursing Management*, **16**(8), 30B, 30F, 30H.

Southard R (1989) COBRA legislation: complying with ED provisions. *Journal of Emergency Nursing*, **15**(1), 23–25.

UKCC (1992a) *Code of Professional Conduct for the Nurse, Midwife and Health Visitor*, 3rd edn. London: UKCC.

UKCC (1992b) *The Scope of Professional Practice*. London: UKCC.

Wheeler SQ, Siebelt B (1997) Calling all nurses – how to perform telephone triage. *Nursing*, **27**(7), 37–41.

UKCC (1993) *Standards for Records and Record Keeping*. London: UKCC.

Chapter 35

Nurse Practitioners

Stuart Cable & Brian Dolan

- Introduction
- Development of the nurse practitioner role in A&E
- The activities of nurse practitioners
- Education needs of nurse practitioners
- Audit and evaluation
- Conclusion

Introduction

Interest in the nurse practitioner concept has stimulated fertile debate in recent years, particularly in A&E settings. The emergency nurse practitioner's role provides a new complementary minor injury service to that currently provided by A&E medical staff (Cooper & Robb 1996). The nurse practitioner may be described as a nurse acting as a health care worker who can assess, diagnose, treat and discharge a patient without reference to a medical practitioner. The influential Audit Commission (1996) has endorsed their use as an alternative approach to delivering care in A&E departments and minor injuries units.

This chapter will consider the development of the nurse practitioner role in A&E, the range of activities nurse practitioners perform, their educational needs, and the audit and evaluation of their role.

Development of the Nurse Practitioner Role in A&E

The term 'nurse practitioner' has been in common usage in the USA since the mid-1960s and in the UK since the early 1980s (Winson & Fox 1995). The nurse practitioner role in the USA was originally focused on community care and derived from a serious shortage of doctors working in the community in the 1960s and 1970s. The hospital sector soon realised that it, too, could make greater use of nurse practitioners and the role has now developed within that area.

In the A&E setting, the first formal emergency nurse practitioner service in the UK was established in Oldchurch Hospital, Romford, Essex in the mid-1980s (Head 1988). While further sporadic developments of the role took place over the following few years, with Read *et al.* (1992) reporting 6% of A&E departments in England and Wales providing a nurse practitioner service, by the beginning of 1994 this figure had risen sharply to 33% in England (Crinson 1995), with an anticipated rise, by the end of 1995, to 63% in England and Wales (Meek *et al.* 1995). A postal survey in 1996 of senior nurses in all major A&E departments in the UK (Tye *et al.* 1998) found that 36% of their sample of 274 departments provided a formal service, with a further 33% planning to introduce nurse practitioners within the year. Considerable regional variation was found, with 27% of A&E departments in Wales planning to introduce nurse practitioners by the end of 1996, rising to 76% of English A&E departments.

A review of use of the nurse practitioner title in A&E departments in one regional health authority demonstrated widespread use of the term (Cable 1994a). However, inconsistencies were evident in the role, collegial support, resourcing, educational preparation and service provision, a finding supported by work undertaken in five A&E departments and minor injuries units in west London (Dolan *et al.* 1997). If it is to have a meaningful part to play in developing cost-effective, high-quality, consumer-friendly health care, then the name must portray a certain standard of care, a level of ability and a clarity of purpose that is meaningful to nurses, allied health care colleagues and patients alike. The terminology remains unclear and continues to confuse and divide those with an interest in the 'nurse practitioner' concept. Indeed, the final draft report on post-registration education and practice (PREP) criticised the term as both 'ambiguous and misleading' (UKCC 1993).

Bowling & Stilwell (1988) proposed that nurse practitioner practice is not exclusively about skill in a range of tasks, diagnosis and treatment. Rather, the developing role represents a philosophy of autonomous practice with accountability for that practice. Individual departments normally set the role parameters through formal protocols which list the range of patient conditions to be managed.

Barker *et al.* (1995) suggested that much development in nursing has been due to the shortfall in doctor service provision, and often under the auspices of the medical profession. This argument is supported by Crinson (1995) who believes the development of an expanded role to provide a service for the management and treatment of patients with minor trauma is service-led and not professionally driven. But is this because gaps in medical provision represent the most pressing health care need? Trnobranski (1994) believes that morbidity changes continue to increase the demand for skilled nursing care and that problems associated with affluence and social behaviour, prominent demographic changes, increased numbers of elderly people and a policy of care in the community are all likely to raise the need for developed nursing practice in primary and secondary care facilities.

The Activities of Nurse Practitioners

The activities of nurse practitioners in A&E departments varies widely with no nationally agreed parameters of practice. Much of the current nurse practitioners' practice is governed by protocols (see Box 35.1), which have been defined as 'an agreement to a particular sequence of activities that assist healthcare workers to respond consistently in complex areas of clinical practice' (Royal College of Nursing 1993). Written practice protocols assure consistent practice of a high quality by specifying:

Box 35.1 – *Range of protocols used by nurse practitioners*

- Epistaxis
- Nasal injuries
- Trauma (isolated eye injury)
- Foreign body in nose
- Foreign body in throat
- Foreign body in ears
- Eye (non-trauma)
- Ocular foreign body
- Minor burns
- Hip injury
- Knee injury
- Whiplash
- Limb injuries
- Mallet finger
- Upper limb trauma
- Foot trauma
- Ankle injuries
- Postcoital pill
- Insect bites
- Allergic reaction
- Facial lacerations/bites
- Foreign body in skin
- Head injury (no loss of consciousness)
- Shoulder injury

- what history must be obtained
- what physical findings must be examined
- what laboratory tests must be performed
- what plan must be implemented.

Protocols also provide a useful audit tool and include protocols for suturing, prescription of antibiotics and analgesia, tetanus toxoid immunisations and requesting and interpretation of X-rays (Freij *et al.* 1996). Cable (1995) warned, however, that if the value of protocols is to be sustained, they must be dynamic documents that are constantly reviewed and updated. Many protocols are developed by, or in conjunction with, medical practitioners. Walsh (1995) has expressed concern that this 'mass of rules and red tape' could 'limit the nurse's role so tightly, that the notion of being an independent practitioner becomes fallacious'. Indeed, Dolan *et al.* (1997) found that the scope of individual nurse practitioners' practice was significantly affected by the support of medical staff in that unit.

Fawcett-Hennessy (1991) described seven characteristics of nurse practitioners practice.

- direct access for patients
- choice for patients (nurse practitioner vs. doctor)
- diagnostic and prescribing skills
- authority for referral
- personal attention during consultation
- adequate time for consultation
- counselling and health education.

The role and activities of the nurse practitioner are governed in the UK by the principles outlined in the UKCC *Code of Professional Conduct* (UKCC 1992a) and *Scope of Professional Practice* (UKCC 1992b). The *Code of Conduct* rules that nurse practitioners are personally responsible for their practice, must acknowledge any limitations in knowledge and/or competence and decline any duties or responsibilities if not able to perform them in a safe and skilled manner. The usual situation is that a nurse practitioner is medicolegally accountable to the health authority/Trust if practising within competence limits.

The dimensions of nurse practitioner practice are defined by an integrated framework comprising professional standards of practice, a code of ethics, health care policies, educational preparation and the health care needs of the population. The nurse may extend his skills through training and experience, and while these are essential prerequisites for role expansion, a move Mechanic (1988) suggested is essentially a cognitive development, the focus is health, practice is based on caring (rather than curing), the collegial relationship is collaborative and the professional need is for autonomy.

The development of practice, while evidently needed, is fraught with difficulties. Particularly among the nursing profession, an element of fear appears to exist that work undertaken that is not covered by policy may result in disciplinary action and even dismissal (Walsh & Ford 1989). Practices that have been taken on in the past have often sheltered under the misconception that the medical profession and their protection societies would take responsibility for anything done by nurses. This misapprehension has no basis in law (Kloss 1989). The adoption of advanced skills by nurses should not be seen as taking on someone else's workload at the expense of nursing care, but rather as the opportunity to provide more holistic care centred on the patient's individual needs, rather than on the convenience of the care providing system and its different workers.

The most frequently cited benefits are decreased waiting times, and this finding appears to be the principal motivation for the introduction of nurse practitioners in A&E (Woolwich 1992). This 'fast-tracking', as it is frequently termed, has been developed in the US as an expanded function of the triage role, 'to include definitive treatment of simple, straightforward problems under pre-approved protocols' (Pardee 1992). Dolan *et al.* (1997) identified a number of perceived benefits of having nurse practitioner services, and these are listed in Box 35.2.

In a study by Cable (1994a) on the way in which nurse practitioners are viewed by doctors, generalist nurses, patients and nurse practitioners themselves, the perceived role benefits based around the nursing skills of nurse practitioners – skills including 'expert nursing advice', health education, 'individualised care',

---

Box 35.2 – *Positive themes relating to service developments*

- Reductions in waiting times
- Reduction in pressure/workload on A&E medical, nursing and administration staff
- Improved patient care and satisfaction
- Improved accessibility to services
- Improved quality and appropriateness of service
- Reductions in levels of aggression towards staff
- Reductions in patient complaints/increases in patient compliments
- Improved image of the A&E departments
- More effective service provision at the hospital/primary care interface

and time and empathy – were found to be unsubstantiated. Minor injury management was almost the exclusive function of the nurse practitioner. This seems insufficient for those who wish to develop a service more oriented towards the needs of underserved areas of the population; areas, incidentally, where the incidence of complex biopsychosocial problem is higher and where people have a greater need for education, support, advice and time from health care professionals. Cable's study indicated that the facility was popular with junior doctors and increased team spirit, whilst one doctor described 'greater collegial equality' as a benefit. This seems a likely finding if nurses are taking on much of the 'minor' work of the department. But it may do little to address nurses' and patients' expressed frustration at their inability to deal with, or have dealt with, complex social problems.

A constraint on practice cited by some of the nurse practitioners was personal self-confidence (Cable 1994a). While it should be noted that there are important differences between UK and US nursing practice, inhibitors identified in US research included a lack of job description, medicolegal issues and resistance from other health providers (Hayden *et al.* 1982, Widhalm & Anderson 1982). This appears to be stifling nurse practitioners' health promotion activities, particularly of a psychosocial nature, encouraging patient throughput and reinforcing an idea that the current type of service is adequate for all, but merely lacking in medical clinicians to execute the practices (Cable 1993). Beales (1994) and Baker (1993) both supported the idea of nurses being capable of providing a minor injuries facility. With experience there seems little reason why such a facility could not be provided by all A&E nurses with the appropriate training.

Education Needs of Nurse Practitioners

Nurse practitioners need to be competent and confident in physical examination and diagnosis, be able to distinguish normal from pathological anatomy and be able to interpret various investigations, e.g. X-rays (Senior 1999). The first formally accredited qualification for nurse practitioners validated by the English National Board aimed to prepare skilled, politically aware, professionally competent nursing 'generalists', i.e. nurses who could monitor, screen, support, advise, refer, prescribe and diagnose, within the limits of their professional capabilities (Royal College of Nursing 1992).

The RCN A&E Association's Emergency Nurse Practitioner Special Interest Group (Royal College of Nursing 1992) identified four main areas of educational need to be addressed in emergency nurse practitioner training courses:

- assessment and diagnosis
- treatment and prescription of care
- communication skills
- health promotion and prevention of injury and illness.

Nurse practitioner schemes for A&E nurses are frequently developed independently along different models. Some nurse practitioners are trained 'on the job' by medical practitioners, others undertake more formal in-house courses designed for A&E staff, while yet others may be sent on intensive courses at hospitals which sell their educational package to other health authorities and Trusts. Currently, the title nurse practitioner is being used by staff who have undertaken courses which range from a few days in length to a BSc(Hons) degree provided by bodies such as the RCN. Dolan (1996) argued that the nurse practitioner title needs to be one that is registerable with the UKCC, like district nursing or health visiting, so the profession and the public can be assured of minimum education and quality standards for those on the nursing register.

Transatlantic comparisons suggest a willingness to enter into nurse practitioner training programmes because of a desire for more autonomy and to learn skills coupled with current job dissatisfaction and employer encouragement. While employer encouragement appears to be widespread in the UK (Read *et al.* 1992), further research is needed to identify which skills emerging nurse practitioners in A&E departments wish to learn. Retrospective analysis of areas in which nurses wish to extend their practice indicates that it would be technical rather than communication or supportive skills in which advancement would be sought (Jones 1986).

In the US, programmes are rather more extensive and curricula from certificate to Masters level include (Price *et al.* 1992):

- advanced technical skills associated with performing and interpreting findings from the history and physical examination
- information specific to disease management
- content on nursing theory, diagnosis, health promotion, disease prevention, lifestyle counselling and family systems theory
- dynamics and care during chronic phases of illness
- emphasis on holistic approaches to care; and clinical judgement and clinical decision-making.

Doctors may argue that they too can provide these services. However, it has been suggested that nurse practitioner development is often argued on two questionable assumptions: first, that doctors will not or cannot provide health maintenance and care, and secondly that cure and care are mutually exclusive. Rather, it is suggested, a continuum exists along which medicine and nursing oscillate, and by combining both cure and care in the same health care provider, both process and outcome measures, such as patient satisfaction, may be maximised.

Changes will require assessment, planning and evaluation of interventions for a range of patient needs in diverse social and clinical environments. Education will be required to support this innovation and explore ways in which the practice–theory gap may be bridged to facilitate improved care (Cable 1994b). This, as Hawkett (1990) identified, 'poses a challenge to create a learning environment where skills such as compassion, empathy and imagination are given equal importance with clinical objectives'. As Price et al. (1992) argued:

> It has become increasingly clear that in addition to basic nursing education, there is a need for a sufficiently sophisticated and competitive advanced practice level that is based on theory and research.

An educational programme designed to teach nurses to examine bodies and write up histories could be brief and task-oriented. This may, in fact, be very popular with A&E nurses who historically cling to the delegated tasks. However, nurse practitioner practice is underpinned by a cognitive development. The learning process takes time, demands reflection on practice, emphasises the importance of empowerment of patients and mutual goal-setting and aims to potentiate the available resources for achievement of optimal patient objectives. Ford (1992), after almost 30 years of involvement with US nurse practitioner developments, argued the need for a specific training course in order to avoid the 'chaos and confusion' generated by lack of educational standards or common definition of a credential. She also advocates this common approach in order to promote acceptance by nurses, allied health professionals and patients. One innovative Masters degree programme in the United States provides students with both cognitive and clinical skills at a high level, incorporating nursing research, epidemiology, pharmacology, pathophysiology, physical examination and differential diagnosis, and primary prevention in the individual, family and community (Cole et al. 1998).

Evidence from the US also supports the idea that clinical judgement/decision making abilities are dev-

eloped through high level, baccalaureate and Masters level study. Tanner (1987) found that performance was related positively to the academic degree held and noted:

> The idea that nurses can provide a safe and acceptable minor injury service seems to be evident from its recent growth, however, what does appear to be lacking from most educational programmes is a focus on decision-making, information-giving, 'holistic' assessment and health promotion, which appear to be implicitly accepted as skills possessed by experienced A&E nurses.

Many educational packages show scant evidence of consultation skills training/attitude development. While this is lacking for nurses, King's A&E Primary Care Service (1994) emphasises this as essential for the preparation of medical staff. Although knowledge and skills are key educational aims, a great emphasis is also placed on attitude development. Additionally, the management of uncertainty, exploration of problem-solving and decision-making are also emphasised. Perhaps, once again, a lack of such education is one explanation of why A&E nurse practitioners concentrate on minor injury management. Such problems are well differentiated, as compared with medical and psychosocial conditions, which may be avoided due to an inability or an unwillingness to cope with uncertainty. This area, however, warrants further investigation.

Audit and Evaluation

Audit and evaluation of nurse practitioner performance has generally involved the comparison of nurse practitioners with physicians, generally A&E SHOs. Constant comparison with doctors' practice, while necessary in terms of safety and cost-effectiveness for equitable provision, may disguise some of the value of skilled nursing (Prescott & Driscoll 1979). Rather than basing practice on task performance, Stilwell (1985) identified five generic areas of work for which the nurse practitioner could take responsibility:

- acting as an alternative consultant for the patient
- detecting serious disease by physical examination
- managing minor and chronic ailments and injuries
- providing health education
- counselling.

The dimensions or variables on which nurse practitioners and physicians have been compared can broadly be categorised into three types (Prescott & Driscoll 1979):

- *Structural variables.* These include organisational, administrative or setting characteristics often considered influential in the provision or delivery of care, e.g. case mix, time allocated for patient visits, and number and types of provider(s).
- *Process variables.* These concern the ways in which health care is provided, e.g. the type/thoroughness of histories and physical examinations, the accuracy of the diagnoses, the types of laboratory tests conducted and the types of management plans devised.
- *Outcome variables.* These are the end results of care, e.g. patients' health status, satisfaction with care and patient hospitalisation rates.

Commonly used measures in A&E departments and minor injuries units include:

- patient tracking time–time of arrival, triage time, time seen by nurse practitioner, discharge time
- patient referral pattern – self-referral, GP, A&E etc.
- triage category
- analgesia administration at triage
- protocol used and protocol adherence
- treatment management
- disposal – home, other hospital, GP, district nurse, occupational health etc.
- ratio of complimentary/complaint letters
- reported incidents of violence.

Nurse practitioners may be called upon to care for those 'difficult' patients with whom compliance is particularly poor. It is therefore necessary that the time is provided for problems to be explored, but also that nurse practitioners are aware of their own potential for prejudicial practice because (Jasmin & Trygstad 1979):

> ...the nurses' attitudes, values, beliefs and opinions regarding health and illness affect the way she interacts with her patients. If the nurse places a high value on health, she will find it frustrating and difficult to understand those patients who continually refuse to follow prescribed medical and nursing treatment plans.

One innovation outside nursing, but perhaps with useful lessons for practice, was undertaken by Dale *et al.* (1991). General practitioners (GPs) were introduced into an A&E department, with the result that consultations utilized fewer diagnostic tests, there was greater emphasis on listening and more flexible use of time than among their casualty officer colleagues, and there was no raised incidence of patient dissatisfaction or evidence of undertreatment. One interesting finding from this study for the emerging nurse practitioner was that very few consultations by either GPs or A&E SHOs included discussion of a patient's lifestyle, such as issues of smoking, diet or exercise. Nurse practitioner consultations may address a number of these issues.

Salisbury & Tettersell (1988) suggested that the nurse practitioner provides an extra service rather than acting as a doctor substitute. Doctors train with an illness perspective emphasising physical disease and treatment, whilst nurse training places greater emphasis on practical teaching and advice. Both are necessary and are complementary in providing comprehensive health care facilities in any setting. The relative status in society of doctors and nurses may also affect the consultation relationship.

Evidence appears to suggest that patients can talk more easily with nurses, while they fear that too much questioning of a doctor may be a waste of his time (Stilwell 1985). Certainly, the literature suggests that medical audit on the efficacy of the nurse practitioner is the norm and that little recognition of the nurse's distinctive role is included in evaluation (Curry 1994, Howie 1992, Morris *et al.* 1989). Ryan & McKenna (1994) highlighted the different care/cure orientation of nursing and medical students, the significantly different values placed on nursing assessment and the varying perception of nurses as independent practitioners by the two groups. Thus, it may be that nurses have to demonstrate the value of their own practices on patient care whilst current methods of audit may prove inadequate for this purpose (Prescott & Driscoll 1980). Means of evaluating nurse practitioner effectiveness are identified in Box 35.3.

Box 35.3 – *Evaluating nurse practitioner effectiveness*

- Activities representing the full range of the nurse practitioner role should be included in any comprehensive evaluation of nurse practitioners
- Explicit criteria with adequate sensitivity should form the basis of comparison between nurse practitioners and physicians
- Empirically established relationships between process and outcome variables should form the basis for establishing non-arbitrary performance standards whenever possible
- Random sampling of nurse practitioners and physicians should be used when possible. When random sampling is not possible, providers should be selected using variables known to correlate with quality of care
- Use of multiple data sources is recommended to decrease the current heavy reliance on audits
- Conclusions should point out differential findings, identifying those which favour physicians, those which favour nurse practitioners and those with no differences between providers

Outcomes in certain areas of practice have been shown to be equitable with doctors, but the process of patient–nurse practitioner interaction is little researched. The nurse practitioner offers an opportunity for different attitudes and skills, increased patient time, a more equitable nurse–patient relationship and a more supportive/advisory role that is moulded by autonomous, innovative nurses.

Patient satisfaction with nurse practitioners has attracted some attention from researchers. The high levels of satisfaction shown for both doctors and nurse practitioners show that patients find nurse practitioners acceptable and are willing to consult them. However, Avis & Bond (1995) counselled against overreliance on the use of patient satisfaction surveys as a potentially superficial indicator of quality. Stilwell *et al.* (1987) stated that where patients had a choice as to whether to consult a nurse practitioner or a GP, they chose to consult the nurse practitioner with conditions and health problems appropriate to the service the nurse practitioner could provide and took other more medical problems to the GP.

Patients are unlikely to have to decide whether the nurse practitioner or A&E doctor is most appropriate as this decision is likely to be made on their behalf by the triage nurse. With the increasing trend of setting up trauma systems (Davis & Wood 1994) and more minor injury units around some major A&E sites, patients may well have to make decisions about where to seek the most appropriate treatment, in order to avoid lengthy waiting times. In order to develop nurse practitioner services, a range of issues need to be addressed, as listed in Box 35.4.

From the evidence available, clinical decisions made by nurse practitioners compare favourably with decisions taken by medical practitioners. Unfortunately, British nurse practitioners are not seeing enough patients on a regular basis, at present, to make a proper randomised controlled trial feasible (Read & George 1994). Studies which have been undertaken show that, with suitable patient selection criteria in place, it is unlikely that patients would receive unsuitable care.

Conclusion

The American Nurses Association (1980) consider as highly significant the following abilities in nurse practitioners:

- to tolerate uncertainty
- to demonstrate respect for the patient's autonomy, including religious and cultural beliefs
- to value staff and patient's time and make judicious use of health service resources
- to maintain flexibility and good humour.

Box 35.4 – *Issues to be addressed in developing nurse practitioner services*

- **Commissioning services** – greater clarity and agreement between purchasers and providers about the philosophy, aims and objectives of each service development

- **Needs and demands** – needs assessment should be closely linked to service development

- **Service development** – the introduction of uniform triage classification system to enable more reliable and consistent planning and provision of services, as well as comparison between service activities

- **Performance measures and quality standards** – sharing of information across sites to avoid duplication/replication of work; broad agreement between purchasers and providers about performance and quality standards in relation to service developments

- **Community support** – information about the range of services available should be produced for the public

- **Costs** – the cost-effectiveness of the services needs consideration in light of local purchasing strategies

---

The inclusion of such training also appears vital to nurses, particularly in the light of abundant evidence of the negative attitudes held by many A&E nurses towards certain client groups (Kemp & Larson 1997).

The evidence appears overwhelming that medical colleagues, patients and nurses consider it acceptable and appropriate that nurses can expand their practice. The question, however, remains: what direction should developments take and what is the educational route to their achievement? As Robinson (1993) pointed out:

We do the patients as well as ourselves a disservice by this continued lack of clarity. The A&E nurse's role is one that has been identified for change; let the change be that desired and initiated by nurses in the interests of the patients.

The nurse practitioner has become an important provider of care in A&E departments. However, the pace of development has highlighted the need for coherent educational, audit and evaluation strategies to further enhance their practice. While acknowledging that the driving forces behind the development of this role have been service-rather than patient-driven, the need for a coherent, specialist nursing role to enhance the care of patients and their families must remain the prime objective in A&E.

References

American Nurses Association (1980) *Nursing: a Social Policy Statement*. Kansas: ANA.

Audit Commission (1996) *By Accident or Design: Improving Emergency Care in Acute Hospitals*. London: HMSO.

Avis M, Bond S (1995) Satisfying solutions? A review of some unresolved issues in the measurement of patient satisfaction. *Journal of Advanced Nursing*, **22**, 316–322.

Baker B (1993) Model methods. *Nursing Times*, **89**(47), 33–35.

Barker PJ, Reynolds W, Ward T (1995) The proper focus of nursing: a critique of the 'caring' ideology. *International Journal of Nursing Studies*, **32**(4), 386–397.

Beales J (1994) Why are they waiting? *Emergency Nurse*, **2**(1), 23–34.

Bowling A, Stilwell B (eds) (1988) *The Nurse In Family Practice: Practice Nurses and Nurse Practitioners in Primary Health Care*. London: Scutari Press.

Cable S (1993) Health promotion breaks the mould. *Emergency Nurse*, **1**(2), 23–24.

Cable S (1994a) *A Complement to Medical Practice: Defining the Role of the Nurse Practitioner in the Accident and Emergency Department*. [Unpublished] London: Primary Care Development Fund, Department of General Practice, United Medical and Dental School of Guy's and St Thomas's Hospitals, University of London.

Cable S (1994b) What is a Nurse Practitioner. *Primary Health Care*. **45**, 12–14.

Cable S (1995) Minor injuries clinics: dealing with trauma. *British Journal of Nursing*, **4**(20), 1177–1182.

Cooper M, Robb A (1996) Nurse practitioners in A&E: a literature review. *Emergency Nurse*, **4**(2), 19–22.

Cole F, Ramirez E, Mickanin J (1998) ENP education: a United States perspective. *Emergency Nurse*, **6**(4), 12–14.

Crinson I (1995) Impact of *The Patient's Charter* on A&E departments 2: the emergency nurse practitioner. *British Journal of Nursing*, **4**(22), 1321–1327.

Curry JL (1994) Nurse practitioners in the emergency department: current issues. *Journal of Emergency Nursing*, **20**, 207–215.

Dale J, Green J, Glucksman E, Higgs R (1991) *Providing for Primary Care. Progress in A&E*. London: Department of General Practice and Primary Care, King's College School of Medicine and Dentistry.

Davis S, Wood I (1994) Trauma centres in the UK: a nursing perspective. In: Sbaih L, ed. *Issues in Accident and Emergency Nursing*. London: Chapman and Hall.

Dolan B (1996) Editorial. *Emergency Nurse*, **4**(2), 3.

Dolan B, Dale J, Morley V (1997) Nurse practitioners: role in A&E and primary care. *Nursing Standard*, **11**(17), 33–38.

Fawcett-Hennessy A (1991) Setting the scene for the revolution. *Nursing Standard*, **4**(21), 35.

Ford LC (1992) Advanced nursing practice: future of the nurse practitioner. In: Aiken L, Fagin C, eds. *Charting Nursing's Future*. Philadelphia: Lippincott.

Freij RM, Duffy T, Hackett D, Cunningham D, Fothergill J (1996) Radiographic interpretation by nurse practitioners in a minor injuries unit. *Journal of Accident and Emergency Medicine*, **13**(1), 41–43.

Hawkett A (1990) A gap which must be bridged: nursing attitudes to theory and practice. *Professional Nurse*, **6**(3), 166–170.

Hayden ML, Davies LR, Clore ER (1982) Facilitators and inhibitors of the nurse practitioner role. *Nursing Research*, **31**(5), 294–299.

Head S (1988) The new pioneers. *Nursing Times*, **84**(26), 27–28.

Howie P (1992) Development of the Nurse Practitioner. *Nursing Standard*, **6**(27), 10–11.

Jasmin S, Trygstad LN (1979) *Behavioural Concepts and the Nursing Process*, St Louis: CV Mosby.

Jones G (1986) Behind the times. *Nursing Times*, **82**(42), 30–33.

Kemp S, Larsen D (1997) Provision of needle exchanges in A&E. *Emergency Nurse*, **4**(4), 23–25.

King's A&E Primary Health Care Service (1994) *King's A&E Primary Care Service Activity Report*. London: Department of General Practice and Primary Care, King's College School of Medicine and Dentistry.

Kloss D (1989) Uncharted Territory. *Nursing Times*, **85**(3), 40–41.

Mechanic HF (1988) Redefining the expanded role. *Nursing Outlook*, **36**(6), 280–284.

Meek SJ, Ruffles G, Anderson G, Ohiorenoya D (1995). Nurse practitioners in major accident and emergency departments: a national survey. *Archives of Emergency Medicine*, **9**, 19–22.

Morris F, Head S, Holkar V (1989) The nurse practitioner: help in clarifying clinical and educational activities in Accident and Emergency departments. *Health Trends*, **21**: 124–126.

Pardee DA (1992) Decreasing the wait for emergency department patients: an expanded triage nurse role. *Journal of Emergency Nursing*, **18**(4), 311–315.

Prescott PA, Driscoll L (1979) Nurse practitioner effectiveness: a review of Physician-Nurse Comparison studies. *Evaluation and the Health Professions*, **2**(4), 387–418.

Prescott PA, Driscoll L (1980) Evaluating nurse practitioner performance. *Nurse Practitioner*, **5**(4), 28–31, 53.

Price MJ, Martin AC, Newberry YG, Zimmer PA, Brykczynski KA, Warren B (1992) Developing national guidelines for nurse practitioner education: an overview of the product and the process. *Journal of Nursing Education*, **31**(1), 10–15.

Read S, George S (1994) Nurse practitioners in accident and emergency departments: reflections on a pilot study. *Journal of Advanced Nursing*, **19**, 705–716.

Read SM, Jones NMB, Williams BT (1992) Nurse practitioners in accident and emergency departments: what do they do? *British Medical Journal*, **305**, 1466–1470.

Robinson DK (1993) Nurse Practitioner or mini-doctor? *Accident and Emergency Nursing*, **1**, 53–55.

Royal College of Nursing (1992) *Nurse Practitioner Diploma Curriculum Document*, London: RCN.

Royal College of Nursing (1993) Protocols: guidance for good practice. *Nursing Standard*, **8**(8), 29.

Ryan AA, McKenna HP (1994) A comparative study of the attitudes of nursing and medical students to aspects of patient care and the nurse's role in organizing that care. *Journal of Advanced Nursing*, **19**, 114–123.

Salisbury CJ, Tettersell MJ (1988) Comparison of the work of a nurse practitioner with that of a general practitioner. *Journal of the Royal College of General Practitioners*, **38**, 314–316.

Senior K (1999) ENP scheme: highlighting the barriers. *Emergency Nurse*, **6**(9), 28–31.

Stilwell B (1985). Opportunities in general practice. *Nursing Mirror*, **161**(19), 30–31.

Stilwell B, Greenfield S, Drury M, Hull FM (1987) A nurse

practitioner in general practice: working style and pattern of consultations. *Journal of Royal College of General Practitioners*, **37**, 154–157.

Tanner CA (1987) Teaching clinical judgement. *Annual Review of Nursing Research*, **5**, 153–173.

Trnobranski PH (1994) Nurse practitioner: redefining the role of the community nurse? *Journal of Advanced Nursing*, **19**, 134–139.

Tye C, Ross F, Kerry SM (1998) Emergency nurse practitioner services in major accident and emergency departments: a United Kingdom postal survey. *Journal of Accident and Emergency Medicine*, **15**, 31–34.

UKCC (1992a) *Code of Professional Conduct*, 3rd edn. London: UKCC.

UKCC (1992b) *The Scope of Professional Practice*. London: UKCC.

UKCC (1993) Final draft report on the future of professional education and practice. London: UKCC.

Walsh M (1995) The A&E Department and the nurse practitioner. *Nursing Standard*, **4**(11), 34–35.

Walsh M, Ford P (1989) *Myths and Rituals in Nursing*. Oxford: Butterworth Heinemann.

Widhalm SA, Anderson LA (1982) Emergency nurse practitioners: motivators, barriers, and autonomy in role performance. *Journal of Emergency Nursing*, **8**(2), 67–74.

Winson G, Fox J (1995) Nurse practitioners: the American experience. *British Journal of Nursing*, **4**(22), 1326–1329.

Woolwich C (1992) A wider frame of reference. *Nursing Times*, **88**(46), 34–36.

Part 8

Professional Issues in A&E

36. Clinical Leadership and Supervision   **497**

37. Clinical Reasoning   **505**

38. Ethical Issues   **513**

39. Law   **521**

40. Maintaining a Safe Environment   **529**

Clinical Leadership and Supervision

Andrew Cook & Lynda Holt

- Introduction
- Clinical leadership
- Clinical supervision
- Conclusion

Introduction

This chapter will consider two complementary dimensions of managerial practice: clinical leadership and clinical supervision. While the concept of leadership has been used in organisational developments for over 50 years (Huczynski & Buchanan 1991), clinical supervision has a more recent history (Sloan 1998). The chapter will consider leadership activities and how nurses can develop them for use in the A&E environment. It will also offer guidance on how A&E nurses can introduce and sustain clinical supervision in their workplace.

Clinical Leadership

Leadership within nursing has moved slowly, but reflects the trends demonstrated by theorists of organisational leadership (McDaniel & Wolf 1992). No longer can a nurse expect to become a leader because of social background, appearance or domineering personality. In A&E, effective clinical leadership is of prime importance. Leadership skills are essential, for team-building requires the leader to be responsible, confident and to have respect for others (Fincke 1993). The nature of A&E work is such that priorities and pace can change dramatically over a very short period, with a potential for staff to feel threatened by the perceived chaos. The clinical leader needs to foster an environment where care delivery has some structure, staff have guidance and security and trust can develop (Cook 1996).

Garbett (1995) described leaders as people who have a vision; they make things happen, and at the same time they strengthen and support their followers, inspiring them to trust the leader. These appear to be the core qualities needed to lead the nursing team in A&E. To help nurses develop these skills, a simple model can be developed (Fig. 36.1). Leadership consists of three key activities (Manthey 1992):

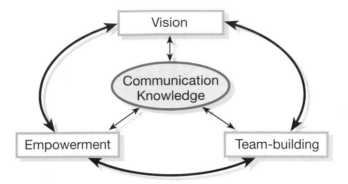

Figure 36.1 – *Key activities of clinical leadership.*

- vision
- empowerment
- team-building.

To fulfil these activities successfully, the nurse must have a sound knowledge base and the ability to communicate effectively (Fincke 1993).

Vision

This is the ability of the leader to see a finished product, which may be as simple as prioritising and organising the nursing work to ensure all demands are met. In terms of leadership, however, vision is often the ability to take an external directive, e.g. the *Patient's Charter* (Department of Health 1991), and find creative ways of achieving expected targets while keeping the activity acceptable to the nurses delivering care.

Vision is the ability to see a way forward to the desired outcome. Selling that vision with enthusiasm, realism and commitment creates followers. It is important to remember that vision is a fluid concept and open to change. Opinions and ideas of followers can help to mould a vision to ensure success.

Empowerment

If the leader wants commitment from the followers, she must be able to pass on knowledge and information about goals. This way the team is empowered, not simply doing as it is told. It is sometimes difficult to imagine this taking place in a busy A&E department when decision-making is necessarily rapid. Empowerment of individuals or a team is a lengthy process. The clinical leader needs to be credible and able to work with nurses on an individual basis. She needs to understand and appreciate the nurse's contribution, give constructive feedback and invest in the nurse's individual development. This way when rapid decisions do need to be made, the followers are more

likely to trust their leader and accept and support the action proposed.

Empowerment does not mean a lack of managerial control. The clinical leader must set boundaries on what are acceptable standards and behaviours and what are unacceptable. These must be communicated to followers and should remain constant. This way the team is free to participate in decision-making within a preset structure. For most people, boundaries provide a sense of stability and security. This can be particularly important when trying to maintain a departmental direction and vision (Senior 1999). Using a named nurse structure of care delivery is a good example of this: the standards are agreed and act as boundaries for nurses working individually within a team structure.

Team-building

The ability to build and sustain a team is fundamental to being an effective leader. Part of the role of the leader is to draw people together, create common goals and encourage a sense of collaboration. This way a team can be formed that will face challenges together. This is best demonstrated by a well-run resuscitation – the team comes together, each member has a role, and a comprehensive package of care is given.

These teams last only for a short while. In building a team which is expected to work closely for a sustained period of time, such as a project group within a department, the leader must have an understanding of group dynamics. This means knowing the characteristics of the group members, matching team roles to ability, and building a team with members whose skills will complement each other.

A crucial factor in team-building is the function of the leader. To be successful, this person must remain part of the team, giving direction and support to the other team members. The leader must be secure enough in her own knowledge to encourage and utilise the abilities and knowledge of other team members without being threatened. Dean (1995) believes it is important for leaders to recognise their own limitations.

Effective communication

Becoming a clinical leader is a time of great personal vulnerability. The leader's knowledge, ability to organise and sustain direction, and skills in supporting others will all come under scrutiny before followers decide to adopt the leader's vision. Effective communication is fundamental to gaining acceptance as a leader. Most A&E nurses have experienced a shift where the nurse in charge keeps information about patient progress to herself and does not keep staff informed of activity. This results in a withdrawal from the situation; nurses continue to function under direction, but they have no ownership of the activity and offer little support to the leader. Conversely, where communication is good and ideas are welcomed from other nurses, staff work as a team, supporting each other and the leader (Haire 1998, Kacperek 1997).

In addition to clinical and organisational knowledge, a leader needs to have a good level of self awareness. She can then capitalise on leadership strengths and build on potential weaknesses. The model identified in Figure 36.1 can help leaders to increase awareness of the key activities of clinical leadership of vision, empowerment and team-building. The successful achievement of these relies on the ability to communicate effectively with other staff members. This means the leader is able to give direction and feedback to staff, but also can receive feedback, air ideas and develop strategy.

In order to sustain leadership, the clinical leader should have a sound clinical and professional knowledge. The leader should be able to use this knowledge to create an environment in which staff feel secure and can trust her judgement. A&E demands a variety of approaches to nursing work and similarly leadership skills should be diverse and creative enough to match the patterns of work. A leader who uses a rigid approach may find it successful in some situations, but inappropriate in others. A leader who can cultivate a flexible but equitable attitude to team members will gain respect and support from followers.

Clinical Supervision

While clinical supervision is a buzzword that hit the nursing profession in the mid-1990 s, its ultimate aim is to improve patient care. Holt (1996) argued that a dilemma exists when interpreting the term clinical supervision in relation to the realities of nursing practice. She asked: 'How can clinical supervision be implemented when so many ambiguities still exist about its true purpose and its effect on nurses?' For the UKCC (1995), clinical supervision provides legitimacy for an activity in which nurses can turn round some of their anxieties and find innovative ways of developing themselves and their nursing practice.

The importance of clinical supervision was emphasised in the light of serious concerns identified by the Allitt Inquiry (1991). The Health Service Ombudsman at that time repeatedly raised concerns about a number of flaws identified in the delivery of nursing care, including the quality of record-keeping. Clinical supervision offered a potential solution to some of the difficulties being encountered by the nursing profession on an individual and organisational basis. Clinical supervision was increasingly viewed as a mechanism by which to safeguard standards and support development in the quality of care that the professions wanted to provide (Marrow *et al.* 1998).

Like many good ideas in nursing, however, clinical supervision has become entangled with jargon and ended up as a series of models remote from the reality of everyday nursing practice. The Department of Health (England), in its document *A Vision for the Future* (NHS Management Executive 1993), stated that the implementation of clinical supervision was a key target as it would help address stress and provide development for staff. Some areas of nursing, such as psychiatry, have used supervision for many years; however, in acute nursing the concept has been underdeveloped.

The King's Fund (1994) has described clinical supervision as a formal arrangement in which nurses can discuss work with another professional colleague. It has been promoted as a support mechanism for nurses, a tool for professional development and a method of quality control. The UKCC (1995) identified several key factors for the success of clinical supervision:

■ It is a clinically focused professional relationship.
■ It is necessary to establish and maintain standards, and promote innovation in practice.
■ The practitioner must have formally identified access to a supervisor.
■ The process should be determined to suit local need.
■ It should be evaluated to see how it contributes to establishing, maintaining and improving patient care.

The message from the UKCC (1995) is that clinical supervision is an activity which links practitioner awareness as an accountable professional for everyday clinical work. For this to happen, managers and clinicians must value the contribution of nurses and invest time and resources in their professional development (Bond & Holland 1998).

For its introduction to be successful in any clinical environment, it is essential for participants to share a common understanding of their interpretation of clinical supervision. One approach to this is for A&E nurses to explore the many activities and skills in nursing work, including:

- caring
- curing
- supporting
- empowering
- teaching.

These activities all involve interaction with others, such as patients and their relatives or friends, and are not without personal risk. In A&E, patient stay is (usually) short and the onus is on the nurse to develop a therapeutic relationship quickly, but how do nurses maintain this relationship when someone is off sick, the shift is busy or the relative has complained about the ever-increasing waiting times?

Types of supervision

Clinical supervision must be clearly separated from issues relating to pay, promotion or discipline. Only then can a trusting relationship be fostered. Several ways of addressing supervision have emerged. These include:

- one-to-one supervision with an expert from a nursing or related background
- one-to-one supervision with a line manager
- one-to-one supervision within a peer group
- group or network supervision.

In A&E, the most likely methods are supervision from a line manager, such as the sister/charge nurse, or supervision from a peer. There are advantages and disadvantages with both methods. With a line manager, clinical supervision could be more successful because of the management commitment, increased time and communication, and the developing relationship. For the nurse seeking supervision, however, it may be harder to build a trusting relationship because of the perceived power of the manager. There is a possibility of a conflict of interest between the nurse's development needs and those of the A&E department, and access to the supervisor may be limited.

Peer supervision means the supervisor and supervisee are involved in similar clinical work, and possibly face similar challenges. The advantages are increased awareness, potentially greater trust and a relationship which is less threatening to the supervisee. The disadvantage is that without effort and commitment from both parties, the activity can become purely one of support and not development. Group and network supervision have been developed in some areas of health care, particularly in community settings. This involves a group of similar professionals sharing experiences and developing their practice using one another. For this to be successful, a large degree of trust and commitment is needed from participants. It does have disadvantages in that some members of the group can remain non-participative or dominate activity. It is perhaps organisationally easier to facilitate than one-to-one supervision.

Whichever method of supervision is adopted, it is essential that the clinical supervisor remains clinically challenging. When introducing clinical supervision, a type should be chosen, then a gentle process of learning and development commenced to establish a practitioner-led activity which is non-hierarchical, and open to all clinical nursing activity. The success of clinical supervision relies on its perceived value to the department, and therefore agreeing the aims and process before implementation is imperative. Bishop (1994) provided three overall aims which act as a bedrock for supervision activities:

- to facilitate professional expertise
- to improve patient care
- to safeguard standards of care.

To achieve these objectives, clinical supervision should be seen as a continuum along with mentorship and preceptorship. A mentor helps to develop clinical competence by guiding a nurse through learning a new skill, such as cannulation. A preceptor helps the nurse gain confidence in that role. A clinical supervisor aids professional development from acquisition of new skills. But for clinical supervision to be successful it is important to consider the impact of the nurse as a whole and not as a technician. This does not mean the supervision will not focus on specific activities of care at any one time, but the supervisor must ensure development of activities of nursing and growth of the individual nurse as a result.

The philosophical approach to clinical supervision does not have to be complicated. Proctor (1986) suggested a simple tripartite approach to supervision (see Fig. 36.2). The formative role is one of education, supplementing the supervisee's knowledge and facilitating growth. The restorative aspect relies on

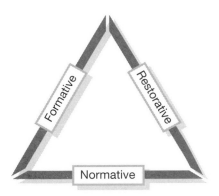

Figure 36.2 – *Functions of clinical supervision.*

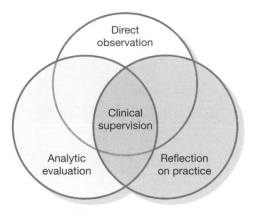

Figure 36.3 – *Activities of a supervisor.*

support, exploring anxieties or critical incidents and allowing the supervisee to resolve stress. The normative function is one of quality control, looking at actual practice and challenging methods to maintain high standards of patient care.

The success of clinical supervision relies on its perceived value to the department and staff commitment. The activities of clinical supervision revolve around the provision of regular space for reflection on the content and process of work. Its functions are to develop the understanding and skills of the supervisee, to ensure quality nursing care and to provide space to explore and express distress about work. Done effectively this results in the supervisee feeling valued and validated both as a person and as a nurse, as she is able to receive feedback and therefore gain new perspectives on her work. This empowers the nurse to plan and utilise personal resources and become proactive and innovative. Clinical supervision is not a forum for self-congratulation or self-destruction, and cannot become personal therapy. Clinical supervision must not be allowed to become a management tool, a substitute for individual performance review (IPR) or a means of controlling nurses. The supervisor can facilitate this by observation of practice, encouraging retrospective reflection and participation in evaluating outcomes (see Fig. 36.3).

Getting clinical supervision

Clinical supervision is not without personal risk, because the nurse is being asked to expose anxieties or perceived areas of weakness to a close colleague. Trust and confidentiality are therefore pivotal to a successful relationship. The nurse has a responsibility to seek supervision actively by going into a meeting with identified areas for support. She must ask for help in these areas and not rely on the supervisor to

work it out. For supervision to succeed, the nurse needs to be able to share her feelings and be open to feedback, monitoring any tendencies to defend practice, but also monitoring what feedback is useful. Perhaps most important to the success of the relationship is the ability to be creative about clinical practice.

Self-awareness helps to minimise the impact of any 'blocks' the nurse may have towards supervision, such as negative past experiences, inhibition, misunderstandings or relationship problems such as personality clashes. Much of this can be overcome if the nurse being supervised has a choice of who acts as supervisor. In making this choice it is important that the supervisee chooses a supervisor based on that person's ability to challenge and develop nursing practice and not because of popularity with the supervisee. This person is most likely to be another nurse from the same or a similar speciality. The supervisor needs to apply clinical knowledge in a manner which promotes innovation, is constructive and creative, and facilitates the professional growth of the supervisee. It is not enough to be more senior or more experienced; the supervisor also needs advanced skills in listening, giving positive and negative feedback, facilitating reflection and defusing distress.

Before clinical supervision is established in a department, its ground rules should be identified and agreed by participants (Simms 1993); for example, it should be agreed that any acceptable breach of the *Code of Professional Conduct* (UKCC 1992) may need to be taken outside the supervisory relationship. These ground rules are outlined in Box 36.1. A robust audit tool is useful to measure quantitative data about activity such as the frequency and duration of supervision sessions. Marrow *et al.* (1998) suggested that one important area to audit would be patient

---

Box 36.1 – *Ground rules of clinical supervision*

- Confidentiality and its limits
- Professional responsibility
- Frequency and length of meetings
- Boundaries, i.e. work issues only
- Criteria for supervisor
- Termination routes if sessions become destructive
- Record-keeping

Box 36.2 – *Potential benefits of clinical supervision*

Benefits to the nurse
- Offers support and aids in confidence building
- Invests in staff and acknowledges the value of nurses and nursing
- Helps to develop nursing practice
- Allows nurse to review practice creatively and critically
- Can aid objective setting at IPR and reveal deficits
- Allows practice to change
- Promotes critical reflection on and in practice
- Develops individual accountability
- Aids personal and professional growth
- Helps link theory and practice
- Increases self-awareness

Benefits to the manager
- Helps monitor/maintain standards
- Promotes innovation
- Facilitates professionally accountable practitioners
- Links with organisational audit
- Challenges poor practice
- Strengthens collegiate relationships
- Maximises training resources
- Creates a dynamic, changing environment
- Improves communication systems

---

complaints; not just the number of complaints but the nature of the complaints. It is much harder, however, to measure the effectiveness of clinical supervision, in terms of enhancement of patient care, while retaining the confidentiality of sessions. Evidence of its value to nurses is largely subjective, but potential benefits are outlined in Box 36.2.

The cost of clinical supervision should not be underestimated. If it is to be effective, staff time out to participate must be protected, and the only sure way of guaranteeing this is to ensure a replacement in the clinical area or to pay staff to hold supervision in their off-duty time. A place where supervision meetings can be held must be available; sometimes this is an added cost. Training for supervisors and their time out of the clinical area must be taken into account. Finally, there is the hidden expense of any subsequent practice development.

A confidential record of the content of sessions should be kept by the supervisee, for use in subsequent sessions and, for instance, in her professional profile as it helps to demonstrate professional development. Statistics of activity should be available to organisations for audit purposes and to assist with costing clinical supervision as an activity. Clinicians or managers should not be put off by this apparent outlay; well developed, motivated nurses are becoming a decreasing commodity in all areas of nursing, not just the NHS, and the time is right to invest in staff. Clinical supervision offers a mechanism for nurses to quantify their development by keeping a record of supervision activities in their professional profile. It facilitates the development of their clinical practice and provides quality patient care. Perhaps most importantly, clinical supervision provides a forum for innovation and creativity to flourish.

Clinical supervision is a complex activity. Its implementation has been hampered by misunderstanding of its function, not aided by the inference of its title 'supervision'. It is, however, a real opportunity for nurses to develop their nursing practice further, challenge professional boundaries and celebrate the value of nursing.

Conclusion

This chapter has identified a range of clinical leadership and supervision issues which A&E nurses should consider when developing themselves and their practice. In an increasingly complex emergency service, support for and by those responsible for developing services is needed in order to recruit, retain and value that most precious commodity – the staff.

References

Bond M, Holland S (1998) *Skills of Clinical Supervision.* Buckingham: Open University Press.

Bishop V (1994) Clinical supervision for an accountable profession. *Nursing Times*, **90**(39), 35–37.

Cook A (1996) Effective clinical leadership in A&E. *Emergency Nurse*, **4**(3), 24–25.

Dean D (1995) Leadership: the hidden dangers. *Nursing Standard*, **10**(13), 54–55.

Department of Health (1991) *The Patient's Charter.* London: HMSO.

Fincke MK (1993) Orchestrating team building for harmonious leadership. *Accident & Emergency Nursing*, **1**, 229–233.

Garbett R (1995) Leading questions. *Nursing Times*, **91**(27), 26–27.

Haire J (1998) Communication and trauma management. *Emergency Nurse*, **6**(5), 24–30.

Holt L (1996) Clinical supervision in nursing practice. *Emergency Nurse*, **3**(4), 21–23.

Huczynski A, Buchanan D (1991) *Organisational Behaviour: an Introductory Text.* London: Prentice Hall.

Kacperek L (1997) Non-verbal communication – the importance of listening. *British Journal of Nursing*, **6**(5), 275–279.

King's Fund (1994) *Clinical Supervision: an Executive Summary.* London: King's Fund Centre.

McDaniel C, Wolf GA (1992) Transformational leadership in nursing service: a test of theory. *Journal of Nursing Administration*, **22**(2), 60–65.

Manthey M (1992) Leadership: a shifting paradigm. *Nurse Educator*, **17**(5), 5–14.

Marrow C, Yaseen T, Cook M (1998) Caring together: clinical supervision. *Nursing Standard (RCN Nursing Update)*, **12**(22), 4–22.

NHS Management Executive (1993) *A Vision for the Future: the Nursing, Midwifery and Health Visiting Contribution to Health and Healthcare.* London: Department of Health.

Proctor B (1986) Supervision: a co-operative exercise in Accountability. In: Marken M, Payne M, eds. *Enabling and Ensuring.* Leicester: Leicester Youth Bureau and Council for Education and Training in Youth and Community Work.

Senior K (1999) ENP scheme: highlighting the barriers. *Emergency Nurse*, **6**(9), 28–32.

Simms J (1993) Supervision. In: Wright H, Giddey M, eds. *Mental Health Nursing.* London: Chapman & Hall.

Sloan G (1998) Clinical supervision: characteristics of a good supervisor. *Nursing Standard*, **12**(40), 42–26.

The Allitt Inquiry (1991) *Independent Inquiry Relating to Deaths and Injuries on the Children's Ward at Grantham and Kesteven General Hospital During the Period February to April 1991.* London: HMSO.

UKCC (1992) *Code of Professional Conduct.* London: UKCC.

UKCC (1995) *Position Statement on Clinical Supervision for Nursing and Health Visiting.* London: UKCC.

Chapter 37

Clinical Reasoning

Bernie Edwards

- Introduction
- Nursing process
- Intuitive reasoning
- Hypothetico-deductive approach
- Conclusion

Introduction

The role of the nurse within the A&E department is unique. In no other clinical setting is the nurse called upon to respond to the needs of such a wide range of patients and patient concerns. Every day A&E nurses are required, without prior warning, to assess and meet the immediate health needs of individuals of whom they have no prior knowledge. Unlike all other areas of the acute hospital, the range of patients is not defined by age, sex or diagnosis, or even classification as to whether a problem is 'medical' or 'surgical'. Not for nothing is A&E often said to stand for 'anything and everything'.

The sudden and unanticipated nature of the presenting problems means that clinical judgements are often based on the minimum of information and frequently executed prior to medical assessment, notably in triage. Because these decisions shape the priority and nature of the clinical care provided, they can have a profound impact on the well-being of the patient.

In addition, many of these problems require immediate nursing intervention, which necessitates nurses having to think and act at the same time. From these situations of tremendous uncertainty the nurse must be able to extract the most relevant pieces of information and use them in order to make a rapid yet accurate clinical judgement. Clinical decisions in this context are frequently made in an environment of crisis, which demands a speed of assessment. Yet the skills which are used by nurses to assess and initiate the management of clients under conditions of uncertainty are not fully understood. As a result, this major area of A&E nursing expertise has gone largely undescribed.

Clinical decision-making can be defined as the process nurses use to gather patient information, to evaluate that information and to make a judgement that results in the provision of patient care (White *et al.* 1992). This process involves a complex mixture of observation, critical thinking and data gathering. This chapter will explore three theories of clinical reasoning derived from other areas of nursing and consider the extent to which they may relate to the practice of assessment in A&E:

■ Rationalist perspective – nursing process
■ Intuitive reasoning
■ Hypothetico-deductive.

Nursing Process

Of the three models, the nursing process is the one with which nurses are most familiar. Although called the nursing process, it is not exclusive to nursing, being primarily a problem-solving cycle in which the main elements of assessment, planning, implementation and evaluation are common to all scientific approaches.

Central to this method is the reliance placed upon the complete gathering of data prior to the identification of patient problems (see the case study in Box 37.1). It is argued that only when this occurs can nursing care be planned in a logical manner and that in doing so nurses will be able to provide a complete and rational explanation for their actions. In this model, mistakes in the decision process are usually attributed to the failure to obtain adequate information and the tendency to look for quick solutions.

Box 37.1 – *Case study: the nursing process – complete gathering of data*

Ethel, a 68-year-old widow was brought into hospital by her daughter following a fall in which she injured her left wrist. The wrist, although bruised, showed no obvious deformity or loss of neurovascular function. Mindful of the possible difficulties Ethel and her family might face on discharge, the nurse undertook a full assessment of her background, normal function and social circumstances.

In the case study described in Box 37.1, to do anything other than obtain a complete picture of the patient could expose her to considerable risk. The advice and support provided need to be rationally planned. However, what of situations where speed is essential?

Taken to its logical conclusion, when confronted with a patient with severe chest pain or abdominal trauma, the rationalist approach argues that a nurse should only act when all the information pertinent to the problem has been obtained. To do otherwise, according to the rationalist model, would put the patient at risk by exposing her to hasty and therefore potentially erroneous decisions.

In reality, not only is rapid intervention vital, but it is normally carried out in an efficient, accurate and methodical manner. Therefore, it can be seen that the use of this formal strategy of judgement is limited, being, by definition, inappropriate in situations requiring rapid intervention or conditions of uncertainty where key information specific to the problem is incomplete.

In situations such as A&E, where action precedes rational thought, alternative explanations of the decision making process are required.

Intuitive Reasoning

This can be defined as an immediate understanding of a clinical situation occurring without conscious reasoning (Radwin 1990). According to Benner & Tanner (1987) these judgements or 'gut feelings' that nurses experience are not isolated bursts of inspiration, but are recurring skilled capacities which result from the internalisation of education and experience.

Experience exposes nurses to a wide variety of clinical presentations, which cause nurses to view a situation in terms of past situations. As the frequency with which nurses encounter a particular patient problem increases, so they learn to recognise patterns and similarities within these presentations. This ability to see the whole picture enables the nurse to discriminate rapidly between potential causes of an initial problem and to focus on the specific cause. They develop what is termed a 'common-sense' understanding (Harbison 1991) (see the case study in Box 37.2).

Box 37.2 – *Case study: intuitive reasoning*

Rita Smith came into the department with an arm injury sustained by a fall. Despite heavy bruising, the X-rays showed no fracture. All the time Rita was in the department she was very pleasant and polite. However, the nurse looking after Rita had a feeling that something else was wrong. She couldn't say why, but something about Rita reminded her of previous, more traumatic situations. The nurse felt that Rita was being a bit too polite and that something other than the arm was upsetting her. When Rita was asked by the nurse whether there was anything else that she wanted to say, she burst out crying and stated that she had not fallen – her husband had, in fact, pushed her down the stairs.

The regularity with which nurses witness the impact of specific problems on clients, and also how these clients normally respond to interventions, enables experienced nurses to anticipate the way in which a person with a particular problem should progress. They are thus able to notice even the most subtle deviations from the norm and thereby recognise when the client's condition is about to deteriorate even before the physiological changes manifest themselves (Benner 1984) (see the case study in Box 37.3).

The concept of intuitive judgement is attractive in that it explains how experienced nurses are able to bypass the conscious thought processes and make accurate decisions at a very early point in time, a skill well known to A&E nurses. It also underlines what practising nurses have realised all along: that the knowledge needed to make clinical decisions is already embedded in clinical practice. Nonetheless, there are drawbacks limiting the practical use of the concept of intuition.

Because the skills are internalised, they are essentially unknown. The contextual cues in clinical situations are so numerous, and the time span involved so compact, that it is all but impossible for nurses to articulate reasons for their decisions. How many times have nurses expressed concern to medical staff that a particular patient may be deteriorating, only to say, when asked to explain why: 'I don't know why, I just know.'?

According to Radwin (1990), intuitive skills can be viewed as a 'black box', being recognisably present in those nurses whom we may regard as experts, yet unable to be passed on directly to inexperienced staff.

Two profound criticisms are levied by Farrington (1993), who stated that the fact that an experienced nurse makes decisions intuitively does not, of itself, make that nurse an expert: he could be intuitively wrong! Indeed, experience can sometimes hinder as well as promote accurate decision-making. Moreover, Farrington stated that intuition can be equally well explained as a form of rapid reasoning, or heuristics. In other words, what is described as intuition is merely rapid reasoning which because it is performed unconsciously, is experienced by the nurse as intuition.

Hypothetico–Deductive Approach

This theory suggests that, when interacting with a patient, the nurse will selectively attend to the signs and symptoms (cues) presented by that patient. These cues will vary in significance to the nurse and their importance will be greatly influenced by the context of the situation (Jones 1988). Having attended to these cues, the nurse will immediately and automatically formulate in his mind a range of possible causes. In order to confirm which of these initial tentative thoughts, or hypotheses, is the most probable, he must accumulate further data. As more information becomes available, the nurse will continue to modify his ideas as to the source of the problem until such time that he is persuaded that only one cause is plausible, (see the case study in Box 37.4).

It is thought that this automatic reasoning process works by reducing the cognitive strain clinicians in situations of uncertainty experience. In considering the most probable causes for the patient's problems, the range of possible responses is narrowed, thereby providing immediate direction to inquiry and action. The process is thought to occur in stages as illustrated in Figure 37.1.

Pre-encounter data

This refers to information about the patient that may be available to the nurse prior to meeting him or her. At first glance much of the pre-encounter data open to

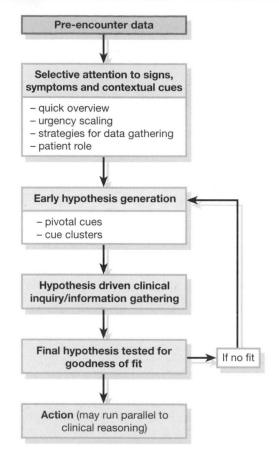

Figure 37.1 – *Model of clinical reasoning. (After Carnevali et al. 1984.)*

colleagues on the wards, such as medical diagnosis, hospital notes, laboratory results, handover from colleagues etc., appears to be denied to A&E nurses. However, various clues may be present that are not consciously articulated. Information from ambulance control that a 'collapse' is on the way already makes it more likely that the patient will be suffering from a non-traumatic condition. Information about the mechanism of a road traffic accident will assist in the anticipation of possible injuries.

The age, time of day and location may also be influential in nurses' thinking. For example, a call at 10.30 p.m. warning of the arrival of a 20-year-old male found collapsed outside the 'Dog and Duck' will arouse a different set of possibilities in the mind of the nurse from that of an 80-year-old lady found collapsed at home in the afternoon. A study by Hughes (1980) discovered that ambulance crews sometimes made judgements about the urgency of the cases they handled purely on the basis of the location of the casualty.

Activating diagnostic hypotheses and information gathering

This is the process whereby the nurse links together apparently dissimilar cues into clusters of interrelated information from which a diagnostic hypothesis is formed. These clusters are formed in the nurse's mind by associating the presenting cues with patterns of clinical features already held in the nurse's memory. These patterns are then used as a basis for labelling the problem (see the case study in Box 37.5).

> **Box 37.5** – *Case study: forming a diagnostic hypothesis*
>
> A young male patient admitted following a road traffic accident had profound tachycardia and gasping respirations. Upon exposing the patient, the nurse noticed pattern bruising on the lower abdomen. The nurse hypothesised that these three cues taken together were probable indicators of internal abdominal bleeding.

The way in which the nurse subsequently gathers information will be determined by the significance that he attaches to the cues encountered. Two classical studies on the reasoning process in physicians (Elstein *et al.* 1972, Kassirer & Gorry 1978) suggested that diagnoses were generated according to:

- probability – the prevalence of the problem within a given population
- seriousness or degree of threat – irrespective of likelihood
- amenability to health care intervention
- novelty.

Referring to the case study of the patient with chest pain (Box 37.4), as the incidence of myocardial infarction is relatively common in a 40-year-old, it would be considered more likely to occur in someone aged 40 than in someone aged 20. It is more serious than a muscular strain, as is a possible pneumothorax, and so should not be discarded as a possibility unless it can clearly be shown that it is not applicable. Both a myocardial infarction and pneumothorax are amenable to treatment. The presence of chest pain radiating down the left arm may be considered a sufficient enough 'classical' sign that the nurse may care for the patient on that basis alone until proven otherwise.

Hammond *et al.* (1966) argued that nurses use the information before them in three ways:

- to determine the presence or absence of an abnormal state on the basis of a single cue

- to determine the presence or absence of an abnormal state on the basis of many cues
- to differentiate between two or more abnormal states.

How effectively this is carried out will depend on the extent of the nurse's knowledge.

By contrast, in situations where the implications of the cues are not immediately apparent or where the nurse is uncertain how to proceed, two other methods of clinical reasoning may be employed (Putzier *et al.* 1985, Tanner *et al.* 1987). First, there is the systematic approach, which follows a review of the body system of functional area; this method would appear to be similar to that of the nursing process model. Secondly, there is a 'hit and miss' approach where the nurse moves from one aspect to another without any plan or pattern, a type of random grouping.

The initial hypotheses are continuously evaluated in the light of each new piece of information. This process may be considered as establishing a threshold whereby, if the probability of a given hypothesis existing exceeds a certain level, it is accepted by the practitioner as a basis for action (Benner *et al.* 1999, Tanner 1984). What this level may be, as with most aspects of this reasoning process, may be unknown to the practitioner. It needs to be remembered that what has been described may take place in a matter of seconds and at a mainly unconscious level. However, it is the very rapidity at which reasoning takes place that renders it vulnerable to error.

Possible sources of error

- *Confirmation bias.* This is where practitioners attend to information that supports their initial or favourite hypotheses. The result is that cues which offer other explanations are ignored unless they become overwhelming (Jones 1992).
- *Personal bias.* This is linked to the above and can be illustrated by the treatment often provided to 'regulars', which can be based on knowledge of previous presentations rather than upon a proper assessment, with potentially detrimental results (Dingwall & Murray 1983).
- *Considering too few hypotheses.* The probability of making an accurate diagnosis depends to a large extent on whether it was included in the initial range of possibilities considered. Lack of knowledge can lead to a problem being ignored, and to incorrect or even dangerous advice being given (Crouch 1992). In other words, the inexperienced nurse does not know what he does not know!

There appears, therefore, to be a thin line between the ability to effect accurate decisions rapidly and merely jumping to conclusions. Two major influences on the nurse help to differentiate these: extrapersonal and intrapersonal factors.

Extrapersonal factors

The main influences here are the physical characteristics of the clinical setting. An A&E department that is full to overflowing and understaffed will increase the pressure to think quickly. Under these conditions the nurse may be forced into adopting a routinised approach to care which may lead to non-recognition of the atypical case.

The frequency with which nurses encounter a given situation is also going to influence the way they think. A nurse having recently come from a ward with numerous diabetic patients may well consider hypoglycaemia as a likely cause of collapse in a 20-year-old man outside a pub, whereas A&E nurses who regularly work nights would probably consider a different cause! Nurses tend to draw on their most recent or dramatic experiences for comparison (Woolley 1990). This is not detrimental provided other possible causes, e.g. overdosage or epilepsy, in the 20-year-old patient's collapse are not excluded from the nurse's initial thoughts.

Information received from others such as ambulance personnel may bias the focus of care. Hughes (1988) illustrated the extent to which medical staff are influenced in their judgements by the information they receive from nurses. Such information is, of course, absolutely vital and should be given credence. However, it does need to be remembered that even the best of information may be incomplete.

Intrapersonal factors

Degree of specialist knowledge. The greater the amount of knowledge the nurse possesses, the more likely he will be to appreciate the relative significance of the items of clinical information available. This will enable the nurse to be selective about which items of clinical information are attended to, to generate a broader range of initial hypotheses and to link these items together in an efficient and meaningful way. The ability to do this is considered a characteristic of expertise (Cholowski & Chan 1992, White *et al.* 1992).

Corcoran *et al.* (1988) argued that the nurse requires a combination of textbook (formal) and experiential knowledge. However, while formal knowledge is essential to provide an overall framework, it may be insufficient to provide information regarding the atypical presentation. It cannot account for the social context in which the problem occurs nor assess its impact on the individual. This social knowledge is regarded by Hughes (1988) as central to the whole process of clinical management. Theoretical knowledge alone does not facilitate the clinical sensitivity necessary to discriminate between all the cues confronting a nurse. While clinical experience does not guarantee expertise and can be a possible source of bias, expertise cannot arise without it.

Personal representation of the problem. This implies that nurses using legitimate critical thinking processes can arrive at different interpretations of the same situation (Jones & Brown 1991). This is because a situation is viewed in the context of the individual nurse's own experiences and philosophical approach. Clinical reasoning is not purely analytically driven.

This is particularly pertinent in A&E nursing where there is no consistent or explicit agreement on an appropriate model. When caring for a patient, the nurse's clinical reasoning will be dependent on what is viewed as important, which may sometimes coincide with the medical framework, at the expense of other issues. This could lead to a patient being labelled as an 'inappropriate attender' if the medical diagnosis is not one that could be considered either an accident or an emergency.

Degree of confidence. In an emergency, nurses need to act decisively and confidently. Yet clinicians often erroneously equate confidence with competence. If this occurs, nurses may become overconfident and less likely to evaluate their own actions. This can give a false sense of security and lead to the possibility that alternative diagnoses and actions are not always fully evaluated, thus leading to confirmation bias (Baumann *et al.* 1991). Benner (1984) argued that a residual sense of uncertainty is a characteristic of expertise; it

is also a tacit acknowledgement that uncertainty is an unavoidable characteristic of clinical decision-making.

The role of uncertainty was highlighted in a study into how experienced nurses made triage dispositions via the telephone (Edwards 1994). It was found that nurses' perceptions of their professional and personal vulnerability caused them to ask the question 'What if …?' and thereby take action to cover themselves and account for even the most unlikely eventuality.

The research also revealed that when making the final triage decision, as well as determining the most likely cause of the presenting problem, nurses also considered the impact of the problem on the caller, the accessibility of alternative sources of health care, and their own ability to control the reactions of the caller. This suggests that the reasoning process is more complex and the experiential knowledge which the nurse draws upon more wide-ranging than is currently acknowledged.

The differences between the reasoning processes of expert and non-expert nurses are summarised in Table 37.1.

Implications for practice

In A&E, the prime focus of nursing judgement is the determination of the impact the presenting problem has, or may have, on patients' physiological and/or emotional well-being and their capacity for self-care. It differs from medical diagnosis, which is primarily concerned with identifying the cause of a pathological process and its treatment. However, the majority of patients present with anatomical injuries or disruption

Table 37.1 – *Comparison of the characteristics of expert and non-expert decision-making*

Expert	Novice
■ Can distinguish and discriminate between significant and irrelevant cues	■ Cannot appraise significance of cues – all appear equally valid
■ Recognises relationships between cues	■ Cannot interrelate cues
■ Selectively utilises theoretical knowledge	■ Reliance on 'textbook' presentations
■ Draws the correct inferences from the cues	■ Clinical inquiry will be unfocused
■ Generates a wide range of possible hypotheses	■ Range of hypotheses will be narrow – unaware of all possibilities
■ Flexible – prepared to re-evaluate initial hypothesis in the light of new information	■ Displays overconfidence in an effort to reduce uncertainty
■ Can tolerate ambiguity	■ Needs to see things in black and white terms
■ Aware of sources of bias	■ Unduly influenced by most recent or profound experiences

to a physiological system, and therefore nurses have to reason and make treatment decisions in both medical and nursing domains (Carnevali 1984, Jones 1990).

As most of the studies utilising the hypothetico-deductive framework have focused on the reasoning processes adopted by physicians and nurses to label clinical symptoms, it would appear reasonable to suppose that where nursing judgements overlap with medical diagnosis, this model of reasoning may hold. If this is so, clinical reasoning in A&E can be improved by methods which enable the nurse to:

- recognise significant cues
- efficiently cluster interrelated cues
- generate a wide range of hypotheses
- utilise methods of data gathering that will rapidly discriminate between competing hypotheses.

In order to do this effectively, it is necessary to use methods which draw on both theoretical and practical knowledge.

Courses such as advanced trauma life support, which focus on the ability to interpret presenting cues and their significance in terms of threat to the individual, are more relevant than traditional clinical education, which tended to take a given disease or pathology and subsequently consider the signs and symptoms that may arise out of it. This principle needs to be expanded to incorporate other areas of practice.

Similarly the use of decision trees or protocols may enable nurses to use questions more effectively in situations where more than one hypothesis presents itself. However, it must be remembered that protocols cannot account for individual variations or the context in which the situation occurs, which form a major component of nurses' experiential knowledge.

Benner (1984) suggested that experienced nurses can make this knowledge explicit by providing reflections on critical incidents, particularly those where nursing intervention made a difference, and making them available to junior staff. Molitor (1985) argued that similar results can be obtained by analysing experienced nurses' reasoned responses to written case studies.

Simulations may also be rich source of material, particularly those which can be recorded. Thus a library of 'model' simulations by experts could be built up. Simulations in which the novice is recorded could form the basis for analysis by the novice and expert together. The effectiveness of these methods would be enhanced if the participants were to be encouraged to 'think aloud' whilst participating, thereby making the components of reasoning more visible (Corcoran *et al.* 1988).

Conclusion

Further research is required into how A&E nurses, *specifically*, make decisions. Failure to elicit what expertise already exists will result in a lack of recognition of the unique character of emergency nursing and a continuing tendency to draw on knowledge derived from other disciplines or areas of practice, delaying still further the realisation of true professional autonomy.

Further reading

Carnevali D, Thomas M (1993) *Diagnostic Reasoning and Treatment Decision Making in Nursing.* Philadelphia: Lippincott.

Edwards B (1998) Seeing is believing – picture building: a key component of telephone triage. *Journal of Clinical Nursing,* **7**(1), 51–57.

Higgs J, Jones M (eds) (1995) *Clinical Reasoning in the Health Professions.* Oxford: Butterworth-Heinemann.

References

Baumann A, Deber RB, Thompson GG (1991) Overconfidence among physicians and nurses: the 'micro-certainty, macro-certainty phenomenon'. *Social Science & Medicine,* **32**(2), 167–174.

Benner P (1984) *From Novice to Expert: Excellence and Power in Clinical Nursing.* Menlo Park, California: Addison Wesley.

Benner P, Hooper-Kyriakidis P, Stannard D (1999) *Clinical Wisdom and Interventions in Critical Care: a Thinking-in-action Approach.* Philadelphia: WB Saunders.

Benner P, Tanner C (1987) How expert nurses use intuition. *American Journal of Nursing,* **87**, 23–31.

Carnevali D (1984) The diagnostic reasoning process. In:

Carnevali D, Mitchell P, Woods N, Tanner C, eds. *Diagnostic Reasoning in Nursing.* Philadelphia: Lippincott.

Carnevali D, Mitchell P, Woods N, Tanner C (eds) (1984) *Diagnostic Reasoning in Nursing.* Philadelphia, Lippincott.

Cholowski K, Chan L (1992) Diagnostic reasoning among second year nursing students. *Journal of Advanced Nursing,* **17**, 1171–1181.

Corcoran S, Narayan S, Moreland H (1988) Thinking aloud as a strategy to improve clinical decision making. *Heart and Lung,* **17**(5), 463–468.

Crouch R (1992) Inappropriate attender in A&E. *Nursing Standard, (Emergency Nurse* supplement), **6**(27), 7–9.

Dingwall R, Murray J (1983) Categorisation in accident departments: 'good' patients, 'bad' patients and 'children'. *Sociology of Health and Illness*, **5**(2), 127–145.

Edwards B (1994) Telephone triage: how experienced nurses make decisions. *Journal of Advanced Nursing*, **19**, 717–724.

Elstein A, Kagan N, Shulman L, Jason H, Lovpe M (1972) Methods and theory in the study of medical inquiry. *Journal of Medical Education*, **47**, 85–92.

Farrington A (1993) Intuition and expert clinical practice in nursing. *British Journal of Nursing*, **2**(4), 228–233.

Hammond K, Kelley K, Schneider R, Vancini M (1966) Clinical inference in nursing: analyzing cognitive tasks representative of nursing problems. *Nursing Research*, **15**(2).

Harbison J (1991) Clinical decision making in nursing. *Journal of Advanced Nursing*, **16**, 404–407.

Hughes D (1980) The ambulance journey as an information generating process. *Sociology of Health & Illness*, **2**(2), 115–131.

Hughes D (1988) When nurse knows best: some aspects of the nurse/doctor interaction in a casualty department. *Sociology of Health & Illness*, **10**(1), 1–22.

Jones G (1990) *Accident and Emergency Nursing: a Structured Approach*. London: Faber & Faber.

Jones J (1988) Clinical reasoning in nursing. *Journal of Advanced Nursing*, **13**, 185–192.

Jones M (1992) Clinical reasoning in manual therapy. *Physical Therapy*, **72**(12), 875–884.

Jones S, Brown L (1991) Critical thinking: impact on nurse education. *Journal of Advanced Nursing*, **16**, 529–533.

Kassirer J, Gorry G (1978) Clinical problem solving: a behavioural analysis. *Annals of Internal Medicine*, **89**, 245–255.

Molitor L (1985) Triage dilemmas and decisions: a tool for continuing education. *Journal of Emergency Nursing*, **11**(1), 40–42.

Putzier D, Patrick K, Westfall VE, Tanner CA (1985) Diagnostic reasoning in critical care nursing. *Heart and Lung*, **14**(5), 430–437.

Radwin L (1990) Research on diagnostic reasoning in nursing. *Nursing Diagnosis*, **1**(2), 70–77.

Tanner C (1984) Factors Influencing the Diagnostic Process. In: Carnevali D, Mitchell P, Woods N, Tanner C, eds. *Diagnostic Reasoning in Nursing*. Philadelphia: Lippincott.

Tanner C, Padrick KP, Westfall UE, Putzier DJ (1987) Diagnostic reasoning strategies of nurses and nursing students. *Nursing Research*, **36**(6), 358–363.

White J, Nativo DG, Kobert SN, Engberg SJ (1992) Content and process in clinical decision-making by nurse practitioners. *Image*, **24**(2), 153–158.

Woolley N (1990) Nursing diagnosis: exploring the factors which may influence the reasoning process. *Journal of Advanced Nursing*, **15**, 110–117.

Chapter 38

Ethical Issues

Kevin Kendrick

- Introduction
- Duty as a moral endeavour
- Applying the imperative to practice
- Duty as a moral problem
- Above all, do no harm
- Consent as an ethical process
- Conclusion

Introduction

Perceptions of ethics are as varied as the mores that inform individual behaviour. Some people see ethics as an esoteric abstraction that belongs firmly in the ivory towers of academia; others see it as an ethereal subject that parliamentarians manipulate in matters of political controversy. There are elements of truth in both these perspectives; ethics is, however, much more than this.

Unlike many words, the nature and essence of ethics cannot be succinctly reflected in a single definition. Taking this further, Sparkes (1992) questioned the usefulness of dictionaries and argued that the best which can be offered for ethics is a semantic interpretation; this is given as 'the philosophical study of moral conduct and reasoning'.

Sparkes' interpretation gives direction and focus to the essential themes of ethics. In essence, it is concerned with the way in which reason can clarify situations that have a moral dimension. This last point gives a *prima facie* rationale for placing ethics at the centre of the nursing equation, since the focus of that profession is steeped with issues that demand ethical enquiry and a moral response. Mirroring the vibrancy ethical analysis can offer nursing, Tschudin (1993) asserted:

> *Ethics is not only at the heart of nursing, it is the heart of nursing. Ethics is about what is right and good. Nursing and caring are synonymous, and the way in which care is carried out is ethically decisive. How a patient is addressed, cared for and treated must be right not only by ordinary standards of care, but also by ethical principles.*

The purpose of this chapter is to use philosophical reasoning to examine some areas of moral concern that frequently confront practitioners in accident and emergency departments. These areas will provide a philosophical adjunct to the legal issues that are covered in Chapter 39, e.g., a duty of care, consent. The reason for this is to conduct an ethical examination of concepts central to health care law in this country.

This exercise will also usefully show that what may be legal may not be moral and what may be moral may not be legal. History abounds with examples that support this position: it was once illegal for women to have the vote or for gay men to give physical expression to their sexuality. A pressing example from the contemporary arena is euthanasia; proponents argue it is both a moral and humane concept that liberates an individual's self-governance about the manner and time of death – it has, however, no legal standing.

Given that nurses have a legally enforced duty of care towards patients within the A&E department, its seems fitting that a chapter dealing with ethics should begin by considering the notion of 'duty' as a central theme in the development of a school of ethical analysis called 'deontology'. During this process, strong parallels will be drawn between deontology, duty as a traditional motivational force in nursing and, also, the *Code of Professional Conduct* (UKCC 1992a).

Duty as a Moral Endeavour

The historical dimensions of nursing are engulfed by the notion of duty; this tradition is succinctly entwined in the most central of nursing edicts, 'a duty of care'. Within contemporary nursing there remains a strong allegiance to this theme. This approach is based upon the intrinsic and inalienable relationship that exists between 'rights' and 'duties'. Broadly speaking, once a duty of care has been established, the patient has a right to be cared for and the nurse must facilitate care giving – this is both a legal and moral theme.

The UKCC *Code of Professional Conduct* (UKCC 1992a) encourages high standards during professional endeavours and expects all practitioners to operate within its framework and guidelines. This is reflected in the following extract:

> *The Council is the regulatory body responsible for the standards of these professions and it requires members of the professions to practice and conduct themselves within the standards and framework provided by the code.*

Statements of this nature serve to reinforce notions of duty and the maxims within the code provide motivational guidelines for nursing actions. Basing actions upon duties, rules or motives has a long history in ethics and is known as deontology. Kendrick (1993) made the following comment about this method of moral thinking: 'This school of ethical analysis maintains that being moral entails acting from a sense of moral duty, respecting others' rights and honouring one's obligations.'

This interpretation clearly aligns itself with the themes of the professional *Code of Conduct* and the onus which it places upon registered practitioners. The person most closely associated with deontology is the philosopher Immanuel Kant; he was a prolific writer and fervently advocated that people had intrinsic worth and value. Furthermore, he argued that an essential part of being human was the ability to use reason in deliberating over the moral worth of an action. For Kant, this ability invariably found itself rooted in a sense of duty.

There are many attractive elements of Kantian ethics. In particular, it places a great deal of emphasis upon respect amongst persons and encourages a fervent sense of individual duty. Tschudin (1986) summarised these themes by stating:

> *A right action is only so if it is done out of a sense of duty, and the only good thing without qualification is a person's good will: the will to do what one knows is right.*

Kant devised a complex moral theory, consisting of three formulations, that he called the categorical imperative. Their precise interpretation and mutual relations are a matter of controversy. Kendrick (1993) simplified the different formulations as follows:

- An action is only moral if you are willing for it to be applied to everyone, yourself included, as a universal law.
- For an action to be moral it must never lead to people being seen just as 'means to an end' but always as 'ends' in their own right.
- In wishing to be moral, individuals must act as members of a community where everybody is seen as having intrinsic worth (ends in their own right).

The essence of the categorical imperative can be readily applied to the duty based nature of nursing; this will now be discussed with particular relevance to A&E practice.

Applying the Imperative to Practice

The first part of the imperative indicates that all people have intrinsic worth and should attribute respect to each other; for example, most societies would agree that it is intrinsically wrong to murder another person. The implications of Kant's theory are that persons wishing to undertake such acts should be willing to accept the same being done to themselves – as if they were governed by a universal law that related to that given activity. Expressed simply, the first principle is a moral edict that requires us to ask: 'Would I like this act to be done either to myself or those close to me?' If the answer is 'no' then Kant would have serious reservations about the moral worth of the motives underpinning the action.

These themes are often introduced to the novice nurse who is asked to care from a basis of duty. While this may initially seem a little simplistic, it can act as a strong image for mental reinforcement and maintaining standards during the delivery of care throughout a nurse's career. The second of Kant's principles further emphasises the notion of equal respect amongst persons and resolutely argues that individuals should never be seen or treated solely as means to an end. This does not mean that people cannot work together or help each other – the key theme is that this should involve some degree of mutual reciprocity.

An example of this is the staff nurse who needs to attain the skills of suturing. Obviously, to be able to perform this task safely and competently requires the cooperation of a willing patient. While a patient may be used as a means to an end – the end being the nurse suturing competently – this does not echo the full essence of this part of the imperative. Suturing an open wound also offers some therapeutic worth to the patient; thus the process has benefited the nurse through the acquisition of a skill and the patient through the closure of a wound. Kant did not object to individuals being used as a means to an end as long as they are also valued as ends in their own right.

The essence of the second principle in the imperative does not just apply to the nurse/patient relationship but extends to all interaction within the professional milieu. Not only are nurses required to respect patients as being of equal worth, but this must also govern the professional ethos in dealing with colleagues. This duty to enact the principle of respect for persons is a cogent thread throughout the *Code of Professional Conduct*, but it finds particular relevance in clauses 6 and 7 (UKCC 1992a)

- Clause 6: *Work in a collaborative and co-operative manner with health care professionals and others involved in providing care, and recognise their particular contributions within the care team.*

- Clause 7: *Recognise and respect the uniqueness and dignity of each patient and client, and respond to their need for care, irrespective of their ethnic origin, religious beliefs, personal attributes, the nature of their health problems or any other factor.*

Such themes are vitally important given that recent years have seen the blurring of roles between doctors and nurses. If practitioners from both professions are to have shared working practices, it must be through mutual respect and the fervent desire to embellish the care that is offered to patients. Such notions offer the opportunity to embrace the themes of shared governance and create an organisational milieu where all concerned can achieve their potential. Such themes were given sharp focus for nursing by the introduction of the *Scope of Professional Practice* (UKCC 1992b) and the associated concept of advanced practice (Kendrick 1997).

Respect is a central element in Kantian thinking and the word appears frequently throughout the *Code of Conduct* (UKCC 1992a). A strong emphasis upon respect emerges from the third and final part of the imperative; its essential message is that persons form a community where each member has equal worth as a moral decision-maker. As nurses, we meet colleagues or patients who may have very different values or beliefs from our own. Sometimes these differences are informed by cultural or religious diversity. Kantian ethics suggests that the key issue is to respect the freedom of other individuals to hold moral perspectives and to act upon them – this is part of what it means to treat others as ends.

If this is applied to the professional setting, it asks that all people have equal authority to express and defend their respective positions. Once again, it can be suggested that this theme runs throughout the *Code of Professional Conduct*. However, clause 5 specifically supports this notion:

> *Work in an open and co-operative manner with patients, clients and their families, foster their independence and recognise and respect their involvement in the planning and delivery of care.*

To this point it has been seen that duty-based approaches to ethical thinking and analysis have a long history in moral theory. This has been supported with reference to deontology and the philosopher most closely associated with it, Immanuel Kant. Moreover, clear links have been drawn between the deontological approach and the duty-based themes that run throughout nursing. The *Code of Professional Conduct* provides a series of guidelines and principles that inform a practitioner's professional obligations and preserve the traditional emphasis upon duty-based care-giving. However, while it may be suggested that principles of duty provide indications that can help give directions about professional conduct, there are problems with such approaches that demand clarification and analysis.

Duty as a Moral Problem

A glaring problem with duty-based approaches to morality and Kantian ethics in particular is that they tend to portray certain maxims as absolute, universal and all-encompassing. There are many examples from the real world which highlight an unquestioning bond to duty-based dictums; for example, certain religions require their members not to accept whole blood products during medical treatments. There is much room for debate about whether or not a principle/duty can ever be thought to be ubiquitous and applied as a categorical tenet.

Within nursing there are certain rules which are perceived, as has already been discussed, as absolute; principal among these is the duty of care. However, sometimes the maxims within a duty of care can be at variance with each other. Consider the following principles:

- a duty to do good (beneficence)
- a duty to do no harm (non-maleficence).

At first glance these principles seem closely related. However, further analysis does reveal distinct differences between the two themes. Nurses always try to ensure that their actions promote good and preserve the best interests of the patient. This leads nurses to an interesting and penetrating question: 'Can we say that nursing actions always promote good results for patients?' It is very doubtful that nurses can say 'yes' to this question; to a large extent this is because harm is an intrinsic part of some nursing actions.

The simplest example of this is when a nurse gives an intramuscular injection. Every time the syringe is introduced, it causes pain which, even to a very small degree, can be equated with harm. Many other nursing interventions carry the same ethos: antibiotics can cause an irritating rash; aspirin can cause gastric erosion; and diamorphine or other opiate derivatives can cause chronic constipation. Some of the more advanced nursing practices, e.g. intubation or cannulation, carry a host of risks that can, if realised, greatly harm the patient. Given the amount of harm which can result from some of our actions, the nurse needs to ask if the principle of non-maleficence is appropriate and applicable as a universal tenet in nursing.

Above All, Do No Harm

Believing the absolute notion that nursing actions will never do any harm is impractical because it can never be totally achieved within the professional role. We have already been seen some of the 'harm' which can be induced by nursing actions. This theme has been explored and analysed by Illich (1975), with particular reference to the medical profession, but may be applied with equal resonance to nursing, especially now that advanced practice involves nurses performing tasks that formally fell under the sole auspices of medics.

Illich (1975) used the word 'iatrogenesis' to describe the harmful results and illnesses that can result from the intervention of doctors. For example, Illich made the following claims:

It has been established that one out of every five patients admitted to a typical research hospital acquires an iatrogenic disease, sometimes trivial, usually requiring special treatment, and in one case in thirty leading to death. Half of these episodes resulted from complications of drug therapy; amazingly, one in ten comes from diagnostic procedures. Despite good intentions and claims to public service, with a similar record of performance a military officer would be relieved of his command and a restaurant or amusement centre would be closed by police.

Illich has been criticised for not placing enough emphasis upon the amount of good which medicine achieves. This is a valid criticism and it leads to the centre of the debate about absolute duties as all-encompassing principles. It can be stated with a degree of certainty that the primary intention of practitioners is to promote beneficence and to strive to achieve non-maleficence. However, to place these two themes in the language of absolute duties is no more than an exercise in rhetoric and cannot be upheld in the 'real' world of delivering care.

The key issue is not to insist that health professionals abide unquestioningly by a duty to do good and a duty to do no harm – clearly the two duties are not always reconcilable as consummate themes. The essential worth of the two principles is found in balancing them both together, not viewing them as isolated absolutes. Returning to the example of the intramuscular injection, while the initial result may be pain or harm, this is usually outweighed by the amount of good which results from the therapeutic worth of the injected drug. This serves to highlight that the balance between beneficence and non-maleficence can help practitioners to reflect upon the worth of an action.

The essential problem with this is that the consequences of an action cannot always be forecast beforehand – crystal ball gazing is a poor basis for moral analysis. Despite this drawback, trying to weigh the moral worth of an action against the harm which it may produce at least asks for a degree of questioning, reflection and analysis; this is surely more acceptable than a passive acceptance of absolute, but conflicting, duties.

Practitioners at the 'cutting edge' of health care delivery have always had an intuitive awareness of the precarious balance between beneficence and non-maleficence. Unfortunately, the power relationship between doctors and nurses has usually resulted in the nurse handing issues of a moral nature over to the doctor, who then tries to deal with them through the value-free objectivity of a 'clinical decision'. Contemporary practice challenges such themes; 'teamwork' and parity in the decision-making process demand input from all interested parties; the author has supported such themes elsewhere (Kendrick 1998):

> In the UK, doctors need to stop seeing situations that are ethically relevant as something to be subsumed under the broad notion of a 'clinical decision'. In essence, this should mean shared governance with other practitioners – after all, ethics belongs to us all and is not the sole domain of medics.

This section has presented an argument which highlights the inadequacies of duty-based principles as moral panaceas which can be applied and invoked for all ethical 'ills'. Emerging from this is a clear theme that moral duties can rarely stand as absolute and isolated 'ends'. Moral duties, whatever their nature, remain rhetorical unless they give clear and non-conflicting directions for the pathways of practice.

Chapter 39 gives a focused and cogent overview of the legal themes that inform a 'duty of care'. In comparison, this section has given an adjunct to the legal scenario and shown that using duty-based approaches to moral reasoning is often self-limiting. Taking this further, duty has been considered here in relation to such themes as: duty as a traditional force in nursing, the *Code of Professional Conduct* (UKCC 1992a), the nurse/patient relationship, inter-professional relationships and, finally, the moral conflict that results when duties conflict. However, and this is vital, while nurses may liberally question the philosophical foundation of duty-based methods of ethical analysis, our legal requirement to fulfil a duty of care to patients, once established, remains absolute (Jones 1997).

It has been seen that the duties of beneficence and non-maleficence must have value as means to an end if they are to have meaning and essence for practitioners. This can be said with equal efficacy about the principles embodied in the UKCC *Code of Professional Conduct*. In essence, they provide the starting point for discussion, analysis and professional discernment but they are not categorical absolutes. Chadwick & Tadd (1992) pursued this line of enquiry and commented: 'A code of conduct or ethics should perhaps be seen, not as the last word on ethics, but as a stimulus to moral thinking'. Such themes are vital when considering the moral milieu of nursing practice in A&E units. What is

also essential is an understanding of the ethical issues that engulf the notion of consent. In Chapter 39, consent is considered within a legal framework; the next part of this chapter will explore the moral dimensions of that concept.

Consent as an Ethical Process

Informed consent, by its very nature, demands that nurses give patients all the information needed to make an informed decision. This theme is reflected by Gillon (1985) who argued that consent can be defined as:

> ...a voluntary and uncoerced decision made by a sufficiently competent or autonomous person, on the basis of adequate information and deliberation, to accept rather than reject some proposed course of action that will affect him or her.

However, a key issue is: how do nurses define 'adequate information'? For example, how many nurses would divulge to a male patient, brought into A&E with acute urinary retention, the remote possibility that catheterisation may result in a perforated urethra? Intrinsic to this notion is a complex and controversial question: how much information should be given to patients before an informed consent can be given to the treatment or intervention offered? (Kendrick 1994).

Broadly speaking, there are two opposing perspectives towards this question, Kendrick (1991) argued that:

> ...at one end of the spectrum there are those who believe that the patient should have access to every conceivable issue involved in their treatment or care. This is based on the understanding that a patient who is privy to both negative and positive aspects of their treatment or care will be able to make an informed and valid consent. In contrast to this perspective is the paternalistic view that a nurse has the necessary insight and professional knowledge to judge when the giving of certain information would be harmful to the patient.

Both of these positions contain elements which make a valid argument and deserve further examination. This demands an exploration of the key ethical principles which support the notion of a full and informed consent.

The myth of self-governance

In its most basic form, autonomy is concerned with an individual's level of self-government. Faulder (1985) broadened this to offer an interpretation which can be directly applied to nursing practice: 'the individual's freedom to decide her or his goals and to act according to these goals'. However, the idea of absolute autonomy is something of a myth – nobody can be fully independent and self-governing. Consider the term 'autonomous nurse'; it is facile to think of an individual's practice as something which is free of constraints. Nurses have to work within a framework which is influenced by a *Code of Professional Conduct* (UKCC 1992a), the organisational milieu and the needs of patients; thus, total autonomy is not reconcilable with the limitations of the real world. These themes are reflected by Henry & Pashley (1990) who stated:

> *Full autonomy is an ideal notion and we can only approximate to it. It is obvious that, in reality, some situations, states and circumstances will diminish a person's autonomy, such as the ability to control his or her actions, or both, through being restricted in some way, for example, illness, psychological impairment, physical or mental disability.*

However, despite many practical difficulties, nurses must always strive to eliminate barriers which may hinder a patient's autonomy and freedom of choice.

Freedom to choose

There is a close relationship between autonomy and informed consent, the former being concerned with freedom and choice, the latter being the key which unlocks and enables their expression. Taking this further, it would be extremely difficult for patients to take an active part in decisions relating to care if they did not have the necessary information on which to make choices.

If autonomy is respected in practice, then patients should feel uninhibited about identifying their own needs and actively deciding how these should be met. However, a problem with discussing autonomy is that it can create an impression that all patients want to take part in such a full and dynamic role. A missing element here is that patients are, by definition, sick and often vulnerable; this may be particular relevant to the patients you meet in A&E – especially given the often shocking nature of sudden illness or trauma. This may conjure up different images for different people. Some patients may see it as a place of safety where their illness or trauma will be addressed, while others see it as a reflection of their own mortality and hear the ringing of the death knell.

For patients who see the A&E department as a symbol of fear, it may be inappropriate to expect them to take an active role in the decision-making process. This is not parentalism; if, after the choice has been offered, patients express no wish to take an active role in their care then it should be accepted as an expression of autonomy. Kendrick (1991) supported this notion and stated:

> *The patient should be given the freedom to say to the nurse that he wishes to surrender any role within the decision making process. This agreement may be temporary or permanent in nature. What must be emphasised here, is that when a patient gives the nurse responsibility for decisions he does not relinquish autonomy, but gives acknowledgement of it.*

Such approaches indicate the patient's right to freely decide what may or may not be done to his body. Indeed, irrespective of ethical considerations, performing an act without the patient's permission may, as is discussed in Chapter 39, constitute negligence in legal terms. All of this reflects an ethicolegal emphasis which is intended to protect the vulnerable status of patients. Such themes, however, frequently place practitioners in A&E in very precarious positions; perhaps the most telling example of this is when an unconscious person is brought into the department after taking an overdose. Practitioners do not usually have the benefit of time and must act quickly if life is to be preserved. This is frequently when the maxim 'act first, ask questions later' comes into its own. What happens, however, when a patient is semi-conscious and gives the expressed desire to be left to die? There is no time to get a psychiatrist's opinion, no time to think about the patient's level of competence – just a very real dilemma that needs an immediate decision. This is where ethics finds its most cutting edge.

The legal grounds for acting without the patient's consent could well be based on urgency and necessity – remembering also that failing to act holds the risk of being accused of negligence (see Ch. 39) It is an unfortunate aspect of contemporary practice that practitioners may be 'damned if they do and damned if they don't'. Proponents of a literal and absolute interpretation of autonomy (self-governance) may argue that, irrespective of legal defences, health care professionals never have a sufficient moral mandate to override the expressed wish of a patient to be left to die; Brown *et al.* (1992) offered a brief and cogent comment on such themes: 'We cannot solve the dilemmas by saying that we should always do what the patient wishes.'

Such sober insights give buoyancy to the essential elements of moral reasoning in health care; ethics is not about providing panaceas for all the moral ills of practice. It can, however, offer a focused means of reaching rational decisions about the issues that confront practitioners in A&E departments.

Conclusion

This chapter has critically explored two major ethical themes that continually challenge practitioners in A&E departments: duty and consent. Within these broad concepts, a host of other issues have also been considered that often cause moral concern. It would be impossible, in a chapter of this size, to do justice to all the dilemmas that confront practitioners in A&E; such an endeavour would command a book in its own right. However, it is hoped that this chapter has charged the reader with enough creative energy to read further and explore other areas that confront one's own practice.

Further reading

Kohner N (1996) *The Moral Maze of Practice: a Stimulus for Reflection and Discussion*. London: Kings Fund.

Reed J, Ground I (1997) *Philosophy for Nursing*. London: Edward Arnold.

Thompson IE, Melia KM, Boyd KM. (1994) *Nursing ethics*, 3rd edn. Edinburgh: Churchill Livingstone.

Tschudin V (1994) *Deciding Ethically: a Practical Approach to Nursing Challenges*. London: Baillière Tindall.

References

Brown JM, Kitson A, McKnight TJ (1992) *Challenges in Caring: Explorations in Nursing and Ethics*. London: Chapman and Hall.

Chadwick RF, Tadd W (1992) *Ethics and Nursing Practice: a Case Study Approach*. Basingstoke: Macmillan.

Faulder C (1985) *Whose Body is it?: the Troubling Issues of Informed Consent*. London: Virago.

Gillon R (1985) Autonomy and consent. In: Lockwood M, ed. *Moral Dilemmas in Modern Medicine*. Oxford: Oxford University Press.

Henry C, Pashley G (1990) *Health Ethics*. Lancaster: Quay Books.

Illich I (1975) *Medical Nemesis: the Expropriation of Health*. London: Calder and Boyers.

Jones G (1997) Liability in A&E nursing. *Emergency Nurse*, **5**(5), 18–20.

Kendrick KD (1991) Partners in passing: ethical aspects of nursing the dying person. *International Journal of Advances in Health and Nursing Care*, **1**(1), 11–27.

Kendrick KD (1993) Ethics and Nursing Practice. *British Journal of Nursing*, **2**(18), 920–926.

Kendrick KD (1994) Freedom to choose: the ethics of consent. *Professional Nurse*, **9**(11), 739–742.

Kendrick KD (1997) What is advanced nursing? (Editorial) *Professional Nurse*, **12**(10), 689.

Kendrick KD (1998) Ethical Issues in Critical Care. In: Tadd W, ed. *Nursing Ethics: a European Perspective*. Basingstoke: Macmillan.

Sparkes AW (1992) *Talking Philosophy: a Workbook*. London: Routledge.

Tschudin V (1986) *Ethics in Nursing: the Caring Relationship*. London: Heinemann Nursing.

Tschudin V (1993) *Ethics: Aspects of Nursing Care*. London: Scutari Press.

UKCC (1992a) *Code of Professional Conduct for the Nurse, Midwife and Health Visitor*, 3rd edn. London: UKCC.

UKCC (1992b) *The Scope of Professional Practice*. London: UKCC.

Chapter 39

Law

Ann Young

- Introduction
- An outline of law in the UK
- Classification of law
- Attendance
- Assessment
- Treatment and care
- Death and organ donation
- Patient property
- Consent to treatment
- Detention of patients
- Confidentiality, the police and the press
- Staff health and safety
- Conclusion

Introduction

This chapter introduces the main areas of law of relevance in the A&E department. It highlights the key issues where a knowledge of law is essential and discusses some of the legal dilemmas that may arise. Attendance, assessment, treatment and care, consent to treatment, detention of patients, confidentiality, the police, the press and staff health and safety are considered.

An Outline of Law in the UK

Although the UK is one state, it is made up of four countries whose laws originally developed separately. England and Wales have identical legal systems, the law in Northern Ireland has developed along similar lines, but Scottish law has different roots. Some law is made specifically for each country; one example relating to health care is the absence of an Abortion Act in Northern Ireland. In this chapter, the law stated applies to England and Wales. Where marked differences exist in Northern Ireland and Scotland, these will be mentioned. Otherwise, the reader can assume that the law is broadly applicable across the whole of the UK.

Statute law is created through Acts of Parliament or through a system of delegated legislation which is becoming increasingly important due to the pressures on parliamentary time. Statutory Instruments, or Rules, form part of delegated legislation. They empower statutory bodies to expand or amend law for enactment by the Secretary of State. An example of this was the creation by the UKCC of parts 12–15 on the nurse registrar to enable Project 2000 nurses to register their qualification.

Old law and statute sometimes needs clarification. This happens through the judicial system and case law has developed as judges make decisions on the interpretation of law within the court setting. Once an outcome has been reached then a precedent is set for all other judges to follow in similar circumstances.

Decisions made are binding on all courts below that where the precedent was set. For example, the House of Lords is binding in the UK, but can overturn its own decisions. The European Court of justice can set precedent for other member states. Case law is of particular relevance to health care (Montgomery 1997).

Department of Health circulars and UKCC codes of practice, including the *Code of Conduct* (UKCC 1992a), are not legally binding but they are recommended practice. While the UKCC has legal status and authority under the Nurses, Midwives and Health Visitors Act (1979) to prepare rules that carry the weight of law, the *Code of Conduct* is issued for 'guidance and advice', laying a moral responsibility rather than a statutory duty on members of the profession. A marked failure to abide by the *Code* could, in turn, lead to the UKCC using its disciplinary function, with legal implications of removal of the nurse's name from the register.

Classification of Law

Of particular relevance in health care is the division into criminal and civil law. Criminal offences are committed against the state and are punishable by the state. Examples of relevance include drug offences and theft. Civil law is concerned with the rights and duties of individuals towards each other. Legal action is taken by a private citizen rather than the state, and a successful outcome results in an award of monetary compensation only, e.g. a patient suing a hospital for damages following some harm that has resulted from treatment or the lack thereof. Some civil wrongs can also be crimes, e.g. assault and battery, and gross negligence which could become manslaughter.

The concept of a legal defence is an important one. This is a legally recognised reason for the act committed not to have been a criminal or civil wrong. The most widely met example of this is the giving of consent as a defence against assault and battery. Civil law is probably the area of law of greatest significance to the A&E nurse. Negligence, or delict in Scotland, is the underpinning for the standard of care given to the patient, and the law on assault and battery, in civil law, for much of the reasoning behind patients' rights.

Negligence

For negligence of any kind to be proved, it must be shown that all four of the following components exist (Knight 1992):

■ that the defendant (nurse) owed a duty of care to the plaintiff (patient)

■ that the defendant was in breach of that duty
■ that the plaintiff suffered damage
■ that the damage was caused by the breach of duty of care.

The Bolam case (Pannett 1992) laid down the principle of how to judge the standard of care that must be given as that of the 'reasonably skilled and experienced doctor as accepted by a responsible body of medical men skilled in that particular art' (Bolam *v* Friern Hospital Management Committee 1957). The Wilsher case (Wilsher *v* Essex AHA 1988) made it clear that the standard of care required was that of the post held not of the post-holder (Tingle 1988). These precedents are applicable to all health care workers (see Box 39.1).

> **Box 39.1** – *Negligence checklist (Carson & Montgomery 1989)*
>
> 1. Did the nurse have a duty of care? If 'yes' continue. If 'no' there can be no liability.
>
> 2. Was there a breach in the appropriate standard of care? If 'yes' continue. If 'no' there can be no liability.
>
> 3. Did the breach of the standard cause the losses? If 'yes' continue. If 'no' there can be no liability.
>
> 4. Are the losses of a kind recognised by law? If 'yes' continue. If 'no' there can be no liability.
>
> 5. Were the losses too remote? If 'yes' continue. If 'no' there can be no liability.
>
> 6. Did the patient contribute to the happening or extent of his or her losses? If 'yes' there has been contributory negligence and the damages will be proportionately reduced.

Clinical documentation can be pivotal in cases of negligence (Green 1999). A&E nurses should be scrupulous in the documentation of their actions to reduce the risk of legal difficulties should a case be brought against them or their colleagues.

Assault and battery

The civil wrong of trespass can be committed to land, goods or the person. This last category is also known as assault and battery. Assault is an attempt or threat to apply unlawful force to the person of another, whereby that other person is put in fear of immediate violence or at least bodily contact. Battery is the actual application of force, however slight, to the person of another against his or her will.

> **Box 39.2** – *Legal defences to a civil action for assault and battery*
>
> ■ Consent
>
> ■ Urgency and necessity
>
> ■ Acting under a statutory power, e.g. the Mental Health Act
>
> ■ Patients' 'best interests'

There are a number of important defences against a legal action for trespass to the body (Box 39.2). Success in suing for trespass is not high and a number of patients have a better outcome using the law on negligence, e.g. in relation to inadequate information given in order to gain consent (Brazier 1992).

Attendance

There is a clear legal duty on the hospital running an A&E service to see and treat all those who attend. Purely by virtue of their coming within its doors, the hospital accepts responsibility, even without formally admitting them. A failure to treat those who present themselves could be negligence as demonstrated in Barnett *v* Chelsea and Kensington HMC (1969). In this particular case, three men attended having been vomiting for 3 hours. The nurse phoned the casualty officer (who was in bed) who told the nurse to send them home with instructions to call their own doctors. One of the men died within a few hours and his widow proved that the hospital doctor was careless in not coming to A&E to examine him, although there was no negligence as he would have died anyway (Morgan 1998).

People who bring alcoholic drinks with them and who are intoxicated also pose a dilemma. While it is possible to have some sympathy for the A&E staff in this situation who order the removal of these individuals by security staff, the law would not support such actions. In addition to the duty to see and treat those presenting themselves, there is also the possibility of assault and battery in their physical removal.

The situation would be different if those causing these difficulties were not there as patients, but as friends or relatives, or if the patient had already been seen and treated. In this case, the individuals can be asked to leave; a failure to do so would mean they were then trespassing on hospital property and can be evicted. Only reasonable force can be used and health carers should avoid involvement. All incidents of this kind should be documented.

Assessment

Most A&E departments have a system of assessing the urgency of patients' conditions on arrival. The criteria used to allocate patients to certain treatment groups largely relies on some degree of diagnosis. For the nurse, the legal significance of undertaking triage is whether he has sufficient knowledge to undertake this assessment competently. Assessing a patient as less critically ill than in fact is the case, with a subsequent delay in treatment, could result in negligence.

The UKCC's *Scope of Professional Practice* (UKCC 1992b) makes a nurse undertaking such roles personally accountable for his practice and for the maintenance and development of his knowledge and competence. It is tempered by the *Code of Professional Conduct* (UKCC 1992a) which states the nurse must 'acknowledge any limitations in her knowledge and competence and decline any duties or responsibilities unless able to perform them in a safe and skilled manner'.

If the nurse is required to carry out triage, the manager must provide the necessary training and carry the legal responsibility of delegating appropriately as there can be negligence in delegation. In addition, where triage is seen as part of the nurse's role, the employer will be vicariously liable for any negligence of the employee. This principle applies to any advanced practice agreed by the nurse and employing body. This employer liability arises from the old law of master and servant relationship, where the employer has to carry this legal responsibility by dint of having a contract with the employee. Vicarious liability may also exist with agency staff, but its extent may depend on the exact nature of the contract.

Under Section 2 of the Limitation Act (1980), a case for negligence must be commenced within 3 years of the date of the cause of the action or when the effects become apparent to the plaintiff (Pannett 1992). It may be considerably longer before the case comes to court. Section 14 of the Act also requires that the injury is significant and relates this to the plaintiff's knowledge of the injury. The lengthy timescale underlines the importance of A&E record-keeping for nursing and medical staff.

Treatment and Care

A vitally important question is: what is the standard of care that is expected and must be reached in the A&E department in order to avoid legal repercussions? From a number of legal cases relating to medical care, it is clear that the standard must be safe care and one which is accepted as proper by a responsible body of medical opinion (Mason & McCall-Smith 1987). Reasonable, rather than excellent, skill is considered sufficient. The standard in the A&E department will be that considered acceptable and reasonable in the conditions and circumstances in which nursing care is given.

The standard must relate to the speciality to which it is applied. Thus, nurses new to A&E work must be aware that inexperience can never be an excuse for negligence. This was stated very clearly in Wilsher *v* Essex AHA (1988), when inexperience in the work of the neonatal intensive care unit was put forward as a reason for the doctor's mistake in taking the wrong blood from Baby Wilsher and subsequently prescribing the wrong level of oxygen (Tingle 1988). Both Appeal Judges were emphatic that the standard of care must be that of the post held, not of the post-holder. The lesson to be learned from this is that adequate training and supervision are vital until the nurse is competent in the skills required.

The legal significance of the above applies to both the varied nature of the work as well as the range of skills of the workforce. For example, a number of people presenting to an A&E department are mentally ill, but there are a limited number of registered mental nurses (RMNs) employed in these areas and there may not be one on duty when needed. The registered general nurses therefore have to manage these patients to the best of their ability. In these circumstances, the standard is probably not that of the RMN, but of a nurse experienced in dealing with the range of circumstances presented by the mentally ill in this particular setting.

The importance of multidisciplinary teamwork is recognised in most patient care settings and is particularly relevant to A&E where a number of different professionals work together. Legally, the doctor has to take overall responsibility for a patient's care, but care roles have become blurred. In order to safeguard the different members of the team, care must be taken in delegating tasks to different members, whether it is across professional boundaries or from more senior members of the nursing team to those more junior.

Three checks can be made in order to avoid negligence (Young 1991):

- the extent of the nurse's knowledge
- the level of skill in the task delegated either through asking about past experience or through direct observation
- through teaching and supervision over a period of time.

Death and Organ Donation

A number of other different legal issues surround death in the A&E department. The first is the legal definition of death. Although this still stands as the total stoppage of circulation of blood and cessation of animal and vital body functions, the concept of brain stem death seems to be accepted by the courts. There will not, therefore, be a difficulty in turning off a life support system once brain stem death has been diagnosed. In addition, in situations where death has not occurred but prognosis and quality of life are so poor that to continue with treatment seems to have no useful purpose, the law accepts decisions not to do so.

Organ donation can create legal as well as ethical dilemmas in an A&E department (Sweet 1996). Under the Human Tissue Act (1961), consent for organ removal needs to be gained from the next of kin, if possible. The hospital staff are required to make such reasonable enquiry as may be practicable. If the deceased is identified and the parents, siblings or indeed any relative expresses an objection to the organs being used, then this will effectively prevent their use. While the letter of the Act states 'any surviving relative', in reality this can involve many people (Dimond 1990). The existence of a donor card, although not automatically giving consent, may be used as evidence of the deceased's wishes if relatives are not readily available (Young 1992). In these circumstances, the legal onus would be on the relatives to prove that the deceased had changed her mind, but in practice it is rare for organs to be removed if the relatives object. In all sudden deaths, the coroner's consent for organ removal must be obtained.

Patient Property

The same rules apply for the care of property in the A&E department as in a ward, but the clinical condition of some patients demands the nurse to become 'bailiff' for the property of those unable to take this responsibility themselves (Dimond 1990). The task of checking property soon after arrival in these cases is important, due to the open nature of the environment and the high risk of theft. Preferably, two people should together check, list, sign and ensure valuables are locked away safely. When death occurs, valuables should not be given to relatives, but again the proper hospital procedures should be followed.

In an emergency, such as cardiac arrests, clothing may have to be cut off, but this should only be done as a last resort. If clothes are heavily contaminated by blood or parasites and need to be destroyed, the patient's permission should be sought where possible and documentation of items destroyed should be made.

Consent to Treatment

For treatment to be given, a patient's consent must be gained in order to avoid being sued for assault and battery. For this consent to be legally effective, the patient must be able to understand and come to a decision about what is involved (Skegg 1984). Under common law, the patient has the right to give or withdraw consent for treatment or a procedure at any time.

Consent can be given in writing, orally or be assumed from the patient's actions, e.g. from the fact that the patient voluntarily attends the A&E department. Written consent is usually reserved for those treatments or investigations carrying a marked risk and is usually obtained by the doctor. It is important that the nurse does not take on this responsibility where it is not his role to do so. The nurse may be able to help clarify a patient's lack of understanding or assist the patient in finding out the information required, but taking on the medical role and giving inaccurate information means the nurse could be negligent.

For most nursing actions, consent will be gained orally. This is probably better practice professionally than assuming consent. It is not an unusual occurrence for patients to be brought into the department who are either unable or unwilling to give consent to treatment. As shown in Box 39.2, there are a number of legal 'defences' or reasons that treatment can be given, apart from consent, without there being a case for assault and battery.

When a patient cannot give a valid consent due to a lack of understanding, treatment that is urgent and necessary can still be given. Thus the unconscious, semiconscious or mentally confused patient can be treated on this basis. Nonetheless, in law, the health professionals' care for patients in the absence of consent is part of their duty to care for them out of necessity in an emergency and they would have to defend any subsequent action for trespass to the person on that basis (Young 1991). Those suffering the effects of alcohol or drugs could also be included in this category.

With a child it is usual, if the child is under 16, for the consent of the parents or guardian to be sought. If only one parent is available, clearly this is the one taken even if the parents are separated. If the situation is too urgent to await the arrival of a parent, the child can give consent if she has sufficient understanding or the urgency and necessity rule can be used. The Children Act (Department of Health 1989) also makes it clear that the child's wishes are paramount and no court direction overrides the child's right of refusal to be examined provided she has sufficient understanding (Oates 1993). A 'Gillick aware' minor is capable of full understanding and appreciation of the intended consequences of treatment and possible side-effects and also the anticipated consequences of failure to treat. The degree of maturity required will depend on the treatment proposed. Simple treatment needs a simple decision requiring little maturity, while complex matters require a mature mind (Montague 1996).

Predicaments can arise in any of these situations when relatives either take a different view from the patient or claim that the patient, if mentally capable, would have refused consent. The often quoted example is of the unconscious patient who is a Jehovah's Witness and requires a blood transfusion. The A&E team can still proceed on the basis that, as this is an unforeseen emergency, it would be impossible to know the patient's wishes if faced with possible death.

Relatives may also expect to be in the position of giving consent on behalf of an adult patient unable to do so. There is no legal basis for asking relatives for their consent in these circumstances. They may be consulted, but the decision to proceed with treatment will be a medical one on the basis of urgency and necessity. The law also supports the notion of proceeding if it is in the patient's 'best interests' (NHS Management Executive 1990), although this is not usually applied to emergency situations.

Health carers also face a difficulty when caring for a patient who is still conscious but is refusing treatment following a drug overdose. The patient could be put under the emergency section of the Mental Health Act (1983) and treatment then given against her will, but it would be wrong to assume all those attempting suicide are mentally disordered under the terms of the Act. Castledine (1994) argued that an apparently irrational refusal can still be a competent one and the decision whether to treat or not may then become an ethical one. Proceeding against the patient's will lays the carers open to an action for assault and battery, but this is unlikely to be implemented. If the patient recovers, she may be so relieved to be alive, she would rather thank the staff than sue them. Conversely, the patient may be so determined to die that she will make sure the next attempt is successful without waiting for the case to go to court. Abiding by the patient's wishes, on the other hand, while legally correct, may leave the carers wondering whether they should have done more.

In many of these predicaments, the legal difficulty may be one of balancing patients' rights against a possible accusation of negligence in failing to act. Whatever is decided, both arguments should be considered and, if particularly contentious, a written record made of how the decision was reached.

Detention of Patients

As well as times when it is legally acceptable to treat without the patient's consent, there are also occasions when individuals can be detained against their will (Young 1989). Of relevance to the health care worker in the A&E department are the following. Patients may be detained under Section 4 of the Mental Health Act 1983. Admission to hospital for assessment in cases of emergency lasts for 72 hours. The grounds for using this order are an urgent necessity that the patient should be admitted and detained for assessment and that compliance with the normal procedure would involve undesirable delay. The recommendation of only one medical practitioner is required. There will be arrangements made for an on-call psychiatrist to attend the A&E department.

The only other section likely to be met is Section 136. This order can be invoked by the police on finding a person in a public place who appears to be suffering from a mental disorder and in immediate need of care or control. Occasionally, such a person may be brought to the A&E department, although more often she may be held at the police station, which is designated as a 'place of safety' under the Act, for examination by the police surgeon prior to further action. Some patients may be mentally confused due to physical illness, e.g. hypoxia following heart failure. The patient can be detained in the short term for emergency treatment, the law accepting the necessity for this. A failure to do so could be deemed negligence.

Much rarer is the situation of an individual with a certain infectious disease potentially dangerous to others who refuses to stay for treatment. An order made by a magistrate or sheriff can be issued to detain the person who will then be rapidly transferred to an appropriate unit.

The police may detain a person in the A&E department. For example, the patient may have been injured at the time of arrest. In this case it is the police's responsibility to detain, never the nurse's. Even if the police request the nurse to assist them in preventing the patient leaving the department, he should refuse to become involved. The fact that someone is a detained prisoner does not lessen her right to treatment, confidentiality or refusal to consent to procedures.

Confidentiality, the Police and the Press

Professionally, nurses are required to respect confidentiality, but a number of situations arise in A&E that can pose difficulties for those concerned. For example, the UKCC (1987) advice on confidentiality cites the example of staff who found that the unconscious patient they were treating had a gun on his person.

Although patients should be able to expect staff to maintain confidentiality, there are times when that expectation must be broken. If the nurse has to give evidence in court, privilege on the basis of professional position cannot be claimed and the nurse will have to give the information required. The courts can also order the release of medical and nursing notes prior to the court case. In most circumstances, however, there is no legal requirement for the nurse to make statements to the police when asked, although carers in the A&E department should aim to cooperate with the police as far as possible. Staff sometimes feel pressurised by the police to give information that they would prefer not to provide. The nurse should refer police either to the doctor, if the query involves a diagnosis or fitness of the patient to be interviewed, or to a senior manager.

The situation of the gun poses more of an ethical problem than a legal one. Legally, the nurse can maintain confidentiality, but may want to share this information in case the gun is being used illegally and, potentially, to harm others. The *Code of Professional Conduct* (UKCC 1992a) suggests that breach of confidentiality may be necessary 'in the public interest', and the nurse may judge that the situation of the patient with a gun falls into this category. The UKCC (1987) is quite clear that the individual practitioner must make the decision. The nurse should discuss the situation with others and record how the decision was reached, in case of later repercussions.

There is one situation where disclosure of confidential information to the police is required. Under the Prevention of Terrorism Act (Temporary Provisions Act 1984) it is an offence for any person having information which he or she believes may be of material assistance in preventing terrorism or apprehending terrorists to fail, without reasonable cause, to give that information to the police (Dimond 1990). Other circumstances where disclosure of confidential information to the police in the patient's interests may be considered are where child abuse is suspected. Most departments will have clearly laid down guidelines to follow if symptoms point to abuse. The disastrous consequences of not taking action have been well publicised, as has the distress caused to both child and parents when action has been taken on grounds that are later found to be unsubstantiated. A team approach is usually seen as essential.

The health care worker in the A&E department is sure to have a certain amount of contact with the police and, possibly, the press. It is important to be aware of the respective rights of patients, hospital employees and police in these circumstances. The police have a number of powers regarding search and arrest and these will apply to a hospital in the same way as a private dwelling because hospitals are Crown property, not public property. Police can enter premises without a search warrant if the person they wish to search for is suspected of an arrestable offence. An intimate search of body orifices can be authorised if the person concerned is likely to have concealed an item to injure herself or others, or for drugs. Police are entitled to use reasonable force in carrying out an intimate search.

In relation to arrest, police may arrest without a warrant if they suspect that an arrestable offence has been, is being or is about to be committed. Examples of an arrestable offence are unlawful possession of drugs, rape and most offences of violence (English & Card 1985). If the police suspect that an individual who is currently a patient in A&E has committed a serious offence, the staff should not hinder the police in their work, but should ensure the medical condition of the individual is not jeopardised.

A final situation where patient confidentiality may be put at risk is through press enquiries. Most hospitals will have strict rules on which staff are allowed to talk to the press. It is wise for staff always to refer these enquiries to the appropriate senior member of staff.

Staff Health and Safety

Both verbal abuse and physical violence against staff are not unusual occurrences in the A&E department. Police attendance at such incidents can be requested. The nurses involved will need to make statements to the police. However, quite often no charges will be brought against the individual.

The law can be relevant in a number of ways. First, violent actions could be the crime of assault, battery or causing grievous bodily harm. However, the police are often unable to charge a person on the basis of these crimes as there is often some doubt as to whether the person intended to commit the crime. Proving intention is necessary for a successful prosecution. If the patient is mentally ill, drunk or under the influence of drugs, she could claim that she could not form the necessary intention. Increasingly, however, courts take a poor view of acts of violence carried out under the influence of drink or drugs which offenders have taken to deprive themselves of their self-control or their knowledge of what they were doing.

For most criminal charges, not only is self-induced intoxication no defence, but if the offender claims that she only did it because of intoxication, the prosecution are absolved from proving any mental element and need simply prove that the act was done. It is thus easier to obtain a conviction (Montague 1996). It also underlines the need for clear, contemporaneous notes to be taken by staff and witnesses in case of legal action being taken. If injuries are sustained, the statement will provide evidence of the event and the nurse may be able to claim from the Criminal Injuries Compensation Board even in the absence of a successful prosecution.

Assault and battery are also civil wrongs. This means the nurse could sue the individual through the civil courts for damages. In this context, intention does not have to be proved, so evidence of the incident would lead to a successful legal action. It is rare, however, for nurses to take this route. Finally the nurse could complain to the employer that there has been a failure to provide a safe working environment, under common law, the Occupiers Liability Act (1957) and the Health and Safety at Work Act (1974). However, the employer only has to take reasonable steps to ensure the health, safety and welfare of the employees. It is difficult for the employer to create a totally safe environment in A&E, because of the nature of the work undertaken and the open access of the department to the public. If the employee considers further measures should be taken, she should consult with the health and safety representative of her trade union or professional body (see also Ch. 40).

Other health and safety issues in the A&E department are very similar to those elsewhere, e.g. infection risks, moving and handling patients and fire hazards. European Union Directives, laid out in a number of UK Health and Safety Regulations (1992), have resulted in the broadening of the requirements and improved protection of staff in the area of safety. The provision of training and adequate equipment are key elements of any statutory requirements.

Conclusion

In the medicolegal sense, A&E has been described as the most dangerous part of a hospital (Knight 1992). It is important, therefore, for A&E nurses to have a working knowledge of the law if they are to prevent legal problems arising in the first place. This chapter has introduced the main areas of law of relevance in A&E and discussed the implications for A&E practitioners. Like practice, however, the law is constantly evolving and it is in the nurse's interest to keep abreast of these developments.

Further reading

Byrne P (1990) *Ethics and Law in Health Care and Research*. Chichester: Wiley.

Dyer C (1992) *Doctors, patients and the Law*. Oxford: Blackwell.

Faulder C (1985) *Whose Body is it?* London: Virago.

Gostin L (1983) *A Practical Guide to Mental Health Law*. London: MIND.

Hodgson J (1992) *Employment Law for Nurses*. Lancaster: Quay.

Kennedy I, Grubb A (1989) *Medical Law and Ethics*. London: Butterworth.

Kennedy I (1991) *Treat me Right: Essays in Medical Law and Ethics*. Oxford: Oxford University Press.

Montgomery J (1997) *Health Care Law*. Oxford: Oxford University Press.

Pyne R (1992) *Professional Discipline in Nursing*, 2nd edn. Oxford: Blackwell.

References

Brazier M (1987) *Medicine, Patients and the Law*. Harmondsworth: Penguin Books.

Brazier M (1992) *Medicine, patients and the Law*, 2nd edn. Harmondsworth: Penguin Books.

Carson D, Montgomery J (1989) *Nursing and the Law*. Basingstoke: Macmillan.

Castledine G (1994) Ethics and the law in A&E. *Emergency Nurse*, **2**(1), 25.

Department of Health (1989) *The Children Act*. London: HMSO.

Dimond B (1990) *Legal Aspects of Nursing*. Hemel Hempstead: Prentice Hall.

English J, Card R (1985) *Police Law*. London: Butterworths.

Green C (1999) The Nurse and professional negligence. *Nursing Times*, **95**(8), 57–59.

Health and Safety at Work Act (1974) London: HMSO.

Health and Safety (General Provisions) Regulations (1992) London: HMSO.

Human Tissue Act (1961) London: HMSO.

Knight B (1992) *Legal Aspects of Medical Practice* 5th edn. Edinburgh: Churchill Livingstone.

Limitation Act (1980) London: HMSO.

Mason JK, McCall-Smith RA (1987) *Law and Medical Ethics*, 2nd edn. London: Butterworths.

Mental Health Act (1983) London: HMSO.

Montague A (1996) *Legal Problems in Emergency Medicine*. Oxford: Oxford University Press.

Montgomery J (1997) *Health Care Law*. Oxford: Oxford University Press.

Morgan J (1998) Establishing medical negligence. *Emergency Nurse*, **6**(5),

NHS Management Executive (1990) *A Guide to Consent for Examination or Treatment*. London: NHS Management Executive.

Nurses, Midwives and Health Visitors Act (1979) London: HMSO.

Oates M (1993) Children Act 1989: the essential issues. *Emergency Nurse*, **1**(1), 21–22.

Occupiers Liability Act (1957) London: HMSO.

Pannett AJ (1992) *Law of Torts*, 6th edn. London: Pitman.

Prevention of Terrorism Act (Temporary Provisions Act) (1984) London: HMSO.

Skegg PDG (1984) *Law, Ethics and Medicine*. Oxford: Clarendon Press.

Sweet A (1996) Organ donation in A&E. *Emergency Nurse*, **3**(4), 6–9.

Tingle JH (1988) Negligence and Wilsher. *Solicitors Journal*, **132**(25), 910–911.

UKCC (1987) *Confidentiality, Advisory Paper*. London: UKCC.

UKCC (1992a) *Code of Professional Conduct*, 3rd edn. London: UKCC.

UKCC (1992b) *Scope of Professional Practice*. London: UKCC.

Young AP (1989) *Legal Problems in Nursing Practice*, 2nd edn. London: Chapman and Hall.

Young AP (1991) *Law and Professional Conduct in Nursing*. London: Scutari Press.

Young AP (1992) *Case Studies in Law and Nursing*. London: Chapman and Hall.

Chapter 40

Maintaining a Safe Environment

Sheelagh Brewer

■ Preventing accidents
■ Legislation
■ Legislation since 1992
■ Infection control
■ Working time
■ Framework for maintaining a safe environment
■ Conclusion

Introduction

It seems incongruous that a service set up to provide emergency care sometimes causes harm to the staff involved in delivering that care. Accident statistics (Chard 1993) show that the physical and mental health of nurses is put at risk within their working environment to an extent where permanent disability and subsequent loss of career are possible. Regulations and requirements to provide a safe environment exist to protect employees and others, such as patients, visitors, contractors' employees and agency staff. This chapter considers various aspects of accidents at work, describes the legal responsibilities of employers and employees, and also how this legislation is applied to hazards found in A&E departments.

Preventing Accidents

The Health and Safety Executive (1993) use the term 'accident' to refer to any unplanned event that results in injury or ill health of people, or damage or loss to property, plant, materials or the environment, or a loss of business opportunity. Before any action can be taken to prevent accidents, the causes must be identified. Causes can be divided into unsafe conditions (e.g. wet floors, trailing cables, insufficient lifting aids, faulty equipment) or unsafe acts (e.g. nurses' failure to wear protective equipment or ignoring safety instructions). Unsafe acts arise from lack of training or nurses' attitudes towards their own safety. Workplaces should be regularly inspected to check that hazards do not exist and, although trade union safety representatives have this as part of their role, it should be a cooperative process between staff, managers and safety representatives. Local policies should encourage nurses to report hazards before accidents occur so that preventive action may be taken.

If an accident does occur, accurate records are needed. From the employer's point of view there is a duty to report certain types of accidents defined within the Reporting of Injury, Diseases and Dangerous Occurrence Regulations (RIDDOR) (1995) to the Health and Safety Executive. Failure to do so is a criminal offence. The employer needs information about an accident so the event can be investigated to prevent its recurrence. Employees are obliged to report accidents and it is in their interests to accurately complete accident forms and accident books to protect themselves in the event of future loss of income or long-term effects of injury or disease.

It has always been difficult to arrive at the true costs of accidents and yet this information could provide an incentive to tackling the problem of workplace accidents, by providing a measurement against which financial loss can be judged. In 1989, the HSE's Accident Prevention Advisory Unit carried out a series of five case studies with the aim of developing a methodology to accurately identify the full costs of accidents (Health & Safety Executive 1993). One such study looked at a hospital employing 200 people. Over a period of 13 weeks the cost of accidents totalled just under £100 000, equating on an annual basis to 5% of the hospital's running costs (Health & Safety Executive 1993). More recently, the National Audit Office (1996) carried out a survey of health and safety in the NHS Acute Hospital Trusts in England. As a result, the estimate of the immediate costs of accidents in NHS Acute Hospital Trusts in England was £12 million. When the longer-term costs are taken into account, this figure rises to £154 million. The cost of an accident is directly related to the outcome of that accident. This, however, can be difficult to predict; a needlestick injury may or may not result in a nurse contracting hepatitis B. The total cost of accidents must include the cost of maintaining a safe environment. A relationship exists between underlying safety control and accident occurrence.

Implementing safety control will involve some cost, such as staff communication and training, physical protection (alarm systems), publicity campaigns, time spent in risk assessment, inspecting the workplace for hazards and maintenance of equipment (Royal College of Nursing 1998). These costs will be offset by the direct and indirect costs resulting from accidents and ill health, such as occupational sick pay, equipment damage, disruption in patient care, damage to the environment, costs of replacement staff and costs of litigation. The management responsibility is to decide how much to spend on controlling the causes of accidents in order to minimise their financial impact.

Legislation

The health service was not covered by any health and safety legislation until 1974 when the Health & Safety at Work etc. Act was passed. This is still the major legislative power and any new regulations come under its framework. Its provisions applied to all health care premises although the NHS enjoyed Crown Immunity at the time and could not be prosecuted for any breaches of health and safety law. A trade union campaign to remove Crown Immunity began in the 1980s and this, combined with the outbreak of food poisoning in 1984 at Stanley Royd Hospital, Wakefield, in which 19 patients died, resulted in the removal of Crown Immunity from both the Health & Safety at Work Act (1974) and the Food Hygiene Regulations (1970). Since 1987, the NHS has been subject to the same processes of enforcement as any other employer.

The Health & Safety at Work Act (1974) specifies the duties of the employer with the general requirement to 'ensure, so far as is reasonably practicable, the health, safety & welfare at work of all his employees' (Section 2(1)). The Act then specifies the particular areas where this duty applies. (see Box 40.1)

Another section of the Health & Safety at Work Act

Box 40.1 – *Duties of employer in the Health & Safety at Work Act 1974*

■ The provision of plant and systems of work that are without risk to health and safety. In addition, the equipment must be maintained so it remains safe. This could include systems of handling and moving patients, infection control procedures or extraction systems to remove hazardous fumes

■ Making arrangements in the use, handling, storage and transport of articles and substances so that the risk is minimised. The safe disposal of clinical waste including sharps would be covered by this requirement

■ Providing information, instruction, training and supervision so that employees are kept safe at work. General training on health and safety must be provided along with specific training on particular hazards of handling of loads and fire procedures

■ Providing and maintaining a safe place of work so that there is adequate heating, lighting, ventilation and fire exits

■ Provision of adequate welfare facilities. Welfare is a very broad area but could include access to occupational health services, vaccination against hepatitis B, facilities for changing, showers and toilets and a smoke-free working environment

(1974) defines the duty of the employer to non-employees, including patients, visitors and contractors' employees, to ensure these people are also protected from harm whilst they are on the premises. Systems of work must be developed to protect these groups. Floor cleaning is an example of the need to ensure that staff and others are prevented from walking on wet, slippery floors by the use of coned areas and warning signs.

The approach to health and safety legislation is to involve both employers and employees. The Health & Safety at Work Act (1974) specifies that all employees must take reasonable care for the health and safety of themselves and others who may be affected by their acts or omissions and cooperate with the employer to enable compliance with statutory requirements. If the employer provides any protective equipment, such as gloves, goggles or aprons, the employee must wear it. This presumes the employer has defined the need for the equipment and has trained staff in the correct use.

The Health & Safety at Work Act (1974) is a wide-ranging piece of legislation and one which permits further regulations to be developed which refer to specific aspects of health and safety. In 1992, six new sets of regulations were enacted which were based on EC Directives, but prior to that, in the period 1974–1992, other regulations included:

■ Safety Representatives & Safety Committees Regulations (1977) which define the rights and functions of trade union appointed safety representatives and the arrangements for safety committees.
■ Health & Safety (First-Aid) Regulations (1981) which provide a framework for the provision of first aid arrangements for employees. Even in A&E departments procedures need to be defined for staff who suffer an accident.
■ Reporting of Injuries, Diseases & Dangerous Occurrences Regulations (1995) which specify the duty on the employer to report to the Health & Safety Executive certain categories of injuries, dangerous occurrences and designated diseases.

In the case of disease, the nature of the work is specified. Hepatitis B is a reportable disease for anyone who comes into contact with blood, blood products or body secretions. The regulations specify the type of dangerous occurrences which must be reported, whether or not anyone has been injured. Similarly, the specific types of injury are defined along with a broad category of any injury which results in absence from work for 3 days or more. These regulations were amended in 1995 to cover injuries that result from a violent assault. In addition to a fatal injury, the other reportable major injuries are outlined in Box 40.2.

Box 40.2 – *Reportable major injuries under RIDDOR (1995)*

■ Fracture other than to fingers, thumbs or toes

■ Amputation

■ Dislocation of the shoulder, hip, knee or spine

■ Loss of sight (temporary or permanent)

■ Chemical or hot metal burn to the eye or any penetrating injury to the eye

■ Injury resulting from an electric shock or electrical burn leading to unconsciousness or requiring resuscitation or admittance to hospital for more than 24 hours

■ Any other injury leading to hypothermia, heat-induced illness or unconsciousness or requiring admittance to hospital for more than 24 hours

■ Acute illness requiring medical treatment or loss of consciousness arising from absorption of any substance by inhalation, ingestion or through the skin

■ Acute illness requiring medical treatment where there is reason to believe that this resulted from exposure to a biological agent or its toxins or infected material

---

Control of Substances Hazardous to Health Regulations (1994)

The Control of Substances Hazardous to Health (COSHH) Regulations (1994) were implemented in response to concerns about the effect on health of exposure to hazardous substances and replaced and revoked the earlier COSHH Regulations (1988). Dangerous substances must be categorised in terms of hazard and risk. A hazardous substance is one which has the potential to cause harm. The risk is the likelihood that it will cause harm in the actual circumstances where it is used. The regulations require the employer to carry out an assessment of the risk and subsequently to establish a safe system of work. The definition of a hazardous substance is any solid, liquid, gas, fume, vapour or microorganism that can endanger health by being absorbed or injected through the skin or mucous membranes, inhaled or digested. One exclusion is substances administered as part of a medical treatment, although the impact on the health care worker would need to be assessed.

Once the assessment has been carried out, steps must be taken to prevent or at least control exposure.

Prevention is the ideal solution to the problem but there will be circumstances where this is not reasonably practicable. Glutaraldehyde is the most effective cold disinfectant available and may not be substituted by other chemicals. It is, however, an eye and nasal irritant and can cause dermatitis, asthma and eczema. There is a maximum exposure limit of 0.05 parts per million (ppm) over an 8 hour time-weighted average, but it is difficult to monitor airborne glutaraldehyde. In these circumstances careful measures of control must be devised and implemented. Glutaraldehyde must be used in closed systems such as automated washers, but the very minimum is a trough with a lid. Goggles and nitrile gloves should also be worn. Whenever glutaraldehyde is in use there should be an efficient ventilation system. The regulations require the control measures to be properly used and maintained and for employees and non-employees to be informed, instructed and trained in what the risks are and how to control them.

Where nurses have been exposed to risk there is a requirement to carry out health surveillance. Health surveillance is needed to protect the health of individuals by detecting adverse changes attributed to exposure to hazardous substances at the earliest possible stage. This will help in assessing the effectiveness of control measures. Where health surveillance is carried out, the employees' health records must be kept for 30 years.

Within A&E departments and fracture clinics there are three main areas of risk where COSHH assessments should be carried out. The first is chemical exposure including drugs and plaster of Paris dust. The assessment and subsequent control measures should consider storage, local ventilation, waste disposal, need for personal protective equipment, training and air monitoring. Special attention should be paid to the type of environment and the potential for patients, accompanying relatives and children to gain unauthorised access to materials such as antiseptics.

The second group of substances comprises the disinfectants such as phenolics, hypochlorites, glutaraldehyde alcohol mixtures and idophors. Many of these can be irritant to the skin and eyes. The third group of hazards involves the microbiological hazards from contact with body fluids such as blood, vomit and urine. Every patient must be regarded as a potential biohazard and it is impossible to identify all those who are seropositive to HIV or hepatitis B. Clear infection control procedures must be adhered to by nurses and routine barrier methods used to prevent contamination by blood or body fluids. The RCN information sheet on universal precautions gives clear guidance (Royal College of Nursing 1987a).

Chlorine-releasing disinfecting agents used in spillages of urine can be used as an example of the application of COSHH. The indiscriminate use of powdered or granular products designed to disinfect and contain spills of body fluids can lead to ill effects in staff and patients through exposure to chlorine. The use of such a substance must be controlled so it does not become a greater danger than the risk of infection. A COSHH assessment in this instance would consider both microbiological and chemical hazards. It would take into account the urgency of any situation, the nature of the spillage, the quantities that might be spilt and the degree of ventilation. With this information a system of work may be defined to cover storage, handling and use of any disinfecting agent, the procedure for dissolving or diluting it before use and the need for any personal protection for the user.

Legislation since 1992

Health and safety is an issue which has featured prominently in European legislation. Article 118A of the Single European Act 1986 (EU 1986) states that member states shall pay particular attention to encouraging improvements especially in the working environment as regards the health and safety of workers and shall set as their objective the harmonisation of conditions in this area, whilst maintaining the improvements made.

Directly arising out of this article was a Framework Directive (EC Directive 1989) on health and safety with a number of so called 'daughter directives' covering manual handling, personal protective equipment, work equipment, the workplace, temporary workers and display screen equipment. Once these directives were agreed, European Union member states were required to include the provisions of the directives into their own law by 1992. In the UK, this resulted in a set of regulations often referred to as 'the six pack', comprising:

■ the Management of Health & Safety at Work Regulations 1992 (Health & Safety Commission 1992)
■ the Display Screen Equipment Regulations 1992 (Health & Safety Executive 1992a)
■ the Manual Handling Operations Regulations 1992 (Health & Safety Executive 1992b)
■ the Personal Protective Equipment Regulations 1992 (Health & Safety Executive 1992c)
■ the Work Equipment Regulations 1992 (Health & Safety Executive 1992d) (replaced by The Provision and Use of Work Equipment Regulations 1998 and the Lifting Equipment Regulations 1998)

- the Workplace Regulations 1992 (Health & Safety Executive 1992e).

Although all of these have relevance in A&E departments, the first two are considered in more detail.

The Management of Health & Safety at Work Regulations 1992

These regulations build on and make more explicit the duties of employers and employees defined in the Health & Safety at Work Act (1974). The main requirement is the need to carry out a risk assessment for every hazard in the workplace (see Box 40.3). All of the activities and processes carried out within the A&E service should be subjected to the process of risk assessment.

Box 40.3 – *Some possible hazards in the workplace*

- Chemical hazards, e.g. glutaraldehyde and formaldehyde

- Biological hazards, e.g. blood-borne and airborne infections

- Electrical hazards

- Manual handling

- Physical hazards, e.g. violence

- Psychological hazards, e.g. stress

- Equipment, e.g. autoclaves, sharp instruments, computers

- Ionising radiation, e.g. diagnostic X-rays

- Hot and cold working conditions

- Poor lighting

- Fire

- Workplace layout and design

Risk assessment

Nursing staff should be involved in risk assessment because they are familiar with the environment, the procedures and equipment used. Risk assessment is the starting point for total risk management. The aim is to identify where things could go wrong and what the effect would be. Risk may arise from physical hazards, e.g. unsafe flooring, poor lighting, no alarm systems, or working practices, e.g. failure to dispose of sharps safely, failure to wear gloves, failure to alter bed heights when moving patients. Risk assessment then identifies:

- probability of exposure to risk
- frequency of exposure to risk
- maximum probable effect which could range from minor injury to fatal injury
- number of persons at risk.

Some risk assessment procedures apply numerical values to these items which are multiplied together to produce an overall risk score. This can be used to introduce greater objectivity and to look at relative risks from hazards, but in some cases it may be misleading. With manual handling, for example, an uncooperative patient will have an impact on the assessment. A skilled assessor, sensitive to all the variables, may produce a more useful assessment than the application of numerical values.

The process of risk assessment should result in a decision as to whether the risk is acceptable or not. If not, further work is required to control the risk. Elimination is the ideal solution but may not be always possible. Other methods of control are:

- to substitute a less hazardous process or substance
- to use engineering methods such as ventilation systems
- to redefine systems of work
- to provide personal protective equipment
- to immunise staff where possible
- to define emergency procedures.

The results of the risk assessment must be written and all staff affected must be informed about the risks and about the preventive measures or controls to be used (Clough 1998).

There are specific requirements relating to pregnant employees which were incorporated as a result of the EU Pregnant Workers Directive (1992). The risk assessment must cover any risks to the health and safety of a new or expectant mother from physical, biological or chemical agents. Where the risk cannot be avoided, the employer must alter the individual's working conditions or hours of work. If it is not reasonable to do so or if it would not avoid the risk, the employer must offer suitable alternative employment or suspend the employee from work. Furthermore, if the employee works nights and medical evidence states that this is a health risk, the employer must provide other employment or suspend her from work.

In addition to the requirement to carry out risk assessment, the Management of Health & Safety at Work Regulations (1992) contain other important duties. If the assessment identifies that nurses will be exposed to risk, it may be necessary to provide health surveillance. This is needed where there is an identifiable disease related to the work and where the techniques exist to detect indications of the disease. If a nurse is exposed to glutaraldehyde, it may be appropriate to carry out lung function tests. Under these regulations the employer must appoint one or more competent persons to provide health and safety assistance. This could be one person or a team depending on the size of the organisation. They may be appointed from existing employees or brought in on a consultancy basis. In any event they must have adequate time and resources to carry out their functions.

The employer must take account of employers' capabilities, training and knowledge experience when allocating work. Training on health and safety must be given in working practices and systems introducing new equipment. The training must be repeated periodically and carried out during the employees' working hours. Specific reference is made to temporary staff. Where agency or bank staff are used, essential information must be provided about the workplace and about any particular risks to health and safety. These regulations clearly define what is needed to develop an organisational safety culture and provide the framework within which departmental approaches are developed.

Employees duties

The duty of the employee to cooperate includes the use of equipment, dangerous substances, transport equipment, means of production or safety device and the need to operate these in accordance with training and instruction received. Additional duties are specified; each employee must inform the employer of any work situation which represents a serious and immediate danger to health and safety and any shortcoming in the protection arrangements for health and safety believed to exist by the employee.

This duty can be considered in the light of provisions within the Employment Rights Act (1996) which gives employment protection to employees in relation to health & safety. Employees and safety representatives have the right not to have action short of dismissal or be dismissed in the following circumstances:

■ where they have been designated by the employer to carry out activities to prevent or reduce risks to health and safety and have done so or are proposing to do so
■ where the employee is a safety representative and is acting in that capacity
■ where the employee left the workplace because of serious and imminent danger
■ where the employee took steps to, or proposed to take appropriate steps to, protect himself or others from the danger. The protection applies regardless of length of service.

Nurses are able to combine their responsibilities in the UKCC *Code of Professional Conduct* (1992) with health and safety regulations to take action to secure a safe working environment. Staff are an expensive resource and staffing costs are now closely monitored and reduced wherever possible. If a nurse believes staffing levels are insufficient to provide safe standards of practice, she has a responsibility to report this. It is also likely that such staffing levels would pose a risk to the health and safety of other staff and so the nurse would be compelled under health and safety legislation to report this also.

Manual Handling Operations Regulations 1992

The impact of manual handling on the health of nurses has long been recognised, but these are the first set of regulations to address the problem specifically. In health care, 50% of all accidents reported to the Health and Safety Executive are related to manual handling and, of these, 70% are as a result of patient handling (Royal College of Nursing 1996). A survey undertaken on behalf of the Royal College of Nursing (Smith & Secombe 1996) showed that, of those surveyed, 32% reported having had time off work due to back pain or injury. As far as recent absence was concerned, the survey found that 5% of respondents reported that they had taken time off in the previous 6 months as a consequence of back pain or injury. Extrapolating the figures suggests that no less than 14 000 nurses had time off in the 6 months preceding the study. It is estimated that at least 93 000 nurses have had time off due to back pain or injury at some time during their career.

The Manual Handling Operations Regulations (Health & Safety Executive 1992b) require the employer to avoid the need for employees to undertake any manual handling operations at work which involve a risk of injury. This is qualified by the phrase 'so far as is reasonably practicable' and where this applies the employer must carry out an assessment to reduce the risk to the lowest level reasonably practicable. The approach in the risk assessment is based on ergonomic principles of optimising the fit between the nurse and her work.

The guidance to the regulations identifies four factors for the assessment:

■ the task
■ the load
■ the environment
■ individual capability.

These factors are interrelated and may not be considered in isolation. What is required is a completely new attitude to the manual handling of patients which starts from an approach that no nurse should be required to manually lift any patients and that systems of work must be developed which enable this to happen. In 1996, the Royal College of Nursing revised its code of practice for patient handling. The aim is to eliminate hazardous manual handling in all but exceptional or life-threatening situations.

Examples of the risk factors under the four headings are summarised in Box 40.4. Once the risk factors have been identified, the next stage is to take steps to eliminate or reduce the risk. Possible control measures are summarised in Box 40.5.

Box 40.4 – *Risk factors in lifting patients*

Patients
- Weight
- Cooperation
- Dependency
- Consciousness level
- Condition
- Pain
- Comprehension
- Behavioural problems

Task
- Frequency
- Repetition
- Job rotation
- Holding loads away from trunk, reaching upwards long distances
- Restrictions by uniform twisting/stooping
- Awkward posture
- Urgency of task

Environment
- Space to move freely
- Floor slippery, uneven, lightly adequate
- Other tripping hazards, equipment available, equipment in good repair

Employee
- Training
- Danger to pregnant staff
- Danger to those with health problems, stress levels

Box 40.5 – *Control factors when lifting patients*

Patient
- Use mechanical equipment
- Involve patient
- Explain to patient
- Consider patient's dignity
- Consider any attachments to patient

Task
- Sufficient number of staff
- Improved design of task
- Rest breaks for staff
- Decreased distances for moving patient, improved equipment
- Adjustable heights on equipment

Environment
- Use of ranges for easier movement
- Harmonise heights of work surfaces, location of equipment
- Improve lighting, temperature, noise levels
- Improve tidiness and cleanliness

Employee
- Improve individual technique
- Report unsafe systems
- Provide training
- Consider individual situations, e.g. pregnancy
- Increase level of supervision to eliminate poor practice

The assessment will take place at two levels. First, the workplace itself must be assessed by the department manager in conjunction with any specialist help. This assessment will take into account departmental accident and absence statistics, layout, availability of handling aids and training of staff. Once completed, the risk-reducing actions are likely to have been identified and action plans developed.

The particular needs of the nature of the work make a difference to the assessment. In A&E areas, it would be appropriate to develop generic assessments for many of the transfers which take place, e.g. trolley to bed, wheelchair to bed. In emergency situations, an on-the-spot assessment is needed by skilled staff to judge whether the generic assessment is relevant. The risk assessment must be written and should be available to staff who need the information. If circumstances change so that the assessment is no longer valid, it must be updated. The next level of assessment is in relation to individual patients. In wards or in the community, a manual handling assessment would be incorporated into the patient care plan. Within A&E, a system should exist which would enable an initial manual handling assessment to be carried out; this would need updating as the patient's condition and treatment are known.

The duties of the employee under these regulations are to make full and proper use of the systems provided by the employer. Nursing staff have a responsibility for their own actions and their own competence. Where training on manual handling is available the nurse should attend. If the training is not provided, the nurse should be requesting that she has the opportunity to receive this training.

Infection Control

Infection control is particularly important within A&E because the status of each patient arriving in the department will not be known and treatment may be necessary before there is any indication that the patient may present a risk. Specific local infection control policies are needed in relation to cleaning the workplace, use of disinfectants, hand washing, dealing with laundry, protective clothing, disposal of waste and transport of specimens.

Contact with patient's blood/body fluids now carries with it the risk of occupational exposure to blood-borne infections such as HIV or hepatitis B. Health care workers need to follow universal precautions to prevent contamination by blood/body fluids. These precautions include covering any abrasions to exposed skin, wearing disposable powder-free latex gloves and plastic aprons, thorough hand washing between procedures, and wearing eye protection if there is any risk of blood splashes or flying contaminated debris. The use and disposal of sharps are sources of potential risk. Extreme care is needed and sharps should never be resheathed prior to disposal. Approved sharps boxes must also be available for disposal and these must be used in accordance with instructions about the amount of sharps the container will hold. Boxes should never be overfilled.

In the event of a needlestick injury, the immediate action is to make the puncture wound bleed by gentle squeezing of the area. Wash thoroughly with soap and water and apply a waterproof dressing. If the source patient is known, a record should be kept with the name of the patient. In any event, contact should be made with occupational health and an accident form completed. Procedures should be defined for spillages of blood and body fluids using sodium dichloro-isocyanurate granules or paper towels with 10 000 ppm sodium hypochlorite solution. Household gloves and plastic apron should be worn and these disposed of with the spillage as clinical waste.

HIV/AIDS

HIV is infectious, not contagious, and the only method of transmission to A&E staff would be though inoculation of infected blood by a sharps injury or exposure of mucous membranes to blood. This reinforces the need for staff to adhere to the universal precautions. All patients attending A&E should be approached in the same way as far as infection control is concerned. If it becomes clear that the patient is HIV antibody-positive and there is extensive haemorrhage or severe diarrhoea, the need for isolation must be considered. If a nurse suffers a needlestick injury, blood samples for storage and possible testing for HIV antibodies must not be taken from the injured nurse or the source patient without informed consent and pre-test counselling.

Hepatitis B

Hepatitis B has been known to be a problem to health care staff for over 20 years, and recently other strains of hepatitis have been identified. Hepatitis B is a stable virus, resistant to common antiseptics, and is therefore highly infectious. Hypochlorite, glutaraldehyde, chlorine and autoclaving at 134°C for a minimum of 3 minutes are known to destroy the virus (Royal College of Nursing 1987b).

In A&E departments it is most unlikely that there will be any indication that a patient is infected with hepatitis B. It is advisable that all staff are vaccinated with the hepatitis B vaccine in accordance with Department of Health guidance (UK Health Departments 1993). This guidance specifies that anyone who is HBeAg-positive must not be involved in exposure-prone procedures. These are defined as those where there is a risk that injury to the worker may result in the exposure of the patient's open tissues to the blood of the worker. These procedures include those where the worker's gloved hands may be in contact with sharp instruments, needle tips and sharp tissues, such as spicules of bone or teeth, inside a patient's open body cavity, wound or confined anatomical space where the hands or fingertips may not be completely visible at all times.

Staff who are hepatitis B surface antigen (HBsAg) positive but not HBeAg-positive will not be a risk to patients and need not be barred from any area of work. It must be emphasised that good routine infection control procedures are the key to preventing transmission of blood-borne viruses.

Working Time

It is clear that the organisation of work in A&E departments, which normally provide a 24-hour service, is a factor that can have an impact on the health of staff. Working time had not been covered specifically by health and safety legislation until the European Directive on Working Time was agreed in 1993. Member states were due to implement the requirements of the directive by November 1996. The UK government's view was that the European Commission was wrong in using health and safety processes to regulate working hours and they challenged the directive. The challenge was not successful and the UK introduced regulations to implement the directive in 1998.

Doctors in training are excluded from the directive and the government has the opportunity to apply some flexibility in relation to some parts of the directive for health care workers. The basic provisions of the directive are outlined in Box 40.6.

Box 40.6 – *Basic provisions of Working Time Directive*

- Entitlement to a rest break of 11 consecutive hours per 24-hour period

- Entitlement to an uninterrupted rest period of at least 24 hours per 7-day period. These provisions may be varied for health care workers provided that equivalent compensatory periods of rest are arranged

- Weekly working time including overtime must not exceed 48 hours. This can be averaged out over a period of 17 weeks or longer by agreement

- Normal hours of night work may not exceed an average of 8 hours in any 24-hour period. This can be averaged out over a period of time as agreed through collective bargaining

- Night workers are entitled to a free health assessment prior to starting night work and then at regular intervals

- Night workers suffering from health problems recognised as being connected with the fact that they perform night work are to be transferred to day work wherever possible

- Records of night workers are to be maintained and provided to competent authorities on request

---

All workers are entitled to 4 weeks paid annual leave. The implementation of the Working Time Directive (EC Directive 93/104/EC 1993) is likely to mean that working patterns and hours of work will be the subject of negotiation between employers and their employees, but the key purpose is to ensure that the arrangements do not have a detrimental effect on the health of staff.

Framework for Maintaining a Safe Environment

Health and safety is covered by extensive legislation aimed at producing working environments that are safe for both nurses and patients. The legislation must be translated into practical policies which are known and understood. The main employer must have an overall safety policy but particular areas should have departmental policies which address problems in those areas. In A&E departments, specific policies may be needed for manual handling, dealing with violence and aggressive behaviour, disposal of clinical waste and, infection control. Each member of staff, whether clinical or not, should be clear about her responsibility for health and safety.

Procedures should be defined in the event of any accident taking place, from immediate first aid to the reporting procedures. The policy should specify the consultative arrangements which may exist. Normally this would be a safety committee with management and trade union safety representatives, along with specialist support such as occupational health safety adviser, infection control and radiation protection adviser. Safety problems which cannot be resolved within the department should be addressed by the safety committee.

Conclusion

Professional competence must now include a positive attitude to health, safety and welfare. High standards of care can only be provided in an environment which is not going to cause harm to the nurse or the patient. Health and safety legislation is developing and is driven by European Directives. Nurses need a good basic knowledge of the statutory requirements and a thorough understanding of how these apply to their own workplace. Principles of health and safety should be incorporated in the culture of the department and not be considered as a separate issue. Managers should be regularly reviewing policies, setting performance standards and reviewing progress. All staff must take responsibility for identifying hazards and taking appropriate action. The majority of accidents are foreseeable and therefore preventable. Accident prevention will reduce costs, both direct and indirect, and will lead to a healthier, more productive workforce.

Further reading

Health and Safety Commission, Health Services Advisory Committee (1993) *Getting to Grips with Handling Problems.* London: HMSO.

Health and Safety Commission, Health Services Advisory Committee (1992) *Guidance on the Manual Handling of Loads in the Health Service.* London: HMSO.

Health and Safety Commission, Health Services Advisory Committee (1992) *Safe Disposal of Clinical Waste.* London: HMSO.

Rogers R, Savage J, Cowell R (1999) *Nurses at Risk.* London: Mcmillan

Royal College of Nursing (1994) *Guidance on Infection Control in Hospitals.* London: RCN.

Royal College of Nursing (1996) *Introducing a Safer Patient Handling Policy.* London: RCN.

Royal College of Nursing (1998) *Dealing With Violence Against Nursing Staff.* London: RCN.

UK Health Departments (1994) *AIDS/HIV – Infected Health Care Workers: Guidance on the Management of Infected Health Care Workers.* London: HMSO.

References

Chard C (1993) *Health and Safety for Nurses.* London: Chapman and Hall.

Clough J (1998) Assessing and controlling risk. *Emergency Nurse*, **6**(3), 33–39.

Control of Substances Hazardous to Health Regulations (1994) London: HMSO.

The Control of Substances Hazardous to Health, Guidance for the Initial Assessment in Hospitals (1994) London: HMSO.

EC Directive 89/391/EEC (1989) *Council Directive of the 12th June 1989 on the Introduction of Measures to Encourage Improvements in the Safety and Health of Workers at Work.* Luxembourg: EC.

EC Directive 92/85 EEC (1992) *Pregnant Workers Directive.* Luxembourg: EC.

EC Directive 93/104/EC (1993) *Concerning Certain Aspects of the Organisation of Working Time.* Luxembourg: EC.

Employment Rights Act (1996) London: HMSO.

EU (1986) Single European Act. Luxembourg: EC.

Food Hygiene Regulations (1970) London: HMSO.

Health & Safety Commission (1992) *Workplace Health, Safety and Welfare Approved Code of Practice and Guidance L24.* London: HMSO.

Health & Safety Executive (1992a) *Display Screen Equipment Work Guidance on Regulations L26.* London: HMSO.

Health & Safety Executive (1992b) *Manual Handling Operations Regulations Guidance on Regulations L23.* London: HMSO.

Health & Safety Executive (1992c) *Personal Protective Equipment at Work Guidance on Regulations L25.* London: HMSO.

Health & Safety Executive (1992d) *Work Equipment Guidance on Regulations L22.* London: HMSO.

Health & Safety Executive (1992e) *Workplace Guidance on Regulations.* London: HMSO.

Health & Safety Executive (1993) The costs of accidents at work. *Health & Safety series booklet HS(G) 96.* London, HMSO

Health and Safety at Work etc Act (1974) London: HMSO.

Health and Safety (First Aid) Regulations (1981) London: HMSO.

National Audit Office (1996) *Health and Safety in NHS Acute Hospital Trusts in England.* London: HMSO.

National Back Pain Association/Royal College of Nursing (1992) *The Guide to the Handling of Patients.* Middlesex: NBPA.

Reporting of Injuries, Diseases and Dangerous Occurrences Regulations (1995) London: HMSO.

Rogers R, Savage J, Cowell R (1999) *Nurses at Risk,* London: Macmillan.

Royal College of Nursing (1987a) *Universal Precautions.* London: RCN.

Royal College of Nursing (1987b) *Introduction to Hepatitis B and Nursing Guidelines for Injection Control.* London: RCN.

Royal College of Nursing (1996) *Code of Practice for the Handling of Patients,* 2nd edn. London: RCN.

Royal College of Nursing (1998) *Dealing With Violence Against Nursing Staff.* London: RCN.

Safety Representatives and Safety Committees Regulations (1977) London: HMSO.

Smith G, Seccombe I (1996) *Manual Handling: Issues for Nurses.* Brighton: Institute for Employment Studies.

The Management of Health and Safety at Work Regulations (1992) London: HMSO.

UKCC (1992) *Code of Professional Conduct,* 3rd edn. London: UKCC.

UK Health Departments (1993) *Protecting Health Care Workers & Patients from Hepatitis B.* London: HMSO.

Working Time Regulations (1998) (SI 1998 No. 1833). London: The Stationery Office.

Appendix

Normal values 541

Normal Values

Haematology

Haemoglobin
    Male $14.0–17.7 \text{ g dL}^{-1}$
    Female $12.0–16.0 \text{ g dL}^{-1}$

Mean corpuscular haemoglobin (MCH) $27–33 \text{ pg}$

Mean corpuscular haemoglobin concentration (MCHC) $32–35 \text{ g dL}^{-1}$

Mean corpuscular volume (MCV) $80–96 \text{ fL}$

Packed cell volume (PCV)
    Male $0.42–0.53 \text{ L L}^{-1}$
    Female $0.36–0.45 \text{ L L}^{-1}$

White cell count (WCC) $4–11 \times 10^9/\text{litre}$
    Basophil granulocytes $<0.01–0.1 \times 10^9/\text{litre}$
    Eosinophil granulocytes $0.04–0.4 \times 10^9/\text{litre}$
    Lymphocytes $1.5–4.0 \times 10^9/\text{litre}$
    Monocytes $0.2–0.8 \times 10^9/\text{litre}$
    Neutrophil granulocytes $2.0–7.5 \times 10^9/\text{litre}$

Total blood volume $60–80 \text{ ml kg}^{-1}$

Plasma volume $40–50 \text{ ml kg}^{-1}$

Platelet count $150–400 \times 10^9/\text{litre}$

Serum B_{12} $160–925 \text{ ng L}^{-1}$ ($150–675 \text{ pmol L}^{-1}$)

Serum folate $4–18 \text{ μg L}^{-1}$ ($5–63 \text{ nmol L}^{-1}$)

Red cell folate $160–640 \text{ μg L}^{-1}$

Red cell mass
    Male $25–35 \text{ ml kg}^{-1}$
    Female $20–30 \text{ ml kg}^{-1}$

Reticulocyte count $0.5–2.5\%$ of red cells ($50–100 \times 10^9/\text{litre}$)

Erythrocyte sedimentation rate (ESR) $<20 \text{ mm in 1 hour}$

Coagulation

Bleeding time (Ivy method)   2–7 min

Partial thromboplastin time (PTTK)   24–31 s

Prothrombin time   12–16 s
    International Normalized Ratio (INR)   1

Biochemistry

Acid phosphatase	1–5 UL^{-1}
Alanine aminotransferase (ALT)	5–40 UL^{-1}
Albumin	36–53 g L^{-1}
Alkaline phosphatase	25–115 UL^{-1}
Amylase	<220 U L^{-1}
Angiotensin-converting enzyme	10–70 U L^{-1}
α_1-Antitrypsin	1.1–2.1 g L^{-1}
Aspartate aminotransferase (AST)	7–40 U L^{-1}
Bicarbonate	22–30 mmol L^{-1}
Bilirubin	<17 µmol L^{-1} (0.3–1.5 mg dL^{-1})
Caeruloplasmin	0.20–0.61 L^{-1}
Calcium	2.20–2.67 mmol L^{-1} (8.5–10.5 mg dL^{-1})
Chloride	95–106 mmol L^{-1}
Cholinesterase	2.25–7.0 U L^{-1}
Copper	11–20 µmol L^{-1} (100–200 mg dL^{-1})
C-reactive protein	<10 mg L^{-1}
Creatinine	0.06–0.12 mmol L^{-1} (0.6–1.5 mg dL^{-1})
Creatine kinase (CPK)	
Female	24–170 U L^{-1}
Male	24–195 U L^{-1}
CK-MB fraction	25 U L^{-1} (<60% of total activity)
C3	0.55–1.20 g L^{-1}
C4	0.20–0.50 g L^{-1}
Ferritin	
Female	6–110 µg L^{-1}
Male	20–260 µg L^{-1}
Post menopausal	12–230 µg L^{-1}
α-Fetoprotein	<10 k U L^{-1}
Glucose (fasting)	4.5–5.6 mmol L^{-1} (70–110 mg dL^{-1})
Fructosamine	up to 285 µmol L^{-1}
γ-Glutamyl transpeptidase (γ-GT)	
Male	11–50 U L^{-1}
Female	7–32 U L^{-1}
Glycosylated haemoglobin (HbA$_{1c}$)	3.8–8.5%
Hydroxybutyric dehydrogenase (HBD)	40–150 U L^{-1}
Immunoglobulins (11 years and over)	
IgA	0.8–4 g L^{-1}
IgG	7.0–18.0 g L^{-1}
IgM	0.4–2.5 g L^{-1}

Iron	13–32 µmol L^{-1} (50–150 µg dL^{-1})
Iron binding capacity (total) (TIBC)	42–80 µmol L^{-1} (250–410 µg dL^{-1})
Lactate dehydrogenase	240–460 U L^{-1}
Lead	<0.7 µmol L^{-1}
Magnesium	0.7–1.1 mmol L^{-1}
β_2-Microglobulin	1.0–3.0 mg L^{-1}
Osmolality	280–296 mosmol kg^{-1}
Phosphate	0.8–1.5 mmol L^{-1}
Potassium	3.5–5.0 mmol L^{-1}
Prostate-specific antigen	up to 4.0 µg L^{-1}
Protein (total)	62–80 g L^{-1}
Sodium	135–146 mmol L^{-1}
Urate	0.18–0.42 mmol L^{-1} (3.0–7.0 mg dL^{-1})
Urea	2.5–6.7 mmol L^{-1} (8–25 mg dL^{-1})
Vitamin A	0.5–2.01 µmol L^{-1}

Vitamin D

25-hydroxy	37–200 nmol L^{-1} (0.15–0.80 ng L^{-1})
1,25-dihydroxy	60–108 pmol L^{-1} (0.24–0.45 pg L^{-1})
Zinc	7–18 µmol L^{-1}

Lipids and lipoproteins

Cholesterol	3.5–6.5 mmol L^{-1} (ideal <5.2 mmol L^{-1})

HDL cholesterol

Male	0.95–2.15 mmol L^{-1}
Female	0.70–2.00 mmol L^{-1}
Lipids (total)	4.0–10.0 g L^{-1}

Lipoproteins

VLDL	0.128–0.645 mmol L^{-1}
LDL	1.55–4.4 mmol L^{-1}

HDL

Male	0.70–2.1 mmol L^{-1}
Female	0.50–1.70 mmol L^{-1}

Non-esterified fatty acids

Male	0.19–0.78 mmol L^{-1}
Female	0.06–0.9 mmol L^{-1}
Phospholipid	2.9–5.2 mmol L^{-1}

Triglycerides

Male	0.70–2.1 mmol L^{-1}
Female	0.50–1.70 mmol L^{-1}

Blood gases (arterial)

Pa_{CO_2}	4.8–6.1 kPa (36–46 mmHg)
Pa_{O_2}	10–13.3 kPa (75–100 mmHg)
$[H^+]$	35–45 nmol L^{-1}
pH	7.35–7.45
Bicarbonate	24–28 mmol L^{-1}

Urine values

Calcium	7.5 mmol daily or less (<300 mg daily)
Copper	0.2–1.o µmol daily
Creatinine	0.13–0.22 mmol per kilogram body weight, daily
5-Hydroxyindole acetic acid	<75 µmol daily; amounts lower in females than males
Protein (quantitative)	<0.15 g per 24 hours

Reproduced with permission from Kumar P, Clark M (1998) *Clinical Medicine*, 4th edn. Edinburgh: WB Saunders

Index

Numbers in bold refer to tables or figures

A&E Nursing Association, RCN, 3, 4, 8, 482, 488
A-beta fibres, 326
A-delta fibres, 326
Aaron's sign, 401
ABC principle, 344
Abdomen
    anatomy and physiology, 137–138, 393-395
    examination, 30
    see also Acute abdomen
Abdominal injuries, 137–144
    assessment 30, 141–144
        primary survey, 142
        secondary survey, 142–143
        special diagnostic studies, 143–144
    children, 144
    Munchausen's syndrome, 207
    types and patterns of injury, 138–141
    uncontrolled haemorrhage, 141
Abdominal pain
    assessment, 395–396
    children, 254–255
Abdominal wall, 395
Abrasions, scalp, 54
Abruptio placentae, 423, 424
Abscesses
    peritonsillar, 456
    tooth, 455
Absorbable sutures, 317
Acceleration/deceleration injuries, 57
Access, restricting, major incidents, 40
Accidents at work, prevention, 529–530
Accommodation reflexes, 150
Accountability, 480, 523
Acetabular fractures, 74, 75
Acetazolamide, 445
Achilles tendon rupture, 104
Acid burns, eye, 436
Acid-base balance, 381
Acidosis, near drowning, 379
Acromion fractures, 88
Acting without consent, 518
Activated charcoal, 242
Acute abdomen
    emergencies, 398–401
        appendicitis, 400–401
        bowel obstruction, 398–399
        peritonitis, 399–400
    examination, 396–397
    management principles, 398
    nursing assessment, 395–398
Acute confusional states, 176
Acute organic reactions, 201–202
Acute radiation syndrome, 166
Adenosine diphosphate (ADP), 303
Adenoviral conjunctivitis, 443, 444
Adhesions, bowel, 398
Adhesive strips, 318
Adolescence, 257–266
    caring for adolescent in A&E, 258
    personal fable, 258–259
    psychiatric emergencies, 211

risk-taking behaviour, 259–261
substance misuse, 261–265
    Misuse of Drugs Act, 1971, penalties, 260–261
Adrenaline, nebulised, 239
Advanced Trauma Life Support (ATLS) system, 26, 45
Advanced Trauma Nursing course, 8
Advanced triage, 477
Affective puerperal disorder episode, 204
Afferent nerve fibres, 325–326
Age 5 to puberty, 251–256
    abdominal pain, 254–255
    child development, 251–252
    consent, 255
    environment, 252
    fractures, 253–254
    health promotion, 255–256
    pain relief, 252–253
    sports injuries, 254
Age
    and outcome, head injuries, 45
    wound healing, 312
Agency staff
    health and safety issues, 534
    vicarious liability, 523
Aggression, 175–181
    defusing, 178–179
    legal issues, staff health and safety, 527
    prevention, 177–178
    reason for, 176–177
    recognising potential, 178
    violent patients, 210
        follow-up care, violent incident, 180–181
        management of individual, 179–180
'Air hunger', 304
Airway management
    trauma patients, 26–27
        burn-injured patients, 160–161
        chest injuries, 123–124
        facial injuries, 149
        head injuries, 61
        pre-hospital care, 21
        spinal injuries, 113
    see also Obstructed airway
Akathesia, 212
Akinesia, 212
Alarm reaction, 184
Alcohol intoxication, 206–207
    adolescents, 258, 259, 261
    aggression, 176
        defusing tension, 179
    legal considerations, 523
    proving intention, violent actions, 527
    young adults, 271–272
Alcoholic coma, 271–272
Aldosterone, 302
Alerting stage, major incidents
    A&E response, 37–38
    hospital response, 40
Alginates, 321

Alkali burns, eye, 436
    use of pH paper, checking irrigation, 437
Allergy
    asthma, 374
    conjunctivitis, 444
    rhinitis, 453
Allitt Inquiry, 499
Alveoli, gaseous exchange, 296–297
Ambulance incident officer (AIO), 18
Ambulance liaison officer facilities, major incidents, 35
Ambulance service, 15, 16, 21, 37
    information to be recorded from major incidents, 38
American Nurses Association, nurse practitioner's abilities, 491
Amphetamine abuse, 264
Anaemic hypoxia, 373
Anaerobic metabolism, 397
Anal canal, 394
Anaphylactic shock, 303–304, 379
    aetiology and management, 455
Anatomy and physiology
    abdomen, 137–138, 393–395
    brain, 48–51
    chest, 120–122
    ear, 448
    elbow, 91–92
    eye, 429–433
    female reproductive organs, 411–413
    foot, 84, 85
    hand, 99
    heart, 120, 121, 341–343
    hip, 75
    nose, 451, 452
    pelvis, 72
    radius and ulna, 94
    shoulder, 87
    skeleton, 67–71
    skin, 307–309
    skull, 46, 47
        facial bones, 147–148
    spinal, 109–110
    throat, 454
    wrist, 95
    see also Physiology for practice
Angina, 276, 277, 360–361
    classification, 361
    management, 361
Angioneurotic oedema, 238
Angiotensin, 381
Angle recession, 439–440
Anistreplase (ASPAC), 364
Ankle injuries
    dislocation, 84
    fractures, 81–84
        classification, 82, 83
    sprains, 104
Annual leave entitlement, 537
Anoxic drive, 299
Anterior chamber, eye, 433
    examination, 435
Anteroposterior compression fractures, pelvis, 72, 73

Anti-emetics
  children, 253
  myocardial infarction, 363
Antibiotics
  meningitis, 225
  pancreatitis, 279
  pelvic ring injury, 74
Anticonvulsants, 224
Antidepressants, accidental
    poisoning, 242
Antidiuretic hormone (ADH), 302, 381
Antiseptic solutions, wound cleansing,
    315
Anxiety, pain perception, 327
Anxiety states, 205–206, 273
Aortic aneurysm, 403–405
  differential diagnosis, 404
  dissection, 404
    pain, 276, 277
  management, 405
  pulsation, 396, 404
Aortic rupture, 132–133, 141
Apgar score, 425, **426**
Appearance, mental state examination,
    200
Appendicitis, 254, 399, 400–401
  assessment, 400–401
  differential diagnosis, 401
Appendicular skeleton, 67
Appetite, assessment, 395
Aqueous humour, 433
Arachnoid mater, 48
Arrestable offences, 527
Arrhythmias, 132, 353–357
  elderly patients, 284–285
  hypothermia, 301
Arterial embolism, 405–406
Arteries
  head and neck, 51, **52**
  walls of, 404
Artifical tears, 444
Aspiration, knee haemarthrosis, 104
Aspirin, 253
  accidental poisoning, 242
  myocardial infarction, 364
Assault and battery, 522, 523, 525, 527
Assessment, 6–7
  cardiac emergencies, 344–345
    acute left ventricular failure, 366
    angina, 360, 361
    atrial ectopics, 355
    atrial fibrillation, 356
    cardiogenic shock, 366
    cardiomyopathy, 368
    endocarditis, 367
    myocardial infarction, 362, 363,
      480
    pericarditis, 367
    supraventricular tachycardia, 355
    third degree heart block, 358
    ventricular ectopics, 353
    ventricular tachycardia, 354
  children
    abdominal pain, 254
    accidental poisoning, 241–242
    asthma, 235–236

viral croup, 237–238
elderly patients, 284–285
  confusion, 290
  hypothermia, 285–287
  risk assessment, 291
gynaecological emergencies, 413,
    414
infants, 217–219
legal considerations, 523
medical emergencies
  asthma, 374–375
  blood sugar, 388
  body temperature, 385
  carbon monoxide poisoning, 380,
    381
  chronic obstructive airways
    disease (COAD), 375–376
  dehydration, 384
  haematological assessment, 390
  ischaemic brain injury, 387–388
  near drowning, 379–380
  neurological assessment, 386–387
  pulmonary embolism, 378
  pulmonary oedema, 377
  renal colic, 382, 383
  renal system assessment, 382
  respiratory assessment, 372–373
  urinary tract infection, 382
ophthalmic conditions, 433–436
pain, 328–329
  abdominal in children, 254
  chest pain, 276–277
  pre-hospital care, 21–23
  psychiatric patients, 200–201
surgical emergencies
  acute abdomen, 395–398
  aortic aneurysm, 404
  appendicitis, 401
  arterial emboli, 405
  bowel obstruction, 399
  oesophageal varices, 402
  peritonitis, 400
  testicular torsion, 408
  urinary retention, 406
trauma victims
  abdominal injuries, 141–144
  burns, 159–164
  femoral fractures, 80
  head injuries, **58**, 59–61
  hip injuries, 77
  limb injuries, 78, 79
  pelvic ring injuries, 74
  spinal cord injury, 110, 111–112
  wound assessment, 313–314
  see also Triage
Asthma, 374–375
  children, 235–237
    assessment, 235–236
    life-threatening signs, 236
    management, 236–237
Asystole, 350, 352
Atherosclerosis, 404
Atmospheric pressure
  at altitude, 299
  at sea level, 296
Atonic bladder, 406

Atrial ectopic beats, 355–356
Atrial fibrillation, 356, 405
Atrial flutter, 356, **357**
Atrioventricular valves, 343
Atropine, 352
Attendance at A&E 2, 3, 476
  adolescents, 258
  legal considerations, 523
  legitimacy of, 461–462
  reducing re-attendances, 7
Audit
  in clinical supervision, 501, 502
  and evaluation, nurse practitioner
    performance, 489–491
  triage system and staff, 481–482
Audit Commission report, 1996
  patient attendance, 3
  patient re-attendance, 7
Auscultation, acute abdomen, 396–397
Autodigestion, pancreatic tissue, 278
Autonomic reflex activity, 51
Autonomy, 517–518
Autopsy, 195
Autoregulation, 52, 54, 61
Avulsion fractures
  ankle, 82, 104
  limbs, 78
  navicular, 86
  pelvis, 74
Axial skeleton, 67
Axillary artery damage, testing, 89
Axillary nerve
  nerve block, 336
  testing for damage, 89
Axonal injury see Diffuse axonal injury

Babinski sign, 116
Back, examination, 29
Bacterial infection
  conjunctivitis, 443
  corneal ulcers, 445
  endocarditis, 368
  meningitis, 225
Bag-valve-mask system, 27
Ball and socket joints, 71
Bank staff see Agency staff
Barnett v Chelsea and Kensington
    HMC (1969), 523
Baroreceptors, 381
Barotrauma, tympanic membrane, 451
Bartholin's glands, 412
  cysts, 416
Basal ganglia, 49
Basal layer, epidermis, 309
Base of metacarpal fractures
  second to fifth, 101
  thumb, 100
Base of skull
  anatomy, **47**
  fractures, 30, 55, 149
Basic life support, **349**
Basic triage, 477
Battery see Assault and battery
Battle's sign, 55, 149
Beating heart donors, 195

Beattie, models of health promotion, 469, **470**
Beck's suicide risk scale, 208, 209
Beck's triad, 130
Behaviour
  in A&E, adolescents, 258
  risk-taking
    adolescents, 259–261
    children, 252
  see also Aggression
Beneficence, 516, 517
Benner's model of skill acquisition, 479
Bennett's fracture, 100
Bereavement care, 189–197
  background, 189–190
  breaking bad news, 192–194
    infant death, 229
    telephone notification, 194
  legal and ethical issues, 195–196, 524
  organ donation, 195, 524
  preparing for receiving patient and relatives, 190
  staff support, 196, 230
  sudden infant death syndrome, 228–230
  viewing the body, 194
  witnessed resuscitation, 190–192
Beta-agonists, asthma attack, 236, 237
Bier's block, 336–337
  wrist fracture reductions, 96
Bimalleolar fractures, 82
Bipolar disease, 205
Bite wounds, 322
'Black eye', 438
Black stools, 397
Bladder, injury to, 140
Blast injury, 140
Blepharitis, 442, 443
Blink reflex, loss of, 337
Blisters, burn injuries, 167–168
Blood, 389–390
  cross-matching, 28
  in vomit, 397
  see also Haematemesis
Blood alcohol concentration (BAC), 206
Blood analysis
  arterial blood gas analysis, 373
  cardiac patients, 345
    myocardial infarction, 362
  hypothermic patients, 286–287
Blood pressure
  burns patients, 164
  infants, 221
  left ventricular failure, 365
  maintenance of, 381
  myocardial infarction, 362
  in shock, 398
Blood samples, 28
Blood transfusion, acute abdomen, 398
Blow-out fractures, 152–153, 439
Blunt trauma
  abdomen, 140–141, 143
  chest, 119–120
    cardiac trauma, 132

Body cavities, effects at altitude, 299
Bolam case, 522
Bone, 67, 69
  cell types, 70–71
  healing of, 78, **79**
  pain, 70
Bowel obstruction, 398–400
Bowel sounds, 142–143, 396–397
Bowlby, *Child Care and the Growth of Love*, 234
Bowman's layer, 431
Boxer's fracture, 101
Brachial artery, 92
Brachial plexus
  nerve blocks, 336
  testing function, 89
Bradycardia, infants, 362
Brain
  anatomy and physiology, 48–51
  injuries, 55–59
    ischaemic, 387–388
  tumours, headache, 387
Brain stem, 50–51
  death, 524
Breaking bad news, 192–194
  infant death, 229
Breathing
  asthma attack, 235, 236
  breathlessness with chest pain, 277
  infants, 220
  pre-hospital care, 22
  trauma patients, 27
    head-injured patients, 61
Bridging veins, rupture, 51, 56
British Association for Accident and Emergency Medicine (BAEM)
  bereavement care study, 189–190
  standard five-point triage scale, 482
British Association for Immediate Care (BASICS), 19
Bronchi, injuries to, 133
Bronchial hyperreactivity, 374
Bronchial tone, 373
Bronchiolitis, infants, 222, 223–224
Bronchitis, 375–376
Bronchoscopy, burns patients, 161
Bruits, 397
Budesonide, nebulised, 239
Bullying, 256
Bupivacaine, pharmacology, **334**
Burn-out, 184, 185
  responses to, 187–188
  signs of, 185
Burns, 105, 159–172
  assessment, 159–164
  chemical, 165
  cold, 165–166
  electrical, 165
  escharotomies, 168
  ocular, 436–438
  pain control, 168
  pharyngeal, 456
  psychological considerations, 169
  radiation, 166
  thermal, 160, 164–166
  transfer to specialist unit, 169–170

wound care, 166–168
  dressings, 320
  minor burns, 170–171
Bursitis, 103

C fibres, 326
Caecum, 394
CAGE questionnaire, 207
Calcaneus, fractures, 86
Calcium regulation, 302
Calcium salts, cardiac arrest, 352
Calculi, renal, 382, 383
Calf squeeze test, 104
Call-in procedure, major incidents, 38
Calorie intake, wound healing, 312
Cancellous bone, 70
Candida albicans, **416**
Cannabis, 264
Carbon dioxide transport, 298
Carbon dioxide/oxygen homeostasis, 298–299
Carbon monoxide poisoning, 373, 380, 381
Carboxyhaemoglobin, 381
Cardiac contusions, 30
Cardiac emergencies, 341–369
  acute chest pain, 360–365
    angina, 360–361
    myocardial infarction, 361–365
  acute heart failure, 365–357
    acute left ventricular failure (LVF), 365–366
    cardiogenic shock, 303, 366–367
  anatomy and physiology, 341–343
  assessment, 344–345
  basic ECG interpretation, 345–348
  cardiac arrest, 348–353
    asystole, 350, 352
    drug therapy, 352
    electromechanical disassociation, 352
    ethical considerations, 353
    infants and children, 219–220
    universal algorithm, **351**
    ventricular fibrillation, 349–350
  cardiac cycle, 343–344
  heart block, 357–359
    first degree, 357
    second degree, 357, 358
    third degree, 358, **359**
  pacing, 359–360
  rhythm disturbances, 353–357
    atrial ectopics, 355, **356**
    atrial fibrillation, 356
    atrial flutter, 356, **357**
    supraventricular tachycardia, 354, 355
    ventricular ectopics, 353–354
    ventricular tachycardia, 354
  viral/inflammatory conditions, 367–368
Cardiac enzymes, 277, 345, 363
Cardiac tamponade, 28, 129–131
  assessment, 129, 130
  management, 130–131

Cardiac-related pulmonary oedema, 376–377
Cardiogenic shock, 303
    assessment, 366
    management, 367
Cardiomyopathy, 368
Cardiopulmonary arrest, infants, 219, 220
Carpal fractures, 97–99
Carpopedal spasm, 205
Cartella shield, 438
Cartilaginous joints, 71
Cascading system of alert, major incidents, 40
Casualty clearing station, 18
Casualty departments
    from casualty to accident and emergency, 2
    historical background, 1–2
Cataracts, 440
Categorical imperative, moral theory, 514
    applying to practice, 514–515
Categories, triage, 480
Catgut, 317
Cauliflower ear, 156
Central chemoreceptors, 298
Central venous pressure
    burns patients, 164
    left ventricular failure, 365
Cerebellum, 49, 50
Cerebral circulation, 51, **52, 53**
Cerebral contusions, 55
Cerebral hemispheres, 48, 49, **50**
Cerebral oedema, 62
Cerebral perfusion pressure (CPP), 52
Cerebrospinal fluid (CSF), 48
    circulation, **49**
    leakage, 30, 55, 151, 453
Cervical spine injuries, 110, 111, 114–115
    spinal immobilisation, 26–27, 30, 112–113
    pre-hospital care, 21–22
Cervix, 411
Cetrimide, wound cleansing, **316**
Chalazia, 430
Challenging the Boundaries, RCN, 8
Charcoal, activated, 242
Charity hospitals, 1
Checklist, preoperative, 409
Chemical injury
    burns, 165
        ocular, 436–437
    inhalation injury, 160
Chemical/radioactive contamination, 39–40
Chemoreceptor trigger zone (CTZ), 330
Chemoreceptors, 298, 299, 372
Chemoregulation, 52, 54
Chest
    anatomy, 120–121
    examination, 30
Chest drains, 127

Chest injuries, 119–134
    immediately life-threatening injuries, 123, 125–131
    mechanisms of injury, 119–120
    physiology of respiration, 121–122
    principles of care, 122–125
        assessment, 123
        initial management, 123–125
        the trauma team, 122
    serious chest injury, 131–134
Chest leads, ECG, 346
Chest pain, 275–278, 360–365
    causes, 276
    Munchausen's syndrome, 208
Child abuse, 243–246
    breaching confidentiality, 526–527
    common indicators, 244
    management of suspected, 245–246
    Munchausen's syndrome by proxy, 207, 243, 246, 247
    prevalence, 245
    sexual abuse, 244, 246, 247
Child Care and the Growth of Love, Bowlby, 234
Childbirth, emergency, 424–426
    first stage of labour, 424–425
    second stage of labour, 425–426
    third stage of labour, 426
Children, 8
    adolescence, 211, 257–266
    age 5 to puberty, 251–256
    consent issues, 525
    core temperature, 300
    pre-school, 233–248
    psychiatric emergencies, 211
    trauma, 31
        abdominal injuries, 144
        burns, maintenance fluid requirements, **163**
        facial injuries, 148
        hip fractures, 77
        scalp lacerations, 54
    see also Infants
The Children Act, 1989, 8
    child protection, 246
    consent issues, 255, 525
Children's Charter, 252
Chin lift, 124, 149
    spinal-injured patients, 113
Chlamydia trachomatis, **416**
Chloramphenicol, 440, 443
Chlorhexidine, wound cleansing, **316**
Chlorine-releasing disinfecting agents, 532
Choroid, 432–433
Choroid plexus, 48
Chronic respiratory disease, 372
    chronic obstructive airways disease (COAD), 375–376
Ciliary body, 432
Ciliary muscle spasm, 440
Circle of Willis, 51
Circulation
    infants, 220
    trauma patients, 28
    burns patients, 161

chest-injured patients, 124–125
head-injured patients, 61
pre-hospital care, 22
Circumferential full-thickness burns, 161, 168
Civil law, 522
Clavicular fractures, 88–89
Clingfilm, burn wounds, 168
Clinical leadership *see* Leadership
Clinical nurse managers, 9
'Clinical portraits', 479
Clinical practice, 7–8
Clinical reasoning, 505–511
    hypothetico-deductive approach, 507–511
    intuitive reasoning, 506–507
    nursing process, 506
Clinical Standards Advisory Group, 8
Clinical supervision, 499–502
    benefits, 502
    ground rules, 502
    obtaining, 501–502
    types of, 500, 501
Clostridium tetani, 322
Clotting screen, cardiac patients, 345
Cluster headaches, 387
Cocaine
    misuse, 265
    pharmacology, **334**
    topical anaesthesia, 335–336
Coccyx, fracture, 74
Code of Professional Conduct, UKCC, 480, 481, 514, 518, 522, 534
    acknowledging limitations in competence, 523
    breach of, 501
    confidentiality issues, 526
    nurse practitioners practice, 487
    principle of respect, 515
'Cognitive model of stress', Lazarus, 184
Cognitive state, mental state examination, 200
Cold burns, 165–166
Cold compresses, 331
Collagen, 309, 310
Collars, semi-rigid, 26–27, 112, 113
Colles' fracture, 96
Colloids, 22, 28
    burn-injured patients, 163
Colon, 394
Colour codes, standard triage scale, 482
Command hallucinations, 203
Comminuted fractures
    limbs, 78
    skull, 55
Common bile duct, 394
'Common-sense' understanding, 506
Communication issues, 6
    aggression in A&E, 176–177
        defusing tension, 178–179
    breaking bad news, 192–194, 229
    clinical leadership, 499
    language difficulties, 480

Communication issues (*contd*)
  what to say to relatives witnessing
    resuscitation, 192
Community development, health
    promotion, 472–473
Compact bone, 67, 69
Compartment syndrome, 105–106
  tibial shaft fractures, 81
Competence, acknowledging
    limitations, 523
Complaints
  audit of patient, 501, 502
  from relatives, 6
Compliance, 'difficult' patients, 490
Components of Life model, Jones, 5
Compound fractures, limbs, 78
Compression fractures, limbs, 78
Compression injury, spine, 110, **111**
Computed tomography (CT) scanning
  abdominal injuries, 143
  head-injured patients, 60–61
Computer-based decision support,
    telephone triage, 466
Concussion, 57
  post-concussion symptoms, 63, 64
Cones (photoreceptors), 133
Confidence, forming diagnostic
    hypotheses, 510
Confidentiality, 526–527
Confirmation bias, 509, 510
Confusion
  acute confusional states, 176
  detention of patients, 526
  elderly people, 288–290
Conjunctiva, 431
  abrasion, 440
  examination, 435
Conjunctivitis, 443–444
Consciousness
  burns patients, 164
  Glasgow Comma Scale, 19, 29, 59, 60
  infants, 221
  see also Unconscious patients
Consensual light reaction, 60, 150
Consent
  as an ethical process, 517–519
    freedom to choose, 518–519
  children, 255, 525
  examination following sexual
    assualt, 417
  for organ removal, 524
  surgical emergencies, 408–409
  to treatment, legal issues, 525–526
Constipation
  children, 255
  complete, 399
Consultation
  nurse practitioners, 490
  skills training, 489
  style of, 464
    GPs, 463
Contact burns, 164
Contact lenses, 435–436
Contra-coup injuries, 152
Contraception, emergency, 272, 416,
    417

Contraction phase, wound healing, 310
Control of Substances Hazardous to
    Health (COSHH) Regulations
    (1994), 531–532
Contusions
  brain, 55
  cardiac, 30
  pulmonary, 131–132
  scalp, 54
  soft tissue, 103
Convulsions
  alcoholic coma, 271
  eclampsia, 423
  epilepsy, 388
  febrile, 224
  head-injured patients, 62
Coordinated spinal lift, 114–115
Coping, 184
Copper deficiency, 311
Coracoid process fractures, 88
Core rewarming, 287
Core temperature, 300
  burns patients, 164
  homeostasis, 300
  hypothermia, 285, **286**
Cornea, 131, 132
  abrasion, 440
  donated, 195
  examination, 435
  perforation, 438
  ulcers, 445
Coronary circulation, 343, **344**
Coronary heart disease, 275, 341
  see also Cardiac care; Chest pain
Coroner
  consent for organ removal, 524
  investigation of a death, 195
Coroner's officer, 195
Costs of
  accidents at work, 530
  clinical supervision, 502
  initial nursing assessment, 6
Counselling
  patients, health promotion, 473
  staff, post-traumatic, 180, 181
  see also Nurse counsellors
County emergency planning officers
    (CEPOs), 39
Courses, 2, 8, 37, 511
  Advanced Trauma Nursing course,
    8
  British Association for Immediate
    Care (BASICS), 19
  ENB course 199, 2
  nurse practitioners, 488–489
  Pre-hospital Emergency Care
    Course (PHEC), 20
  Pre-hospital Trauma Life Support
    (PHTLS), 20
  Trauma Nursing Core course, 8
Crack, 265
Creatine kinase, 277, 363
Cremaster muscle, 407
Crescendo angina, 361
Cribriform plate fractures, 30, 149, 453
Cricoid pressure, 61

Cricothyroidotomy, emergency, 27,
    149
Criminal Injuries Compensation
    Board, 527
Criminal law, 522
Critical incident stress debriefing
    (CISD), 181, 187
Croup, 237–239
  differentiation from epiglottitis, **240**
Crown Immunity, removal from NHS,
    530
Crush injuries, 105, 321
  chest, 120, 128
Crystalloids, 22, 28, 74
  burn-injured patients, 163
Cultural background, pain perception,
    327
Cushing's triad, 60, 61, 62

Dantrolene, 263
Dartos muscle, 407
'Dead space', 296
Dead/expectant category, major
    incidents, 18
Death
  abdominal injuries, 141
  burns, 159
    age and percentage of body
      burned, **163**
  confirming, at major incidents, 18
  head injuries, 45
  hypothermic individuals, 287
  incidence in major injury, 25
  legal issues, 524
  pancreatitis, 278
  pelvic injuries, 72
  road traffic accidents, 270, **271**
  sudden death see Sudden death
  trajectory of, 190
Debriefing sessions, serious incidents,
    20
Decision trees, 511
Deep vein thrombosis (DVT), 377
Defibrillation, 350
  infants, 221, 222
  universal algorithm, **351**
Defusion, 186
Dehydration, 383, 384
  infants, 226
  wound healing, 312
Delirium, 288, 290
  clinical features, **289**
Delusions, 202, 203, 204
Dementia, 288
  clinical features, **289**
  psychiatric emergencies, 211
Demobilisation, 186–187
'Dendritic' ulcers, 445
Deontology, 514
Department of Health circulars, 522
Depressed skull fractures, 54–55
Depression, 203–204
  clinical features, **289**
  postnatal, 273
Dermis 309, 316

Descemet's membrane, 432
Desferrioxamine, 243
Desloughing solutions, 315
Detention of patients, 526
Development of child
    adolescence, 257
    age 5 to puberty, 251–252
    normal infant, 218
    pre-school child, 234
Diabetes mellitus, 388–389
    adolescent patients, 259
Diabetic ketoacidosis (DKA), 389
Diagnostic hypotheses
    activating, 508–509
    possible sources of error, 509–510
Diagnostic peritoneal lavage (DPL),
    30, 139, 143
Diamorphine, 330
Diaphragm, ruptured, 133, 140
    excluding, 128
Diaphragmatic breathing, spinal
    injuries, 116
Diastole, 343
Diazepam
    alcoholic coma, 271
    eclampsic fitting, 423
    rectal administration, 224
Diencephalon, 49
Diffuse axonal injury, 57, 59
    mild, 64
Diffuse injuries, brain, 55, 57–59
Diffusion, 121
Dinner-fork deformity, 96
Diphtheria, 238
Diplopia, 149
Direct triage, 475, 477–478
Disciplinary action, fear of, 487
Disinfectants, COSHH regulations,
    532
Dislocations
    ankle, 84
    elbow, 93–94
    forefoot, 86
    hip, 77
    Lisfranc, 86
    patellar, 81
    perilunate and lunate, 98–99
    radial head, 94
    shoulder, 89–90
    temporomandibular joint, 153–154
Displaced fractures, limbs, 78
Dissecting aortic aneurysm, 276, 277,
    404
Disseminated intravascular
    coagulation
    ecstasy, 262, 264
    shock, 305
Distraction techniques, pain relief, 331
District health authorities, major
    incident planning, 36
Diverticulitis, 399
Doctor service provision, shortfall, 486
Documentation
    accidents at work, 529–530
    psychiatric patients assessment, 200
    scrupulous recording, 522

suspected child abuse, 245–246
trauma patients, 31
    burns patients, 170
    major incidents, 38, 39, 41
    triage, 480–481
Donor cards, 524
Doppler ultrasound, spermatic cord,
    408
Dressings, 319–320
    burn wounds, 171
    optimum, 319
    types, 320–321
Drowning *see* Near drowning
Drug intoxication
    adolescents, 258, 259, 261–265
    aggression, 176
        defusing tension, 179
    clinical effects, **263**, **264**
    Misuse of Drugs Act, 1971,
        penalties, 260–261
    proving intention, violent actions,
        527
Drug overdose, 208, 209
    adolescents, 259, 265, 266
    ethical issues, 518
    legal issues, 525
Drugs, COSHH regulations, 532
'Dry' drowning, 379
Duodenum, 394
    rupture, 140
Dura mater, 46, 48
Duty, 517
    as moral endeavour, 514
    as moral problem, 515–516
Dysmenorrhoea, 414
Dyspnoea, 362
Dystonia, 212

Ear
    anatomy, 448
    examination, 149
    foreign bodies, 450
    infection, 448–450
    injury, 156, 447
    mechanical obstruction, 450
Ear drum, 448
    perforation, 156, 449–450, 450–451
Ear wax, 448
    impacted, 450
Eating disorders, 211, 273
Ecchymosis, 438
ECG monitoring, 345–348
    12-lead ECG, 345, **346**
        analysis, summary, 348
        normal complex, single heartbeat,
            347
        normal trace, **348**
    angina, 360, **361**
    asystole, **352**
    atrial ectopic beats, **355**
    atrial fibrillation, **356**
    atrial flutter, **357**
    basic rhythm recognition, 348
    chest pain, 277
    during pericardiocentesis, 131

heart block
    first degree, **357**
    second degree, **358**
    third degree (complete), **359**
hypothermia, 286
left ventricular failure, 365
myocardial infarction, 362, **363**
non-invasive temporary pacing, **360**
pericarditis, 367
pulmonary embolism, 378
supraventricular tachycardia, **355**
trauma patients, 28, 30
ventricular ectopic beats, **353**
ventricular fibrillation, **349**
ventricular tachycardia, **354**
Echolalia, 234
Eclampsia, 423
Ecstasy, 261, 262, 263, 264
Ectopic pregnancy, 415, 421–422
    differential diagnosis, **422**
Educational Exchange Scheme, 464
Egocentricity, pre-school child, 234
Einthoven triangle, 346
Elastic recoil, arteries, 403
Elbow injuries, 91–94
    dislocation, 93–94
    radial head fractures, 84
    supracondylar fractures, 92–93
Elderly patients, 283–291
    assessment, 284–285
    confusion, 288–290
    elder abuse, 284, 287–288
    falls, 290–291
    hypothermia, 285–287
    physiology of old age, 283–284
    psychiatric emergencies, 211
'Electric shock' feelings, 111
Electrical burns, 165
Electrical system model (Hills), health
    promotion, 471
Electrolytes, 301
    cardiac patients, 345, 363
Electromechanical dissociation
    (EMD), 28, 352
Electronic tympanic thermometers,
    385
Elevation, musculoskeletal injuries, 331
Ellipson joints, 71
Embolectomy, 406
Embolism, 405–406
    mesenteric, 398
    pulmonary, 276, 277, 377–378
Emergency contraception, 272, 416,
    417
Emergency protection order, 246
Emotional abuse, 244
Emotional disturbances, psychiatric
    patients, 202
Emphysema, 376
Employees duties, health and safety,
    534
Employer's duties, Health and Safety
    at Work Act, 530
Empowerment, leadership skills, 498
ENB course 199, 2
Encephalins, 326

Endocarditis, 367–368
Endocardium, 343
Endometriosis, 414
Endorphins, 326
Endoscopic sclerotherapy, 403
Endothelium, corneal, 432
Endotracheal intubation, 27
    facial injuries, 149
    indications, 61, 124
    spinal-injured patients, 113
Enophthalmus, 150, 153
Entonox, 29, 330–331
    burns patients, 168
    children, 253
    emergency childbirth, 424
Entrapment, mobile team assistance, 19
Environment
    children, 235, 252
    control of, trauma victims, 29
        pre-hospital care, 22–23
    prevention of aggression, 177
Epidermis, 307, **308**, 309
Epigastric pain, 279–280
Epiglottitis, 239–240, 456
Epilepsy, 388
Epistaxis, 154, 452–453
Epithelialisation, 310, 319
Epithelium of cornea, 431
Erythrocyte sedimentation rate (ESR),
        cardiac patients, 345, 363
Escharotomies, 168
Ethical issues, 513–519
    applying the imperative to practice,
        514–515
    definition of ethics, 513
    doing no harm, 516–517
    duty as moral endeavour, 514
    duty as moral problem, 515–516
    informed consent, 517–519
European Court of Justice, 522
European Union Directives, health
        and safety, 527, 531
    EU Directive on Working Time
        (1993), 537
    EU Pregnant Workers Directive
        (1992), 533
    Framework Directive (1989), 532
Eusol (Edinburgh University solution
        of lime), 315
Evacuation of retained products of
        conception (ERPC), 420, 427
Exophthalmus, 150
Expert decision-making, **510**
Expiration, 372
External cardiac massage, 28
External ear, 448
Extracellular fluid, 301, 302
Extradural haematomas, **55**, 56
Extrapersonal factors, influence on
        diagnostic hypotheses, 509
Extremities, examination, 31
Extrication devices, 21
Eye
    anatomy and physiology, 429–433
    examination

following facial trauma, 150
    ophthalmic conditions, 433–436
    see also Ophthalmic emergencies
Eye contact, defusing aggression, 179
Eye opening, Glasgow Coma Scale, 60
Eyebrow injuries, 156
Eyedrops, 441, 442
Eyelids, 430
    examination, 435
    injuries, 155
Eyepads, 441, **442**

Face, examination, 30
Faces pain scales, 328, 329
Facial bones, 46, **47**, 147, **148**
Facial injuries, 147–157
    assessment, 148–150
    facial wounds, 155–156
        burns, 171
    frontal sinus fractures, 154
    Le Fort fractures, 150–152
    mandibular fractures, 152
    mechanism of injury, 148
    nasal fractures, 154–155, 453
    orbital floor fractures, 152, 153, 439
    temporomandibular joint
        dislocations, 153–154
Facial nerve
    damage, 149, 150
    testing, 150
Faculty of Emergency Nursing, 8–9
Faeces, 397
Failure to thrive, 226–227
Fallopian tubes, 412
Falls, elderly patients, 290–291
False localising, 59
Fasciotomy, 106
Fast pain system, 326
Fast-tracking patients, 9, 364, 365, 487
Fauces, injury to, 156
Febrile infants, 224
    convulsions, 224–225
Femoral bruits, 397
Femoral fractures, 79–80
    see also Neck of femur fractures
Femoral nerve blocks, 253
Femoral pulse, 74
Fertilisation of ovum, 412–413
Fever, 301
    infants, 224
Fibrin clot, 303
Fibrinolysis, 303
Fibroblast growth factor (FGF), 310
Fibroblasts, 309, 310
Fibrous joints, 71
Fibular fractures, 81
Fifth metatarsal fractures, 87
Fight or flight response, 326
Film dressings, 319, 320
Financial/material abuse, 287–288
Fire hazards, oxygen equipment, 22
Fire-retardent suits, mobile teams, 17
First aid
    burns, 159–160
    nurse triage, 478

First metacarpal fractures, 99
First metatarsal fractures, 87
Fish bones, inhalation, 456
Flail chest, 27, 128–129
Flash burns, 164, 165
Flexion injury, spine, 110, **111**
Flexor tendon injury, 314
Flight physiology, 299–300
Floor cleaning, health and safety, 531
Fluid and electrolyte balance, 301–302,
        381
Fluid replacement, 28
    acute abdomen, 398
        bowel obstruction, 399
    burns patients, 161, 162, 163, 164
    head-injured patients, 62
    pelvic ring injuries, 74
    pre-hospital care, 22
Fluorescein drops, 435
'Flying squads', non-major incidents,
        19–20
    see also Mobile medical/nursing
        teams
Focal injuries, brain, 55–57
Foot injuries, 84–87
    burns, 171
Footwear, mobile teams, 17
Forearm injuries, 94–95
Forefoot, 86–87
Foreign bodies
    conjunctival, 440
    in ear, 450
    inhalation, 454
        croup, 238
        infants, 222
    in nose, 451–452
    in rectum or genitalia, 272
    subtarsal, 441
Forensic evidence, 142
    major incidents, 41
    sexual assault, 417, 418
Forensic medical examiner (FME),
        417, 418
Foreskin entrapment, 272
Fourth ventricle, 48
Fractures
    children, 253
    facial
        blow-out, 152–153, 439
        frontal sinus, 154
        Le Fort, 150–152
        mandibular, 152
        nasal bones, 154–155, 453
    hip, 75–77
    limb, 77–78
        ankle, 81–84
        elbow, 91–94
        femoral, 79–80
        foot, 84–87
        forearm, 94–95
        hand, 99–101
        lower, leg 81
        upper arm, 89, 90–91
        wrist, 95–99
    pelvis, 72–75, 140, 142
    rib, 134, 140, 142

Fractures (*contd*)
    flail chest, 128–129
    shoulder, 87–89, 134
    skull, 30, 54–55, 63, 149
    spine, 110, **111**, 112, 114–115
Frontal sinus fractures, 154
Frostbite, 165–166
Frusemide, 366
Full-thickness burns, 167
    circumferential, 161
    healing, 170, 171
Fungal endocarditis, 368

Gag reflex, 124
Galeazzi fractures, 95
Gamgee dressings, 320, 321
Garden's classification, neck of femur
        fractures, 75–76
Gardinerella vaginalis, **416**
Gas-permeable dressings, 320
Gastric distension, 396
Gastric lavage, 242
Gastritis, 279
Gastro-oesophageal reflux, 227
Gastroenteritis, infants, 227
Gate control theory, 327–328
Gauze dressings, 320, 321
Gelofusine, 22
'General adaptive syndrome' (GAS),
        Selye, 183–184
General practitioners (GPs), 1–2, 3
    X-ray requests, 463
    in A&E departments, 490
    consultation style, 463
    GP cooperatives, 466
Genital warts, **416**
Genitalia
    examination, 31
    injuries, 272
Genitourinary disorders, 406–409
Geudal airway, 27, 124
'Gillick aware' minors, 525
Girth measurement, 142
Glasgow Coma Scale, 29, **58**, 59
    major incidents, 19
    scores, 60
Glaucoma, acute, 433, 439, 444–445
Glenohumeral joint dislocations, 89
Glenoid fossa fractures, 88
Gliding joints, 71
Gloves, pre-hospital care, 20
Glucagon, 388
Glucose regulation, 388–389
Glutaraldehyde, 532, 534
Goals for A&E nurses, 5
'Golden hour', 20
Granulating wounds, 170, 171, 320
Granulation tissue, formation, 310,
        319, 320
Greater omentum, 395, 400
Greenstick fractures, 78, 253–254
    children, 81
Grey matter
    brain, 49, 51
    spinal cord, 110

Grief, symptoms of, 190
Ground substance, 309
Group crisis intervention, 186
Group supervision, 500
Guarding, abdominal, 143
Gunshot injuries, abdominal, 139–140,
        141
Gynaecological emergencies, 413–418
    assessment, 413
    Bartholin's cyst, 416
    emergency contraception, 272, 416,
        417
    history, 413, 414
    menstrual pain, 413–414
    ovarian cysts, 414–415
    pelvic inflammatory disease, 255,
        415–416
    sexual assault, 417–418, **419**
    sexually transmitted diseases, 416

Haemarthrosis, knee, 81, 104
Haematemesis, 397, 452
    oesophageal varices, 402
Haematocrit, burns patients, 164
Haematology, 389–391
Haematoma, 103
    ears, 156
Haematoma block, wrist fracture
        reductions, 96
Haematuria, 142
Haemoglobin, 297
Haemopericardium, 120, 121
Haemophilus influenzae, 239, 240
Haemorrhage
    abdominal, 141
    brain, 55–57, 387
    control of, 28
    Munchausen's syndrome, 207
    oral, 454
    postpartum, 426–427
    subconjunctival, 440, 442
Haemorrhagic pancreatitis, 278
Haemostasis, 302–303
    in wound healing, 309
Haemothorax, massive, 127, 128
Haire splints, 80
Hallucinations, 202, 203
'Halo test', 30, 55
Hand
    examination, acute abdomen, 396
    injuries, 99–101
        burns, 171
Hartmann's solution, 28
Haversian canals, 70
Hazards
    at accident scenes, 20
    COSHH regulations, 531–532
    work-related
        possible hazards, 533
        reporting, 529
Head
    anatomy and physiology, 46–51
    examination, 30
Head injuries, 45, 54–64
    assessment, **58**, 59–61

brain stem death, 62–63
classification, 54–59
infants, 228, 229
management
    minor head injury, 63–64
    serious head injury, 61–62
raised intracranial pressure,
        physiology, 51–54
transfer to specialist neurosurgical
        unit, 62
Headaches, 386–387
Healing
    burn wounds, 170–171
    fractures, 78, **79**
Health care assistants (HCAs), 477
The Health of the Nation (DOH), 5–6,
        341, 469
    accidents, pre-school children, 241
Health promotion, 469–473
    children, 255–256
    community development, 472–473
    health persuasion techniques,
        470–471
    legislative action for health, 471–472
    nurse practitioners, 488
    personal counselling for health, 473
Health and Safety at Work Act (1974),
        527, 530, 531
Health and Safety Executive, 529, 530
    Accident Prevention Advisory Unit,
        530
Health and Safety (First Aid)
        Regulations (1981), 531
Health surveillance, 532
Heart
    anatomy, 120, 121, 341, **342, 343**
    blunt trauma, 132
    heart valves, 343
        donated, 195
    see also Cardiac
Heart block, 357–359
    first degree, 357
    second degree, 357, 358
    third degree, 358, **359**
Heart failure, 365–367
    acute left ventricular failure (LVF),
        365–366
    cardiogenic shock, 303, 366–367
Heart rate
    elderly patients, 284–285
    infants, 221
Heat exhaustion, 385
Heat stroke, 385, 386
Heimlich manoeuvre, 454
    children, 222
Helicobacter pylori, 279
Helmets, mobile teams, 17
Hepatitis B, 531, 535
Herbert's classification, scaphoid
        fractures, 98, 99
Heroin, 265
Herpes simplex, **416**
    corneal ulcers, 445
High Fowler's position, 151
High-visibility fluorescent jackets,
        mobile teams, 17, 20–21

Hindfoot, 84, 85, 86
Hinge joints, 71
Hip injuries, 75–77
    management, 77
Histamine release, burns patients, 161
Historical background, casualty
        departments, 1–2
History, taking
    chest pain, 277
    obstetric, 419
    ophthalmic conditions, 433–435
    psychiatric patients, 200
    sexual assault, 418
    suspected child abuse, 245–246
    trauma patients, 29
        abdominal injuries, 141–142
        head injuries, 59
        spinal injuries, 110, 111–112
Histotoxic hypoxia, 373
HIV/AIDS, staff safety, 536
Home circumstances elderly patients,
        assessment, 291
Homelessness, 280
Homeostasis, 183, 295–296
    compensatory mechanisms in
        shock, 304–305
    haemostasis, 302–303
    oxygen/carbon dioxide, 298–299
    temperature, 300
Hospital closures, 476
Hospital control centre, major
        incidents, 40
Hospital coordination team, major
        incidents, 36
Hospital information centre, major
        incidents, 35
Hospital major incident plan (HMIP),
        36, 37, 41
Hot fat injuries, 164
House of Lords, 522
Human Needs Model, 4
Human Tissue Act (1961), 524
Humeral fractures, 89, 90–91
Humidification therapy, viral croup, 239
Hydrocolloid dressings, 171, 320
Hydrofluoric acid burns, eye, 436
Hydrogen peroxide, wound cleansing,
        315, **316**
Hygiene, elderly patients, 285
Hyperbaric oxygen therapy, 381
Hypercapnia, 62
Hyperglycaemia, cardiac patients, 345
Hyperpyrexia, 224, 301
Hypertension
    head-injured patients, 61
        with pyrexia, 60
    hypertensive crisis, MAOI-induced,
        212–213
Hypertrophic scarring, 311
Hyperventilation
    anxiety states, 205
    differentiation from asthma, 375
    induced, head–injured patients, 54,
        61, 62
    as result of shock, 304
Hyphaema, 438–439

Hypocalcaemia, 279
Hypoglycaemia, 389
Hypomania, 204–205
Hypotension
    head-injured patients, 60
    neurogenic shock, 116
Hypothalamus, 49
Hypothermia, 301, 379, 398
    elderly patients, 285–287
        management, 287
    homeless people, 280
    near drowning, 379
    trauma patients, 29
        children, 31
        pre-hospital situations, 22
Hypothetico-deductive approach,
        clinical reasoning, 507–511
    activating diagnostic hypotheses,
        508–509
    implications for practice, 510, 511
    possible sources of error, 509–510
    pre-encounter data, 507–408
Hypovolaemic shock, 303, 404
Hypoxia, 373
    altitude above 10,000 ft, 299
    brain injury, 59
    types, 373
    viral croup, 239
Hypoxic hypoxia, 373

Iatrogenesis, 516
    drug-induced psychosis, 212
Ibuprofen, 253
Ideas of reference, 202
Ileocaecal sphincter, 394
Ileum, 394
Iliac wing fractures, 74
Immobilisation, musculoskeletal
        injuries, 331
Impacted neck of femur fractures, 75,
        76
Impulse control, mental state
        examination, 201
Inadine, 320
'Inappropriate attenders', 3, 461, 462
Incident forms, 180, 181
Incontinence, spinal injuries, 111
Incus, 448
Indirect triage, 475
Individual case review, 481–482
Infants, 217–230
    assessment, 217–219
    critically ill, 219–222
    dehydration, 226
    failure to thrive, 226–227
    febrile, 224
        convulsions, 224–225
    injured infants, 228
    meningitis, 225, 226
    oxygen therapy, 299
    respiratory difficulty, causes, 222,
        223–224
    sudden infant death syndrome,
        228–230
    vomiting infants, 227–228

Infection
    control of, 476–477, 536
    ear, 448–450
    eye, 443–444
    wound, 313, 321–322
Infectious disease, detention of
        patient, 526
Inflammatory phase, wound healing,
        309–310
Informed consent see Consent
Infraorbital nerve damage, 151
Initial Assessment standard, 6
Inner city A&E departments, 178
Innominate bones, 72
Insect in ear, 450
Insight and judgement, mental state
        examination, 200
Inspiration, 372
Insulin, 388
Intercerebral haemorrhage, 387
Intercostal nerve block, 129, 134
Intercostal recession, 236, 373
Intermediate triage, 477–478
Internal carotid arteries, 51
Internal respiration, 371
Interrupted box sutures, 317
Interstitial fluid, 302
Intertrochanteric fractures, 76–77
Intimate searches, police
        authorisation, 527
Intracellular fluid, 301, 302
Intracerebral haematomas, 56–57
Intracranial pressure see Raised
        intracranial pressure
Intractable angina, 361
Intraoperative local anaesthesia, 337
Intrapersonal factors, influence on
        diagnostic hypotheses, 509–510
Intrauterine contraceptive device, 417
Intravenous access, trauma patients, 28
Intravenous regional anaesthesia, 96,
        336–337
Intuitive reasoning, 506–507
Intussusception, 227, 399
Ipecacuanha, 242
Ipratropium, nebulised, 375
Iridodialysis, 439
Iris, 432
    examination, 435
Iron
    accidental poisoning, 243
    deficiency, 311
Irrigation of wounds, 315
Ischaemia
    brain injury, 387–388
    chest pain, 276

Jackets, mobile teams, 17, 20–21
Jaw thrust, 124, 149
    spinal-injured patients, 113
Jehovah's Witness, unconscious
        patient, 525
Jejunum, 394
Jewellery, removal after death,
        195–196, 524

Joints, 71
see also Dislocations
Jones, Components of Life model, 5
Jugular venous pressure (JVP), elevated, 128, 130

Kantian ethics, 514–515
Kehr's sign, 141
Keloid scarring, 311
Kendrick Extrication Device (KED), 21
King's College Hospital primary care research project, 3, 463
King's Fund
    clinical supervision, 499
    response to major incidents report, 17
Knee injuries, 81
    soft tissue, 103–104
Kocher's technique, 90
Kussmaul's sign, 130
Kyle's classification, intertrochanteric fractures, 76

Lacerations
    cerebral, 55
    scalp, 54
Lacrimal bones, 147
Lacrimal system, 430, 431, **432**
Lactate dehydrogenase, 277, 363
Lange-Hansen classification, ankle injury, 82, **83**
Language development, pre-school child, 234
Laparoscopy
    appendectomy, 401
    salpingostomy, 422
Laparotomy
    eclampsia, 423
    exploratory, 139, 141
Large intestine, 394–395
    obstruction, 398, 399
Large-scale major incident exercises, 36
Laryngeal oedema, 455
Laryngeal trauma, 133
Laryngopharynx, 454
Laryngotracheobronchitis, 237–239
    admission criteria, 239
    assessment, 237–238
    differentiation from epiglottitis, **240**
    discharge advice, 239
    management, 238–239
    physiology, 237
Lateral compression fractures, pelvis, 72, **73**
Lateral malleolus fractures, 82
Lateral ventricles, 48
Law, 521–528
    attendance at A&E, 523
    classification, 522–523
    confidentiality, the police and the press, 526–527
    consent to treatment, 525–526

death and organ donation, 195–196, 524
    detention of patients, 526
    health promotion legislation, 471–472
    health and safety legislation, 530–536
    outline of UK law, 521–522
    patient assessment, 523
    patient property, 524–525
    staff health and safety, 527
    treatment and care, 523–524
Lazarus, 'cognitive model of stress', 184
Le Fort fractures, 150–152
    clinical evidence, 151
    management, 151–152
Lead aprons, 26
Leadership, 497–499
    key activities, **498**
    vision, 498
Learning disability clients, 210–211
    local anaesthesia, 335
Left ventricular failure (LVF), 365–366, 376
Legal defence, concept of, 522
Legislative action, health promotion, 471–472
Lens of eye, 433
    luxation/subluxation, 439
Lesser omentum, 395
Life outside work, 188
Ligaments, 71
    sprains, 102
Lignocaine
    local infiltration, 336
    pharmacology, **334**
    use in cardiac arrest, 352
Limb leads, ECG, 346
Limbs
    anatomy, 77
    ankle injuries, 81–84
    assessment, 78, 79
        head-injured patients, 59
    classification of fractures, 77–78
    elbow injuries, 91–94
    examination, 79
    femoral fractures, 79–80
    foot fractures, 84–87
    forearm injuries, 94–95
    hand injuries, 99–101
    lower leg injuries, 80–81
    upper arm injuries, 89, 90–91
    wrist injuries, 95–99
Limitation Act (1980) Section 2, 523
Line manager, clinical supervision, 500
Linear skull fractures, 54
Lip injuries, 156
Lipids, cardiac patients, 345, 363
Lisfranc dislocation, 86
'Listed' hospitals, 36
Listening, 185
Lithium carbonate, 204–205
Litmus testing, chemical burns, 165
Liver, injury to, 140
Lobbying policy makers, A&E nurses, 472

Local anaesthetics
    benefits, 334, 335
    classification, 334
    disadvantages and limitations, 335
    eyedrops, 441, 442
    nursing implications, 337
    pharmacology, 333–334
    potential toxic effects, 335
    types and uses, 335–337
Log roll, spinal-injured patients, 113–114
Longitudinal skin traction, 75
Lower leg injuries, 80–81
Lumbar puncture, infants, 225, 226
Lumbar spine fractures, 86, 110
Lumbosacral injuries, 110
Lunate
    dislocation, 98–99
    fractures, 98
Lund and Browder charts, 161, **162**
Lungs, anatomy, 120

McBurney's point, 401
Macrophages, 309, 310
Magnesium trisilicate, 277–278
Major incidents, 16–17, 33
    A&E department response, 37–40
        alerting stage, 37–38
        chemical/radioactive contamination, 39–40
        receipt of casualties, 38–39
        treatment of casualties, 39
    aftermath, 41
    definition, 33–34
    exercises, 19, 36–37
    hospital response, 40
    medicolegal issues, 41
    mobile medical/nursing teams, 16
        defining role, 18–19
        equipping, 17
        hospitals providing, 17
        training and experience, 17–18, 19, 37
    planning, 34–36
        functions of emergency management planning, 35
        reasons for, 34
        responsibility for, 35–36
Mallet finger, 105
Malleus, 448
Malnutrition, effect on wound healing, 311
Management of Health and Safety at Work Regulations (1992), 533–534
Manchester Triage Group, 482
Mandible, 148
Mandibular fractures, 152
Mania, 204–205
Mannitol, 62
Manual handling, 533
    Manual Handling Operations Regulations (1992), 534–536
Marfan's syndrome, 439
Marginal ulcers, cornea, 445

Maslach burn-out inventory (MBI), 185
Mast cells, 309
Masters degree course, nurse practitioner, 489
Maturation phase, wound healing, 310–311
Maxilla, 147
Mechanical ventilation, 27
    flail chest, 129
    pre-hospital care, 21–22
    pulmonary contusion, 132
The media, 527
    major incidents, 40
Medial malleolus fractures, 82
Median nerve, assessing function, **93**
Mediastinum, 120
Medical emergencies, 371–391
    anaphylaxis, 303–304, 379, 455
    asthma, 235–237, 374–375
    carbon monoxide poisoning, 373, 380–381
    chronic obstructive airways disease (COAD), 375–376
    dehydration, 226, 312, 383, 384
    glucose regulation, 388–389
    haematology, 389–391
    near drowning, 379–380
    nervous system, 386–388
    overhydration, **384**
    pulmonary embolism, 276, 277, 377–378
    pulmonary oedema, 376–377
    renal disorders, 381–382
    respiration, 371–373
    thermoregulation, 384–386
    urinary tract infection, 382
Medical incident officer (MIO), 18
Medical model of care, 5, 470
Medulla, 51
Meibomian glands, 430, 431
Meninges, 46, 48
Meningitis, 225, 226
Menstruation, 412
    pain, 413–414
Mental Health Act (1983)
    detention of patients, 526
    treatment against patient's will, 525
Mental state examination, 200–201
Mentorship, 500
Mesenteric adenitis, 254–255
Mesenteric embolus, 399
Mesentery, 395
Mesocaval shunt, 403
Metabolic acidosis, 122, 379
Metabolism, excretion of by-products, 382
Metacarpal fractures
    second to fifth, 101
    thumb, 99, 100
Metatarsal fractures, 86, 87
Methadone, 265
Metronidazole, 279
Microbiological hazards, COSHH regulations, 532
Midbrain, 50, 51

Middle years, 275–280
    chest pain, 275–278
    epigastric pain, 279–280
    homelessness, 280
    pancreatitis, 278–279
Midfoot, 86
MIG welder, ocular burns, 437–438
Migraine, 386–387
Minor injuries, 3
    head injuries
        Glasgow Coma Score, 60
        indications for hospital admission, 64
        management, 63–64
    nurse practitioner role, 488
Miosis, traumatic, 439
Miscarriage, 419–420, 421
    categorisation, **420**
    management, 420, 421
    threatened, differential diagnosis, **422**
Misuse of Drugs Act, 1971, penalties, 260–261
Mitral valves, 343
Mittelschmerz disease, 413–414
Mobile medical/nursing teams, 16
    defining role, 18–19
    equipping, 17
    hospitals providing, 17
    major incidents, 16–17
    non-major incidents, 19–20
    training and experience, 17–18, 19, 37
Mobitz type heart block, **358**
'Model' simulations, library of, 511
Models of nursing, 4–5
Moderate head injuries, 60
Monoamine oxidase inhibitors (MAOIs), 212–213
Monocytes, 310
Monofilament polyglyconate polymers, suture material, 317
Monteggia fracture, 94
Mood, mental state examination, 200
Moral theory, Kant's formulations, 514
Morphine, 330
Mortuary, temporary, major incidents, 35
Motor disturbances, psychiatric patients, 202
Motor function
    assessment, head-injured patients, 59
    transient loss of, 337
    wound assessment, testing nerves, 314
Motor response, Glasgow Coma Scale, 60
Mouth, injury to, 156, 454–455
Muir and Barclay fluid replacement formula, 162, 163
Multidisciplinary case review, 481
Multidisciplinary teamwork, avoiding negligence, 524
Multiply-injured patients, 25
    preparation for arrival, 26
Munchausen's syndrome, 207–208

Munchausen's syndrome by proxy, 207–208, 243, 246–247
Muscles, 71
    spasm, shoulder dislocation, 89
    strains, 102–103
Musculoskeletal pain, 276
Mydriasis, traumatic, 439
Myocardial infarction, 361–365, 376
    assessment, 362, 363, 480
    cardiac enzyme release, 277
    management, 363–365
    pain, 276, 277
    signs of reperfusion, 364
Myocardium, 343
Myogenic relfex, 302
Myoglobin in urine, 165

NAIR scheme, 39
Naloxone, 330
Named nurse, 5, 6, 190
Narcotic drugs, accidental ingestion, 242–243
Nasal bones, 147
    fractures, 154–155, 453
Nasogastric tube insertion
    contraindications, 30
    stomach decompression, 30, 142
Nasopharyngeal airway, 27, 124
Nasopharynx, 454
National Audit Office
    accidents at work, costs survey, 530
    patient attendance report, 1992a,b, 3
National triage scale, 482–483
Navicular avulsion fractures, 86
Near drowning, 379–380
Nebulised medications
    adrenaline, 239
    budesonide, 239
    ipratropium, 375
    salbutamol, 236, 237, 375
    terbutaline, 375
Neck, examination, 30
Neck of femur fractures, 75–76, 291
    fast-tracking patients, 9
    nursing care issues, 7
Needlestick injuries, 530, 535
Negative evaluation of patients, 462
Neglect
    of children, 243
        common indicators, 244
    of elderly people, 288
Negligence, 518, 522, 524, 526
    checks to avoid, 524
    failure to treat, 523
    Limitation Act (1980) Section 2, 523
Neisseria gonorrhoea, **416**
Nerve fibres, diameter, 334
Nerve function, wound assessment, 314
Network supervision, 500
Neural control of respiration, 372
Neurogenic shock, 116, 303
Neurological assessment
    medical emergencies, 386–387
    trauma patients, 28–29

Neurological assessment (*contd*)
  head injuries, 59
  pre-hospital care, 22
Neurological type, Munchausen's
  syndrome, 207
Neurotransmitters, 326
Neurovascular integrity, wounds, 313,
  314
Neutrophils, 309–310
The New NHS white paper, 9
NHS Direct, 9, 465–466
NHS Executive regional offices, major
  incident planning, 36
Night workers, EU Working Time
  Directive, 537
Nitrous oxide *see* Entonox
Nociceptors, 325, 326
Non-absorbable sutures, 317, 318
Non-accidental injury *see* Child abuse
Non-allergic asthma, 374
Non-beating heart donors, 195
Non-expert decision-making, **510**
Non-invasive temporary pacing, 359,
  360
Non-maleficence, 516, 517
Non-professional triage, 477
Non-toxic agents, ingestion, 242
Non-verbal communication, 6,
  176–177, 179
Non-VF/VT (asystole,
  electromechanical
  dissociation), infants, 221
Northern Ireland
  abortion, 521
  major incident planning
    guidelines, 34
Nose
  allergic rhinitis, 453
  anatomy, 451, **452**
  epistaxis, 154, 452–453
  foreign body, 451–452
  nasal bones, 147
    fractures, 154–155, 453
  rhinorroea, 453
NSAIDS, 331
  pericarditis, 367
Nuclear accidents, 39
  radiation burns, 166
Nurse counsellors, 185–186
Nurse practitioners, A&E, 4, 7, 178,
  465, 485–491
  activities of, 486–488
  audit and evaluation, 489–491
  development of role, 485–486
  education needs, 488–489
  issues to be addressed in
    developing services, 491
Nurse specialist, A&E, 8, 9
Nurse triage *see* Triage
Nurse-run clinics, minor injuries,
  3
Nurse/patient relationship, 5–6
Nursing incident officer (NIO),
  18
Nursing process, 506
Nutrition and wound healing, 312

Obstructed airway, 27, 122, 454
  asthma attack, 374
  epiglottitis, 239–240
  facial injuries, 149
  indicators, 124
  infants, 219
  see also Airway management
Occulogyric crisis, 212, 253
Occupiers Liability Act (1957), 527
Ochsner's test, 92
Oedema, burns patients, 161
Oesophageal pain, 276
Oesophageal varices, 401–403
  assessment, 402
  management, 402–403
Oesophagus
  anatomy, 393, 394
  injury, 134
Open pneumothorax, 127
Ophthalmic emergencies, 429–445
  anatomy and physiology of eye,
    429–433
  assessment, 433–436
    contact lenses, 435–436
    equipment to aid, 435
    examining eye, 434–435
    history, 433–434
    visual acuity, 434
  chemical injuries, 165
  eyedrops, 441, 442
  eyepads, 441, **442**
  health promotion, 445
  major closed trauma, 153, 438–440
  minor trauma, 440–441
  ocular burns, 436–438
  penetrating trauma, 438
  red eye, 442–445
Ophthalmoscopes, 435
Opiates, 326, 330
  angina attack, 361
  burns patients, 168
  children, 253
    accidental poisoning, 242, 243
  contraindications in pancreatitis, 278
  myocardial infarction, 363
  pulmonary oedema, 377
  trauma patients, 29, 75
Opposing factions, clashes, receiving
  hospital, 35
Oral injuries, 156, 454–455
Oral rehydration solutions, 226
Orbit, 429, 430
  fractures, 152–153, 439
Orem's model of self-care, 4
Organ donation, 195
  legal issues, 524
Organic illness mimicking psychiatric
  symptoms, 202
Oropharyngeal airway, 27, 124
Oropharynx, 454
Osmoreceptors, 381
Ossicles, 448
Osteoblasts, 70
Osteochondritis, 254
Osteoclasts, 71
Osteocytes, 70–71

Otitis externa, 448–449
Otitis media, 449–450
Otorrhoea, 30, 55
Ottawa ankle rules, 104
Outpatients department, voluntary
  hospitals, 1
Ovaries, 412
  cysts, 414–415
Overflow incontinence, 406
Overhydration, **384**
Overload injuries, 269
Overuse injuries, 269
Oxygen saturation, 297
Oxygen therapy, 122, 299
  asthma attack, 236
  carbon monoxide poisoning, 381
  chest pain, **277**
  chronic bronchitis, 376
  left ventricular failure, 366
  myocardial infarction, 363
  trauma patients, 27
    burns patients, 160
    pre-hospital care, 22
Oxygen transport, 296–298
Oxygen-haemoglobin dissociation
  curve, 298
Oxygen/carbon dioxide homeostasis,
  298–299
Oxyhaemoglobin, 297

P wave, ECG, 347
P-R interval, ECG, 347
Pacing, 359–360
Paediatric advanced life support,
  221–222, **223**
Paediatric basic life support, **222**
Pain
  assessing, 253, 328–329, 482
    acute abdomen, 395–396
  chest, 275–278
  epigastric, 279–280
  eye, 440
  menstrual, 413
  physiology, 325–327
    effects of pain, 326–327
    pain relay systems, 326
    pain transmitters, 326
  theories, 327–328
Pain relief
  children, 252–253
  non-pharmacological, 331
  pharmacological, 330–331
  see also Local anaesthetics; Opiates
Pain scales, 253, 328, 329
Pain thresholds, 326, 327
Palatine bones, 147
Pale stools, 397
Pallor, 277
Pancreas, injury to, 140
Pancreatitis, 278–279, 399
'Panda eyes', 149
Papillary layer, 309
Paracetamol, accidental poisoning,
  242
Paradoxical chest movement, 128

Paraffin tulle dressings, 171
Parainfluenza virus, 237
Paralytic ileus
    abdominal injuries, 142–143
    acute abdomen, 396, 400
    burn-injured patients, 164
    spinal cord injuries, 116
Paramedics, 37
Paraphimosis, 272
Parasuicide see Self-harm
Parathyroid hormone, 302
Parents
    child abuse, 245
    consent issues, 525
    pre-school child, 234, 235
    separation from, adolescents, 258
Paroxysmal supraventricular
        tachycardia, 205
Partial pressure, 296, 297
Partial-thickness burns, 166–167
    healing, 170
Passivity, 202
Patellar fractures, 81
Patient assessment see Assessment
Patient satisfaction, nurse
        practitioners, 491
The Patient's Charter
    named nurse standard, 5
    patient assessment, 6, 475, 477, 483
    waiting times, 7
Peak flow measurement, 236, 374
Pedestrian deaths, 270
Peer pressure, 252
Peer supervision, 500
Pelvic inflammatory disease, 415–416
    children, 255
Pelvic injury, 72–75, 140, 142
    fracture patterns, 72–74
    mechanism, 72
    pelvic ring fracture, 73, **74**
        management, 74–75
Pelvis
    anatomy, 72, 138
    examination, 31
Penetrating injuries
    abdomen, 138–140, 141
    chest, 120, 140
Penis
    bites to, 272
    examination, 74
Peptic ulcers, 279–280, 402
Perceptions, mental state examination,
        200
Percussion, abdominal, 143, 397
Percutaneous transhepatic portal vein
        embolisation, 403
Perfusion, 121
    of tissue, wound healing, 312
Pericardiocentesis, 130–131
Pericardium, 343
    pericardial tears, 140
    pericarditis, 276, 367
Perilunate and lunate dislocation, 98,
        99
Perineum, examination, 74
Periorbital swelling, 150

Periosteum, 70
Peripheral chemoreceptors, 298
Peripheral nerve blocks, 336
Peritoneal compartment, 137, 138
    bleeding, 141, 142, 143
Peritoneum, 395
Peritonitis, 400
Peritonsillar abscesses, 456
Permanent pacing, 360
Personal bias, 509
Personal fable, 258–259
Personal possessions, removal after
        death, 195–196, 524–525
Personal space, 179
Personality types, A&E nurses, 185
Petechial rash, 225
Pethidine, 330
Phalangeal fractures, 87, 101
    thumb, 100
Pharyngoconjunctival fever, 444
Pharynx, 455–456
Phayrngo-tympanic tube, 448
Phentolamine, 212
Phosphate regulation, 302
Photographs
    accident scene, spinal injury, 111
    infant death, 230
    suspected child abuse, 246
Photoreceptors, 433
Physical abuse
    children, 243
    elders, 287, 288
Physiology for practice, 295–305
    carbon dioxide transport, 298
    flight physiology, 299–300
    fluid and electrolyte balance,
        301–302
    haemostasis, 302–303
    homeostasis, 295–296
    oxygen therapy, 299
    oxygen transport, 296–298
    oxygen/carbon dioxide
        homeostasis, 298–299
    pain, 325–327
    raised intracranial pressure, 51–54
    respiration, 121–122
    shock, 303–305
    temperature control, 300–301
Pia mater, 48
Pinna, 448
    trauma, 451
        avulsion injury, 156
Pivot joints, 71
Placenta, 413
    abruptio placentae, 423–424
    delivery of, 426
Plasma, 390
Plaster of Paris dust, 532
Platelets, 390
    plug formation, 302–303
Platinum 10 minutes, 20
Platt Report (Standing Medical
        Advisory Committee 1962), 2, 3
Play, 235, 253
Pleura, anatomy, 120
Pleuritic pain, 276

Pneumatic anti-shock garment
        (PASG), 28, 75
Pneumothorax, 27, 28, 125–127
    classification, 125
Poisoning, pre-school child, 241–243
    assessment, 241–242
    management, 242–243
Police
    detention of patients, 526
    documentation team, major
        incidents, 39
    hospital facilities, 35
    powers of search and arrest, 527
Polyglycolic acid suture material, 317
Pons, 51
Portacaval shunt, 403
Portal hypertension, 396, 402
Post mortem see Autopsy
Post-ictal state, 62
Postcoital contraception, 272, 416, 417
Posterior chamber, eye, 433
Postpartum haemorrhage, 426–427
Postpartum psychiatric problems, 204,
        273
Potassium balance, 302
Povidine-iodine
    soaks, 80
    wound cleansing, 315, **316**
PQRST model of triage assessment,
        479
Pre-eclampsia, 422–423
Pre-encounter data, 507–508
Pre-hospital care, 15–23
    burns
        chemical, 165
        radiation, 166
        thermal, 164
    delivery of care, 20–21
    major incidents, 16–17
    mobile teams
        defining role, 18–19
        equipping, 17
        training and experience, 17–18
    non-major incidents, 19–20
    'nurses' unique role, 23
    patient assessment, 21–23
Pre-hospital Emergency Care Course
        (PHEC), 20
Pre-hospital Trauma Life Support
        (PHTLS) course, 20
Pre-school children, 233–248
    accidental injury, 240–241
    accidental poisoning, 241–243
    acute laryngotracheobronchitis,
        237–239
    asthma, 235–237
    child under stress, 234–235
    epiglottitis, 239–240
    Munchausen's syndrome by proxy,
        243, 246–247
    non-accidental injuries, 243–246
    normal development, 234
    sexual abuse, 246, 247
    understanding illness, 235
Preceptorship, 500
Precordial thump, 350

Prednisolone
asthma attacks, 237
viral croup, 239
Pregnancy, 419–427
abruptio placentae, 423, 424
assessment, 419
eclampsia, 423
ectopic, 415, 421–422
emergency childbirth, 424–427
miscarriage, 419–420, 421
physiological changes, 413
pre-eclampsia, 422–423
staff, safety at work, 533
testing for, 28
Preoperative preparation, 408–409
The press see The media
Pressure waves, gunshot injuries, 140
Prevention of Terrorism Act
(Temporary Provisions Act
1984), 526
Priapism, 112
Prilocaine, pharmacology, **334**
Primary care, 461–466
bridging the gap between A&E and
primary care, 464
changing the culture, 465
future implications, out-of-hours
care delivery, 466
legitimacy of attendance, 3, 461–462
nurse practitioners, 4, 7, 178, 465
primary care role, 464–463
developing, A&E nurses, 463–464
providing for primary care in A&E,
463
telephone consultation, 9, 465–466
Primary health promotion, 470
Primary nursing, 6
Primary survey, 6–7
infants, 220
trauma patients, 26–29
pre-hospital care, 21, 22
Printzmetal's angina, 361
Priority setting, nurse triage, 480
Privacy, adolescents, 258
Prochaska and Diclemente, 'stages of
change' model, 473
Professional profile, clinical
supervision records, 502
Profunda femoris artery, 75, 80
Proliferation phase, wound healing,
310
Property of patient, legal
considerations, 195–196,
524–525
Proptosis, 150
Prostate
high riding, 30, 31, 74, 140, 142
obstruction, 406
Protective clothing
Health and Safety at Work Act, 531
mobile teams, 17, 20
trauma teams, 26
Protein intake, wound healing, 312
Protocols
clinical reasoning, 511
triage assessments, 480

used by nurse practitioners, 486, 487
violent incidents, 177
Pseudo-fits, 207
Pseudologia fantastica, 208
Psoas sign, 401
Psychiatric emergencies, 199–213,
272–273
acute organic reactions, 201–202
acute psychotic episode, 202–205
aetiology, mental illness, 200
alcohol-related emergencies,
206–207
see also Alcohol intoxication
anxiety states, 205–206
assessment of psychiatric patients,
200–201
children and adolescents, 211
eating disorders, 211
elderly clients, 211
iatrogenic drug-induced psychosis,
212
individual at odds with society, 210
learning disability clients, 210–211
monoamine oxidase inhibitors
(MAOIs), 212–213
Munchausen's syndrome, 207–208
Munchausen's syndrome by proxy,
207–208, 243, 246–247
social problems, 211–212
suicide and deliberate self-harm,
208–210, 210, 259, 265, 266, 273,
380, 456
see also Drug intoxication
Psychological abuse, elder abuse, 287
Psychological considerations
burns patients, 168, 169
pre-hospital care, 23
preparation for surgery, 408
staff support following major
incidents, 41
wound healing, 312
Psychosis, drug-induced, 212
Psychotic patients, 202–205
depression, 203–204
hypomania/mania, 204–205
postpartum psychotic problems,
204
schizophrenia, 203
symptoms, 202
Pubic ramus, fractures, 74
Pulmonary contusion, 131–132
Pulmonary embolism, 377–378
pain, 276, 277
Pulmonary oedema, 376–377
Pulse
asthma attack, 236
burns patients, 164
left ventricular failure, 365
myocardial infarction, 362
Pulse oximetry, 27, 297, 373
asthma attack, 236
chest pain, 277
Pupils, assessment, 59, 60
Pyloric stenosis, 228
Pyramidal tract decussation, 51
Pyrexia see Fever

QRS complex, ECG, 347
Questions, triage assessment, 480

'Racoon eyes', 55
Radial fractures, 94, 95
distal radius, 96
radial head, 94
Radial nerve, 92
assessing function following elbow
injury, **93**
Radiation incidents, 39–40
burns, 166
ocular, 437–438
Raised intracranial pressure
head-injured patients, 62
physiology, 51–54
Ranitidine, 279
Rape trauma syndrome (RTS), 418,
419
Rash, petechial, 225
RCN
A&E Nursing Association, 3, 4
Challenging the Boundaries, 8
Emergency Nurse Practitioner
Special Interest Group, 488
standard five-point triage scale,
482
Accident and Emergency Nursing
course, 2
Advanced Trauma Nursing course,
8
aggressive incidents, 175, 176
bereavement care study, 189–190
Children in A&E Special Interest
Group, 8
elder abuse definition, 287
patient handling, 535
time off work survey, 534
Trauma Nursing Core course, 8
Reasonable force, physical restraint,
180
Rebound tenderness, 143, 397, 400
Recombinant tissue-type plasminogen
activator (tPA), 364
Rectum, 394
examination, 31, 74
pelvic injuries, 142
spinal-injured patients, 114
injury to, 140
Red blood cells, 389–390
Red eye, 442–445
differential diagnosis, **443**
Referred pain, shoulder, 141
Refusing care, 462
Regent's Park bombing, 16
Regional anaesthesia
nerve blocks, 96, 129, 134, 335,
336–337
children, 253
Regional health authorities, major
incident planning, 36
Relatives
aggression, 176
of cardiac arrest patients, 352
drunk and intoxicated, 523

Relatives (*contd*)
  giving consent, 525
  of sudden death victims, 6, 8, 190
    breaking bad news, 192–194
    legal and ethical issues, 195–196
    organ donation, 195
    preparing to receive, 190
    viewing the body, 194
    witnessed resuscitation, 190–192
  of trauma patients
    burns patients, 169
    keeping informed, 31–32
    support at accident scene, 23
    witnessing violent incident in A&E,
      180
  see also Parents
Renal bruits, 397
Renal disorders, 381–382
*Report on the Management of Patients
  with Major Injuries*, RCS, 8
Reporting of Injury, Disease and
  Dangerous Occurrence
  Regulations (RIDDOR), 530,
  531
Reports, violent incidents, 180
Reproductive cycle, 412
Respect, principle of, 515
Respiration, 371–373
  assessment of
    gas exchange, 373
    mechanics, 372
    respiratory control, 372–373
  burns patients, 164
  infants, 219, 220
  physiology, 121–122
Respiratory arrest, asthma attack, 374
Respiratory centre, 298, 299, 372
Respiratory rate
  asthma, 235, 236
  infants, 221
Respiratory syncytial virus (RSV), 222,
  224
Restraint, violent individuals, 180
Resuscitation
  effects of failed on staff, 196
  witnessed, 190–192
Retention of urine, 405–406
  urinary catheterisation, 406–407
Retina, 433
  burns, 437–438
Retrolental fibroplasia, 299
Retroperitoneal compartment, 138, 395
Rewarming hypothermic patients, 287
Rhabdomyolysis, 263
Rhinitis, allergic, 453
Rhinorrhoea, 30, 55, 453
Rib fractures, 134, 140, 142
  flail chest, 128–129
Right to refuse treatment, 209
Ring block, digit anaesthesia, 336
Ringer's solution, 74
Risk assessment
  elderly patients, 291
  lifting patients, 535
  Management of Health and Safety at
    Work regulations, 533–534

Risk-taking behaviour
  adolescents, 259–261
  children, 252
Road traffic accidents, 270–271
Rods, 433
Rolando's fracture, 100
Roper's nursing model, 4
Rotational injury, spine, 110, **112**
Rotator cuff injuries, 104, 105
Rovsing's sign, 401
Royal College of Surgeons (RCS), 8
Rule of 'nines', 161
Russel Extrication Device (RED), 21

Sacral fractures, 74, 115
Saddle joints, 71
Safety at work, 527, 529–537
  framework for maintaining safe
    environment, 537
  infection control, 536
  legislation, 530–532
    since 1992, 532–536
  preventing accidents, 529–530
  working time, 536–537
Safety, pre hospital care, 20–21
Safety Representatives and Safety
  Committees Regulations
  (1977), 531
Salbutamol, 236, 237
Saline
  administration, 74–75
  wound cleansing, 315, **316**
    burn wounds, 167
Salpingostomy, laparoscopic, 422
Scalds, 164
Scalp injuries, 54, 149
Scaphoid fractures, 97–98
Scapular fractures, 87–88, 134
Scarring, 311
  multiple abdominal, 208
Schizophrenia, 203, 272–273
Sclera, 432
  perforation, 438
Sclerotherapy, endoscopic, 403
'Scoop' stretchers, 112
Scope of Professional Practice, UKCC,
  480, 481, 515, 523
Scotland, major incident planning
  guidelines, 34
Screening for admission to A&E, lack
  of, 462
Seat belts
  injuries
    abdominal injury, 140, 270
    sternal fractures, 134
    law enforcement, 471, 472
Secondary brain injury, 61, 62
Secondary health promotion, 470, 471
Secondary hypothermia, 29
Secondary survey, 7
  infants, 220
  trauma patients, 29–31
  pre-hospital care, 21
Security measures, inner city
  departments, 178, 179

Sedation, alcoholic coma, 271
Seidal's test, 438
Seizures *see* Convulsions
Self-awareness
  clinical leader, 499
  clinical supervision, 501
Self-confidence, nurse practitioners,
  488
Self-governance, myth of, 517–518
Self-harm, 208–210, 273, 380
  adolescents, 259, 265, 266
  hanging, 456
  mutilation, 210
Self-support groups, coping with
  stress, 186
Selye, 'general adaptive syndrome'
  (GAS), 183–184
Semi-conscious patients
  ethical issues, 518
  legal issues, 525
Semilunar valves, 343
Sengstaken triple-lumen tube, **402**,
  403
Sensation-seeking behaviour,
  adolescents, 259
Septic shock, 303
Serum glutamic oxaloacetic
  transaminase (SGOT), 277, 363
Severe head injuries, 60
  management, 61–62
Sexual abuse
  of children, 244, 246, 247, 255
  of elderly people, 288
Sexual assault, 417–418, 419
Sexually transmitted diseases, 416
  pelvic inflammatory disease, 415
Sharps, use and disposal, 536
Shift handovers, 186
Shivering, 285, 300, 385
Shock, 30, 116, 303–305, 404
  acute abdomen, 397–398, 399
  anaphylactic, management of, 455
  cardiogenic, 303, 366–367
Shoulder
  injuries
    dislocations, 89–90
    fractures, 87–89
    rotator cuff injury, 104, 105
  pain referred to, 141
Sickle cell disease, 390–391
Silk sutures, 317
Silver sulphadiazine cream, 171
Simmonds' test, 104
Simple fractures, limbs, 77
Single European Act (1986), Article
  118A, 532
Sinus rhythm, 345
Sinus tachycardia, 132
Sinusitis, 453–454
'Six pack' regulations, 532–536
Skeleton, anatomy and physiology, 67,
  68–71
Skin
  anatomy, 307, **308**, 309
  assessment, elderly patients 284
  functions, 308

Skin (contd)
  injury, mechanism of, 313, **314**
  perfusion, infants, 221
  preoperative preparation, 409
  temperature, 300, 308
    burns patients, 164
    infants, 221
Skull
  anatomy, 46, **47**
  fractures, 63, 149
    classification, 30, 54–55
    cribriform plate, 30, 149, 453
Slit lamps, 435
Slow pain system, 326
Small intestine
  anatomy, 394
  obstruction, 397, 398, 399
Small-scale major incident exercises, 36
Smith's fractures, 96–97
Smoke inhalation, 160
Smoking and wound healing, 312
Snellen chart, 434
'Snowballing', 265
SOAP model of triage, 478, 479
Social class, 471
Social knowledge, 509–510
Social problems, 211–212
Social worth, perceived by staff, 462
Socioeconomic status, 3
Sociopathy, 210
Sodium bicarbonate, use in cardiac
    arrest, 352
Sodium and water balance, 302
Soft tissue injuries, 101–106
    knee, 103–104
SOLER acronym, 209
Solvent injury, eye, 436, 437
Sore throat, 456
Space blankets, 287
Spacers, pre-school children, 237
Specialist knowledge, forming
    diagnostic hypotheses, 509–510
Specificity theory, pain, 327
Speech and thought
    disturbances, 202
    mental state examination, 200
    pre-school child, 234
'Speedballing', 265
Spillages, blood and body fluids, 536
Spinal boards, 21, 27, 30
Spinal injuries, 109–117
    examination, 112–114
      airway, 113
      primary survey, 113
      secondary survey and log roll,
        113–114
      spine immobilisation, 21, 26–27,
        30, 112–113
    fractures
      cervical spine, 114–115
      thoracolumbar spine, 115
    history-taking, 110, 111–112
    pathophysiology, 110, **111**
    spinal cord injury, 115–116
      neurogenic shock, 116
      spinal shock, 116

Spiritual support, staff, following
    major incidents, 41
Spleen, injury to, 140, 143
Splenorenal shunt, 403
Splinting
  femoral fractures, 80
  hand injuries, 101
Spontaneous abortion see Miscarriage
Sports injuries
  children, 254
  young adults, 269–270
Sprains, 102
  ankle, 104
ST segment, ECG, 347
Stab wounds, abdominal, 138–139, 140,
    141
Stable angina, 361
'Stages of change' model, Prochaska
    and Diclemente, 473
Stagnant hypoxia, 373
Standards of care
  A&E service principles, 2
  children, 8
  Faculty of Emergency Nursing, 9
  Initial Assessment standard, 6
  legal considerations, 523–524
'Standby', major incidents, 38
Stapes, 448
Staples, wound, 318
Status epilepticus, 388
Statutory Instruments, 521
Steam injuries, 164
Sternal injuries, 134
Sternal recession, 236, 373
Steroids
  asthma attack, 237
  viral croup, 239
Stomach
  anatomy, 394
  decompression, 30, 142
Strains, 102–103
Stratum corneum, 307, 309
Stratum lucidum/granulosum/
    spinosum and basale, 309
Streptokinase, 364, 378
Stress, 176, 183–188
  coping, 184
  critical incident stress debriefing
    (CISD), 187
  defusion, 186
  demobilisation, 186–187
  distress in A&E nursing, 9, 184–185
  responses to burn-out, 187–188
  stress-related pain, 276
  support and care, 185–186
    following sudden death, 196
Stress fractures
  children, 254
  fibula, 81
Stridor, 124
  infants, 219
  pre-school children, 238
Stroke, 387–388
Subarachnoid haemorrhage, 55, 56,
    387
Subconjunctival ecchymosis, 150

Subconjunctival haemorrhage, 442
  traumatic, 440
Subdural haematomas, 51, 56
Subgaleal haematoma, 54
Sublingual glyceral trinitrate (GTN),
    277, 361
Substance misuse, 261–265
  language of, **262**
  Misuse of Drugs Act, 1971,
    penalties, 260–261
Substance P, 326
Substantia gelatinosa, 327
Substantia propria, 431
Subtarsal foreign body, 441
Sucking chest wounds, 27, 127
Suction apparatus, 27
Sudden death, 8
  bereavement care, 189–197
  complaints from relatives, 6
  sudden infant death syndrome,
    228–230
    continuing care, 229–230
    initial response, 229
Suicide, 208–210, 273
  strangulation or hanging, 456
Superficial burns, 166, **167**
  healing, 170
Superficial punctate keratitis, 445
Supracondylar fractures
  femur, 80
  humerus, 92–93
Suprapubic aspiration of urine, 406
Supraspinatus injury, 105
Supraventricular tachycardia, 354, 355
Surgical cleaning, wounds, 313, 315
Surgical emergencies, 393–409
  abdomen, anatomy and physiology,
    393–395
  acute abdomen, 395–401
  genitourinary disorders, 406–409
  preoperative preparation, 408–409
  vascular disorders, 401–406
Surgical exploration, abdomen, 143
Suturing, 316–318
  common errors in, 318
  suture removal, 318
Sweating, 277, 300, 385
'Swimmer's ear', 449
'Swimmer's view', 115
Symphyses, 71
Symptom clustering, 479
Synchondroses, 71
Synometrine, 425
Synovial joints, 71
Systematic assessment of triage, 479
Systole, 344

T wave, ECG, 347
Table-top major incident exercises, 36
Tachycardia
  anxiety attacks, 205
  infants, 220
  left ventricular failure, 365
  myocardial infarction, 362
  supraventricular 354, 355
  viral croup, 238

Tachypnoea, 362
Talus, 84, 85, 86
Tampons, lost, 272
Tap water, wound cleansing, 315, **316**
Tarry stools, 397
Tarsal glands, 430, 431
Tattoo scarring, 311
Team leader, managing violent
    individuals, 179, 180
Team nursing, 6
Team-building, 498
Tear film, 430, 431
    recording pH after chemical burns,
      437
Teeth
    abscesses, 455
    examination, 149
    injuries, 156
      bleeding from sockets, 454
Telephone, use of
    NHS Direct, telephone advice
      service, 9, 465–466
    notification of bereavement, 194
    triage, 466, 475
Temperature
    chest pain, 277
    control of, 300–301, 384–386
    elderly patients, 285
    myocardial infarction, 362
    skin, 300, 308
      burns patients, 164
      infants, 221
    wound, speed of healing, 320
    see also Hypothermia
Temporary pacing (transvenous), 360
Temporomandibular joint dislocation,
    153–154
Tendon injury, wound assessment, 314
Tendonitis, 103, 104
    rotator cuff, 105
Tendons, 71
    strains, 102–103
Tensile strength, wounds, 310
Tension headaches, 386
Tension pneumothorax, 27, 28,
    125–127
    assessment, 126
    immediate management, 126–127
Tertiary health promotion, 470, 471
Testicles, examination, 74
Testis, torsion, 407–408
Tetanus prophylaxis, 322–323
Tetany, 205, 279
Thermal injuries, 160, 164–166
    ocular, 437
Thermoregulation, 300–301, 384–386
    see also Temperature
Third ventricle, 48
Thirst centre, 302
Thomas splints, 80
Thoracentesis, 27, 127
Thoracic injuries *see* Chest injuries
Thoracolumbar spine injuries, 110, 115
Thought insertion/blocking/
    broadcasting, 202
Throat, anatomy and physiology, 454

Thrombolytic therapy
    myocardial infarction, 364–365
    pulmonary embolism, 378
Thumb injuries
    fractures, 99–100
    sprains, 105
Thyroid gland, temperature
    homeostasis, 300
Tibial fractures, 81
Tissue adhesive, 318, 319
Tongue
    examination, 395
    injuries to, 156, 454
Tonsillitis, 238
Topical local anaesthetics, 253,
    335–336
Tourniquet time, 336, 337
Toxic agents, ingestion
    drugs, 242, 243
    household products, 243
Toxic shock, 303
Trace element deficiency, 311
Tracheal injuries, 133
Tracheitis, bacterial, 238
Tracheostomy
    facial fractures, 151
Traction, shoulder dislocation, 89
Traction/counter-traction
    shoulder dislocation, 89–90
    wrist fracture reduction, 96
Trade Union Reform and Employment
    Rights Act (1993), 534
Training, 524
    'flying squads', non-major incidents,
      20
    major incidents, 37
      mobile teams, 17–18, 19
    nurse practitioners, 488–489
    nurse triage, 480–481
    see also Courses
Trajectory of death, concept of, 190
Transfer teams, major incidents, 39
Transforming growth factor (TGF),
    310
Transient cells, skin, 309
Transient ischaemic attacks, 387
Transoesophageal ligation,
    oesophageal varices, 403
Transport
    major incident triage, 19
    time-critical injuries, 23
Transport Road Research Laboratory,
    270, **271**
Trauma, 25–32
    abdominal, 137–144
    burns, 105, 159–172
    children, 31
      age 5 to puberty, 253–254
      infants, 228
      pre-school child, 240–241
    definitive care, 31–32
    ear, tympanic membrane
      perforation, 450–451
    facial, 147–157
    genital, 272
    head, 45, 54–64

    hip, 75–77
    limb, 77–79
      ankle, 81–84
      elbow, 91–94
      femur, 79–80
      foot, 84–87
      forearm, 94–95
      hand, 99–101
      lower leg, 80–81
      upper arm, 89, 90–91
      wrist, 95–99
    non-accidental injury, 243–246
    ophthalmic, 438–440
    pelvis, 72–75
    pre-hospital care, 15–23
    preparation, multiply-injured
      patients, 26
    primary survey, 26–29
    secondary survey, 29–31
    shoulder, 87–90, 104, 105
    spinal, 109–117
    sports injuries
      children, 254
      young adults, 269–270
    thoracic injuries, 119–134
Trauma care, 8
Trauma Nursing Core course, 8
Trauma teams, 25, 26
Treatment team, major incidents, 39
Treatment without consent, 209
Trespass, 522, 523
Triage, 6, 177, 178, 462, 464, 475–483
    audit, 481–482
    concept of nurse triage, 475 477
    direct nurse triage, 477–478
    documentation, 480–481
    eye complaints, 436
    legal considerations, 523
    major incidents
      identification of patients at
        hospital, 38, 39
      incident site, 18–19
    national triage scale, 482–483
    patient assessment, 478–479
    providing nurse triage system, 478
    telephone, computer-based decision
      support, 466
    training, 480–481
    the triage decision, 479–480
Trichomonas vaginalis, **416**
Tricuspid valves, 343
Tricyclic antidepressants, accidental
    poisoning, 242
Trigeminal nerve, testing, 150
Trimalleolar fractures, 84
Trimleolar fractures, 98
Triquetrum fractures, 98
TROCARS mnenomic, 396
Tulle dressings, 320
Turbinate bones, 147
Tympanic membrane, 448
    perforation, 156, 449–450, 450–451
Tympany, 397

UKCC
    clinical supervision 499

UKCC (*contd*)
  Code of Professional Conduct, 480, 481, 487, 514, 515, 518, 522, 523, 526, 534
  Scope of Professional Practice, 480, 481, 515, 523
Ulna
  anatomy, 94
  fractures, 94–95
Ulnar collateral ligament injuries, 105
Ulnar nerve, 92
  assessing function following elbow injury, **93**
Ulnar styloid fractures, 96
Ultrasound
  abdominal injuries, 143–144
  Doppler, testicular torsion, 408
  miscarriage, 420
Umbilical cord, care of, 425
Umbilicus, distended veins, 396
Unconscious patients
  ethical issues, 518
  legal issues, 525
  Munchuasen's syndrome, neurological type, 207
Unipolar ECG leads, 346
Universal precautions, 26, 536
Unstable angina, 361
Upper arm injuries, 89, 90–91
Urea, cardiac patients, 345, 363
Urethral catheterization, 30, 74, 142
  catheters, 406–407
  contraindications, 142
Urinary output, burns patients, 164
Urinary retention, 406
  spinal injuries, 116
Urinary tract infection, 382
  children, 255
Urine, darkened, 165
Urometer, 30
US, nurse practitioner courses, 488, 489
Uterus, 411
Uveal tract, 432–433
Uveitis, 444
  traumatic, 439

Vagina, 412
  examination, 31, 74, 142
    in miscarriage, 420
  injury to, 140
Vapour-permeable dressings, 320
Vasoconstriction/vasodilation, temperature homeostasis, 300
Vasopressin, 403
Veins, head and neck, **53**
Ventilation/perfusion ratio, 121, 122
Ventricles, 48, **49**
Ventricular ectopic beats, 353–354
Ventricular fibrillation (VF), 349–350
  infants, 221, 222

Ventricular tachycardia (VT), 354
  infants, 221, 222
Verbal response, Glasgow Coma Scale, 60
Vertebral arteries, 51
Vertebral column, anatomy, 109, **110**
Vicarious liability, 523
Videos in waiting room, 177
Villi, 394
Violent patients, 210
  follow-up care after violent incident, 180–181
  legal issues, 527
  management of individual, 179–180
Viral infection
  conjunctivitis, 443–444
  corneal ulcers, 445
  meningitis, 225
A Vision for the Future, DOH, 7–8, 499
Visual acuity, 150, 434
Visual analogue scales (VAS), 328, **329**
Visual disturbances, migraine, 386
Vitamins
  deficiency, 311
  vitamin D synthesis, 308
Vitreous body, 433
Volkmann's ischaemia, 92
Volume replacement *see* Fluid replacement
Voluntary hospitals, 1
Volvulus, 399
Vomer, 147
Vomiting, 397
  airway management, 27
  bowel obstruction, 399
  induced, 242
  infants, 227–228
Vulva, examination, 74

Waiting areas, 177, 258, 476
  children, 235
  health promotion, 255–256, 470
Waiting times, 7, 476
  and aggression, 176, 177, 178
  decreased, nurse practitioner benefits, 487
Wales, major incident planning guidelines, 34
Warm compresses, 331
Warming fluids, pre-hospital care, 22
Water balance, 302
Weapons, use of objects as, 179
Wedge compression fractures, thorax, 115
Wenckebach type heart block, 357
Wernicke's encephalopathy, 271
'Wet' drowning, 379
Wheezing, 236, 374
White blood cells, 390
  count, cardiac patients, 345, 363

White matter
  brain, 49
  spinal cord, 110
Wilsher *v* Essex AHA (1988), 522, 524
Witnessed resuscitation, 190–192
  guidelines for staff, 192
Wolfe, 'protective reaction pattern', 183
Working time, 536–537
Wound exudate, removal, 320
Wounds, 309–323
  assessment, 313–314
  bite wounds, 322
  burn, 166–168
    minor burns, 170–171
  cleansing, 314–315
    properties of solutions, **316**
  closure, 315, 316–321
    primary, 315, 316–319
    secondary, 319–321
    tertiary, 321
  discharge information, 323
  facial, 155–156
  healing, 309–313
    factors affecting, 311, 312
    wound pain, 311, 312, 313
  infection, 313, 321–322
  tetanus prophylaxis, 322–323
Wrist injuries, 95–99
Written consent, 525

X-rays
  acute abdomen
    bowel obstruction, 399
    peritonitis, 400
  myocardial infarction, 363
  requests for, GPs and registrars/SHO comparison, 463
  trauma patients, 29
    abdominal injuries, 142
    burn-injured patients, 160–161
    cervical spine, 114, 115
    pulmonary contusion, 131
    skull, 60, 63
    tension pneumothorax, 127

Young adults, 269–273
  accidents related to sexual activity, 272
  alcohol-related attendances, 271–272
  psychological illnesses, 272–273
  road traffic accidents, 270–271
  sports injuries, 269–270

Zinc deficiency, 311
Zones, burn wounds, 170
Zygoma, 147